To Jonathan Rhoads
— teacher, investigator,
surgeon statesman —

On the occasion
of your
80th birthday

with my admiration and
highest regards

Jim Thompson

9 May 1987

UTMB
Galveston Tx

Gastrointestinal Endocrinology

Gastrointestinal Endocrinology

edited by

James C. Thompson

George H. Greeley, Jr.

Phillip L. Rayford

Courtney M. Townsend, Jr.

McGRAW-HILL BOOK COMPANY

New York St. Louis San Francisco Auckland Bogotá Hamburg Johannesburg Lisbon London Madrid Mexico Milan Montreal New Delhi Panama Paris San Juan São Paulo Singapore Sydney Tokyo Toronto

NOTICE

Medicine is an ever-changing science. As new research and clinical experience broaden our knowledge, changes in treatment and drug therapy are required. The editors and the publisher of this work have checked with sources believed to be reliable in their efforts to provide drug dosage schedules that are complete and in accord with the standards accepted at the time of publication. However, readers are advised to check the product information sheet included in the package of each drug they plan to administer to be certain that the information contained in these schedules is accurate and that changes have not been made in the recommended dose or in the contraindications for administration. This recommendation is of particular importance in connection with new or infrequently used drugs.

GASTROINTESTINAL ENDOCRINOLOGY

1 2 3 4 5 6 7 8 9 0 HALHAL 8 9 8 7 6

ISBN 0-07-064406-3

The book was set in Zapf Book by TAPSCO, Inc.
The editors were Beth Kaufman Barry and
Stuart D. Boynton.
The production supervisor was Thomas J. LoPinto.
The cover was designed by Edward R. Schultheis.
Arcata Graphics/Halliday was printer and binder.

Library of Congress Cataloging-in-Publication Data

Gastrointestinal endocrinology.

Includes bibliographies and index.
1. Gastrointestinal hormones. I. Thompson, James C., date. [DNLM: 1. Gastrointestinal Hormones.
2. Peptides. WK 170 G2544]
QP572.G35G33 1987 612′.32 86-15187
ISBN 0-07-064406-3

CONTENTS

SECTION SIX: OTHER PEPTIDES

SECTION SEVEN: NONPEPTIDE AGENTS

SECTION EIGHT: REGULATORY INTERRELATIONSHIPS

SECTION NINE: CLINICAL ISSUES

SECTION TEN: APPENDIX

LIST OF CONTRIBUTORS

GUNNAR ALINDER, M.D.
Department of Surgery, Solleftea Hospital, Solleftea, Sweden

ANDERS ALWMARK, M.D., Ph.D.
Department of Surgery, University of Lund, Lund, Sweden

R. DANIEL BEAUCHAMP, M.D.
Resident, Department of Surgery, The University of Texas Medical Branch, Galveston, Texas

CARY W. COOPER, Ph.D.
Professor and Chairman, Department of Pharmacology and Toxicology, The University of Texas Medical Branch, Galveston, Texas

HOWARD R. DOYLE, M.D.
Resident, Department of Surgery, The University of Texas Medical Branch, Galveston, Texas

MASAKI FUJIMURA, M.D.
Department of Surgery, Shiga University of Medical Science, Otsu-City, Shiga, Japan

GUILLERMO GOMEZ, M.D.
Visiting Scientist, Department of Surgery, The University of Texas Medical Branch, Galveston, Texas; permanent address: Universidad Catolica de Chile, Santiago, Chile

GEORGE H. GREELEY, Jr., Ph.D.
Associate Professor, Department of Surgery, The University of Texas Medical Branch, Galveston, Texas

KAREN S. GUICE, M.D.
Department of Surgery, University of Michigan Medical Center, Ann Arbor, Michigan

YAN-SHI GUO, M.D.
Visiting Scientist, Department of Surgery, The University of Texas Medical Branch, Galveston, Texas; permanent address: Department of Physiology, Beijing Medical College, Beijing, China

MICHAEL B. HANCOCK, Ph.D.
Professor, Department of Anatomy, The University of Texas Medical Branch, Galveston, Texas

TALAAT KHALIL, M.D.
Resident, Department of Surgery, The University of Texas Medical Branch, Galveston, Texas

FELIX LLUIS, M.D.
Visiting Scientist, Department of Surgery, The University of Texas Medical Branch, Galveston, Texas; permanent address: Department of Surgery, Hospital Sta. Creu i Sant Pau, Barcelona, Spain

JANOS LONOVICS, M.D.
First Department of Medicine, Szeged University Medical School, Szeged, Hungary

DONALD G. MACLELLAN, M.D.
Department of Surgery, University of Melbourne, Austin Hospital, Melbourne, Victoria, Australia

MARILYN MARX, M.D.
Resident, Department of Surgery, The University of Texas Medical Branch, Galveston, Texas

LASZLO MATE, M.D.
8203 Vermissa Ct #3, Louisville, Kentucky

WILLIAM H. NEALON, M.D.
Assistant Professor, Department of Surgery, The University of Texas Medical Branch, Galveston, Texas

JAN B. NEWMAN, M.D.
Christian Hospital Northeast-Northwest, St. Louis, Missouri

KEITH T. OLDHAM, M.D.
Department of Surgery, University of Michigan Medical Center, Ann Arbor, Michigan

JAMES N. PASLEY, Ph.D.
Professor, Department of Physiology and Biophysics, University of Arkansas for Medical Sciences, Little Rock, Arkansas

GRAEME J. POSTON, F.R.C.S.
Department of Surgery, Hammersmith Hospital, Royal Postgraduate Medical School, London, United Kingdom

PHILLIP L. RAYFORD, Ph.D.
Professor and Chairman, Department of Physiology and Biophysics, University of Arkansas for Medical Sciences, Little Rock, Arkansas

NORMA H. RUBIN, Ph.D.
Research Instructor, Department of Internal Medicine, Division of Hematology-Oncology, The University of Texas Medical Branch, Galveston, Texas

TSUGUO SAKAMOTO, M.D.
The First Department of Surgery, Osaka University Hospital, Osaka, Japan

POMILA SINGH, Ph.D.
Assistant Professor, Department of Surgery, The University of Texas Medical Branch, Galveston, Texas

JAMES C. THOMPSON, M.D.
Professor and Chairman, Department of Surgery, The University of Texas Medical Branch, Galveston, Texas

COURTNEY M. TOWNSEND, Jr., M.D.
Robertson-Poth Professor, Department of Surgery, The University of Texas Medical Branch, Galveston, Texas

J. PATRICK WALKER, M.D.
Chief Resident, Department of Surgery, The University of Texas Medical Branch, Galveston, Texas

ISIDORO WIENER, M.D.
Grupo Medico Lomas, S.C., Mexico City, Mexico

PREFACE

Writing and editing this book has been great instructive fun. We believed that we could provide a service to students of gut hormones by bringing together in one place as much information as we could practically assemble. The evolution of our plan is detailed in the Introduction, Chap. 1.

Development of gastrointestinal endocrinology was slow. After demonstration of secretin and gastrin, a long period of relative inactivity followed. Since 1964, there has been explosive development (Figure). Not all of the agents are true hormones, some have not yet been isolated. We are all greatly indebted to Viktor Mutt who has provided the intellectual stimulus and the substrate for isolation and purification of most recently discovered peptides.

We are grateful to our colleagues in research, visiting scientists and surgical residents, in the Department of Surgery at UTMB, Galveston, and to our colleagues at the University of Arkansas for Medical Sciences and in the Department of Pharmacology and Toxicology, UTMB. We are especially grateful to our superb manuscript secretary, Julie Gips.

Much of our work has been supported by the Research and Development Fund of the Department of Surgery, UTMB. We are grateful to our surgical colleagues for their help. The Hartford Foundation in a previous incarnation supported our studies and we want to thank the Directors. The Moody Foundation has provided generous help that greatly facilitated important initial studies. We want to express our lifelong gratitude to the National Institutes of Health, from whom all Blessings flow. Since 1960, the NIH has supported the studies of our group of investigators. Lastly, we want to thank our wives—Marilyn Thompson, Carol Haase-Greeley, Gerry Rayford, and Mary Townsend.

J.C.T., G.H.G. Jr., P.L.R., C.M.T. Jr.

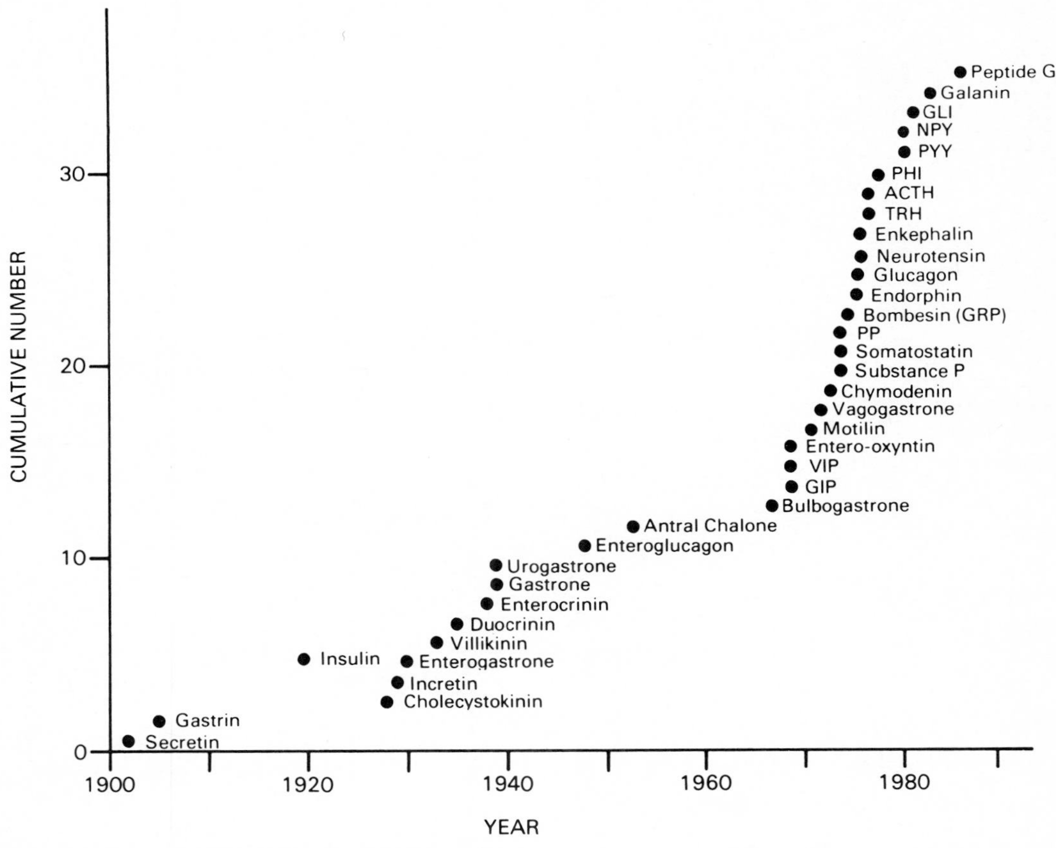

Adapted from Rehfeld JF, in SR Bloom and JM Polak (eds): *Gut Hormones*. New York, Churchill Livingstone, 1981, p. 11. Reproduced with permission.

Gastrointestinal Endocrinology

Section One

Overview

Chapter 1

Introduction

James C. Thompson, M.D.

The entire field of endocrinology began with gut hormones. The beginning can be pinpointed with precision: the time was the afternoon of 16 January 1902, the place, the University College Hospital, London, and the event was the discovery of secretin. W. M. Bayliss and E. H. Starling [1] elicited the brisk secretion of pancreatic juice following the irrigation of a denervated loop of small bowel with dilute HCl. They understood the significance of their finding immediately; they suggested that a chemical messenger was released from the acidified intestine to mediate the response. According to Babkin [2], the word "hormone" was introduced by Starling on the suggestion of W. B. Hardy [3]. The word is from the Greek δρμαω, meaning "I arouse to activity," or, "I excite."

The discovery of secretin activity was followed shortly by Babkin's discovery of gastrin [4,5], but more than 50 years elapsed before the physiologic and pathologic implications of gastrointestinal hormones were realized. The Zollinger-Ellison syndrome [6] was described in 1955, but the actual breakthrough occurred in the early 1960s, when gastrin [7] and secretin [8] were isolated almost simultaneously. Gregory and Tracy [9] announced the constitution and properties of gastrin in 1964, initiating the biochemical era of gut endocrinology. Secretin [10] and cholecystokinin [8] were next isolated and chemically characterized and, by now, a wide variety of new hormones and related substances are recognized [11,12]. New developments in the field have been celebrated and analyzed in conferences at Los Angeles [13], Edmonton [14], Aalborg [15], Stockholm [16], Erlangen [17], Rochester, NY [18], Galveston [19], Asilomar [20], Rome [21], Lausanne [22], Bieto [23], Cambridge [24], Stockholm [25], and Rochester, MN [26], among others. Much of the rapid development of gastrointestinal endocrinology is due to the brilliant contributions of Gregory, Jorpes, Mutt, and Grossman. Important advances have been made by surgeons, especially Dragstedt, Woodward, Zollinger, and Ellison.

Gastrointestinal hormones are chemical messengers that regulate gut function. Most of them—perhaps all, depending on definitions—are peptides. They are secreted by endocrine cells that are widely distributed throughout the gastrointestinal mucosa in such profusion that the gut has been called the largest endocrine organ in the body. Although we call these agents hormones, they do not always function in a truly endocrine fashion, that is, the active peptides are not always discharged into blood vessels to act on a distant site. Sometimes they are discharged and act locally in a paracrine fashion. They also may serve as transmitting agents for nervous impulses, or they may be discharged into blood vessels following nervous stimulation in a true neuroendocrine fashion (Fig 1-1). Gastrointestinal endocrinology includes all of these functions, and we do not always know when an agent acts locally as well as at a distant site.

What about the present volume? More than 2 years ago, my colleagues and I began the periodic ritual of preparation for renewal of the grant that has supported our work for several years (AM-15241), but this time, things were different. Several coinvestigators (my coeditors, as well as Cary Cooper, Ph.D., and Pomila Singh, Ph.D.) and I had been encouraged at this same time to prepare and submit a Program Project Grant, which would provide support for our coordinated efforts in the field of gastrointestinal endocrinology. As part of this combined effort in grant writing, we decided to embark on a review of the literature concerning gastrointestinal hormones; we assigned these reviews to one another and to various visiting scientists and research fellows in our laboratory. The early drafts were concise, and a brief précis of these reviews was published in 1984 [27].

In short order, however, a brisk competition arose regarding the scope of these reviews; they became increasingly definitive. The senior investi-

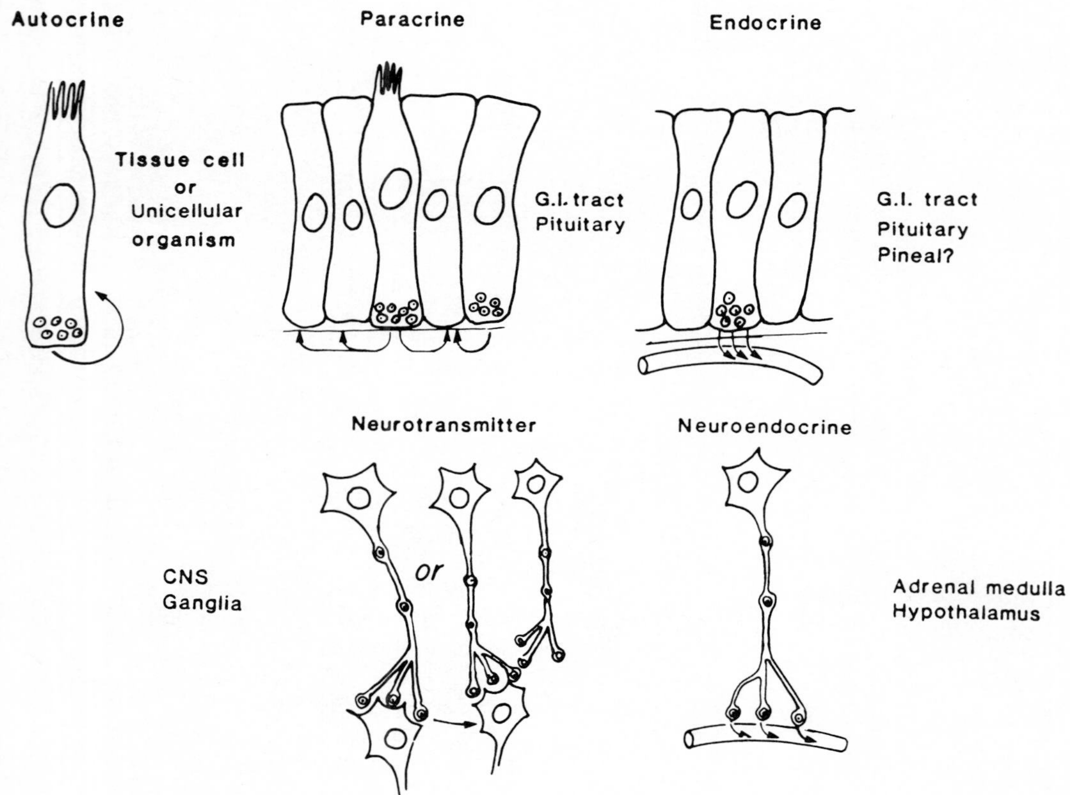

Figure 1-1. Modes of action of regulatory peptides. The secreted autocrine product acts locally on the cell of origin. Paracrine secretion involves local action of a peptide on neighboring cells, either by systems of extracellular fluid transport or by means of gap junctions between cells. Endocrine secretion involves secretion of a regulatory peptide into the bloodstream to affect distant targets. Nerve cells, shown in the lower portion of the figure, may transmit impulses from cell to cell by means of axodendritic or presynaptic axoaxonic synapses (neurotransmitter). Neurohumoral secretion (neuroendocrine) refers to release of a peptide product of the neuron into the bloodstream to act on other tissues. (From Krieger DL, Clin Res 31:342, 1983.)

gators in our group were frankly unprepared for the enthusiastic manner in which our colleagues responded to the challenge of providing a summary of all that is known about our field. We were overwhelmed by searching, thoughtful, critical reviews that appeared to deserve more exposure than to appear in truncated form as a synopsis in a grant request (however vital). We decided to write a book. And here it is.

We have tried to provide fellow students with information of use in the study of gastrointestinal endocrinology. We have provided a summary of the investigative techniques that we use in studying the synthesis, storage, release, transport, actions and interactions, and catabolism of regulatory peptides of the gut. There is a relatively detailed series of descriptions of various surgical procedures that we have found useful. We have discussed in detail some models for study: receptors for gastrin and cholecystokinin, the blood-brain barrier, and the various prototypic actions of gut hormones. Additionally, we have provided information on the ontogeny of gut peptides and on the effects of aging, on the possible role of gut hormones in cancer, and on the effects of circadian rhythms on gut peptides.

We have discussed the classic gut peptides, other agents that have been closely studied, nonpeptide agents, and other peptides that we have arbitrarily called candidates (clearly recognizing that the veil between anointed and nonanointed is constantly in motion).

We have discussed important regulatory interrelationships, the calcium-gut hormone interactions, the brain-gut axis, the entero-insulinar axis, and the gonad-gut axis. We finish with a short section on the clinical significance of gastrointestinal hormones.

At the end is an appendix that provides the amino acid composition and molecular weights of gut hormones and related substances. We provide this information for about 60 peptides, plus histamine, serotonin, and some prostaglandins. These range alphabetically from bombesin to urogastrone, and in familiarity from gastrin to sauvagine.

The editors are grateful to colleagues in our laboratory who have put most of this information together. My coeditors and I have gone over every page in our very best effort to weed out all errors and to include all pertinent information. Long familiarity with such projects forces us to recognize that errors will be present. We apologize for them and invite the reader to notify us so that they can be corrected. We have provided an extensive bibliography that we hope will help any student embark upon further closer study of any area of interest. Interested readers may wish to consult reviews that have been helpful and informative to us [11,12,27–49].

We have found the study of gastrointestinal hormones to be a wonderful, exciting, and highly rewarding field in which to spend a lifetime. We commend it to all potential and fellow students. We hope that this book will provide worthwhile information to gastroenterologists and to surgeons with interest in the gut, as well as to endocrinologists, physiologists, pediatricians, internists, and all clinicians and scientists who are interested in gut function.

Last, I wish to acknowledge the immense contributions of research fellows (listed below), who have come from all over the world to work in our laboratory. Their efforts are responsible—in large part—for whatever has been achieved. 1) B. Guy Clendinnen, F.R.C.S., 1970, UK. 2) B. Michael Jackson, M.D., 1970, USA. 3) Herbert H. Bunchman, M.D., 1970, USA. 4) Jack L. Conlee, M.D., 1971, USA. 5) Larry C. Watson, M.D., 1971, 1976, 1979, USA. 6) J. Robert Searcy, M.D., 1971, USA. 7) Ulf B. E. Hjelmquist, M.D., 1972, Sweden. 8) John C. W. Evans, F.R.C.S., 1972, UK. 9) Melvyn Lerman, M.D., 1972, USA. 10) H. Dieter Becker, M.D., 1972, 1975, 1976, West Germany. 11) Charles S. Clark, Jr., M.D., 1972, USA. 12) Robert A. D. Booth, F.R.C.S., 1973, UK. 13) Takaho Watayou, M.D., 1973, Japan. 14) Hugo V. Villar, M.D., 1973–1975, USA. 15) N. Ian Ramus, F.R.C.S., 1975, UK. 16) H. Roberts Fender, M.D., 1975, USA. 17) Peter J. Curtis, F.R.C.S., 1976, UK. 18) Osvaldo L. Llanos, M.D., 1975–1977, Chile. 19) Janusz S. Swierczek, M.D., 1976, 1977, 1979, 1983, Poland. 20) Reinhard K. Teichmann, M.D., 1977–1978, West Germany. 21) Thomas A. Miller, M.D., 1977, USA. 22) Talaat Khalil, M.D., 1977, 1984, Egypt. 23) J. Tom Peurifoy, M.D., 1977, USA. 24) Anton Schafmayer, M.D., 1977–1978, West Germany. 25) Webster S. Lowder, M.D., 1978, USA. 26) Masahiko Miyata, M.D., 1978, 1980, Japan. 27) Jean-Alain Chayvialle, M.D., 1978, France. 28) Sergio Guzman, M.D., 1977–1979, Chile. 29) Janos Lonovics, M.D., 1979, 1984, Hungary. 30) William A. Banks, 1978, USA. 31) Peter G. Devitt, F.R.C.S., 1980, UK. 32) Amram Ayalon, M.D., 1980, Israel. 33) Raul Yazigi, M.D., 1980, Chile. 34) Patricia M. Simon, Ph.D., 1980, France. 35) Kazumoto Inoue, M.D., 1980, 1981, 1982, Japan. 36) Isodoro Wiener, M.D., 1981, Mexico. 37) Per Lilja, M.D., 1981, Sweden. 38) Gerald M. Fried, M.D., 1982, Canada. 39) Xue-Guang Zhu, M.D., 1982, China. 40) Owen Winsett, M.D., 1982, USA. 41) Beverly Lewis, M.D., 1982, USA. 42) W. David Ogden, M.D., 1982, USA. 43)

Qing-Hao Lu, M.D., 1982, China. 44) Tsuguo Sakamoto, M.D., 1982–1984, Japan. 45) Masaki Fujimura, M.D., 1983–1985, Japan. 46) Laszlo Mate, M.D., 1984, Hungary. 47) Jan Newman, M.D., 1983, USA. 48) Marilyn Marx, M.D., 1982–1984, USA. 49) Anders Alwmark, M.D., 1984, Sweden. 50) J. Patrick Walker, M.D., 1984, USA. 51) Dan Beauchamp, M.D., 1984, USA. 52) Felix Lluis, M.D., 1984–present, Spain. 53) William Nealon, M.D., 1984–present, USA. 54) Gunnar Alinder, M.D., 1984, Sweden. 55) Yan-shi Guo, M.D., 1984–present, China. 56) Guillermo Gomez, M.D., 1985–present, Chile. 57) Isamu Asada, M.D., 1985–present, Japan. 58) J. Robert Upp, M.D., 1985–present, USA. 59) Chong-Zheng Yao, M.D., 1985–present, China. 60) Donald MacLelland, M.D., 1985–present, Australia. 61) Graeme Posten, F.R.C.S., 1986–present, UK. 62) Jin Ishizuka, M.D., 1986–present, Japan.

REFERENCES

1. Bayliss WM, Starling EH: The mechanisms of pancreatic secretion. J Physiol (Lond) 28:325, 1902.
2. Babkin BP: *Secretory Mechanism of the Digestive Glands.* 2nd Ed. New York, Paul B. Hoeber Inc, 1950, p 560.
3. Bayliss WM: *Principles of General Physiology.* 4th Ed. London, Longmans, Green and Co, 1924, p 112.
4. Edkins JS: On the chemical mechanism of gastric secretion. Proc R Soc Lond 76:376, 1905.
5. Edkins JS: The chemical mechanism of gastric secretion. J Physiol 34:133, 1906.
6. Zollinger RM, Ellison EH: Primary peptic ulcerations of the jejunum associated with islet cell tumors of the pancreas. Ann Surg 142:709, 1955.
7. Gregory RA: Memorial lecture: The isolation and chemistry of gastrin. Gastroenterology 51:953, 1966.
8. Jorpes JE: Memorial lecture: The isolation and chemistry of secretin and cholecystokinin. Gastroenterology 55:157, 1968.
9. Gregory RA, Tracy HJ: The constitution and properties of two gastrins extracted from hog antral mucosa. Part I. The isolation of two gastrins from hog antral mucosa. Gut 5:103, 1964. Part II. The properties of two gastrins isolated from hog antral mucosa. Gut 5:107, 1964.
10. Mutt V, Jorpes JE: Secretin: Isolation and determination of structure. Presented at the Fourth International Symposium on the Chemistry of Natural Products. Stockholm, June 1966.
11. Grossman MI and others: Candidate hormones of the gut. Gastroenterology 67:730, 1974.
12. Rayford PL, Miller TA, Thompson JC: Secretin, cholecystokinin and newer gastrointestinal hormones. N Engl J Med 295:1093, 1157, 1976.
13. Grossman MI (ed): *Gastrin: Proceedings of a Conference Held in September 1964.* Berkeley, University of California Press, 1966.
14. Shnitka TK, Gilbert JAL, Harrison RC (eds): *Gastric Secretion: Mechanisms and Control.* Proceedings of a symposium held at the University of Alberta, Edmonton, Canada, September 1965. Oxford, Pergamon Press, 1967.
15. Thaysen EH (ed): *Gastrointestinal Hormones and Other Subjects.* Proceedings of the Fifth Scandinavian Conference on Gastroenterology, Aalborg, Denmark, August 1971. Copenhagen, Munksgaard, 1971.
16. Andersson S (ed): *Frontiers in Gastrointestinal Hormone Research.* Proceedings of the 16th Nobel Symposium, Stockholm, July, 1970. Stockholm, Almqvist & Wiksell, 1973.
17. Demling, L (ed): *Gastrointestinal Hormones.* Proceedings of the International Symposium held in Erlangen, August 1971. Stuttgart, Georg Thieme Verlag, 1972.
18. Chey WY, Brooks FP (eds): *Endocrinology of the Gut.* Proceedings of the International Symposium on Recent Advances in Gastrointestinal Hormone Research held in Rochester, New York, August 1973. Thorofare, NJ, Charles B Slack Inc, 1974.
19. Thompson JC (ed): *Gastrointestinal Hormones.* Proceedings of a Symposium held in Galveston, Texas at The University of Texas Medical Branch, October 1974. Austin, University of Texas Press, 1975.
20. Proceedings of the First International Symposium on Gastrointestinal Hormones, held in Asilomar, California, October 1976. Gastroenterology 72:785, 1977.
21. Grossman MI, Speranza V, Basso N, Lezoche E (eds): *Gastrointestinal Hormones and Pathology of the Digestive System.* Proceedings of a symposium held in Rome, Italy, July 1977. New York, Plenum Press, 1978.
22. Bloom S (ed): *Gut Hormones.* Proceedings of a symposium held in Lausanne, Switzerland, June 1977. New York, Churchill Livingstone, 1978.
23. Myren J, Schrumpf E, Hanssen LE, Vatn M (eds): Proceedings of the Second International Symposium on Gastrointestinal Hormones. Scand J Gastroenterol 13 (Suppl 49):1, 1978.
24. Bloom SR, Polak JM (eds): Proceedings of the Third International Symposium on Gut Hormones held in Cambridge, U.K., September, 1980. Regul Pept Suppl 1:S1, 1980.
25. Mutt V, Uvnas-Moberg K (eds): Proceedings of the Fourth International Symposium on Gastrointestinal Hormones held in Stockholm, Sweden, June, 1982. Regul Pept Suppl 2:1, 1983.
26. Brooks FP, Go VLW (eds): Proceedings of the Fifth International Symposium on Gastrointestinal Hormones held in Rochester, Minnesota, September, 1984. Dig Dis Sci 29 (Suppl):1S, 1984.
27. Thompson JC, Marx M: Gastrointestinal hormones. Curr Probl Surg 21:1, 1984.
28. Thompson JC: Gastrin and gastric secretion. Annu Rev Med 20:291, 1969.
29. Thompson JC: Chemical structure and biological actions of gastrin, cholecystokinin and related compounds, in Holton P (ed): *The International Encyclopedia of Pharmacology and Therapeutics.* Oxford, Pergamon Press Limited, 1973, pp 261–286.

30. Thompson JC, Reeder DD, Villar HV, et al: Natural history and experience with diagnosis and treatment of the Zollinger-Ellison syndrome. Surg Gynecol Obstet 140:721, 1975.
31. Brown JC, Dryburgh JR, Ross SA, Dupre J: Identification and actions of gastric inhibitory polypeptide. Rec Prog Horm Res 31:487, 1975.
32. Rayford PL, Thompson JC: Gastrin. Surg Gynecol Obstet 145:257, 1977.
33. Thompson JC: Gastrointestinal hormones—Introduction. World J Surg 3:389, 1979.
34. Rehfeld JF: Cholecystokinin. Clinics Gastroenterol 9:593, 1980.
35. Hacki WH: Secretin. Clinics Gastroenterol 9:609, 1980.
36. Walsh JH, Lam SK: Physiology and pathology of gastrin. Clinics Gastroenterol 9:567, 1980.
37. Bloom SR, Polak JM (eds): *Gut Hormones*. New York, Churchill Livingstone, 1981.
38. Lonovics J, Devitt P, Watson LC, et al: Pancreatic polypeptide. A review. Arch Surg 116:1256, 1981.
39. Bethge N, Diel F, Usadel KH: Somatostatin—A regulatory peptide of clinical importance. J Clin Chem Clin Biochem 20:603, 1982.
40. Morley JE: Minireview. The ascent of cholecystokinin (CCK)—from gut to brain. Life Sci 30:479, 1982.
41. Said SI (ed): *Vasoactive Intestinal Peptide*. New York, Raven Press, 1982.
42. Krieger DT: Brain peptides: What, where, and why? Science 222:975, 1983.
43. Schwartz TW: Pancreatic polypeptide: A hormone under vagal control. Gastroenterology 85:1411, 1983.
44. Christophe J, Rosselin G, Said SI, Yanaihara N (eds): Proceedings of the First International Symposium on VIP and Related Peptides held in Brussels, Belgium, September, 1983. Peptides 5:141, 1984.
45. Taylor IL: Gastrointestinal hormones in the pathogenesis of peptic ulcer disease. Clinics Gastroenterol 13:355, 1984.
46. Townsend CM Jr, Thompson JC: Surgical management of tumors that produce gastrointestinal hormones. Annu Rev Med 36:111, 1985.
47. Vanderhaeghen J-J, Crawley JN (eds): Neuronal cholecystokinin. Proceedings of a conference on neuronal cholecystokinin, held in Brussels, Belgium, July, 1984. Ann NY Acad Sci 448:1, 1985.
48. Ballesta J, Bloom SR, Polak JM: Distribution and localization of regulatory peptides. CRC Crit Rev Clin Lab Sci 22:185, 1985.
49. Lucas A, Bloom SR, Green AA: Gastrointestinal peptides and the adaptation to extrauterine nutrition. Can J Physiol Pharmacol 63:527, 1985.

Section Two

Methods

Chapter 2

Radioimmunoassay of Gut Peptides

George H. Greeley, Jr., Ph.D.

A radioimmunoassay (RIA) is a biochemical technique in which the concentration of almost any naturally occurring or fabricated substance can be measured quantitatively. Radioimmunoassays, in comparison to most biologic assays, are exquisitely sensitive and highly specific.

The RIA is founded on a simple concept that utilizes the inherent specificity of the immune reaction between an antigen and its antibody [1–3]. In a majority of cases, a fixed amount of antibody is incubated with a standard amount of radioactive antigen (i.e., ^{125}I-peptide) and graded amounts of nonradioactive antigen (reference standard or test sample). During this incubation period, the radioactive antigen and the nonradioactive antigen compete for binding sites on the antibody (Fig 2-1). A dose-response curve can be generated from the reference standard, and this is used to determine the amount of antigen in test samples.

There are three basic requirements for the development of a radioimmunoassay. These are 1) a specific and sensitive antibody; 2) a radiolabeled antigen; and 3) a quick and reproducible method for separating antibody-bound antigen (bound) from unbound antigen (free), since the immune complex does not normally precipitate in a test tube. Parenthetically, the radioactive and nonradioactive ligands need not exhibit identical immunologic behavior. The standard and test samples, however, should compete similarly for antibody sites, but they need not be chemically or biologically identical.

The generation of an antibody in a laboratory animal is usually the first step to establishing an RIA. However, other substances that possess high affinity binding sites for specific biologic molecules, such as a membrane receptor, enzyme, or blood protein (e.g., cortisol-binding globulin, thyroid hormone-binding globulin), can be used in place of a specific antibody. In order to generate an antibody, a semipure antigen is adequate, although a pure antigen is preferred. If the antigen alone is inadequately antigenic, it can be linked chemically to a larger molecule, such as bovine serum albumin, using the carbodiimide or glutaraldehyde conjugation method [4]. If the peptide antigen consists of less than 30 amino acid residues, it is usually advisable to link it to a larger

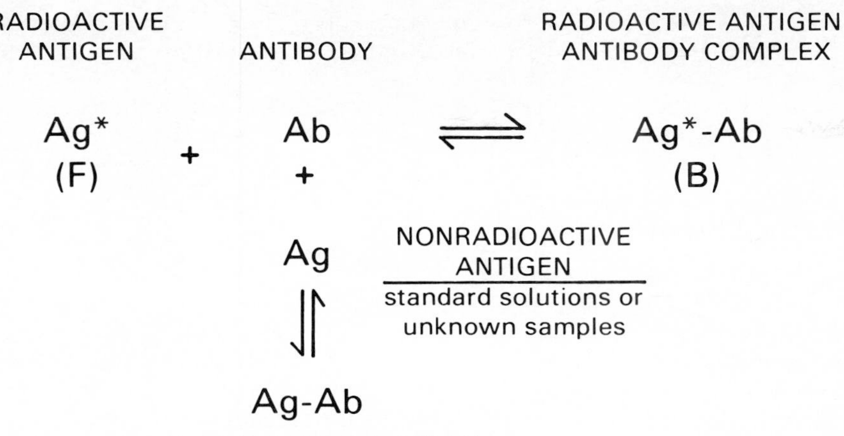

Figure 2-1. The competing reaction that is the basis of a radioimmunoassay. (F) = free; (B) = bound.

molecule. The antigen may also need to be modified chemically, which allows attachment to a larger molecule. Alternatively, a small fragment of the antigen (determinant) can be used in place of the entire antigen.

Antibodies are usually generated in rabbits, guinea pigs, goats, or sheep. There is, however, no set protocol that can be relied upon to ensure success. In our laboratory, the antigen is always emulsified with complete Freund's adjuvant, and pertussis vaccine (0.5 mL) is given along with the antigen. Antigen (100 μg to 1 mg) is injected into 50–100 intradermal sites on the shaved back of a rabbit [4]. It is advisable to collect some preimmune serum, which may be necessary in control experiments. The formula of 1:1 (vol:vol) of antigen to Freund's adjuvant is used. The frequency of booster injections varies from every 2 weeks to every 2–3 months, depending upon the response of the immunized rabbit. The amount of the antigen given in the booster injection also varies, depending upon the response of the rabbit and the purity and availability of the antigen. Blood is collected for titering every week after the second or third booster and checked for antibodies. When blood is collected, an antibody titer curve, using dilutions of 1:100–1:100,000, is constructed. An antibody with a titer of at least 1:500 is desirable at this time. Sometimes the immune response of the immunized animals will drop precipitously after repeated inoculations. If so, it may be better to start over with a different animal. At times, however, better results may be achieved with booster injections with smaller doses of antigen spaced farther apart. Patience is required in this stage of RIA development, as it may take months before a satisfactory antibody is developed. Generation of antibodies is not an exact science.

The second step in establishing an RIA is to obtain a radioactive antigen. This may, at times, be purchased from a commercial source; many radioactive pharmaceuticals, steroids, polypeptides, peptides, neurotransmitters, and vitamins with suitable specific activities are currently available. The radioactive ligand must be pure and stable, and most importantly, one must be confident of its identity. If a radioactive ligand cannot be purchased, it must be prepared. Most frequently, proteins, peptides, or other substances can be iodinated with ^{125}I or ^{131}I.

The Hunter and Greenwood method [5] for iodination is usually used with minor modifications that suit the particular antigen. In brief, a small amount of ligand (2–10 μg) is mixed with chloramine-T and ^{125}I, resulting in a radiolabeled ligand. The presence of a tyrosyl or histyl residue in proteins or peptides is necessary for this method of iodination; otherwise, a modified form of the peptide containing a tyrosine can be synthesized. The iodination reaction is halted with the addition of sodium metabisulfite or a small amount of bovine serum albumin. The next step is to separate the radiolabeled peptide from other contaminants. This can usually be done easily and quickly on a small gel or affinity column. High pressure liquid chromatography (HPLC) may also provide an excellent means to purify the radiolabeled peptide, that is, to separate it from free iodine and fragments of peptides. In fact, the HPLC method may be superior to the gel and affinity chromatography methods, since HPLC can separate monoiodo forms from polyiodo forms of the peptide.

Since chloramine-T is a strong oxidizing agent, use of this method may damage the antigen. Alternate methods include the milder lactoperoxidase method [6], the introduction of ^{125}I onto the antigen using the Bolton-Hunter reagent [7], or the iodogen method [8,9]. For example, Singh et al [10] have used the iodogen method in preparing a ligand for use in a method to measure gastrin receptors.

The next stage in the development of a radioimmunoassay is to decide upon a usable method for separating the antibody-bound antigen from the free antigen. The most frequently used method takes advantage of a second antibody that is generated against the first antibody. In other words, sheep or goats are immunized with rabbit serum (or the gamma globulin fraction) if the first antibody is generated in rabbits. The first antibody might be, for example, a rabbit-antigastrin antibody, and the second, a sheep antirabbit antibody. Other useful methods include the use of polyethylene glycol, dextran-coated charcoal [11], alcohol, and protein A. Protein A (Pansorbin) is a product derived from *Staphylococcus aureus* cells that selectively binds the IgG fraction of blood with a high avidity [12]. Protein A is commercially available from Calbiochem-Behring (San Diego, CA). Using a suitable separation method, the free and bound ligands are separated, and one or both are counted in a gamma or scintillation counter. A standard line is then constructed, and the amount of antigen in the test specimens can be calculated by a direct comparison with the standard line.

In the course of establishing a radioimmunoassay, the method must be validated. Despite the specificity of the immune reaction, a variety of nonspecific factors can interfere and disrupt the immune reaction taking place in the test tube. The specificity of the particular assay must be evaluated by testing all substances with structural similarities. If, for example, a radioimmunoassay for cholecystokinin-33 (CCK-33) is under development, substances related to the antigen-ligand must be examined, since any agent that is chemically related may cause interference immunologically. Whether CCK-8, CCK-4, CCK-12, or gastrin, for example, can compete with CCK-33 for antibody sites must be evaluated. Similar evaluations must be performed in the development of an assay for steroid hormones, certain drugs, polypeptide hormones, and their metabolites. A variety of nonspecific factors that are not related to the antigen can also cause interference, including the ionic environment, pH, or the presence of heparin in the specimen. Temperature also brings about a variable destruction of substances, which is related to the amount of specimen in the tube. One way to avoid this problem is to dilute or purify the test sample before adding it to the antibody-buffer mixture.

Some other aspects regarding a radioimmunoassay deserve comment. Sensitivity can be defined arbitrarily as that amount of antigen that depresses binding of radioactive antigen by 50 or 33 percent. Another more useful definition for sensitivity is the smallest concentration of added ligand that produces a significant inhibition of binding ($p < 0.05$) when compared to total binding of radioactive antigen. This is also called the lower detection limit of the assay. Additionally, serial dilutions of natural endogenous antigen should produce a parallel dilution curve when compared to standard antigen. In other words, dilution curves of blood- and tissue-derived antigen must be parallel to the dose-response line of the standard. Parallelism is not a conclusive test, since there can be substances that behave similarly, if not identically, to the antigen in the radioimmunoassay.

We will not review the numerous published RIAs for multiple gut peptides, since references will be provided in the discussion of each agent. We will, instead, provide some general remarks relative to the development of a radioimmunoassay for CCK-33/39 in order to demonstrate the specific steps in development.

In the process of achieving a specific assay for CCK-33/39 [13–15], rabbits were first immunized with pure or semipure preparations of CCK-33/39. A combination procedure of 16 percent pure CCK-33/39 and 99 percent pure CCK-33 without conjugation to a larger protein was used successfully. The antibody has been shown to be specific for the large variants of CCK with negligible to no cross-reactivity with small forms of CCK (CCK-8, CCK-4) or with any of the multiple forms of gastrin. The antibody that was initially developed by Rayford et al [13] is unique in that it requires the entire CCK molecule for complete cross-reactivity. Further development by Rayford and Greeley has improved this assay [14,15].

In this particular radioimmunoassay procedure, CCK-39 is radioiodinated using chloramine-T. The radiolabeled hormone is usable for 4–6 weeks, with negligible loss of binding to the antibody. Although unextracted plasma samples are used in some laboratories, other laboratories extract and concentrate CCK before measurement. The use of the C_{18} Sep-Pak (Waters Associates, Milford, MA) has proved useful and seems to result in lower basal levels of CCK, although these differences are not fully resolved [16]. On the other hand, other laboratories have used plasma extracts rather than plasma in their assays, and they have reported CCK-33 levels similar to those reported by a laboratory that uses ordinary plasma [17,18]. The use of Sep-Paks in extracting neurotensin from plasma specimens has also proved useful [19]. Extraction of neurotensin and CCK immunoreactivity from plasma specimens results in lower values when compared to unextracted specimens [20]. Another technique that appears promising is the use of HPLC for the isolation and separation of the molecular forms of CCK with subsequent radioimmunoassay [21,22].

REFERENCES

1. Berson SA, Yalow RS, Bauman A, et al: Insulin-I^{131} metabolism in human subjects: Demonstration of insulin binding globulin in the circulation of insulin treated subjects. J Clin Invest 35:170, 1956.
2. Yalow RS, Berson SA: Immunological specificity of human insulin: Application to immunoassay of insulin. J Clin Invest 40:2190, 1961.
3. Yalow RS, Berson SA: General principles of radioimmunoassay, in Hayes RL, Goswitz FA, Pearson Murphy BE (eds): *Radioisotopes in Medicine. In Vitro Studies.* Tennessee, U.S. Atomic Energy Commission, 1968, pp 7–41.
4. Vaitukaitis J, Robbins JB, Nieschlag E, et al: A method for producing specific antisera with small doses of immunogen. J Clin Endocrinol 33:988, 1971.
5. Greenwood FC, Hunter WM, Glover JS: Preparation of ^{131}I labelled human growth hormone to high specific radioactivity. Biochem J 89:114, 1963.
6. Hamlin JL: Radioiodination of polypeptide hormones, in Antoniades HN (ed): *Hormones in Human Blood. Detection and Assay.* Cambridge, Mass, Harvard University Press, 1976, pp 83–86.
7. Bolton AE, Hunter WM: The labelling of proteins to high specific radioactivities by conjugation to a ^{125}I-containing acylating agent. Application to the radioimmunoassay. Biochem J 133:529, 1973.
8. Fraker PJ, Speck JC Jr: Protein and cell membrane iodinations with a sparingly soluble chloroamide, 1,3,4,6-tetrachloro-3α,6α-diphenylglycoluril. Biochem Biophys Res Commun 80:849, 1978.
9. Salacinski PRP, McLean C, Sykes JEC, et al: Iodination of proteins, glycoproteins, and peptides using a solid-phase oxidizing agent, 1,3,4,6-tetrachloro-3α,6α-diphenyl glycoluril (iodogen). Anal Biochem 117:136, 1981.
10. Singh P, Rae-Venter B, Townsend CM Jr, et al: Gastrin receptors in normal and malignant gastrointestinal mucosa: Age-associated changes. Am J Physiol, 249:G761, 1985.
11. Herbert V, Bleicher SJ: Separation of antibody-bound from free hormone by the coated charcoal technique, in Antoniades HN (ed): *Hormones in Human Blood. Detection and Assay.* Cambridge, Mass, Harvard University Press, 1976, pp 115–120.
12. Ying S-Y: Radioimmunoassay of peptide hormones using killed *Staphylococcus aureus* as a separating agent. Methods Enzymol 73:245, 1981.
13. Rayford PL, Schafmayer A, Teichmann RK, et al: Cholecystokinin radioimmunoassay, in Bloom SR (ed): *Gut Hormones.* New York, Churchill Livingstone, 1978, pp 208–212.
14. Fried GM, Ogden WD, Swierczek JS, et al: Release of cholecystokinin in conscious dogs: Correlation with simultaneous measurements of gallbladder pressure and pancreatic protein secretion. Gastroenterology 85:1113, 1983.
15. Lilja P, Fagan CJ, Wiener I, et al: Infusion of pure cholecystokinin in humans. Correlation between plasma concentrations of cholecystokinin and gallbladder size. Gastroenterology 83:256, 1982.
16. Eysselein VE, Bottcher W, Kauffman GL, et al: Molecular heterogeneity of canine cholecystokinin (CCK) in portal and peripheral plasma. Gastroenterology 84:1147, 1983.
17. Chang TM, Lee KY, Berger-Ornstein L, et al: Radioimmunoassay of cholecystokinin. Gastroenterology 82:1031, 1982.
18. Chang T-M, Chey WY: Radioimmunoassay of cholecystokinin. Dig Dis Sci 28:456, 1983.
19. Sakamoto T, Newman J, Fujimura M, et al: Role of neurotensin in pancreatic secretion. Surgery 96:146, 1984.
20. Greeley GH Jr, Thompson JC: Cholecystokinin-8 and neurotensin levels of plasma extracts and unextracted plasma. Fed Proc 43:1072, 1984.
21. Maton PN, Selden AC, Chadwick VS: Large and small forms of cholecystokinin in human plasma: Measurement using high pressure liquid chromatography and radioimmunoassay. Regul Pept 4:251, 1982.
22. Draviam E, Greeley GH Jr, Lluis F, et al: A new high pressure liquid chromatography-radioimmunoassay method for the characterization of cholecystokinin variants in dog plasma. Gastroenterology 88:1369, 1985.

Chapter 3

Immunohistochemistry of Gut Peptides

Masaki Fujimura, M.D., Michael B. Hancock, Ph.D., and George H. Greeley, Jr., Ph.D.

Microscopic studies of the gastrointestinal endocrine cells were initiated by Heidenhain in 1870, when he described chromaffin cells [1]. These chromaffin cells (also called enterochromaffin cells) were found to contain serotonin. Basigranular acidophilic cells that lacked chromaffinity and argentaffinity were described subsequently by Kull in 1913 (described in reference [1]). Much later, with the aid of new histochemical techniques, peptide-containing endocrine cells were also demonstrated [1].

During recent decades, a variety of peptide-containing enteric cells have been described using histochemical and fluorescent histochemical methods [1]. However, the immunohistochemical methods in current use are unequaled for localizing peptides within cells and nerve fibers of the alimentary canal, pancreas, and elsewhere in the body.

Basically, immunohistochemistry exploits the highly specific antigen-antibody reaction to which some type of visible label, such as fluorochromes or enzymes, is linked to the antibody; the labels are used to visualize the exact location of the antigen under a UV microscope. The fluorescent antibody or immunofluorescent technique was first applied in a method in which a fluorogen, such as fluorescein or rhodamine, was coupled to an antibody [2]. The visible reagent was then used to identify antigen-containing sites. Later, in place of a fluorogen, an enzyme, such as horseradish peroxidase, was conjugated to an antibody. This reagent catalyzes a reaction, which produces a substance visible under conventional light microscopic methods. This method is called the enzyme-labeled antibody method [3].

This technique evolved subsequently into the unlabeled antibody enzyme method [4] and then into the peroxidase-antiperoxidase (PAP) method [5,6]. More recently, the avidin-biotin-complex method (ABC method) [7], which is more sensitive than the PAP method, has been used successfully. With the fluorescence immunohistochemical technique, the problem of photochemical degeneration of the fluorochrome coupled to the antibody occurs with time. The fluorescence at immunoreactive sites will fade as it is observed under UV light. Moreover, the enzyme-antibody technique, including the PAP and ABC methods, has some distinct advantages when compared to the fluorescent antibody technique: it can be used at both light and electron microscopic levels; it is possible to preserve stained specimens for long periods; it is not arduous to localize positive (immunoreactive) cells, and the relationship of these cells with surrounding tissue can be observed using the common light microscope. Both the fluorescent and enzyme-antibody techniques consist of direct and indirect methods (Fig 3-1).

The steps involved in the immunohistochemical procedure for tissue staining are identical to the procedures used in classic histochemical staining (tissue fixation, dehydration and embedding, sectioning, deparaffinization and rehydration, staining, dehydration and mounting, observation, and microscopic photography) (Table 3-1). There are several different methods for staining in immunohistochemistry. These methods are discussed.

STAINING METHODS IN IMMUNOHISTOCHEMISTRY

Direct Method

In the direct method (Figs 3-1 and 3-2), the immunohistochemical localization of antigen is accomplished by using a fluorogen- or enzyme-

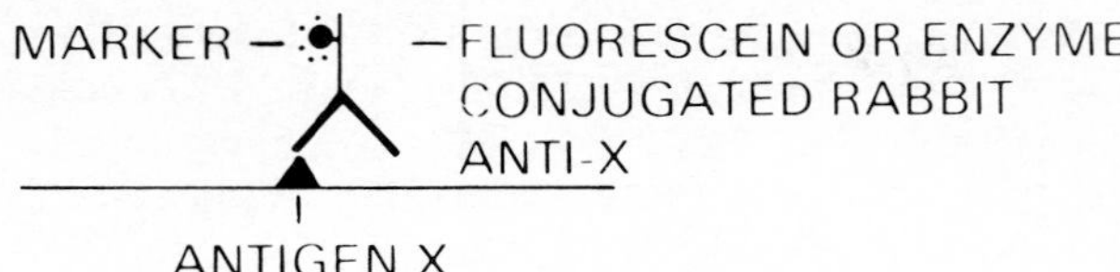

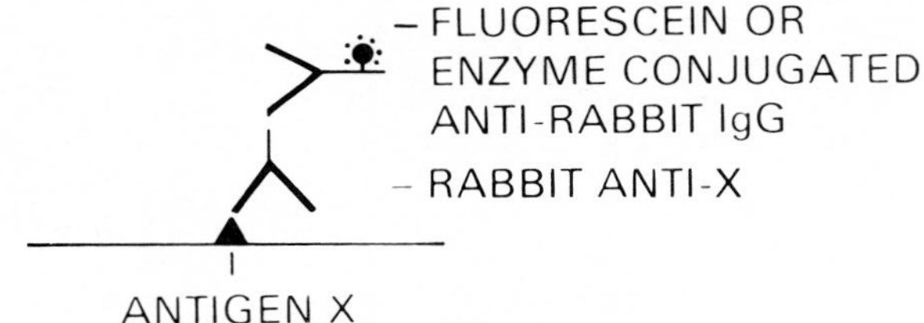

Figure 3-1. Direct and indirect methods

labeled primary antibody. As this procedure involves only a single application of a primary antibody, nonspecific reactions are reduced. A large amount of primary antibody is required to prepare the labeled antibody, and the sensitivity of this method is comparatively low. Today, this method is utilized only when another technique cannot be applied, such as in the study of cell-surface immunoglobulins. In this case, the use of a secondary antibody can react in the absence of a primary antibody.

Indirect Method

This technique (Figs 3-1, 3-3, and 3-4), called the sandwich technique, consists of two distinct antigen-antibody reactions. First, the primary antibody reacts with the antigen that is contained in or found on the cell surface. The primary antibody acts in effect as an antigen and reacts with a fluorogen or enzyme-labeled second antibody. The second antibody is generated against the gamma globulin fraction of the species in which the primary antibody is raised and for most studies, the second antibody is obtained easily from commercial sources. When compared with the direct method, the indirect method is more sensitive, since the primary antibody has many binding sites that provide more attachment sites for the labeled second antibody. In fluorescent immunohisto-

Table 3-1. Immunohistochemical procedure

1. Tissue fixation
2. Dehydration and embedding
3. Sectioning
4. Deparaffinization and rehydration
5. Staining
6. Dehydration and mounting
7. Observation and photography

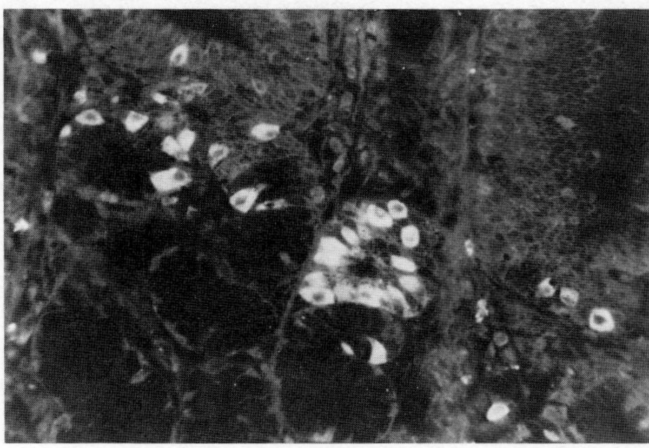

Figure 3-2. Fluorescent antibody technique (direct method). Dog antral mucosa; 10% formalin fixation, stained with gastrin antiserum (at a dilution of 1:2000). Original magnification ×200.

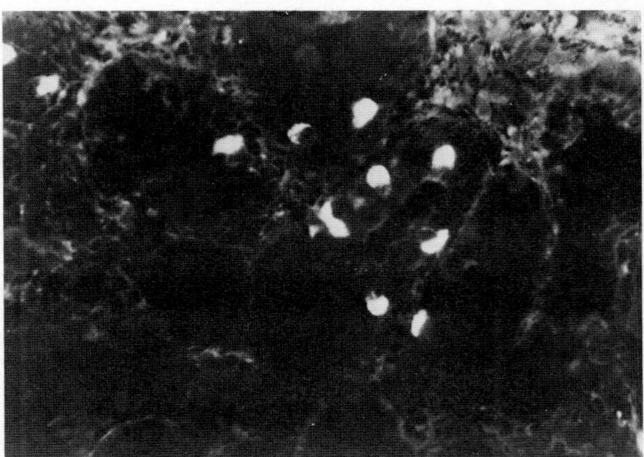

Figure 3-3. Fluorescent antibody technique (indirect method). Dog duodenal mucosa; p-benzoquinone fixation, stained with CCK antiserum (at a dilution of 1:5000). Original magnification ×400.

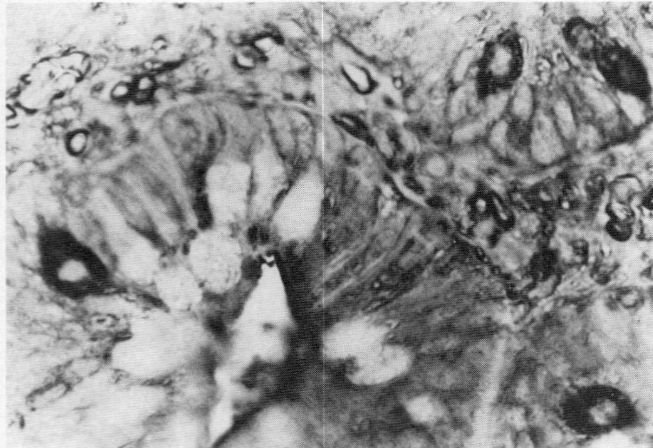

Figure 3-4. Enzyme antibody technique (indirect method). Dog duodenal mucosa; 10% formalin fixation, stained with CCK antiserum (at a dilution of 1:1500). Original magnification ×400.

chemistry, this technique is used widely; in addition to its high sensitivity, this method necessitates only a single preparation of labeled second antibody.

Unlabeled Antibody Method

Several problems arise in the preparation of the enzyme-labeled antibody. First, the labeling process itself can destroy much of the antibody activity. Furthermore, when the labeling process is mild, unconjugated antibody remains and, unless removed, will interfere with uptake of labeled antibodies. Additionally, the labeling process itself can introduce nonspecific background staining. To circumvent these problems, the method has been modified.

In the direct method, enzyme-labeled rabbit antibody (IgG) is applied in the final stage. However, in the unlabeled antibody technique, rabbit IgG generated against purified horseradish peroxidase is applied. Then purified peroxidase is applied and combines with the rabbit antiperoxidase via the antigen-antibody reaction.

In comparison to the enzyme-labeled antibody method, this approach is exceptionally sensitive, but two difficulties still remain. The yield of purified antibody is often less than 2 percent, and peroxidase is lost during the washing stage. Furthermore, procedures for preparing the antibody seem to selectively enhance the preparation of less avid antibodies [5].

PAP Method

The shortcomings of the unlabeled antibody technique have been overcome by the development of the peroxidase-antiperoxidase (PAP) complex (Table 3-2, Figs 3-5 to 3-8). The average PAP complex consists of three molecules of peroxidase and two molecules of antiperoxidase [5]. The PAP complex is usually stable and homogeneous. The PAP method is about 20 times more sensitive than the unlabeled antibody enzyme method, and it is 100 to 1000 times more sensitive than the indirect immunofluorescence technique. Background or nonspecific staining is minimal, since the inherent high sensitivity of this technique permits use of a primary antiserum at a high dilution. The unoccupied binding site of the specific anti-IgG antibody in the second layer possesses equal IgG specificity compared to that bound to the primary antibody.

Table 3-2. **Staining procedure of PAP method applied in our laboratory**

1. **Incubate with 3% normal goat serum (NGS) for 30 minutes: 0.2% Triton X-100; 0.75% gelatin in 0.1 M phosphate buffer; saline (PBS; pH 7.4)**
2. **Incubate with primary antiserum (diluted with 1% NGS, 0.2% Triton X-100, in 0.1 M PBS) overnight at room temperature**
3. **Wash three times with 1% NGS in 0.1 M PBS**
4. **Incubate with 3% NGS; 0.75% gelatin in 0.1 M PBS for 30 minutes**
5. **Incubate with goat antirabbit IgG (diluted 1:100 with 1% NGS in 0.1 M PBS) for 30 minutes**
6. **Wash three times with phosphate buffer (PB; pH 7.4)**
7. **Incubate with 3% NGS; 0.75% gelatin in 0.1 M PBS for 30 minutes**
8. **Incubate with PAP (rabbit) (diluted 1:640 with 1% NGS in 0.1 M PBS) for 30 minutes**
9. **Wash three times with PBS**
10. **Rinse three times with 0.1 M acetate buffer (pH 6.0)**
11. **Incubate in 0.035% diaminobenzidine (DAB) and 2.5% nickel ammonium sulfate in 0.1 M acetate buffer (pH 6.0), which contains H_2O_2 (17 μL/5 mL DAB solution) for 3–5 minutes**
12. **Rinse two times with 0.1 M acetate buffer**
13. **Wash two times with PBS**
14. **Counterstain (or double stain)**
15. **For double stain, repeat steps 2–9. In step 10, delete the nickel salt and use PBS (pH 7.4)**
16. **Rinse in distilled water, dry, and apply coverslip.**

Note: Double-stained slides are not counterstained.

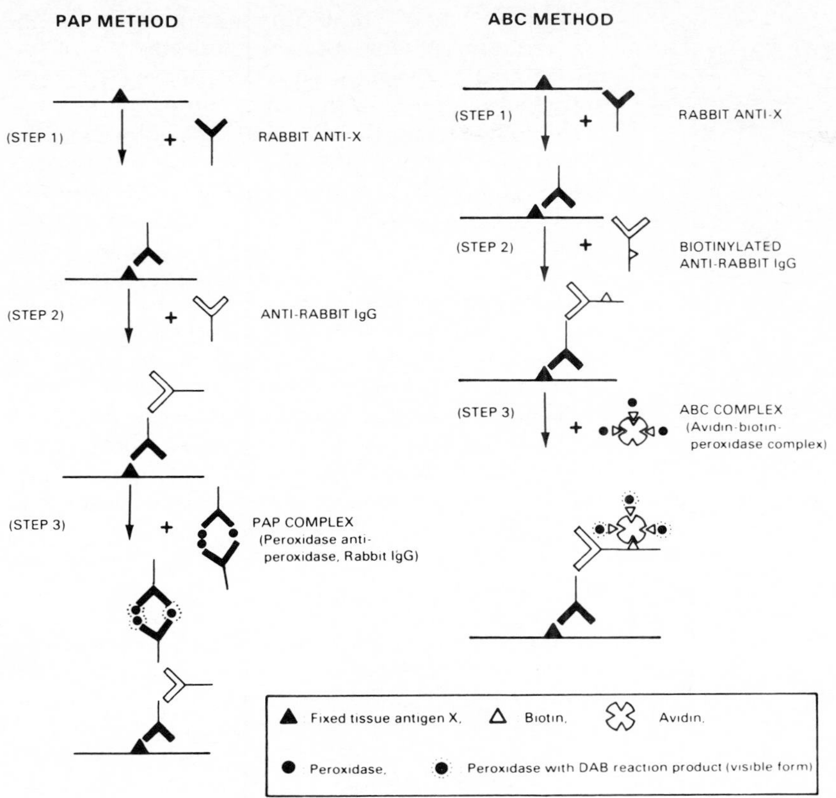

Figure 3-5. PAP and ABC methods

Therefore, it selectively reacts with the PAP reagent. An unoccupied binding site of a nonspecifically attached antibody can react only with a nonspecific component. Since PAP is a pure reagent devoid of such nonspecific components, it does not react with unoccupied antigen binding sites of the nonspecific antibody. If the PAP reagent, in spite of its purification, contains a contaminant also found in the tissue, the bound antibody can react with this nonspecific component. However, such contaminants cannot be an antibody to peroxidase. Therefore, despite its reaction with the (link) antibody, the contaminant is devoid of peroxidase and will not be detected with diaminobenzidine and hydrogen peroxide. Thus, a double amplification of specificity is incorporated into the PAP method. Today, the PAP method is the most popular immunohistochemical method.

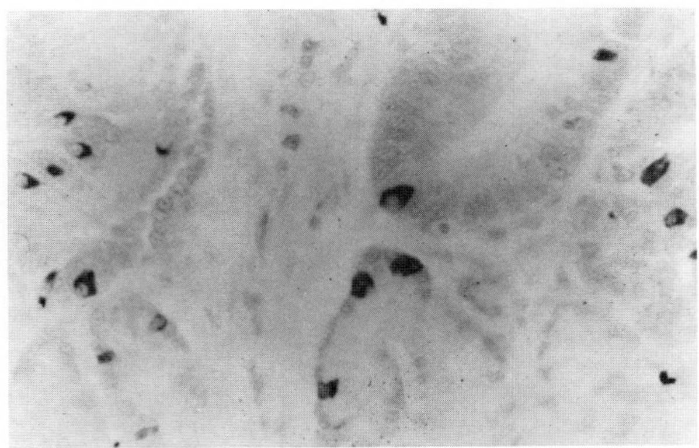

Figure 3-6. Peroxidase-antiperoxidase (PAP) technique. Dog antral mucosa; 4% paraformaldehyde fixation, stained with gastrin antiserum (at a dilution of 1:40,000). Section counterstained with nuclear fast red. Original magnification ×400.

Avidin-Biotin-Peroxidase Complex (ABC) Method

In the PAP method, peroxidase is linked to antiperoxidase by the antigen-antibody reaction to the second antibody. In the ABC method, the high affinity of avidin for biotin is utilized in place of the antigen-antibody interaction (Figs 3-5 and 3-9). This technique consists of three components:

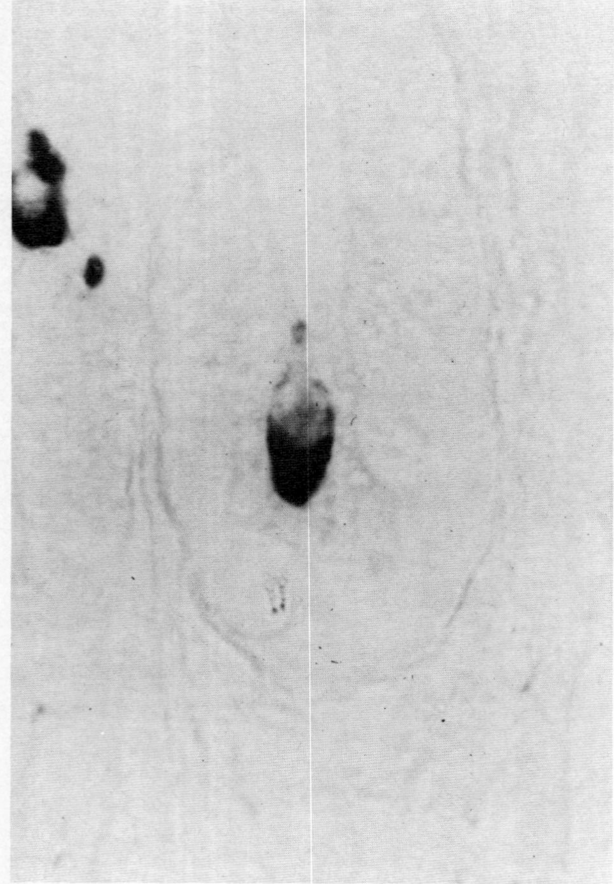

Figure 3-7. Peroxidase-antiperoxidase (PAP) technique. Dog ileal mucosa; 4% paraformaldehyde fixation, stained with neurotensin antiserum (at a dilution of 1:20,000). Original magnification ×500.

1. A primary antibody that is specific for the tissue antigen.
2. Biotin-conjugated second antibody capable of binding to the first antibody.
3. A complex of peroxidase-conjugated biotin and avidin that attaches to the biotin on the second antibody.

Avidin, a glycoprotein, has four binding sites for biotin (vitamin H). The binding affinity of avidin to biotin is extraordinarily higher than most antibody-antigen complexes, and its binding is practically irreversible. The ABC method is 8 to 40 times more sensitive than the PAP method. It is worth noting that endogenous biotin can react with avidin, which results in high nonspecific staining.

Several methods have been devised to identify more than one antigen in the same tissue section simultaneously by combining immunohistochemical procedures. One such method consists of the use of two fluorogens with the fluorescent antibody technique [8]. Different chromogens, such as diaminobenzidine (DAB) and DAB-nickel, can be linked to the same substrate (horseradish peroxidase) [9], or to two or more different substrates in the enzyme-antibody technique [10], or a combination of both immunofluorescence and immunoperoxidase can be used [11]. The enzyme-antibody method has been employed successfully in electron microscopic identification of peptide-containing cells. Conventional thin sections prepared for electron microscopic observation [12], or 1-μm thick epon-embedded sections that are prepared for light microscopy are stained and then correlated with the observations of granule morphology in serial thin sections viewed by electron microscopy [13].

Dual-Color Staining

The relative distributions of different antigens have been determined by staining adjacent tissue sections for single antigens and comparing the sections. However, the use of dual-color immunoperoxidase staining allows the distributions of two antigens to be simultaneously visualized in the same tissue section. The advantage of dual-color immunoperoxidase staining is that it often reveals subtle spatial relations between immunostained elements that may not have been detected on inspection of singly stained adjacent sections. The method was pioneered by Nakane [10], using the peroxidase-labeled antibody method and the chromagens, 3,3′-diaminobenzidine (DAB), alpha-naphthol/pyronin, and 4-chloro-1-naphthol to obtain brown, reddish-pink, and reddish-blue reaction products. In the dual-color immunoperoxidase staining technique, tissue sections are incubated in two sequences of immunoreagents and a different chromagen is used to stain for each antibody-antigen complex. The choice of chromagens, their concentrations, and their sequence of application are critical in avoiding color mixing and obtaining good contrast between stained elements. Elution of antibodies with acidic solutions between stains has been used to prevent color mixing due to residual peroxidase activity [10]; however, this may denature antigens and result in a reduction or complete loss of immunostaining. Sternberger and Joseph [14] developed a dual-color staining procedure using the PAP technique. They found that elution of the first sequence of immunoreagents was not necessary to prevent

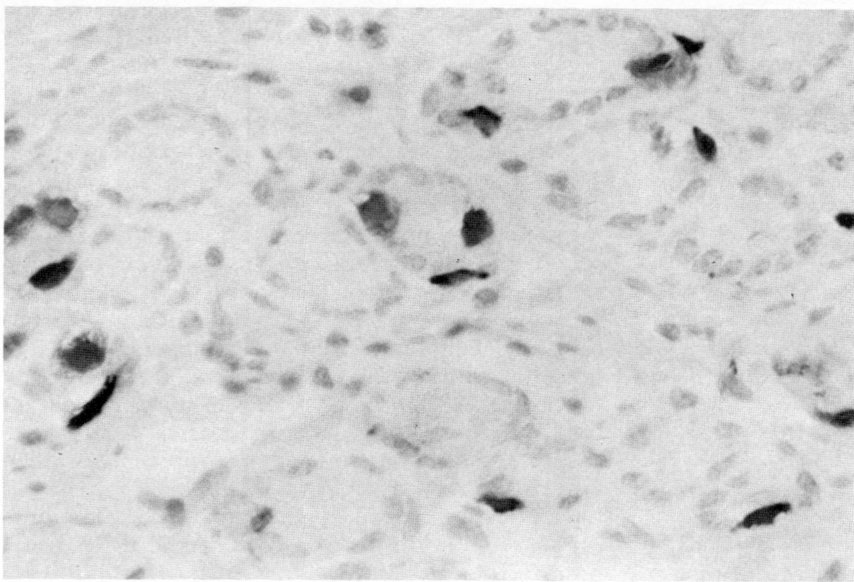

Figure 3-8. Enzyme antibody technique (dual-color immunoperoxidase stain). Hamster antral mucosa was fixed with 4% IV paraformaldehyde perfusion and stained with gastrin antiserum (1:40,000) and serotonin antiserum (1:40,000). Gastrin-immunoreactive cells were stained black using nickle-intensified DAB. Serotonin-immunoreactive cells were stained amber using DAB alone. The section was counterstained with methyl green. Original magnification ×730.

color mixing, provided that the primary antibody and DAB used to localize the first antigen were used in sufficient concentrations. They suggested that the polymeric DAB reaction product masked the antibodies and the peroxidase, so that cross-reactions with the second sequence of antibodies were prevented.

The reaction products obtained with some chromagens are not stable; however, the low solubility of DAB polymeric reaction products in organic solvents makes DAB a chromagen of choice. The addition of a nickel salt to the DAB in a suitable buffer solution has been shown recently to yield a stable black reaction product in the presence of peroxidase and hydrogen peroxide; this product contrasts nicely with the amber-to-brown reaction product obtained with DAB alone [15,16]. These easily distinguishable reaction products have been

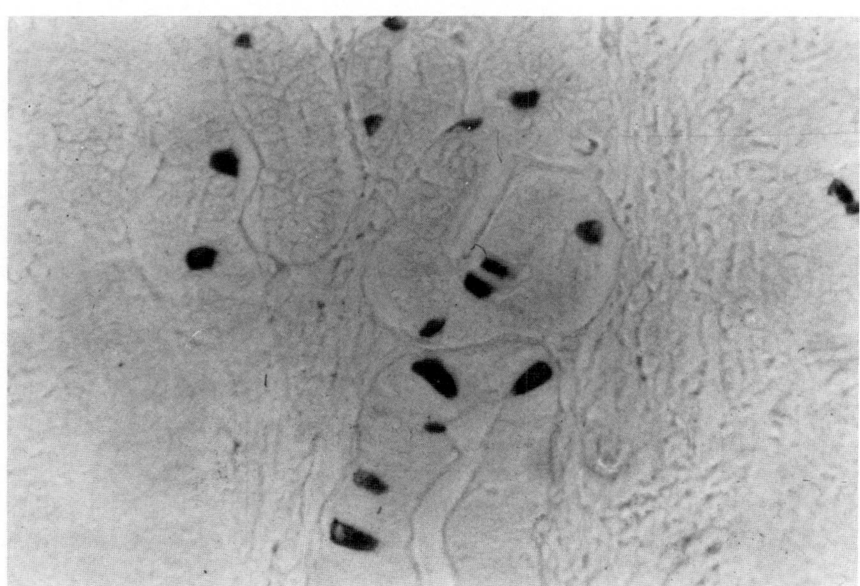

Figure 3-9. Enzyme antibody technique (ABC method). Dog antral mucosa; 4% paraformaldehyde fixation, stained with gastrin antiserum (at a dilution of 1:40,000). Original magnification ×310.

used to visualize black peptide-immunoreactive nerve terminals on amber-stained monoamine-immunoreactive neurons in the central nervous system (CNS) [9], and pairs of immunologically distinct antigens can be localized in cells in the gut using this dual-color immunoperoxidase staining procedure (see Table 3-2 and Fig 3-8). In order to avoid color mixing, it is imperative that the nickel-DAB solution be used to stain for the first antigen; the intense black nickel-DAB reaction product will mask the first-sequence immunoreagents from the second-sequence reagents [14], and antibody elution is not required. In dual-color immunoperoxidase staining, all reactions taking place in chromagen solutions should be monitored under the microscope to obtain optimum contrast.

Precautions in Antibody Application

In order to apply the immunohistochemical technique in identifying cells containing gut peptides, high affinity antibodies that show no cross-reactivity with structurally related peptides are essential. The potential cross-reactivity of the antibody with related peptides should be examined in a radioimmunoassay (RIA) system. However, RIA findings do not always correlate with immunohistochemical features of the antibody, since an antibody that has a negligible cross-reactivity with related peptides in an RIA system is, at times, not useful in immunohistochemistry [17]. In an RIA, a radiolabeled antigen competes with components in the sample for binding sites on the antibody. An antibody unable to cross-react with an antigen rarely occurs. In contrast, in immunohistochemistry, it is possible for an antibody to react with all types of antigens that have an affinity, albeit low, for the antibody. Consequently, positive staining can occur in cells that contain both authentic antigen or structurally unrelated antigens, regardless of the amount of antigen. To increase immunohistochemical specificity, the unique radioimmunocytochemical technique has been utilized [18]. With this method, radiolabeled antigen is incubated with excess antibody. Hence, there will be an unoccupied binding site on the antibody that will attach to the tissue antigen. The tissue antigen is then localized with autoradiography.

Tissue Specimens

An essential ingredient in immunohistochemistry is the preservation of antigenic sites in tissue after fixation or embedding, while maintaining the original tissue structure. Antigenic sites should be intact and exposed so that the antibody can react easily with the tissue antigen. The use of liquid formalin, paraformaldehyde, and Bouin's solution as fixatives is advisable. Bifunctional reagents, such as diethylpyrocarbonate and *p*-benzoquinone, are also recommended [19].

One of the most perplexing problems in immunocytochemistry is obtaining very thin tissue sections while maintaining the antigenicity of the tissue. Frozen sections and sections cut on a Vibratome have been used to maintain antigenicity, but semithin sections (1–2 μm) cannot be obtained with these methods. If the spatial relations between immunoreactive elements in the gastrointestinal tract are to be optimally visualized with the light microscope, semithin sections are required. These can be obtained with embedded material cut on an ultramicrotome, but antigenicity may be lost during the embedding procedure or the embedding medium cannot be penetrated by the immunoglobulins used in immunocytochemical stains. Pre-embedding staining of 25- to 30-μm Vibratome sections followed by embedding and semithin sectioning avoids the loss of antigenicity associated with postembedding immunostaining. For light microscopy, the thick tissue sections are usually treated with a detergent to facilitate the entry of the immunoreagents.

Staining Specificity

It is mandatory to check the specificity of staining results by testing with appropriate controls [20]. There are two controls for specificity: one is to demonstrate the specificity of interaction between the primary antibody and the tissue-bound antigen. This is verified by permitting the antibody to react with varying concentrations of pure native or synthetic peptides (absorption controls). The absorption of an antibody by the pure antigen, but not by related or unrelated peptides, usually results in negative staining. The second staining control serves to exclude autofluorescence, endogenous enzyme activity, and nonspecific binding of the second antiserum. In this control, the primary antibody, the second antibody, the tertiary antibody, or all antibodies are deleted, and blocking tests (only in the direct technique) are used. In these controls, staining should disappear. Several nonspecific reactions have been reported, such as complement-mediated [21], polyvalent immunoreactivities [22], ionic-interaction [23], and fixation-dependent [24].

IMMUNOHISTOCHEMICAL STUDIES ON PEPTIDES IN THE ALIMENTARY CANAL AND PANCREAS

Gastrin-containing cells were first demonstrated as gut endocrine cells in 1968 [25]. Substance P-immunoreactive neurons were demonstrated in 1975 [26]. More recently, many peptide-containing cells and neurons have been reported to exist in all layers and/or the entire length of the alimentary canal, pancreas, and gallbladder [27–29].

Gastrin and Cholecystokinin (CCK)

Gastrin was first demonstrated in human antral mucosa [25] using immunofluorescence and standard light microscopic techniques. Later, electron microscopic and immunohistochemical techniques verified the presence of gastrin in G cell secretory granules [12]. Immunohistochemical studies have shown that the principal site of gastrin is the antropyloric mucosa. Gastrin is also found in the proximal small intestine but not in the oxyntic mucosa, ileum, or colon [30]. It has been suggested that pancreatic D cells also contain gastrin [31]; however, this has not been confirmed by region-specific gastrin antisera [30]. It is conceivable that pancreatic D cells, which contain somatostatin, also contain a peptide that has a primary structure similar to that of gastrin. It is generally believed that gastrin cells do not exist in the adult rat pancreas, although they are found in the fetus [32].

CCK-containing cells have been identified in the mucosa of the dog and human duodenum and jejunum [33]. CCK-containing cells are identical ultrastructurally to the intestinal I cell [34]. Since gastrin and CCK have a common C-terminal primary structure, many of the CCK and gastrin antisera cross-react with both peptides. Hence, the use of a CCK- or gastrin-nonspecific antisera leads to staining of both gastrin and CCK cells [34,35]. Discrimination of enteric CCK-containing cells from gastrin-containing cells has been accomplished successfully by treating CCK antisera with gastrin, and conversely, gastrin cells were shown by using gastrin antisera that were absorbed with CCK [34–36]. By using region-specific gastrin antibodies, gastrin-containing cells were distinguished from CCK-containing cells in the human intestine [37]. Studies with region-specific gastrin antibodies have shown that both gastrin-17 and gastrin-34 appear to be located in the same cell in the antral mucosa, suggesting a pathway of granule maturation [38,39]. The larger clear granules that predominate in antral G cells have been postulated to contain gastrin-17, while gastrin-34 may be present in the smaller dark granules found in antral G cells but predominantly in intestinal G cells [40]. The existence of a third type of related endocrine-like cell (TG cells) has been suggested [41]. These may be found in pancreatic neurons [42]; they appear to cross-react with antisera to the common C-terminal tetrapeptide of gastrin and CCK but fail to cross-react with other gastrin- and CCK-specific sequences. A single study reports CCK-like immunoreactivity existing in the nerves of guinea pig colon [43].

Secretin and Gastric Inhibitory Polypeptide (GIP)

Secretin-containing (or S) cells have been demonstrated in the duodenum and jejunum [44–46]. S cells are scarce in the ileum and are totally absent from the stomach, colon, and pancreas. The presence of secretin-containing cells outside the alimentary tract has been shown in endocrine monolayer cultures of the rat pancreas [47] and in the antral mucosa of several mammalian species [48].

GIP-containing cells have been detected in the duodenum and jejunum [49,50] and GIP-like immunoreactivity has been shown in both pancreatic glucagon (A) cells and in gut glucagon (GLI) cells [51,52], which suggests the presence of a glucagon precursor that shares a primary structure similar to that of GIP [53,54].

Enteroglucagon and Glucagon

Enteroglucagon-containing cells are found in the jejunum, ileum, and colon [55]. Glucagon was found first in both pancreatic A cells and in A cells of the oxyntic mucosa of cats and dogs, but not in humans or the rat [56]. Enteroglucagon antiserum reacts with the N-terminal of glucagon, while pancreatic glucagon antiserum reacts with the C-terminus of glucagon [57]. The possible presence of multiple molecular forms and differences in antisera specificity also complicates interpretations.

Glicentin, a 100 amino acid glucagon-like peptide [57,58], has been shown in both pancreatic A cells and in A cells of cat and dog oxyntic mucosa [59], suggesting that it may be a precursor of glucagon. Glicentin immunoreactivity has also been found in endocrine-like cells of the ileum and colon, which react with NH_2-terminal-specific antibody but not with C-terminal-specific (glucagon-specific) antibody. These cells are referred to as enteroglucagon cells [55] or gut-type glucagon cells [60]. Glicentin-containing, nonglucagon cells of the distal gut might be identical with the L (GLI) cells [61]. The coexistence of glucagon/glicentin-containing cells with GIP [53,54] or pancreatic polypeptide (PP)-containing cells [62] has been shown.

Motilin

Motilin-containing cells have been found in the duodenal and jejunal mucosa of mammals [63], but the specific cell type remains a matter of some dispute. One group indicates that motilin-containing cells are in enterochromaffin cells distinct from substance P-containing cells [13], while another group concludes that motilin is in nonenterochromaffin cells [64,65]. This discrepancy might actually suggest the existence of different molecular forms of motilin that occur in different cells [66,67].

Neurotensin

Neurotensin-containing or N cells have been demonstrated in richest amounts in the ileal mucosa, with smaller concentrations in the jejunum, stomach, duodenum, and colon [68,69]. Neurotensin-containing cells have a typical feature of gut endocrine cells; their villi are in contact with the intestinal lumen, and neurotensin-containing granules are found in the basal portion of the cell (see Fig 3-7). This morphologic evidence supports the suggestion that neurotensin may be released into the general circulation to act as a hormone. Neurotensin-immunoreactive fibers have been reported in rat alimentary canal [70].

PP and Peptide YY (PYY)

PP-containing cells have been demonstrated in pancreatic islets as well as in exocrine parenchyma of the pancreas [71,72]. In the opossum and dog, PP cells are also found in the stomach [71]. PP-immunoreactive cells that occur in the human colon and rectum appear to differ from those that occur in the pancreas. These PP-containing cells in the distal intestine, which were demonstrated in a subpopulation of glucagon/glicentin cells [29], contain a peptide with a primary structure similar to that of PP [73].

Recently, PYY has been isolated from porcine duodenum [74] and localized in endocrine cells of the ileum and colon [75,76]. Hence, it seems reasonable that the PP-immunoreactive cells observed earlier in the colon may actually be PYY cells. Furthermore, coexistence of PYY and glucagon/glicentin has been demonstrated [77]. The icosapeptide fragment of PP isolated from the canine pancreas has been reported to represent a COOH-terminal fragment of the PP precursor [78,79]. Antisera generated against the icosapeptide fragment show PP-immunoreactive cells in the pancreas (which are "true" PP cells), but this antisera does not cross-react with PP-immunoreactive cells in the distal intestine (PYY cells). This finding indicates that PP cells and PYY-containing cells are found in separate regions [80].

Somatostatin

Somatostatin was first found in the CNS as the growth hormone-release-inhibiting factor. Somatostatin has been found in the autonomic nervous system of the gut, in D cells of the pancreas [81], and in the mucosa of the gut [82,83]. Concentrations of somatostatin-containing cells in the gut are especially high in the stomach, and they decrease in a gradient fashion from stomach to lower colon. Somatostatin-containing cells appear to play a paracrine role. This idea has some basis, since somatostatin-containing cells have long cytoplasmic processes that terminate near gastrin and parietal cells in the stomach [84] (Fig 3-10). These cells have the appearance of an interesting intermediate between nerve and endocrine cells. Somatostatin-containing nerve fibers are prominent surrounding the ganglion cells of the myenteric plexus of the small intestine, which suggests that somatostatin may play the role of a neurotransmitter within the enteric nervous system [85]. Somatostatin-containing nerves are seen in the colon, gallbladder, and biliary tract of guinea pigs [86]. Antral somatostatin deficiency in patients with duodenal ulcers has been observed by both radioimmunoassay [87] and immunohistochemistry [88], which suggests that somatostatin deficiency may be one of the causative factors of duodenal ulceration.

Calcitonin Gene-Related Peptide (CGRP)

CGRP, a 37 amino acid peptide, is a product of alternative RNA processing of the calcitonin gene [89]. CGRP is present in the central and peripheral nervous systems of numerous mammals [90].

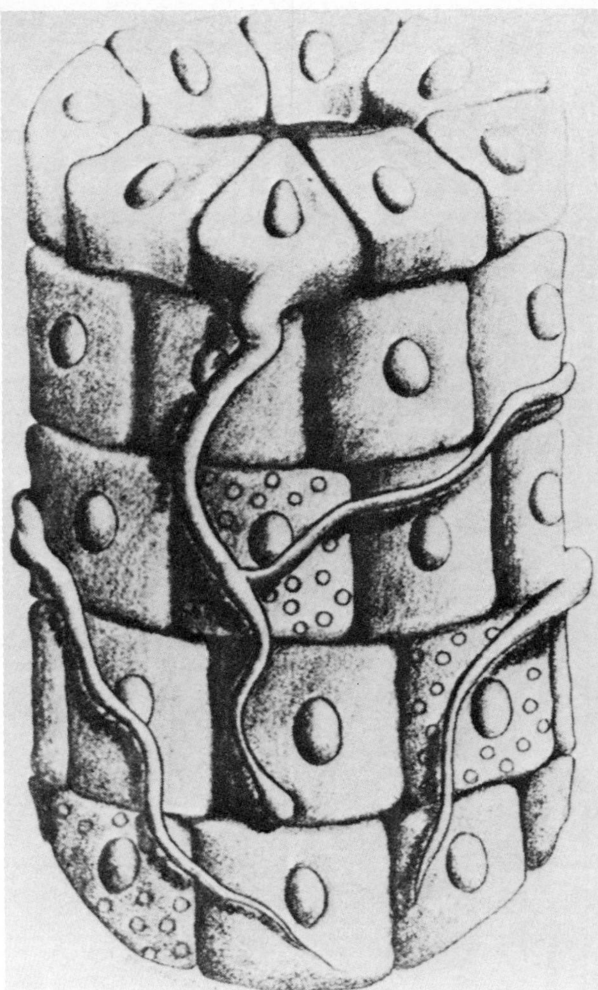

Figure 3-10. Drawing showing the arrangement of somatostatin cells in rat antropyloric glands. (From Larsson L-I [126], by permission of American Association for the Advancement of Science.)

CGRP-immunoreactive cells have been localized in the rat pancreatic islets, and some islet cells exhibit both CGRP- and somatostatin-immunoreactivity [91]. Since CGRP inhibits insulin release from isolated rat pancreatic islets [92], these findings suggest that CGRP has a paracrine role in the regulation of islet cell function.

Vasoactive Intestinal Peptide (VIP)

VIP was initially localized in intestinal endocrine-like cells [93] and then in both endocrine cells and nerves [94]. Another study showed VIP only in neurons [95]. Finally, it was confirmed that at least some of the antisera detecting endocrine cells was directed towards the NH_2-terminal of VIP and could cross-react with secretin and glucagon [96]. Using an antisera with C-terminal specificity, VIP immunoreactivity was shown to exist entirely in nerve fibers and cell bodies [97]. VIP has been shown to be widely distributed in the cerebrovascular nerves of the brain and in nerve fibers and cell bodies throughout the gut. VIP-containing nerves are abundant in the colon and in the intestine [98], in the gallbladder [86,99], in the pancreas [97,100,101], in the wall of the portal vein [102], and in almost all gastrointestinal sphincters [103]. In the alimentary canal, VIP-containing nerve terminals are associated chiefly with blood vessels, smooth musculature, and ganglion cells of Auerbach's and Meissner's plexus [97].

Substance P

Substance P-like immunoreactivity has been demonstrated throughout the gut, mostly in fine nerve fibers in all areas of the gut wall but also in gastrointestinal endocrine cells [26,104,105]. The highest concentrations are in the small intestine, especially in the proximal bowel, and also in the colon. Substance P-containing cells have been identified as a subtype of gastrointestinal enterochromaffin cells (EC_1 cells) [106]. Substance P-containing nerves have also been found in the gallbladder [86] and pancreas [107].

Bombesin

Bombesin, originally isolated from amphibian skin [108], has been identified in CNS and gut of various mammals [109,110] and in the mucosa of the human gastrointestinal tract [111]. In the human gut, bombesin-like immunoreactive cells have been reported to be distributed widely [111] but appear to be localized chiefly in fine varicose nerve fibers in the submucosa and mucosa [112]. Bombesin-containing nerves have been observed in the biliary tract, mainly in the sphincter of Oddi [86]. Gastrin-releasing peptide was recently isolated from nonantral gastric tissue and intestine, and contains 27 amino acid residues, of which nine of the ten C-terminals are identical to bombesin [113]. It is also found in the gut [114].

Enkephalin

Enkephalin-like immunoreactivity has been detected in the human alimentary canal by using met-enkephalin antisera [115]. Met-enkephalin is found in nerve fibers of the myenteric plexus throughout the gut. Enkephalin-containing nerves are observed in the guinea pig gallbladder [86] and in the feline pancreas [107]. Endocrine cells containing enkephalin-like immunoreactivity are identified in the pig antrum and duodenum as enterochromaffin cells [116].

Peptide Histidine Isoleucine (PHI)

PHI, isolated from the porcine intestine [117], has an amino acid sequence similar to that of VIP. PHI-like immunoreactive nerves have been demonstrated in the ileum and colon of the rat and pig, which coincides with VIP nerves, providing the possibility of a common precursor [118].

Neuropeptide Y (NPY)

NPY is a PP analogue isolated from bovine brain [119] and found in both central and peripheral neurons [120]. It is especially rich in neural elements of the gut and pancreas, but not endocrine cells [121], which suggests that NPY is a neurotransmitter. NPY may coexist with noradrenaline fibers in perivascular nerve fibers, which may provide the possible role of NPY in controlling blood flow.

Classic autonomic efferent nerves have been

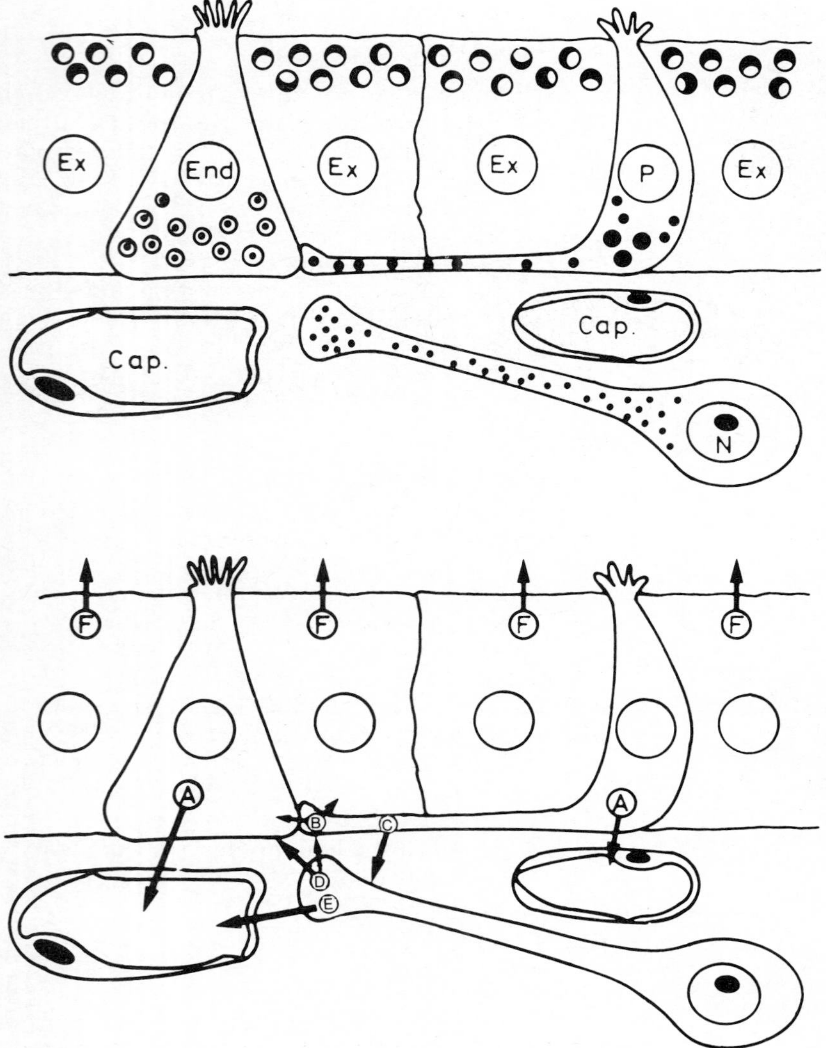

Figure 3-11. Drawing showing the possible interrelationships between exocrine cells (Ex), endocrine cells (End), paracrine cells (P), neurons (N) and capillaries (Cap.). The bottom panel shows some of the putative ways in which these systems may interrelate. A = endocrine secretion; B = paracrine secretion; C = "paracrine" effects on adjacent nerves; D = effects of nerves (neurotransmitter-like effects) on endocrine and paracrine cells; E = possible neuroendocrine secretion; and F = exocrine secretion. (From Larsson L-I [126], by permission of American Association for the Advancement of Science.)

divided into adrenergic and cholinergic, but a large proportion of the autonomic nerve fibers are now considered to be peptidergic. The concept of peptidergic nerves is altering our views of the autonomic nervous system. More recently, the presence of both gastrin and an ACTH-like peptide has been demonstrated in antropyloric gastrin cells [122–124]. Furthermore, some endocrine cells containing multiple peptides have been suggested [115,125]. These findings may change the principle of one cell, one hormone.

Gastrointestinal peptides clearly have multiple roles as endocrine, neurocrine, and paracrine messengers [126] (Fig 3-11). Immunohistochemical techniques may provide valuable help in dissecting the appropriate roles of each peptide.

REFERENCES

1. Solcia E, Capella C, Vassallo G, et al: Endocrine cells of the gastric mucosa. Int Rev Cytol 42:233, 1975.
2. Coons AH, Leduc EH, Connolly JM: Studies on antibody production. I. A method for the histochemical demonstration of specific antibody and its application to a study of the hyperimmune rabbit. J Exp Med 102:49, 1955.
3. Nakane PK, Pierce GB Jr: Enzyme-labeled antibodies: Preparation and application for the localization of antigens. J Histochem Cytochem 14:929, 1967.
4. Sternberger LA, Cuculis JJ: Method for enzymatic intensification of the immunocytochemical reaction without use of labeled antibodies. J Histochem Cytochem 17:190, 1969.
5. Sternberger LA, Hardy PH Jr, Cuculis JJ, et al: The unlabeled antibody enzyme method of immunohistochemistry. Preparation and properties of soluble antigen-antibody complex (horseradish peroxidase–antihorseradish peroxidase) and its use in identification of spirochetes. J Histochem Cytochem 18:315, 1970.
6. Sternberger L: *Immunocytochemistry*. New York, John Wiley & Sons, 1979.
7. Hsu S-M, Raine L, Fanger H: Use of avidin-biotin-peroxidase complex (ABC) in immunoperoxidase techniques: A comparison between ABC and unlabeled antibody (PAP) procedures. J Histochem Cytochem 29:577, 1981.
8. Nash DR, Crabbe PA, Heremans JF: Sequential immunofluorescent staining: A simple and useful technique. Immunology 16:785, 1969.
9. Hancock MB: Visualization of peptide-immunoreactive processes on serotonin-immunoreactive cells using two-color immunoperoxidase staining. J Histochem Cytochem 32:311, 1984.
10. Nakane PK: Simultaneous localization of multiple tissue antigens using the peroxidase-labeled antibody method: A study on pituitary glands of the rat. J Histochem Cytochem 16:557, 1968.
11. Lechago J, Sun NCJ, Weinstein WM: Simultaneous visualization of two antigens in the same tissue section by combining immunoperoxidase with immunofluorescence techniques. J Histochem Cytochem 27:1221, 1979.
12. Greider MH, Steinberg V, McGuigan JE: Electron microscopic identification of the gastrin cell of the human antral mucosa by means of immunocytochemistry. Gastroenterology 63:572, 1972.
13. Polak JM, Pearse AGE, Heath CM: Complete identification of endocrine cells in the gastrointestinal tract using semithin-thin sections to identify motilin cells in human and animal intestine. Gut 16:225, 1975.
14. Sternberger LA, Joseph SA: The unlabeled antibody method: Contrasting color staining of paired pituitary hormones without antibody removal. J Histochem Cytochem 27:1424, 1979.
15. Hancock MB: A serotonin-immunoreactive fiber system in the dorsal columns of the spinal cord. Neurosci Lett 31:247, 1982.
16. Hancock MB: DAB-nickel substrate for the differential immunoperoxidase staining of nerve fibers and fiber terminals. J Histochem Cytochem 30:578, 1982.
17. Larsson L-I: Problems and pitfalls in immunocytochemistry of gut peptides, in Jerzy Glass GB (ed): *Gastrointestinal Hormones*. New York, Raven Press, 1980, pp 53–70.
18. Larsson L-I, Schwartz TW: Radioimmunocytochemistry—A novel immunocytochemical principle. J Histochem Cytochem 10:1140, 1977.
19. Pearse AGE, Polak JM: Bifunctional reagents as vapour- and liquid-phase fixatives for immunohistochemistry. Histochem J 7:179, 1975.
20. van Noorden S, Polak JM: Advances in immunocytochemistry, in Bloom SR, Polak JM (eds): *Gut Hormones*. 2nd Ed. New York, Churchill Livingstone, 1981, pp 80–89.
21. Buffa R, Crivelli O, Fiocca R, et al: Complement-mediated unspecific binding of immunoglobulins to some endocrine cells. Histochemistry 63:15, 1979.
22. Grube D, Weber E: Immunoreactivities of gastrin (G-) cells. I. Dilution-dependent staining of G-cells by antisera and non-immune sera. Histochemistry 65:223, 1980.
23. Grube D: Immunoreactivities of gastrin (G-) cells. II. Non-specific binding of immunoglobulins to G-cells by ionic interactions. Histochemistry 66:149, 1980.
24. Bergroth V, Reitamo S, Konttinen YT, et al: Fixation-dependent cytoplasmic false-positive staining with an immunoperoxidase method. Histochemistry 73:509, 1982.
25. McGuigan JE: Gastric mucosal intracellular localization of gastrin by immunofluorescence. Gastroenterology 55:315, 1968.
26. Pearse AGE, Polak JM: Immunocytochemical localization of substance P in mammalian intestine. Histochemistry 41:373, 1975.
27. Polak JM, Bloom SR: Gastrointestinal hormones: Distribution and tissue localization, in Beers RF Jr,

Bassett EG (eds): *Polypeptide Hormones.* New York, Raven Press, 1980, pp 371–394.
28. Ferri G-L, Adrian TE, Ghatei MA, et al: Tissue localization and relative distribution of regulatory peptides in separated layers from the human bowel. Gastroenterology 84:777, 1983.
29. Sjolund K, Sanden G, Håkanson R, et al: Endocrine cells in human intestine: An immunocytochemical study. Gastroenterology 85:1120, 1983.
30. Larsson L-I: Pathology of the gastrin cell, in Sommers SC, Rosen PP (series eds): *Pathology Annual.* New York, Appleton-Century-Crofts, 1979, pp 293–316.
31. Erlandsen SL, Hegre OD, Parsons JA, et al: Pancreatic islet cell hormones. Distribution of cell types in the islet and evidence for the presence of somatostatin and gastrin within the D cell. J Histochem Cytochem 24:883, 1976.
32. Larsson L-I, Rehfeld JF, Sundler F, et al: Pancreatic gastrin in foetal and neonatal rats. Nature 262:609, 1976.
33. Buffa R, Solcia E, Go VLW: Immunohistochemical identification of the cholecystokinin cell in the intestinal mucosa. Gastroenterology 70:528, 1976.
34. Buchan AMJ, Polak JM, Solcia E, et al: Electron immunohistochemical evidence for the human intestinal I cell as the source of CCK. Gut 19:403, 1978.
35. Larsson L-I, Rehfeld JF: Characterization of antral gastrin cells with region-specific antisera. J Histochem Cytochem 25:1317, 1977.
36. Dubois PM, Paulin C, Chayvialle JA: Identification of gastrin-secreting cells and cholecystokinin-secreting cells in the gastrointestinal tract of the human fetus and adult man. Cell Tissue Res 175:351, 1976.
37. Buchan AMJ, Polak JM, Solcia E, et al: Localisation of intestinal gastrin in a distinct endocrine cell type. Nature 277:138, 1979.
38. Vaillant C, Dockray G, Hopkins CR: Cellular origins of different forms of gastrin. The specific immunocytochemical localization of related peptides. J Histochem Cytochem 27:932, 1979.
39. Varndell IM, Harris A, Tapia FJ, et al: Intracellular topography of immunoreactive gastrin demonstrated using electron immunocytochemistry. Experientia 39:713, 1983.
40. Polak JM, Buchan AMJ, Bryant MG, et al: Intestinal gastrin—Cellular origin, ontogeny and tumour distribution. Gastroenterology 76:1219, 1979.
41. Larsson L-I, Rehfeld JF: A peptide resembling COOH-terminal tetrapeptide amide of gastrin from a new gastrointestinal endocrine cell type. Nature 277:575, 1979.
42. Rehfeld JF, Larsson L-I, Goltermann NR, et al: Neural regulation of pancreatic hormone secretion by the C-terminal tetrapeptide of CCK. Nature 284:33, 1980.
43. Larsson L-I, Rehfeld JF: Localization and molecular heterogeneity of cholecystokinin in the central and peripheral nervous system. Brain Res 165:201, 1979.
44. Bussolati G, Capella C, Solcia E, et al: Ultrastructural and immunofluorescent investigations on the secretin cell in the dog intestinal mucosa. Histochemie 26:218, 1971.
45. Polak JM, Coulling I, Bloom S, et al: Immunofluorescent localization of secretin and enteroglucagon in human intestinal mucosa. Scand J Gastroenterol 6:739, 1971.
46. Larsson L-I, Sundler F, Alumets J, et al: Distribution, ontogeny and ultrastructure of the mammalian secretin cell. Cell Tissue Res 181:361, 1977.
47. Rufener C, Amherdt M, Baetens D, et al: Immunofluorescent localization of secretin in pancreatic monolayer culture. Histochemistry 47:171, 1976.
48. Chey WY, Chang T-M, Park H-J, et al: Secretin-like immunoreactivity and biological activity in the antral mucosa. Endocrinology 113:651, 1983.
49. Buffa R, Polak JM, Pearse AGE, et al: Identification of the intestinal cell storing gastric inhibitory peptide. Histochemistry 43:249, 1975.
50. Buchan AMJ, Polak JM, Capella C, et al: Electron-immunocytochemical evidence for the K cell localization of gastric inhibitory polypeptide (GIP) in man. Histochemistry 56:37, 1978.
51. Smith PH, Merchant FW, Johnson DG, et al: Immunocytochemical localization of a gastric inhibitory polypeptide-like material within A-cells of the endocrine pancreas. Am J Anat 149:585, 1977.
52. Alumets J, Hakanson R, O'Dorisio T, et al: Is GIP a glucagon cell constituent? Histochemistry 58:253, 1978.
53. Smith PH: Immunocytochemical localization of glucagonlike and gastric inhibitory polypeptidelike peptides in the pancreatic islets and gastrointestinal tract. Am J Anat 168:109, 1983.
54. Sjolund K, Ekelund M, Håkanson R, et al: Gastric inhibitory peptide-like immunoreactivity in glucagon and glicentin cells: Properties and origin. An immunocytochemical study using several antisera. J Histochem Cytochem 31:811, 1983.
55. Polak JM, Bloom S, Coulling I, et al: Immunofluorescent localization of enteroglucagon cells in the gastrointestinal tract of the dog. Gut 12:311, 1971.
56. Sasaki H, Rubalcava B, Srikant CB, et al: Gut glucagonoid (GLI) and gut glucagon, in Thompson JC (ed): *Gastrointestinal Hormones.* Austin, University of Texas Press, 1975, pp 519–528.
57. Moody AJ, Thim L: The relationship between glucagon and gut glucagon-like immunoreactants (gut GLIs), in Bloom SR, Polak JM (eds): *Gut Hormones.* 2nd Ed. New York, Churchill Livingstone, 1981, pp 312–319.
58. Sundby F, Jacobsen H, Moody AJ: Purification and characterization of a protein from porcine gut with glucagon-like immunoreactivity. Horm Metab Res 8:366, 1976.
59. Moody AJ, Jacobsen H, Sundby F: Gastric glucagon

and gut glucagon-like immunoreactants, in Bloom SR (ed): *Gut Hormones*. New York, Churchill Livingstone, 1978, pp 369–378.

60. Larsson L-I, Holst J, Hakanson R, et al: Distribution and properties of glucagon immunoreactivity in the digestive tract of various mammals: An immunohistochemical and immunochemical study. Histochemistry 44:281, 1975.
61. Grimelius L, Capella C, Buffa R, et al: Cytochemical and ultrastructural differentiation of enteroglucagon and pancreatic-type glucagon cells of the gastrointestinal tract. Virchows Arch B Cell Pathol 20:217, 1976.
62. Lehy T, Peranzi G, Christina ML: Correlative immunocytochemical and electron microscopic studies: Identification of (entero)glucagon-, somatostatin- and pancreatic polypeptide-like-containing cells in the human colon. Histochemistry 71:67, 1981.
63. Pearse AGE, Polak JM, Bloom SR: The newer gut hormones. Cellular sources, physiology, pathology, and clinical aspects. Gastroenterology 72:746, 1977.
64. Forssmann WG, Yanaihara N, Helmstaedter V, et al: Differential demonstration of the motilin cell and the enterochromaffin cell. Scand J Gastroenterol 11 (Suppl 39):43, 1976.
65. Helmstaedter V, Kreppein W, Domschke W, et al: Immunohistochemical localization of motilin in endocrine non-enterochromaffin cells of the small intestine of humans and monkey. Gastroenterology 76:897, 1979.
66. Polak JM, Buchan AMJ, Dryburgh JR, et al: Immunoreactive motilins? Lancet 1:1364, 1978.
67. Polak JM, Buchan AMJ: Motilin. Immunocytochemical localization indicates possible molecular heterogeneity or the existence of a motilin family. Gastroenterology 76:1065, 1979.
68. Frigerio B, Ravazola M, Ito S, et al: Histochemical and ultrastructural identification of neurotensin cells in the dog ileum. Histochemistry 54:123, 1977.
69. Polak JM, Sullivan SN, Bloom SR, et al: Specific localisation of neurotensin to the N cell in human intestine by radioimmunoassay and immunocytochemistry. Nature 270:183, 1977.
70. Schultzberg M, Hokfelt T, Nilsson G, et al: Distribution of peptide- and catecholamine-containing neurons in the gastrointestinal tract of rat and guinea-pig: Immunohistochemical studies with antisera to substance P, vasoactive intestinal polypeptide, enkephalins, somatostatin, gastrin/cholecystokinin, neurotensin and dopamine β-hydroxylase. Neuroscience 5:689, 1980.
71. Larsson L-I, Sundler F, Hakanson R: Pancreatic polypeptide—A postulated new hormone: Identification of its cellular storage site by light and electron microscopic immunocytochemistry. Diabetologia 12:211, 1976.
72. Orci L, Baetens O, Rufener C, et al: Evidence for immunoreactive neurotensin in dog intestinal mucosa. Life Sci 19:559, 1976.
73. Buffa R, Capella C, Fontana P, et al: Types of endocrine cells in the human colon and rectum. Cell Tissue Res 192:227, 1978.
74. Tatemoto K, Mutt V: Isolation of two novel candidate hormones using a chemical method for finding naturally occurring polypeptides. Nature 285:417, 1980.
75. Lundberg JM, Tatemoto K, Terenius L, et al: Localization of peptide YY (PYY) in gastrointestinal endocrine cells and effects on intestinal blood flow and motility. Proc Natl Acad Sci USA 79:4471, 1982.
76. El-Salhy M, Grimelius L, Wilander E, et al: Immunocytochemical identification of polypeptide YY (PYY) cells in the human gastrointestinal tract. Histochemistry 77:15, 1983.
77. Bottcher G, Sjolund K, Ekblad E, et al: Coexistence of peptide YY and glicentin immunoreactivity in endocrine cells of the gut. Regul Pept 8:261, 1984.
78. Schwartz TW, Gingerich RL, Tager HS: Biosynthesis of pancreatic polypeptide. Identification of a precursor and a co-synthesized product. J Biol Chem 255:11494, 1980.
79. Schwartz TW, Tager HS: Isolation and biogenesis of a new peptide from pancreatic islets. Nature 294:589, 1981.
80. Sundler F, Bottcher G, Håkanson R, et al: Immunocytochemical localisation of the icosapeptide fragment of the PP precursor: A marker for 'true' PP cells? Regul Pept 8:217, 1984.
81. Luft R, Efendic S, Hokfelt T, et al: Immunohistochemical evidence for the localization of somatostatin-like immunoreactivity in a cell population of the pancreatic islets. Med Biol 52:428, 1974.
82. Polak JM, Pearse AGE, Grimelius L, et al: Growth-hormone release-inhibiting hormone in gastrointestinal and pancreatic D cells. Lancet 1:1220, 1975.
83. Canese MG, Bussolati G: Immuno-electron-cytochemical localization of the somatostatin cells in the human antral mucosa. J Histochem Cytochem 25:1111, 1977.
84. Larsson L-I, Goltermann N, de Magistris L, et al: Somatostatin cell processes as pathways for paracrine secretion. Science 205:1393, 1979.
85. Costa M, Patel Y, Furness JB, et al: Evidence that some intrinsic neurons of the intestine contain somatostatin. Neurosci Lett 6:215, 1977.
86. Cai W, Gu J, Huang W, et al: Peptide immunoreactive nerves and cells of the guinea pig gallbladder and biliary pathways. Gut 24:1186, 1983.
87. Chayvialle JAP, Descos F, Bernard C, et al: Somatostatin in mucosa of stomach and duodenum in gastroduodenal disease. Gastroenterology 75:13, 1978.
88. Polak JM, Bloom SR, Bishop AE, et al: D cell pathology in duodenal ulcers and achlorhydria. Metabolism 27 (Suppl 1):1239, 1978.
89. Amara SG, Jonas V, Rosenfeld MG, et al: Alternative RNA processing in calcitonin gene expression gen-

erates mRNAs encoding different polypeptide products. Nature 298:240, 1982.
90. Gibson SJ, Polak JM, Bloom SR, et al: Calcitonin gene-related peptide immunoreactivity in the spinal cord of man and of eight other species. J Neurosci 4:3101, 1984.
91. Fujimura M, Hancock MB, Cooper CW, et al: Immunocytochemical localization of calcitonin gene-related peptide in pancreatic islet cells of the rat. Gastroenterology 88:1390, 1985.
92. Greeley GH Jr, Alwmark A, Cooper CW, et al: Calcitonin and calcitonin-gene related peptide inhibition of insulin secretion in vitro. Fed Proc 44:1391, 1985.
93. Polak JM, Pearse AGE, Garaud J-C, et al: Cellular localization of a vasoactive intestinal peptide in the mammalian and avian gastrointestinal tract. Gut 15:720, 1974.
94. Bryant MG, Bloom SR, Polak JM, et al: Possible dual role for vasoactive intestinal peptide as gastrointestinal hormone and neurotransmitter substance. Lancet 1:991, 1976.
95. Larsson L-I, Fahrenkrug J, Schaffalitzky de Muckadell O, et al: Localization of vasoactive intestinal polypeptide (VIP) to central and peripheral neurons. Proc Natl Acad Sci USA 73:3197, 1976.
96. Larsson L-I, Polak JM, Buffa R, et al: On the immunocytochemical localization of the vasoactive intestinal polypeptide. J Histochem Cytochem 27:936, 1979.
97. Bishop AE, Polak JM, Green IC, et al: The location of VIP in the pancreas of man and rat. Diabetologia 18:73, 1980.
98. Ferri G-L, Botti PL, Vezzadini P, et al: Peptide-containing innervation of the human intestinal mucosa. Histochemistry 76:413, 1982.
99. Sundler F, Alumets J, Hakanson R, et al: VIP innervation of the gallbladder. Gastroenterology 72:1375, 1977.
100. Larsson L-I, Fahrenkrug J, Holst JJ, et al: Innervation of the pancreas by vasoactive intestinal polypeptide (VIP) immunoreactive nerves. Life Sci 22:773, 1978.
101. Holst JJ, Fahrenkrug J, Knuhtsen S, et al: Vasoactive intestinal polypeptide (VIP) in the pig pancreas: Role of VIPergic nerves in control of fluid and bicarbonate secretion. Regul Pept 8:245, 1984.
102. Jarhult J, Fahrenkrug J, Hellstrand P, et al: VIP (vasoactive intestinal polypeptide)—Immunoreactive innervation of the portal vein. Cell Tissue Res 221:617, 1982.
103. Alumets J, Fahrenkrug J, Håkanson R, et al: A rich VIP nerve supply is characteristic of sphincters. Nature 280:155, 1979.
104. Nilsson G, Larsson L-I, Hakanson R, et al: Localization of substance P-like immunoreactivity in mouse gut. Histochemistry 43:97, 1975.
105. Jessen KR, Saffrey MJ, van Noorden S, et al: Immunohistochemical studies of the enteric nervous system in tissue culture and *in situ:* Localization of vasoactive intestinal polypeptide (VIP), substance-P and enkephalin immunoreactive nerves in the guinea-pig gut. Neuroscience 5:1717, 1980.
106. Heitz Ph, Polak JM, Kasper M, et al: Immunoelectron cytochemical localization of motilin and substance P in rabbit bile duct enterochromaffin (EC) cells. Histochemistry 50:319, 1977.
107. Larsson L-I, Rehfeld JF: Peptidergic and adrenergic innervation of pancreatic ganglia. Scand J Gastroenterol 14:433, 1979.
108. Erspamer V, Erspamer GF, Inselvini M, et al: Occurrence of bombesin and alytesin in extracts of the skin of three European discoglossid frogs and pharmacological actions of bombesin on extravascular smooth muscle. Br J Pharmacol 45:333, 1972.
109. Brown M, Tache Y, Fisher D: Central nervous system action of bombesin: Mechanism to induce hyperglycemia. Endocrinology 105:660, 1979.
110. Walsh JH, Wong HC, Dockray GJ: Bombesin-like peptides in mammals. Fed Proc 38:2315, 1979.
111. Polak JM, Bloom SR, Hobbs S, et al: Distribution of a bombesin-like peptide in human gastrointestinal tract. Lancet 1:1109, 1976.
112. Bloom SR, Polak JM: Neuropeptides in the gut and other peripheral tissues, in Gotto AM Jr, Peck EJ Jr, Boyd AE III (eds): *Brain Peptides: A New Endocrinology.* New York, Elsevier/North-Holland Biomedical Press, 1979, pp 103–117.
113. McDonald TJ, Jornvall H, Nilsson G, et al: Characterization of a gastrin releasing peptide from porcine non-antral gastric tissue. Biochem Biophys Res Commun 90:227, 1979.
114. Yanaihara N, Yanaihara C, Mochizuki T, et al: Immunoreactive GRP. Peptides 2 (Suppl 2):185, 1981.
115. Polak JM, Sullivan SN, Bloom SR, et al: Enkephalin-like immunoreactivity in the human gastrointestinal tract. Lancet 1:972, 1977.
116. Alumets J, Hakanson R, Sundler F, et al: Leu-enkephalin-like material in nerves and enterochromaffin cells in the gut. Histochemistry 56:187, 1978.
117. Tatemoto K, Mutt V: Isolation and characterization of the intestinal peptide porcine PHI (PHI-27), a new member of the glucagon-secretin family. Proc Natl Acad Sci USA 78:6603, 1981.
118. Yanaihara N, Nokihara K, Yanaihara C, et al: Immunocytochemical demonstration of PHI and its co-existence with VIP in intestinal nerves of rat and pig. Arch Histol Jpn 46:575, 1983.
119. Tatemoto K, Carlquist M, Mutt V: Neuropeptide Y—A novel brain peptide with structural similarities to peptide YY and pancreatic polypeptide. Nature 296:659, 1982.
120. Lundberg JM, Terenius L, Hokfelt T, et al: Neuropeptide Y (NPY)-like immunoreactivity in peripheral noradrenergic neurons and effects of NPY on sympathetic function. Acta Physiol Scand 116:477, 1982.
121. Sundler F, Moghimzadeh E, Håkanson R, et al:

Nerve fibers in the gut and pancreas in the rat displaying neuropeptide-Y immunoreactivity. Intrinsic and extrinsic origin. Cell Tissue Res 230:487, 1983.

122. Larsson L-I: ACTH-like immunoreactivity in the gastrin cell. Independent changes in gastrin and ACTH-like immunoreactivity during ontogeny. Histochemistry 56:245, 1978.

123. Larsson L-I: Immunocytochemical characterization of ACTH-like immunoreactivity in cerebral nerves and in endocrine cells of the pituitary and gastrointestinal tract by using region-specific antisera. J Histochem Cytochem 28:133, 1980.

124. Larsson L-I: Adrenocorticotropin-like and α-melanotropin-like peptides in a subpopulation of human gastrin cell granules: Bioassay, immunoassay, and immunocytochemical evidence. Proc Natl Acad Sci USA 78:2990, 1981.

125. Solcia E, Buffa R, Capella C, et al: Immunohistochemical and ultrastructural characterization of gut cells producing GIP, GLI, glucagon, secretin and PP-like peptides. Front Horm Res 7:7, 1980.

126. Larsson L-I, Golterman N, de Magistris L, et al: Somatostatin cell processes as pathways for paracrine secretion. Science 205:1393, 1979.

Chapter 4

Bioassay of Gut Peptides

Karen S. Guice, M.D., Felix Lluis, M.D., and James C. Thompson, M.D.

> "Bioassay: The determination of the potency or concentration of a compound by its effect upon animals, isolated tissues, or microorganisms, as compared to a standard preparation." [1]

Before the advent of radioimmunoassay (RIA), bioassay was the only method available for the detection and measurement of hormones. By providing a quantitative relationship between the effect observed and the amount of substance in the sample, bioassay provided a standard by which new, unknown substances could be compared. Today, the technique still provides important and valuable information regarding new hormones, and remains the only test for comparing immunologic reactivity and physiologic activity. Bioassays, although less specific than radioimmunoassays, still remain, in a very real sense, the gold standard of measurement. Each RIA must be validated by bioassay in order to show that the material reacting with the antibody in the RIA does possess the requisite biologic activity, and is not simply a biologically inert fragment that has attracted a specific antibody.

The test system may be in vitro or in vivo; it may use the entire animal, isolated organs or tissues from an animal, or isolated cells or cell cultures. The test effect can be represented as weight or height change, organ response of secretion, excretion or motility, a biochemical response of tissue, or changes in metabolic paths.

Bioassays may be tailored to meet specific needs [2], utilized to study new compounds with clinical or experimental interest, or used to correlate certain hormonal properties with known effects. Bioassays are used to test the specific activity of gut peptides, especially those that are recently isolated. Some bioassays, originally described to measure the effect of a peptide on a specific tissue or animal, can be used in other tissues or species using the same basic techniques, or to detect inhibitory effects of a hormone (that is, its capacity to reverse the stimulatory effects of a known hormone or agent).

Four criteria must be met by each bioassay [3,4]: 1) accuracy, 2) precision, 3) specificity (few false positives), and 4) sensitivity (few false negatives). In performance, attention to assay design, quality control, and statistical analysis must be scrupulous. Ideally, all animals used should be from pure strains raised under standard conditions and obtained from a reliable source. Whenever possible, animals from one shipment should not be mixed with those of another, even if the animals are from the same source. These precautions will minimize seasonal variations and possible environmental changes that may occur. Animals should be studied at the same hour of the day to avert circadian variations. The test compound must be repeatedly compared with a standard preparation, to obtain known effects in the test system used. The design of the assay must be determined as quantitative or qualitative. Finally, quality control should explain the cause of aberrant results.

The following index precedes the bioassay descriptions and gives the organ or tissue under study (in vivo or in vitro), the animal used for the bioassay, and the specific biologic activity or effect to be measured.

Each bioassay has been further organized so that the reader could repeat the experiment in a laboratory setting. Where possible, the earliest references or original description of the specific bioassay have been cited.

Index

Test System	*Animal*	*Effect (Bioassay #)*
Gastric secretion		
In vivo	Dog, rat, cat	Acid secretion (1, 2)
In vitro		
gastric mucosa	Bullfrog	Acid secretion (3)
fundic glands	Guinea pig	Carbonic anhydrase (4)
Pancreatic secretion		
In vivo	Dog, rat	Enzyme and bicarbonate secretion (5, 6, 7)
In vitro (acini)	Guinea pig, rat	Amylase release (8)
Bile secretion	Dog, rat	Bile secretion (9, 10)
Gallbladder motility		
In vivo	Dog, cat, guinea pig	Intraluminal pressure and contraction (11, 12)
In vitro (strips)	Rabbit, dog	Tension (13)
Gut motility		
In vitro	Dog, guinea pig	Tension (14, 15)
In vitro (cells)	Guinea pig	Contraction (16)
Endocrine pancreas		
Isolated pancreas	Pig	Hormone release (17)
Islets of Langerhans	Rat	Hormone release (18)
Organ growth (in vivo)	Hamster, rat, mice, nude mice	DNA/RNA content/synthesis (19); polyamine synthesis (20)
Cell and tumor proliferation (in vivo)	Hamster, rat, mice, nude mice	Tumor growth (21); DNA/RNA content/synthesis (19); polyamine synthesis (20)
Cell proliferation (in vitro)	Neoplastic cell lines from any species	Doubling time (21); polyamine synthesis (20); DNA synthesis (22); ODC synthesis (23); hormone release (24)

***Bioassay 1* [5–8].** Measurement of gastric acid secretion in vivo
See Figs 4-1 and 4-2 (see further description p. 59)

Animal: Male rat (150-400 g), fasted overnight

Equipment
- Rectal thermometer
- Glass cannula
- 4-0 silk suture
- Capillary tubing
- pH electrode, pH meter, recorder
- Warming apparatus (heated table, heat lamp)
- Polyethylene tubing
  - 2 mm E.D., 11 cm long
  - 1 mm E.D., variable length with tip beveled
- Mariotte stock bottle fitted with soda-lime tower in stopper
- Small jacketed warming coil with circulating pump

Solutions
- Normal saline
- 0.1 N HCl
- N/4000 NaOH

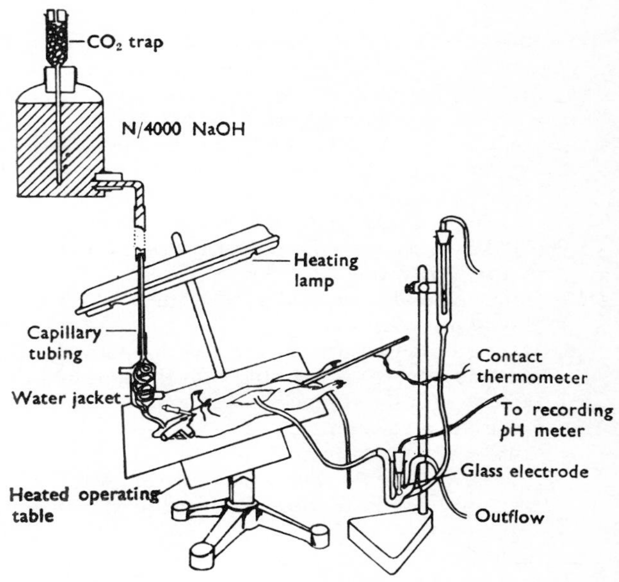

Figure 4-1. Stomach perfusion assembly for a continuous recording of acid secretion in the rat. (From Ghosh and Schild [5], by permission of Macmillan Press Ltd.)

(*Bioassay 1 Cont.*)

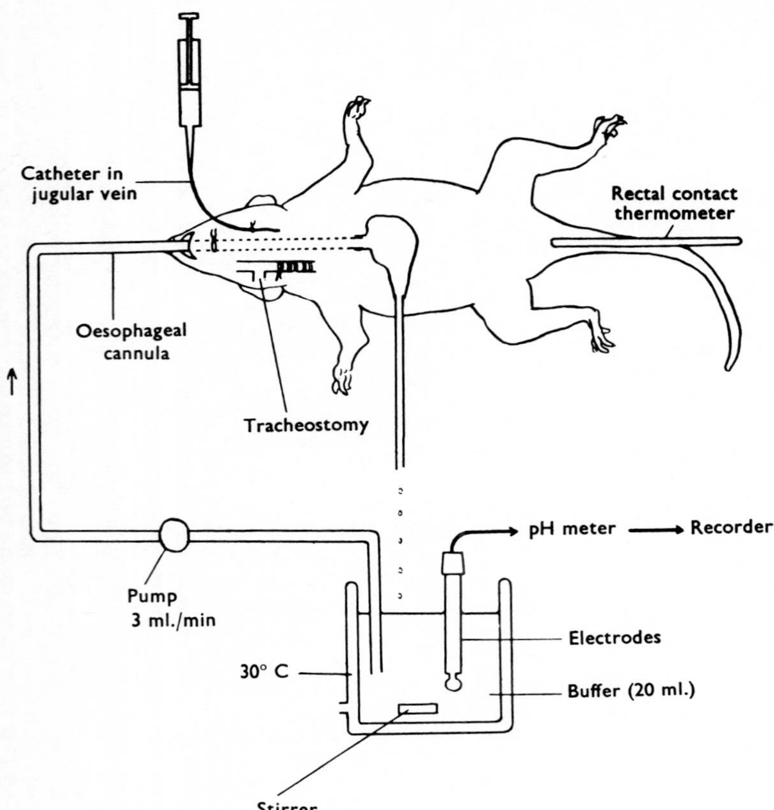

Figure 4-2. Diagram of method of reperfusion. (From Smith et al [7], by permission of Macmillan Press Ltd.)

Procedure (sensitivity: 10–20 ng synthetic human gastrin I)

1. Anesthetize rat until sedation satisfactory.
2. Incise skin over neck; isolate esophagus.
3. Pass the 11 cm length of polyethylene tubing into stomach through the esophagus and tie tubing into place.
4. Expose and cannulate one or both of the jugular veins with the polyethylene tubing; connect this to IV.
5. Open the abdomen and expose the pyloroduodenal junction.
6. Make a small enterotomy in the duodenum and pass the glass cannula into the stomach; tie the cannula in place.
7. Close the abdomen.
8. Connect the esophageal tube to the capillary tubing which has been passed through the warming coil and connected to the Mariotte stock bottle.
9. Begin continuous perfusion of the stomach with dilute NaOH (rate 1 mL/min, pressure 200 cm)*.
10. Connect the duodenal cannula to the pH electrode with a small piece of polyethylene tubing.
11. Position the electrode 15 cm below the plane of the animal to provide a slight negative pressure and to prevent gastric distension.
12. Study drugs are then administered via the jugular cannula and continuous changes in gastric pH measured.
13. Maintain a constant body temperature of 34° throughout the experiment.

* The gastric perfusate can be administered by a recirculating roller pump while the gastric effluent is drained into a reservoir with pH meter.

***Bioassay 2* [*9–12*].** Measurement of gastric acid secretion, in vivo with option of perfusing duodenum

Animal: dog (18–22 kg), male cat (3–4 kg)

Equipment
Gastric and duodenal cannulas

Solutions
NaOH

Procedure
1. After obtaining appropriate anesthesia level, open the abdomen in the midline.
2. Cannulate the stomach anteriorly near the greater curve, 8 cm proximal to the pylorus.
3. Bring the cannula through the abdominal wall and suture.
4. Insert a second cannula into the duodenum 2–4 cm distal to the ampulla of Vater and bring through the abdominal wall.
5. Postoperatively, give benzyl penicillin intramuscularly and normal saline subcutaneously, each for 5 days.
6. Feed animals after 5 days.
7. Two weeks after preparation, the animals are ready for experiments.
8. After fasting for 18 hours, measure basal secretion for 1 hour.
9. The drug to be tested is given intravenously for 15 minutes and volumes of gastric juice are measured for 15-minute periods and titrated against NaOH.
10. If effects of duodenal mechanism for stimulation or inhibition are to be studied, test agents may be infused into the duodenum.

***Bioassay 3* [*13, 14*].** Measurement of gastric acid secretion in gastric mucosa, in vitro

Animal: bullfrog (*Rana catesbiana*)

Equipment
2 Ussing-type chambers
Automatic titrator
Tank 100% O_2
Radiometer pH meter
Tank 95% O_2, 5% CO_2

Solutions
1. Nutrient:
   NaCl 85.3 mmol/L
   KCL 3.4 mmol/L
   $CaCl_2$ 1.8 mmol/L
   $MgSO_4$ 0.8 mmol/L
   KH_2PO_4 0.8 mmol/L
   $NaHCO_3$ 17.8 mmol/L
   Glucose 11.0 mmol/L
2. Secretory:
   NaCl 85.3 mmol/L
   KCL 3.4 mmol/L
   $CaCl_2$ 1.8 mmol/L
   Glucose 11.0 mmol/L
3. 0.1 N NaOH

Procedure (sensitivity: 2.5×10^{-9} mol/L of purified gastrin)
1. Kill frogs by decapitation and pithing.
2. Mount gastric mucosa between the two chambers with an exposed area of 4.5 cm^2: chamber A—nutrient solution, submucosal side; chamber B—secretory solution, mucosal side.
3. Bubble 95% O_2, 5% CO_2 through the solution in chamber A.
4. Bubble 100% O_2 through the solution in chamber B.
5. Incubate at room temperature (22–24°C).
6. Titrate acid formed on secretory side automatically and continuously to pH 5.5, with 0.1 N NaOH.
7. Place test solutions in chamber A, changing nutrient solution after each test.

***Bioassay 4* [*15, 16*].** Measurement of carbonic anhydrase activity in fundic glands, in vitro

Animal: female guinea pig (Hartley), 400–500 g

Equipment
Culture chamber
Bright's cryostat
Vickers M85 microdensitometer
Tank 95% O_2, 5% CO_2
Culture grid
Trough (33 × 18 cm)
Glass tubes and slides
Nitrogen

Solutions
Trowell's T8 medium (Flow Labs)
Human plasma
N-hexane (B.D.H. "free from aromatic hydrocarbons" grade)
Reaction medium:
   5.3×10^{-2} M H_2SO_4
   15.7×10^{-2} M sodium hydrogen carbonate
   3.5×10^{-3} M potassium dihydrogen phosphate
   1.75×10^{-3} M cobalt sulfate
Aqueous hydrogen sulfide
Farrant's medium
1 M HCl
Dry ice

(***Bioassay 4 Cont.***)

Procedure. Sensitivity: 0.005 pg/mL of pentagastrin-like activity.

1. Kill the guinea pig by asphyxiation in N_2.
2. Remove the stomach and wash with T8 medium until clean.
3. Place fundic strips (2 × 3 mm) on the grid in the culture chamber with mucosal side up.
4. Add 10 mL T8 medium with pH 7.0 and gassed with 95% O_2, 5% CO_2 to the chamber until it reaches the grid level.
5. Seal chamber and gas with 95% O_2, 5% CO_2 for 5 minutes; can be maintained for 5 hours.
6. Remove culture medium and replace with fresh T8, with graded concentrations of test solutions or two dilutions of human plasma (1:100, 1:1000) poured over the tissue.
7. Remove the tissue after 5 minutes and chill by precipitate immersion in N-hexane at −65 to −70°C.
8. After 30–60 seconds, pick up the tissue with cold forceps and place in dry glass tube at −70°C.
9. The tissue may be stored up to one week at this point.
10. Section the tissue (18 mm) in a cryostat with cabinet temperature of −25 to −30°C. Chill the sectioning knife to −70°C by packing it in dry ice.
11. Flash-dry the sections onto a warm slide and leave at room temperature for 5–10 minutes.
12. Place the slide into the shallow trough and cover with 40 mL of reaction medium (depth 0.7 mm). The reaction medium *must* be prepared fresh just before this step.
13. Gently agitate the trough for 7.5 minutes.
14. Remove the sections and rinse in tap water and then immerse in aqeous hydrogen sulfide.
15. Again wash the sections in tap water and mount in Farrant's medium.
16. Measure the amount of reaction product in each cell by the microdensitometer.

Bioassay 5 **[*17–19*].** Measurement of pancreatic enzyme and bicarbonate secretion in vivo
See Fig 4-3

Animal: Mongrel dog, 18–25 kg body weight

Equipment
Thomas cannula, Herrera cannula

Solutions

Aprotinin	Sodium heparin
2% Na_2CO_3/0.1 N NaOH	2% Na tartrate
1% $CuSO_4$	Phenol reagent

Procedure

1. After anesthesia, prepare animals with a gastric fistula drained by a Thomas cannula, and a modified Herrera pancreatic cannula.
2. Fast the animals and open the gastric fistulas before the experiment. The gastric fistulas remain open during study to prevent release of secretin from acid stimulation of the duodenum.
3. During a 30-min basal period, sample blood in chilled tubes containing sodium heparin (15 U/mL) and aprotinin (100 U/mL) and pancreatic juice.
4. Give the test substance either ID or IV with sampling every 15 minutes. Measure pancreatic volume.
5. Measure pancreatic bicarbonate content by back titration with 0.1 NaOH, and protein content by the method of Lowry et al [17].

Note: This bioassay may be combined with Bioasay No. 11.

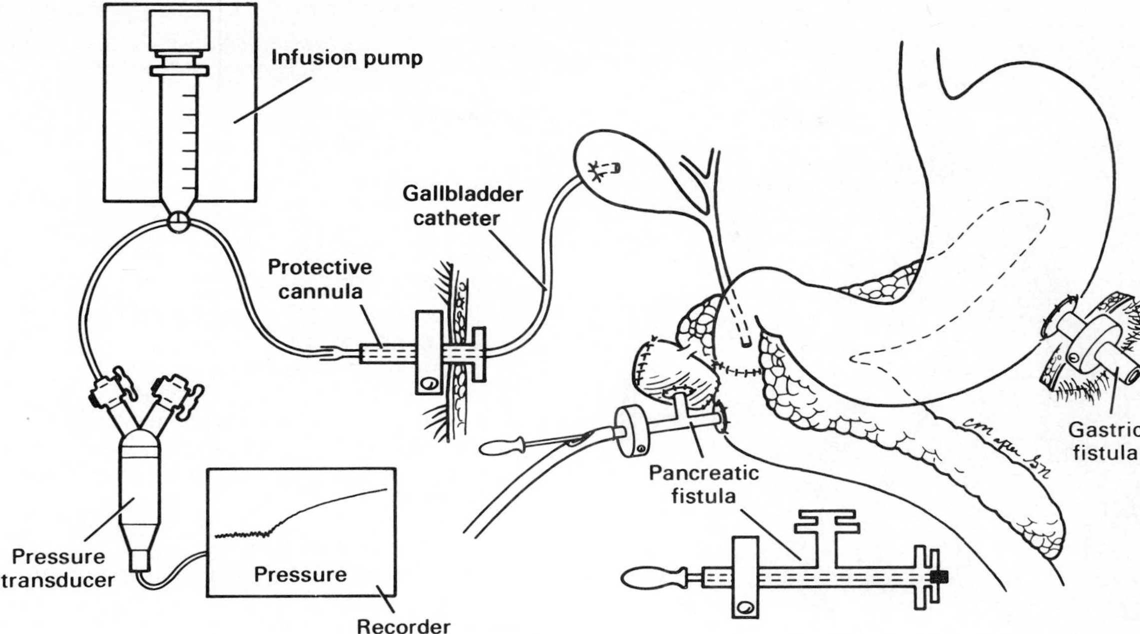

Figure 4-3. Operative preparation in dogs for bioassay of CCK. With an infusion pump, gallbladder catheter is perfused with saline, and pressure is recorded by means of a pressure transducer connected to a polygraph recorder. Pancreatic juice empties into an isolated duodenal segment that is drained by a cannula. During test periods, an obturator occludes the distal duodenal orifice of the cannula, allowing collection of pancreatic juice. Substances can be infused into the duodenum through the hollow obturator. When the cannula is capped, pancreatic juice enters the duodenum. This model combines Bioassays Nos. 5 and 11. (From Fried et al [19], by permission of The CV Mosby Co.)

Bioassay 6 **[*20, 21*].** Measurement of pancreatic enzyme and bicarbonate secretion, in vivo
See Fig 4-4

Animal: male rat, 200 g

Equipment
- Polyethylene tubing (0.024 inches E.D.) 10–20 cm long
- Suture
- Calibrated glass capillary tube

Procedure (numbers in parentheses refer to numbers in Fig 4-4)

1. After the anesthesia, cannulate the femoral vein.
2. Open the abdomen in the midline, place a liver retractor (*2*), and ligate the pylorus (*3*).
3. Pass the polyethylene tubing (*6*) through the abdominal wall using a needle.
4. Pull the duodenal loop up into the wound onto a gauze pad (*4*), loosely knot two sutures around the terminal bile duct (*5*), and place two additional sutures around the proximal end of the bile duct (*7*).
5. Insert the cannula into an incision made in the proximal bile duct and threaded a short distance (5–8 mm) toward the pancreas (*7*).
6. Use another tube (*8*) to convey bile to the duodenum. Place one end of this tube in a more proximal incision in the proximal bile duct (*7*) and the other end in an incision in the duodenum (*9*); tie the sutures to hold the cannulas in place.
7. Use two additional ties in a figure-8 to secure the pieces of tubing together. The ligature (*5*) occludes the pancreatic duct and allows collection of pancreatic secretion via tube (*6*).
8. Secure the exiting pancreatic tube to the skin (*10*) and close the abdomen.
9. Place the external end of the pancreatic cannula over a calibrated capillary tube.

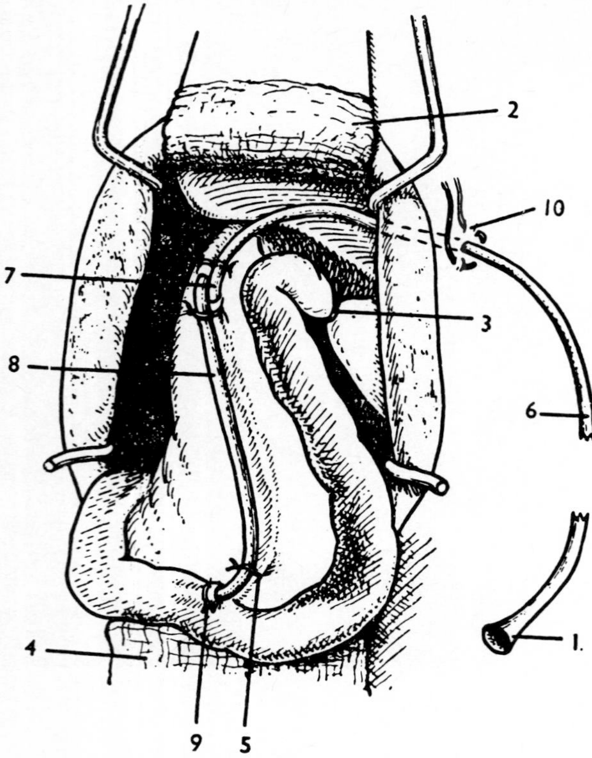

Figure 4-4. Bioassay for secretin in the rat. See text for description. (From Love [20], by permission of Cambridge University Press.)

***Bioassay 7* [22, 23].** Measurement of enzyme and bicarbonate secretion in isolated perfused pancreas, in vivo

Animal: male dog, 12–15 kg

Solutions
- Normal saline
- Heparin

Equipment
- Polyethylene tubing
- Suture

Procedure
1. After sedation, insert a polyethylene tube into the main pancreatic duct.
2. Ligate the accessory pancreatic duct.
3. Isolate the pancreatic circulation.
4. Isolate the gastroduodenal artery and ligate the gastric branches of the splenic artery successively, leaving only the pancreatic branches.
5. Ligate the vascular connections between duodenum and pancreas.
6. Give heparin (500 U/kg) IV, then maintain at 200 μ/kg/hr.
7. Insert an arterial cannula into the gastroduodenal artery and perfuse it with arterial blood pumped from the left femoral artery.
8. Ligate the inferior pancreaticoduodenal artery.
9. Cannulate the splenic artery and perfuse retrograde with femoral artery blood.
10. Ligate the splenic artery at its point of origin, not injuring perivascular nerves and preserving the left gastric artery.
11. Pump arterial blood from the left femoral artery into cannulated arteries. Maintain a constant perfusion pressure of 100 mmHg.
12. Dissolve drugs in saline before IV administration.

***Bioassay 8* [24–27].** Measurement of amylase release from dispersed pancreatic acini, in vitro

Animal: male guinea pig, 350–400 g; and male rat, 150 g

Equipment
- Water bath with oscillator
- Erlenmeyer flask, 25 mL
- Glass pipettes (tip diameter 1.2 mm and 0.9 mm)
- Spectrophotometer for amylase estimation

Solutions

Solution A
- 0.75 mg crude collagenase/mL
- 1.5 mg hyaluronidase/mL
- Krebs-Ringer bicarbonate with added 0.1 mM Ca^{++} and 1.2 mM Mg^{++}

Solution B
- Krebs-Ringer bicarbonate without Ca^{++} and Mg^{++} with 2 mM EDTA

Solution C
- 1.25 mg/mL collagenase
- 2.0 mg/mL hyaluronidase
- Krebs-Ringer bicarbonate, with 0.1 mM Ca^{++} and 1.2 mM Mg^{++}

Crude collagenase 137–200 μ/mg

Crude hyaluronidase 467 U.S.P. U/mg

(*Bioassay 8 Cont.*)

Soybean trypsin inhibitor
Bovine-Plasma albumin, Fraction V.

Incubation medium: Krebs-Ringer bicarbonate equilibrated with 95% O_2, 5% CO_2 (pH 7.4), with 14 mM glucose, L-amino acids, 0.1 mg soybean trypsin inhibitor per mL, 100 U potassium penicillin G per mL, 50 μg streptomycin sulfate per mL.

Procedure

1. Kill animals by a blow to head and quickly dissect pancreas free.
2. Trim the pancreas of fat and inject 4.8 mL of digestive solution A into the interstitium of the gland.
3. Place the distended tissue in 25 mL erlenmeyer flask with excess digestive solution A.
4. Bubble 95% O_2, 5% CO_2 through solutions in flask and incubate flask with tissue at 37° for 15 minutes with agitation of 130 oscillations per minute.
5. Aspirate the solution and discard, leaving partially digested pancreas in flask.
6. Add 8 mL of digestive solution B and incubate for 5 minutes at 37°, aspirate solution, and discard.
7. Repeat step 6.
8. Briefly wash tissue twice with digestive solution A.
9. Add 4.8 mL of digestive solution C and incubate for 45–55 minutes at 37°.
10. Gently dissociate the tissue by sequential pipetting with decreasing size of pipettes (tip diameter 1.2 mm and 0.9 mm).
11. Divide the final solution into two aliquots which are layered over two 8-mL columns of Krebs-Ringer with 4% bovine plasma albumin, 1 mM Ca^{++} and 1.2 mM Mg^{++} in conical centrifuge tubes.
12. Centrifuge tubes at 50 $\times$ g for 5 minutes.
13. Repeat with two more washes of 8 mL each.
14. Suspend acini in 100 mL Krebs-Ringer with 1% bovine-plasma albumin, 2.5 mM Ca^{++} and 1.2 mM Mg^{++}, and prepare aliquots with secretagogue for stimulation of amylase release.
15. Amylase estimation with Phadebas Test kit (Pharmacia Diagnostics) using spectrophotometry [28].

***Bioassay 9* [*29–31*].** Measurement of bile secretion, in vivo
See Fig 6-10

Animal: male dog, 18–22 kg body weight

Equipment

Gastric and duodenal Thomas cannulas
No. 6 French ureteral catheters
Graded plastic tubes
Rubber cork
Infusion pumps

Procedure

1. After anesthesia, perform a cholecystectomy and ligate the accessory pancreatic duct.
2. Insert a duodenal Thomas cannula in the duodenum, opposite to the ampulla of Vater, and a gastric cannula. Allow a 3- to 4-week recovery period.
3. For studies, insert a No. 6 French ureteral catheter 5–6 cm into the common bile duct through the duodenal cannula. Secure the catheter in place and close the duodenal cannula with a rubber cork. Leave the gastric cannula open during the experiments.
4. Collect bile by gravity in graded or preweighed tubes and measure its volume. Save bile samples frozen and in the dark.
5. In experiments with reposition of bile salts, start a constant IV infusion of sodium taurocholate (500 mg/hr), 60–90 minutes after the onset of biliary drainage. Start the infusion of test substances 90–120 minutes after taurocholate infusion, when bile flow is stable.
6. Bile measurements:
   A. Bile flow: bile volume during a given period of time.
   B. Bile acids: 3α-hydroxysteroid dehydrogenase assay [29].
   C. Bile cholesterol: method of Abell et al [30].
   D. Bile phospholipids: method of Fiske and Subarrow [31].

Bioassay 10. Measurement of bile secretion, in vivo

Animal: male rat, 200 g

Equipment
- Polyethylene tubing ID 0.3 mm, OD 0.7 mm (PE-10)
- Warming plates or electric lamps
- Infusion pumps
- Restraining cages
- Preweighed tubes

Procedure
1. After anesthesia, place rats in warming plates or under a lamp to maintain body temperature (37°C). Open abdominal cavity, insert a PE-10 into the proximal bile duct toward the hepatic hilus, and thread it.
2. Ligate the bile duct immediately distal to the tube.
3. Exteriorize the polyethylene tube through the abdominal wall and secure it to the skin.
4. Cannulate the jugular or saphenous veins with PE-10.
5. Place rats in restraining cages after operation.
6. For studies with reposition of bile salts, start an IV infusion of sodium taurocholate (150 mmol/min/100 g body weight).
7. Collect bile in preweighed tubes. Bile volume during a given period of time is calculated by weight differences of the tubes.
8. Bile measurements: same as Bioassay No. 9.

Bioassay 11 **[32, 33].** Measurement of intraluminal gallbladder pressure, in vivo
See Fig 4-3

Animal: dog, cat, guinea pig

Equipment
- Catheter for gallbladder (dog): 30 cm long, 1.19 mm ID, 1.6 mm ED, 1.9 mm side orifice, 1 cm proximal to occluded distal end
- Hollow steel cannula
- Pressure transducer
- Infusion pump
- Chart recorder

Procedure (sensitivity: 1 Ivy dog unit)

Dog
1. Prepare dogs under anesthesia with a catheter cholecystostomy and a duodenal cannula. Experiments are done 3 weeks after operation.
2. Measure gallbladder pressure continuously while perfusing the gallbladder catheter with 0.9% normal saline at 1.25 mL/min using 100 mL glass syringes attached to an infusion pump.
3. Give the test substances either IV or intraduodenally.

Cat and guinea pig
1. Clamp the cystic duct after the animal is anesthetized.
2. Cannulate the fundus of the gallbladder.
3. Now connect the cannula to a pressure transducer.
4. Give the test substances IV.

Note: This bioassay can be combined with Bioassay No. 5.

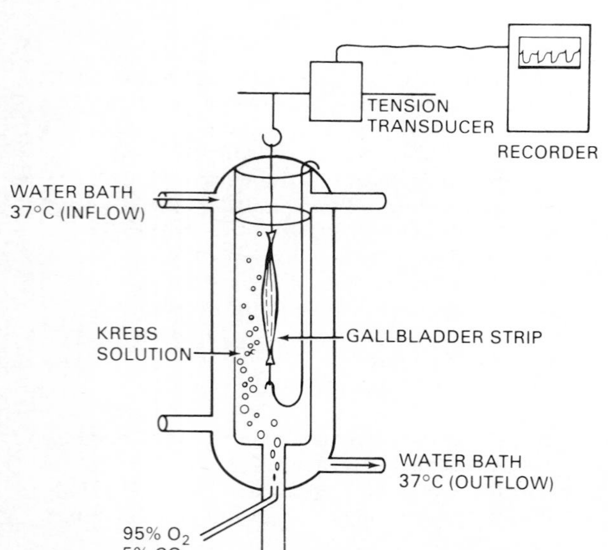

Figure 4-5. Apparatus for measuring gallbladder contraction. A longitudinal strip of gallbladder muscle connected to a strain gauge transducer is suspended in a bath of Krebs solution. Contraction is measured by recording tension in milligrams. (Modification of method of Berry and Flower [36].)

***Bioassay 12* [*34*].** Measurement of gallbladder contraction, in vivo

Animal: male mongrel dogs, 15–20 kg

Equipment
- Three force transducers (Dr. Zen Itoh, Meabashi, Japan)
- Silastic tubing
- Suture
- Canvas protecting jacket
- Polygraph

Procedure
1. Under anesthesia, suture one force transducer to the serosa of the gallbladder body to measure circular muscle contraction.
2. Suture the other force transducers onto the serosa of the gastric antrum, 3 cm proximal to the pyloric ring, and at the mid-duodenum opposite the main pancreatic duct opening.
3. Pull the lead wires from the abdominal cavity through a stab wound; pull them through a subcutaneous tunnel, exiting the skin between the scapulas.
4. Place silastic tubing in a branch of the external jugular vein and fill with heparinized normal saline. It is used for postoperative fluid and blood sampling.
5. Protect the wires and silastic tubing with a canvas jacket.
6. Begin experiments 3–6 weeks postoperatively.
7. During each experiment, use a polygraph to record contractile changes.

***Bioassay 13* [*35–44*].** Measurement of tension changes in gallbladder strips, in vitro
See Fig 4-5

Animal: male New Zealand white rabbit (2–3 kg), or dog (18–22 kg), both fasted for 24 hours

Solutions: Krebs (mmol, in distilled and deionized water): NaCL, 118; KCL, 4.69; $CaCl_2 \cdot 6H_2O$, 2.51; $MgSO_4 \cdot 7H_2O$, 1.17; KH_2PO_4, 1.17; $NaHCO_3$, 24.9; glucose, 5.5

Equipment
- Tanks: O_2, CO_2
- Polygraph
- 20 mL organ bath (Fig 4-5)
- Isometric force displacement transducer

Procedure
1. Remove the gallbladder from the rabbit (killed by cervical dislocation) or from the dog (under general anesthesia).
2. Place gallbladder strips (3–4 cm long and 0.3 cm wide) in the organ bath, containing Krebs solution, constantly bubbled with 95% O_2 and 5% CO_2 at 37°C.
3. Set the transducer to an initial tension of 1 gram. Transducer measurements are made after a 2–3 hour equilibration period and recorded by the polygraph.
4. Bioactivity is compared to the dose-response curves produced by synthetic CCK-8.

***Bioassay 14* [*45*].** Measurement of tension changes in antral muscle strips, in vitro

Animal: male dog, 10–30 kg

Solutions: Krebs

Equipment
- Organ bath
- Strain gauge
- Tank 97% O_2, 3% CO_2
- Polygraph

Procedure (sensitivity: $ED_{50} = 3.5 \times 10^{-10}$ M of CCK-8)
1. After anesthesia, remove the gastric antrum (3–4 cm proximal to the gastroduodenal junction).
2. Dissect the gastric antral muscle from the mucosa including both circular and longitudinal muscle layers.
3. Cut strips (10 × 3 mm) parallel to the long axis of the circular layer.
4. Place the strips in an organ bath of 30 mL Krebs at 37°C and continuously bubble the bath with 97% O_2, 3% CO_2.
5. Measure the isometric tension by connection to strain gauge, one end attached by a stell hook and the other by a jewelry chain.
6. Allow the tissue to equilibrate for 1 hour.
7. Measure the optimum length by contractile response to acetylcholine (5×10^{-6} M).
8. Add the test substance (0.5 mL) to chamber for testing.

***Bioassay 15* [*46–48*].** Measurement of tension and intraluminal pressure changes in ileal segments, in vitro

Animal: guinea pig, 250–300 g

Solutions
Krebs

Equipment
Organ bath
Tank O_2-CO_2
Polygraph
Force displacement and pressure transducers

Procedure
1. Kill the animal by decapitation.
2. Remove a piece of small intestine and place it vertically in an organ bath containing Krebs solution at 37°C and continuously bubbled with 95% O_2 and 5% CO_2.
3. Measure the tension by a force displacement transducer connected to the upper end of the small intestinal segment.
4. Alternatively, tie the small intestinal segment to a glass tubing connected to a container, and measure intraluminal pressure changes by a pressure transducer.
5. Add the test substances in a small volume to the solution in the organ bath for testing.

***Bioassay 16* [*49–51*].** Measurement of contraction from isolated stomach muscle cells, in vitro

Animal: male guinea pig, 300–600 g

Solutions
Krebs
Soybean trypsin inhibitor
Collagenase (150 U/mg, Type II)
Acrolein

Equipment
Tank 95% O_2, 5% CO_2
Nitex filter 500 μm
Hemocytometer
Corkboard
Incubation tubes
Vickers micrometer

Procedure (sensitivity: $ED_{50} = 10^{-11}$ M CCK-8)
1. After anesthesia, open the abdomen and remove the stomach, open along the lesser curvature and place in ice-cold Krebs bicarbonate buffer bubbled with 95% O_2, 5% CO_2.
2. Pin equal halves to frozen corkboard (serosa up).
3. Strip the serosa away with fine scissors.
4. Peel the muscle layer off the mucosa as one sheet.
5. Cut the muscle layer into strips (2 cm long × 2 mm wide).
6. Incubate the strips twice (45 minutes each) at 31° in 15 mL of Krebs with 0.1% collagenase and 0.01% soybean trypsin inhibitor and bubble with 95% O_2, 5% CO_2.
7. After the second incubation, filter the medium through 500 μm Nitex filter.
8. Leave partially digested muscle strips on the filter and wash four times with 50 mL of collagenase-free Krebs solution.
9. Transfer the strips into 15 mL fresh Krebs and let stand for 30 minutes.
10. Harvest the cells by filtration through 500 μm Nitex. No mechanical force is used.
11. Count the cells in hemocytometer (about 10^7 cells per stomach).
12. Add aliquots of 25×10^3 cells in 0.5 mL to 0.1 mL of the solutions to be tested.
13. Stop the reaction in 30 seconds by adding 0.1 mL acrolein to final concentration of 1%.
14. Contractile response taken as decrease in average length as viewed by micrometer with image-splitting eyepiece.

Bioassay 17 **[*52, 53*].** Measurement of pancreatic endocrine secretion from isolated perfused pancreas, in vitro
See Fig 4-6

Animal: pig, 25–35 kg

Solutions
- 4% dextrose in Krebs-Ringer, pH 7.8, with added pyruvate fumarate, glutamate (5 mmol/L of each)
- 0.1% BSA

Equipment
- Perfusion chamber
- Cannula
- Tank 95% O_2, 5% CO_2
- Heat exchanger
- Pump

Procedure
1. After anesthesia, open the abdomen in the midline.
2. Remove the spleen after ligation and division of its vascular supply.
3. After ligating the lumbar branches, free an 8 cm segment of aorta, including celiac and S.M.A.
4. Divide the left gastric artery and vein between ligatures.
5. Dissect the portahepatis, then ligate and divide the common hepatic artery past the gastroduodenal artery take-off.
6. Ligate and divide the common bile duct near the duodenum.
7. Dissect the pancreas from the duodenum.
8. Divide the segment of aorta, along with the portal vein.
9. Place the specimen in an open perfusion chamber with the perfusion fluid at a temperature of 38°C.

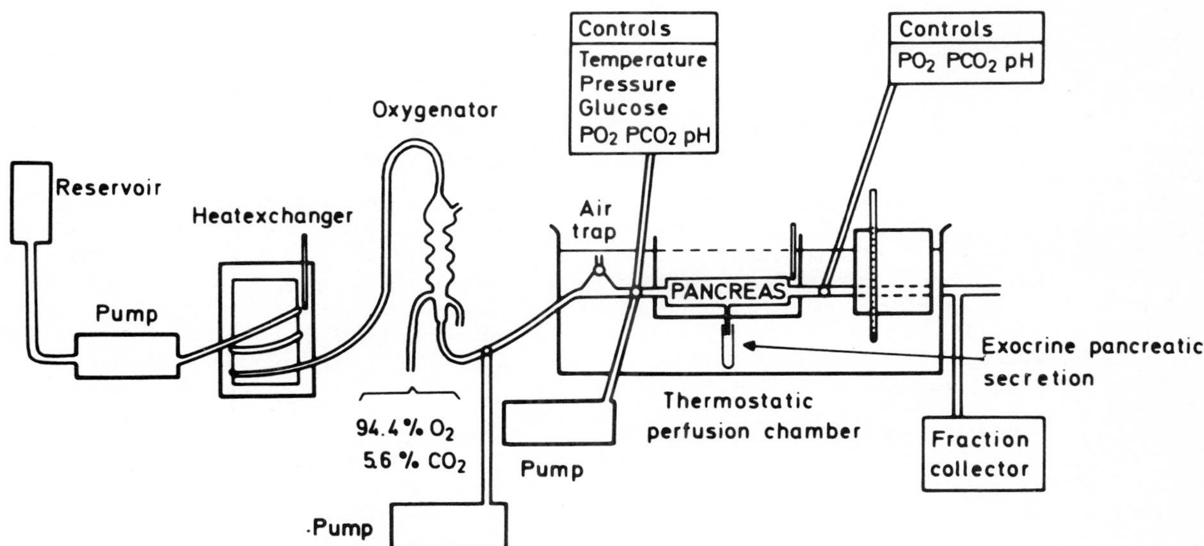

Figure 4-6. Diagram of apparatus for perfusion of isolated pig pancreas. (From Lindkaer Jensen et al [53], by permission of the American Physiological Society.)

***Bioassay 18* [*54, 55*].** Measurement of hormones released by isolated and cultured islets of Langerhans, in vitro

Animal: rat (over 30 days old or newborn 3–5 days old)

Equipment
- 37°C waterbath
- Culture hood
- 20 ml autoclaved vial containing magnet bar
- Autoclaved surgical instrument
- Magnet stirrer with heater
- 5% CO_2/95% air incubator

Solutions
- Ca^{++}- and Mg^{++}-free phosphate buffered saline containing antibiotics
- Antibiotics (streptomycin, 100 U/mL; penicillin G, 100 U/mL; gentamicin, 50 μg/mL; polymixin B, 50 μg/mL; neomycin 50 μg/mL; amphotericin B, 3.0 μg/mL)
- Culture medium: NCTC 135, 45% vol/vol; MEM 199, 45% vol/vol; 10% heat inactivated fetal bovine serum; glucose, 300 mg/dL
- Trypsin solution (1:250 Difco) 2 mg/mL
- Collagenase solution (Class IV) 1.5 mg/mL (1.0 mg/mL in newborns)
- For static incubation study: Krebs-Ringer bicarbonate buffer, dialyzed bovine serum albumin, acid-ethanol (concentrated HCl and 95% ethanol in a 1:50 ratio)

Procedure (rats over 30 days old)
1. Kill the rat by ethyl ether or anesthetics.
2. Excise pancreas with sterile technique.
3. Remove the adipose tissue.
4. Mince finely.
5. Wash in 10 mL Ca^{++}- and Mg^{++}-free PBS for 5 minutes at room temperature, two times.
6. Digestion with 3 mL collagenase solution + 10 mL trypsin solution for 5 minutes with gentle stirring at 37°C, two times.
7. Discard each supernatant.
8. Digestion with 5 mL collagenase solution for 10 minutes with gentle stirring at 37°C, three times.
9. Each supernatant is saved into culture media.
10. Centrifuge at 1500 rpm for 5 minutes at 15°C.
11. Discard the supernatant and resuspend each pellet with culture media.
12. Dispense onto large tissue culture dishes.
13. Incubate for 40–44 hours in 5% CO_2/95% air incubator at 37°C.
14. Save the supernatant and centrifuge at 1500 rpm for 5 minutes at 15°C.
15. Resuspend pellet and dispense onto small tissue culture dishes.
16. Incubate for 3–4 days in 5% CO_2/95% air incubator at 37°C for static incubation.

Procedure (newborn rats)
1. Kill the newborn rat by decapitation.
2. Excise pancreas with sterile technique.
3. Wash in 10 mL Ca^{++}- and Mg^{++}-free PBS for 5 minutes, two times.
4. Digestion with 3 mL collagenase solution + 10 mL trypsin solution for 15 minutes with gentle stirring at 37°C, four times.
5. Last three supernatants are saved into culture media.
6. Centrifuge at 1500 rpm for 5 minutes at 15°C.
7. Discard the supernatant and resuspend pellet with culture media.
8. Dispense onto large tissue culture dishes.
9. Incubate for 4–6 hours in 5% CO_2/95% air incubator at 37°C.
10. Save the supernatant and centrifuge at 1500 rpm for 5 minutes at 37°C.
11. Resuspend pellet and dispense onto small tissue culture dishes.
12. Incubate for 3 days in 5% CO_2/95% air incubator at 37°C for static incubation.

Procedure of static incubation
1. Each dish is preincubated for 1 hour with 1 mL of Krebs-Ringer bicarbonate buffer containing 30 mg/dL glucose and 0.2% dialyzed bovine serum albumin in 5% CO_2/95% air incubator at 37°C.
2. Rinse twice with 2 mL of same buffer as above.
3. Add 1 mL of Krebs-Ringer bicarbonate buffer containing 0.2% dialyzed bovine serum albumin with secretagogue.
4. Incubate for 1–2 hours in 5% CO_2/95% air incubator at 37°C.
5. Each supernatant is saved and each pellet is extracted with acid-ethanol.

***Bioassay 19* [56–58].** Measurement of DNA/RNA content and DNA synthesis, in vivo

Animal

Normal organs of hamsters, rats, mice (pancreas, fundic mucosa, or colon)

Neoplastic cells or solid tumors implanted in hamsters, rats, mice, or nude mice

Equipment

Shaking waterbath

Beakers and magnetic stirrer

Tissue homogenizer

Teflon vortex bars

Centrifuge

Spectrophotometer

Solutions

1.0 and 0.5 N perchloric acid (PCA)

1.6% acetaldehyde: Add 1 mL of 99% acetaldehyde to 50 mL of distilled H_2O (wear gloves and prepare in fume hood).

Diphenylamine reagent (DPA): 1.5 mL DPA + 100 mL glacial acetic acid + 1.5 mL 36 N H_2SO_4. Just before use (preparing tubes for DPA reaction), add 0.1 mL of 1.6% acetaldehyde per 200 mL DPA.

RNA and DNA standards

HCl

$FeCL_3$

0.005 M NaOH

Orcinol

Procedure: Preparation of DNA stock

1. Dissolve 25 mg DNA in 25 mL of 0.005 M NaOH with magnetic stirrer overnight or until completely dissolved.
2. Add 25 mL of 1 N PCA and vortex. Heat, covered with shaking at 70°C for 15 minutes in water bath.
3. Cool and take 100 μL DNA solution and add to 2.4 mL 0.5 N PCA (1 to 25 dilution); check optical density (O.D.) (in duplicate) at 260 nM. Extinction coefficient, 27.8. Multiply O.D. × 27.8 = μg DNA/mL.
4. Record μg DNA/mL (should be 500 μg/mL).
5. Aliquot stock solution in 1 mL amounts and store at −70°C.
6. Recheck O.D. 260 every month.
7. Add 1 mL of stock solution, 5 mL of 1 N PCA, and 4 mL of distilled water to prepare a standard (50 μg/mL in 0.5 N PCA).

Procedure: Preparation of RNA stock

1. Heat RNA standard solution (10 mg RNA dissolved in 100 mL 0.5 N PCA) at 70°C for 20 minutes. After 1:10 dilution in 0.5 N PCA, read O.D. at 261 nM vs 0.5 N PCA. O.D. × 27.8 = μg RNA/mL. Stock solution approximately 100 μg/mL.
2. 0.03% $FeCl_3$: 0.03 g $FeCl_3$ in 100 mL 11.6 N HCl.
3. Orcinol reagent: Add 1 g orcinol per 100 mL $FeCl_3$ solution just before using.

Procedure: DNA/RNA content. Tissue is snap-frozen with liquid nitrogen until extraction.

1. Homogenize tissue to be assayed in 5 volumes of saline.
2. Take 2 samples each of 0.1 mL; add 3.9 mL saline (1:40 dilution); run Lowry [17] protein assay on this.
3. Add 5 volumes of 0.5 N PCA to each original sample.
4. Vortex, centrifuge 10 minutes at 3000 rpm at 4°C, and pour off supernatant.
5. Resuspend in 10 volumes PCA (0.5 N).
6. Centrifuge (10 min at 3000 rpm at 4°C); pour off supernatant.
7. Resuspend each sample in 0.5 N PCA (10 volumes).
8. Heat at 90°C for 10 minutes in a shaking water bath.
9. Centrifuge at 4°C for 10 minutes at 3,000 rpm.
10. Save supernatant for RNA and DNA; measure volume.

Procedure: RNA and DNA standards

1. For standard curves, pipette 1.0 mL of 0.5 N PCA (reagent blank), appropriate RNA standards (0.1, 0.25, 0.5, and 1.0 mL) and DNA standards (0.1, 0.2, 0.3, 0.4, 0.5, 0.6, 0.8, and 1.0 mL) brought to 1.0 mL final volume, and duplicate 1 mL samples.
2. For DNA standard, blanks, and samples, add 2 mL of DPA solution and incubate at room temperature for 16 hours in the dark.
3. Vortex DNA standards and read on the spectrophotometer at 600 nM versus reagent blank.
4. For RNA standards, blanks, and samples, add 1 mL orcinol reagent, and heat in boiling water for 20 minutes (cap tubes with marble to prevent evaporation).
5. Read at 640 nM versus reagent blank on the spectrophotometer.

Procedure: DNA synthesis

1. Inject animals intraperitoneally (IP) 2 hours before killing with 100 μCi (50 Ci/mmol) of [^{3}H]thymidine.
2. Excise the specified organs, weigh, and extract for DNA content (see RNA/DNA content above).
3. Place 1 mL of the extract in a vial with 15 mL of Biofluor and count in a scintillation counter for 5 minutes.
4. Express data as CPM/μg DNA. Data can be converted to disintegrations per minute (DPM), which allows more direct comparison to data from different sources (CPM ÷ efficiency of counter = DPM).

***Bioassay 20* [*59, 60*].** Measurement of polyamine synthesis, in vivo and in vitro

Polyamines (putrescine, spermidine, spermine) are polyionic cations that are essential for DNA synthesis. Polyamine biosynthesis is induced by certain gastrointestinal hormones, such as stimulation by CCK in the rat pancreas.

Animal
- Hamster, rat, mice, human (pancreas, fundic mucosa, or colon)
- Neoplastic cultured cells or solid tumors implanted in hamsters, rats, mice, or nude mice; freshly resected human tumors
- Neoplastic cell lines (in vitro)

Equipment
- Tissue homogenizer
- Sonicator
- Dionex 2110 i high-pressure ion chromatography unit (HPIC)
- Centrifuge

Solutions
- 4% (w/v) sulfosalicyclic acid
- Phosphate buffered saline
- 0.05% trypsin/0.02% EDTA
- Saline
- 0.1 N HCl
- Fetal calf serum
- 50% (w/v) trichloroacetic acid (TCA)
- Fluoropa
  - 1 L borate buffer, pH 10.4 (1.0 M)
  - 800 mg o-phthaldehyde (OPA)
  - 4.5 mL β-mercaptoethanol (βME)
  - 5.8 g KSCN
  - 20 mL methanol
  - 3 mL Brij 30% solution
  - (Put 1 L of buffer in bottle; add βME, Brij, and KSCN; dissolve the OPA in methanol; add OPA/methanol solution to buffer; stir.)
- Potassium chloride/oxalate buffer (K buffer)
  - (Stock buffer solution: 145 g KCl; 31.6 g $K_2C_2O_4$; 5.5 g EDTA. Add this to 1 L of distilled water and bring the pH to 5.65 with HCl or KOH. 1 M KOH must be made fresh.)

Procedure: In vivo extraction
1. Obtain the tissue and weigh (may be snap-frozen and stored).
2. For every 1 g tissue, add 2.0 mL 4% (w/v) sulfosalicyclic acid and homogenize; take 0.1 mL of homogenate and add to 3.9 mL saline for protein assay; incubate on ice 30 minutes.
3. Centrifuge at 10,000 g for 10 minutes.
4. Filter the supernatant, using a 0.45 μm filter, and analyze.

(*Note:* Keep everything on ice; homogenize on ice; store all samples in plastic containers; to run assay on the HPIC, these dilutions must be made: pancreas (rat), 1:30; humans, 1:20; fundic mucosa (rat), 1:10, colon (rat), 1:20)

Procedure: In vitro extraction
1. Wash monolayer of cells once with saline.
2. Trypsinize and inactivate with serum.
3. Obtain a cell pellet in a centrifuge tube using a speed of 2000 rpm for 5 minutes.
4. Wash the cell pellet twice with phosphate buffered saline, centrifuging between washings; always pour off supernatant; be careful not to lose the cell pellet.
5. Add 0.1 N HCl; the amount added depends upon the cell number (0.25 mL for 2×10^6 cells).
6. Sonicate the cells for 15 seconds with microprobe set at 45% power output.
7. Add 50% (w/v) TCA to get a final solution of 10% (w/v) TCA.
8. Put on ice for 30 minutes.
9. Centrifuge at 10,000 rpm for 5–10 minutes.
10. Save the supernatant for polyamine analysis.

Procedure: Polyamine analysis

Polyamines are eluted in the HPIC using a Fluoropa flow rate of 36 mL/hr. Putrescine is eluted with 0.16 M K buffer (1:12 dilution of stock). Spermidine and spermine are eluted with 0.66 M K buffer (1:3 dilution of stock). Data are expressed as nmol/g wet weight or nmol/mg protein.

***Bioassay 21* [*61*].** Measurement of tumor growth (in vivo) or cell doubling time (in vitro)

Animal
- Neoplastic cultured cells or solid tumors implanted in hamsters, rats, mice, or nude mice (in vivo)
- Neoplastic cell lines (in vitro)

Equipment
- In vivo:
  - Syringes
  - Sterile forceps and scissors
  - Calipers
- In vitro:
  - Cell culture
  - Growth medium
  - Pipettes
  - Cell incubator (37°C, 5% CO_2, 95% air)
  - 60 mm tissue culture dishes
  - 0.05% trypsin/0.02% EDTA
  - Coulter counter (Model ZF)

(*Bioassay 21 Cont.*)

Procedure: Tumor doubling time in vivo

1. Inject tissue culture cells subcutaneously into the interscapular region.
2. Transplant solid tumors subcutaneously as 3 mm chunks.
3. Depending upon protocols, administer drugs or peptides to animals IP or drugs orally.
4. Determine tumor doubling time by measuring tumor area. Multiply the two longest perpendicular diameters of tumors measured with calipers (nearest 0.1 mm) biweekly.
5. Determine the rate of occurrence, tumor size, doubling times, and mortality rates.
6. Plot cell counts against time on semilog graph paper and determine cell doubling time during exponential growth.

Procedure: Cell doubling time (T_D), saturation density, and inflection point, in vitro

Basic knowledge in tissue culture techniques is required. The T_D is the time required for the whole cell population to double in number and is equal to the cell cycle time when all cells of the population are proliferating.

1. Harvest culture cells by trypsinization.
2. Determine the type of media to be used; plate 3 $\times$ 10^5 cells per 60 mm dish.
3. Use 20 dishes for each drug dosage and control (two dishes a day for counting).
4. Depending upon protocol, drugs or peptides are added at time of plating or later.
5. At zero hour and every 24 hours thereafter for 8 days, examine cells microscopically (to check for contamination and morphologic changes), remove media, and harvest the cells by trypsinization.
6. Determine total cell number of treated cultures and controls in a Coulter counter.
7. Plot cell counts against time on semilog graph paper and determine T_D during exponential growth.
8. Read the saturation density (the number of cells at the onset of the plateau phase) directly from the graph.
9. Read the inflection point (time at which cells change from a log phase of growth to plateau phase).

***Bioassay 22* [62].** Measurement of DNA synthesis, in vitro

Animal: Neoplastic cell lines

Equipment

- Cell culture
- Repeat Pipetter
- 0.05% trypsin, 0.02% EDTA
- Biofluor vials
- Scintillation counter
- Microharvester
- Incubator (37°C, 5% CO_2, 95% air)
- 96-Well microtiter plates
- Growth medium
- Coulter counter (Model ZF)
- Scintillation vials
- [^{3}H]thymidine (SA 2 Ci/mmol)
- Glass fiber filters

Procedure

1. Harvest culture cells by trypsinization.
2. Plate cells in 200 μL of growth media into designated wells.
3. Place only media in outside wells of the plates to prevent evaporation of experimental wells.
4. Add drugs or peptides in a 10-μL volume; dosages must be calculated to make the appropriate concentration for a final volume of 210 μL.
5. Add drugs or peptides either at initial plating or at time intervals after plating. (Initial trypsinization procedures injure membrane structures such as hormone receptors and adding drugs before cell membrane repair may be ineffective.)
6. Incubate at 37°C, 5% CO_2, 95% air.
7. After the designated treatment period, add [^{3}H]thymidine (2 μCi per well) to each well in a volume of 10 μL of media; incubate cells for a designated period (1–12 hours).

(Steps 8 and 9 can be skipped if cells are easily harvested with pipetting.)

8. Remove media and trypsinize cells with 50 μL per well for 5–10 minutes; gently tap once or twice to achieve complete detachment of cells.
9. Add serum (10% FCS) containing medium (100 μL per well) to block the action of trypsin.
10. Collect cells on glass fiber filters using the microharvester.
11. Rinse wells 10–15 times with distilled water using the microharvester to assure both adequate cell lysis and washing to remove unbound [^{3}H]thymidine.
12. Air dry filters overnight (at least 6 hours).
13. Punch out filter discs and place in vials containing 4 mL of Biofluor.
14. Determine the radioactivity retained on the filter in a scintillation counter; express results as CPM per well or DPM per well.

***Bioassay 23*[63].** Measurement of ornithine-decarboxylase (ODC) synthesis, in vitro

Animal: Neoplastic cell lines

Equipment
- 10 mM dithiothreitol (DTT)
- 0.05% trypsin and 0.025% EDTA in saline
- 0.1 M Na-K phosphate buffer, pH 7.2 mono and dibasic for each (K_2HPO_4, KH_2PO_4, Na_2HPO_4, NaH_2PO_4)
- 1 mg pyridoxal phosphate (Pyr-P) per 10 mL water
- ^{14}C-ornithine 100 μCi/mL (SA) = 52.8 mCi/mmol
- 100 mM phenylmethylsulfonyl fluoride (PMSF) in isopropanol
- 1 M citric acid
- Water shaking bath at 37°C
- Whatman No. 3 filter discs, 2.3 cm
- NCS tissue solubilizer (Amersham)
- Conical centrifuge tubes
- Scintillation fluid
- Wells (Kontes k-882320)
- Stoppers
- Sonicator

Cocktail (10 mL)
- 5 mL buffer
- 1 mL EDTA
- 1 mL DTT
- 10 μL PMSF
- 0.5 mL Pyr-P
- 2.5 mL distilled water

Hot and cold ornithine (5 mL)
- 1.25 mL deionized water
- 1.25 mL hot ornithine
- 2.50 mL cold ornithine

Sample Preparation: Keep all materials on ice.
1. 5.0 × 10^6 cells per sample
2. Wash cells in saline, harvest, and centrifuge to form a pellet.
3. Drain and add 100 μL cocktail per 1 × 10^6 cells.
4. Sonicate to disrupt cell.
5. Add 20 μL of hot and cold ornithine.
6. Add 20 μL of NCS tissue solubilizer to filter paper that has been inserted into the wells by folding into thirds.
7. Cap with stoppers and place in shaking water bath 37°C for 30 minutes.
8. Add 500 μL citric acid to the centrifuge tube to stop reaction, being careful not to let acid absorb on filter paper.
9. Let stand for 90 minutes at room temperature.
10. Remove filter papers and place in a 20 mL scintillation vial that contains 5 mL of scintillation fluid.
11. After the vial equilibrates to refrigeration temperature of the scintillation counter, count for 1 minute.
12. Make sure the hot and cold ornithine are counted by placing 20 μL of it on a filter paper and adding 5 mL of scintillation fluid every time the assay is carried out.
13. Calculate:
    mCi of each sample = sample DPM × 1 mCi ÷ 2.2 × 10^9 DPM mmoles of each sample = mCi sample ÷ 52.8 mCi/mmol
14. Express data as pmol CO_2 per mg protein per 90 minutes.

***Bioassay 24* [61].** Measurement of hormone release, in vitro

Animal: neoplastic cell lines and normal tissue cell lines

Equipment
- Cell culture
- Pipettes
- Test tubes (12 × 75 mm)
- Cell incubator (37°C, 5% CO_2, 95% air)
- 25 cm² tissue culture flasks
- Media
- Coulter counter

Procedure
1. Plate 3 × 10^6 cells per flask in culture media (type depends upon cell line); n = 5 flasks for each group.
2. Incubate 48 hours (depending on cell line).
3. Collect culture media sample for assay.
4. Add test media only and incubate 1 hour.
5. Collect pre-test media sample for assay.
6. Add test media with drugs or peptides and incubate 1 hour.
7. Collect test media sample for assay.
8. Add test media with no drugs as post-test.
9. Incubate 1 hour.
10. Collect post-test media sample for assay.
11. Harvest cells and count on Coulter counter.
12. Measure hormone concentration in the collected media samples using specific radioimmunoassay.
13. Express hormone release as pg per million cells per hour.
14. Measure hormone concentration in extracts from cell pellets.

REFERENCES

1. *Stedman's Medical Dictionary.* 22nd Ed, Baltimore, Williams and Wilkins, 1973, p 155.
2. Hilgar AG, Hummel DJ (eds): *Androgenic and Myogenic Endocrine Bioassay Data.* Entry Nos. 1–1697. Bethesda, Maryland, Cancer Chemotherapy National Service Center, 1964.
3. van Cauwenberge H: Introduction, in van Cauwenberge H, Franchimont P (eds): *Assay of Protein and Polypeptide Hormones.* New York, Pergamon Press, 1970, pp 3–4.
4. van Cauwenberge H, Lefebvre P, Franchimont P: Biological methods, in van Cauwenberge H, Franchimont P (eds): *Assay of Protein and Polypeptide Hormones.* New York, Pergamon Press, 1970, pp 7–11.
5. Ghosh MN, Schild HO: Continuous recording of acid gastric secretion in the rat. Br J Pharmac 13:54, 1958.
6. Lai KS: Studies on gastrin. Gut 5:327, 1964.
7. Smith GM, Lawrence AJ, Colin-Jones DG, et al: The assay of gastrin using the perfused rat stomach. Br J Pharmacol 38:206, 1970.
8. Bugat R, Walsh JH, Ippoliti A, et al: Detection of a circulating gastric secretagogue in plasma extracts from normogastrinemic patients with acid hypersecretion. Gastroenterology 71:1114, 1976.
9. Emås S: Gastric secretory responses to repeated intravenous infusions of histamine and gastrin in nonanesthetized and anesthetized gastric fistula cats. Gastroenterology 39:771, 1960.
10. Uvnas B, Emås S: A method for biological assay of gastrin. Gastroenterology 40:644, 1961.
11. Blair EL, Keenlyside RM, Newell DJ, et al: Assay of gastrin by means of its gastric acid stimulating activity. J Physiol 198:613, 1968.
12. Blair EL, Grund ER, Lund PK, et al: Comparison of gastrin bioactivity and immunoreactivity of antral extracts from man, pig and cat. J Physiol 325:419, 1982.
13. Davidson WD, Lemmi CAE, Thompson JC: Action of gastrin on the isolated gastric mucosa of the bullfrog. Proc Soc Exp Biol Med 121:545, 1966.
14. Ayalon A, Devitt PG, Rayford PL, et al: Electrochemical response patterns to histamine, bombesin, and pentagastrin in isolated bullfrog gastric mucosa. Biochem Biophys Res Commun 103:1186, 1981.
15. Loveridge N, Bloom SR, Welbourn RB, et al: Quantitative cytochemical estimation of the effect of pentagastrin (0.005–5 pg/mL) and of plasma gastrin on the guinea-pig fundus *in vitro.* Clin Endocrinol 3:389, 1974.
16. Askew AR: The biological activity of luminal gastrin. J Surg Res 33:201, 1982.
17. Lowry OH, Rosebrough NJ, Farr AL, et al: Protein measurement with the Folin phenol reagent. J Biol Chem 193:265, 1951.
18. Fried GM, Ogden WD, Swierczek J, et al: Release of cholecystokinin in conscious dogs: Correlation with simultaneous measurements of gallbladder pressure and pancreatic protein secretion. Gastroenterology 85:1113, 1983.
19. Fried GM, Ogden WD, Greeley G, et al: Correlation of release and actions of cholecystokinin in dogs before and after vagotomy. Surgery 93:786, 1983.
20. Love JW: A method for the assay of secretin, using rats. Quart J Exp Physiol 42:279, 1957.
21. Heatley NG: The assay of secretin in the rat. J Endocr 42:535, 1968.
22. Iwatsuki K, Iijima F, Chiba S: Potentiating effects of dipyridamole on the secretion of pancreatic juice induced by secretin in the blood-perfused dog pancreas. Jpn J Pharmacol 32:735, 1982.
23. Hashimoto K, Satoh S, Takeuchi O: Effect of dopamine on pancreatic secretion in the dog. Br J Pharmacol 43:739, 1971.
24. Amsterdam A, Jamieson JD: Structural and functional characterization of isolated pancreatic exocrine cells. Proc Nat Acad Sci USA 69:3028, 1972.
25. Peikin SR, Rottman AJ, Batzri S, et al: Kinetics of amylase release by dispersed acini prepared from guinea pig pancreas. Am J Physiol 235:E743, 1978.
26. Williams JA, Korc M, Dormer RL: Action of secretagogues on a new preparation of functionally intact, isolated pancreatic acini. Am J Physiol 235:E517, 1978.
27. Pan G-Z, Collen MJ, Gardner JD: Action of cholera toxin on dispersed acini from rat pancreas. Postreceptor modulation involving cyclic AMP and calcium. Biochim Biophys Acta 720:338, 1982.
28. Ceska M, Birath K, Brown B: A new and rapid method for the clinical determination of α-amylase activities in human serum and urine. Optimal conditions. Clin Chim Acta 26:437, 1969.
29. Turley SD, Dietschy JM: Re-evaluation of the 3α-hydroxysteroid dehydrogenase assay for total bile acids in bile. J Lipid Res 19:924, 1978.
30. Abell LL, Levy BB, Brodie BB, et al: A simplified method for the estimation of total cholesterol in serum and demonstration of its specificity. J Biol Chem 195:357, 1952.
31. Fiske CH, Subbarow Y: The colorimetric determination of phosphorus. J Biol Chem 66:375, 1925.
32. Ivy AC, Oldberg E: A hormone mechanism for gallbladder contraction and evacuation. Am J Physiol 86:599, 1928.
33. Ivy AC, Janecek HM: Assay of Jorpes-Mutt secretin and cholecystokinin. Acta Physiol Scand 45:220, 1959.
34. Itoh Z, Takahashi I, Nakaya M, et al: Interdigestive gallbladder bile concentration in relation to periodic contraction of gallbladder in the dog. Gastroenterology 83:645, 1982.
35. Amer MS, Becvar WE: A sensitive in-vitro method for the assay of cholecystokinin. J Endocr 43:637, 1969.
36. Berry H, Flower RJ: The assay of endogenous cholecystokinin and factors influencing its release in the dog and cat. Gastroenterology 60:409, 1971.
37. Amer MS: Studies with cholecystokinin *in vitro.* III. Mechanism of the effect on the isolated rabbit gallbladder strips. J Pharmacol Exp Ther 183:527, 1972.

38. Johnson AG, McDermott SJ: Sensitive bioassay of cholecystokinin in human serum. Lancet 2:589, 1973.
39. Yau WM, Makhlouf GM, Edwards LE, et al: Mode of action of cholecystokinin and related peptides on gallbladder muscle. Gastroenterology 65:451, 1973.
40. Vigna SR, Gorbman A: Effects of cholecystokinin, gastrin, and related peptides on coho salmon gallbladder contraction in vitro. Am J Physiol 232:E485, 1977.
41. Simon-Assmann PM, Yazigi R, Greeley GH Jr, et al: Biological and radioimmunological activity of cholecystokinin in regions of mammalian brains. J Neurosci Res 10:165, 1983.
42. Marshall CE, Egberts EH, Johnson AG: An improved method for estimating cholecystokinin in human serum. J Endocr 79:17, 1978.
43. Marshall CE: Automated biological assay of cholecystokinin. Med Biol Engineering 14:327, 1976.
44. Lonovics J, Guzman S, Devitt P, et al: Release of pancreatic polypeptide in humans by infusion of cholecystokinin. Gastroenterology 79:817, 1980.
45. Morgan KG, Schmalz PF, Go VLW, et al: Electrical and mechanical effects of molecular variants of CCK on antral smooth muscle. Am J Physiol 235:E324, 1978.
46. Bortoff A: Electrical activity of intestine recorded with pressure electrode. Am J Physiol 201:209, 1961.
47. Bortoff A: Slow potential variations of small intestine. Am J Physiol 201:203, 1961.
48. Hedner P, Rorsman G: Structures essential for the effect of cholecystokinin on the guinea pig small intestine in vitro. Acta Physiol Scand 74:58, 1968.
49. Bitar KN, Zfass AM, Makhlouf GM: Interaction of acetylcholine and cholecystokinin with dispersed smooth muscle cells. Am J Physiol 237:E172, 1979.
50. Bitar KN, Makhlouf GM: Receptors on smooth muscle cells: Characterization by contraction and specific antagonists. Am J Physiol 242:G400, 1982.
51. Bitar KN, Saffouri B, Makhlouf GM: Cholinergic and peptidergic receptors on isolated human antral smooth muscle cells. Gastroenterology 82:832, 1982.
52. Lindkaer Jensen S, Kuhl C, Vagn Nielsen O, et al: Isolation and perfusion of the porcine pancreas. Scand J Gastroent Suppl 37:57, 1976.
53. Lindkaer Jensen S, Fahrenkrug J, Holst JJ, et al: Secretory effects of secretin on isolated perfused porcine pancreas. Am J Physiol 235:E381, 1978.
54. Lambert AE, Blondel B, Kanazawa Y, et al: Monolayer cell culture of neonatal rat pancreas: Light microscopy and evidence for immunoreactive insulin synthesis and release. Endocrinology 90:239, 1972.
55. Fujimoto WY: Purification of neonatal rat pancreatic monolayer cultures for endocrine cells. Proc Soc Exp Biol Med 162:241, 1979.
56. Munro HN, Fleck A: Recent developments in the measurement of nucleic acids in biological materials. Analyst 91:78, 1966.
57. Solomon TE, Vanier M, Morisset J: Cell site and time course of DNA synthesis in pancreas after caerulein and secretin. Am J Physiol 245:G99, 1983.
58. Morisset J, Chamberland S, Gilbert L, et al: Study of pancreatic DNA synthesis *in vivo* and *in vitro* following caerulein treatment *in vivo*. Biomed Res 3:151, 1982.
59. Seiler N: Ion-pair chromatographic separation of polyamines and their monoacetyl derivatives. Methods Enzymol 94:25, 1983.
60. Tabor CW, Tabor H: Quantitative determination of naturally occurring aliphatic diamines and polyamines by an automated liquid chromatography procedure. Methods Enzymol 94:29, 1983.
61. Freshney RI: *Culture of Animal Cells. A Manual of Basic Technique*. New York, Alan R Liss Inc, 1983.
62. Song M-KH, Krutzsch H, Hankins WD, et al: Rapid determination of DNA synthesis in adherent cells grown in microtiter plates. Exp Cell Res 156:271, 1985.
63. Hayashi S-I, Kameji T: Ornithine decarboxylase (rat liver). Methods Enzymol 94:154, 1983.

Chapter 5

Pharmacokinetics of Gut Peptides

George H. Greeley, Jr., Ph.D.

The term pharmacokinetics refers to the absorption, distribution, metabolism, and excretion of a substance in a biologic system over time [1,2]. This substance can be administered to subjects in a clinical setting or to test animals in a research laboratory. By means of a pharmacokinetic model, an investigator can describe how a particular substance, in this case a gut or pancreatic peptide, behaves in a biologic system.

In order to simplify the biologic system in a pharmacokinetic analysis, the body is represented as a model composed of separate but contiguous compartments. In a compartmental model, the biologic system is described as one or more compartments in which a substance is homogeneously distributed in what is called an apparent volume of distribution (V_d) [3–5]. V_d does not represent an actual anatomic compartment. The rate of passage of substances between these compartments is proportional to the quantity of the substance itself. Obviously, the total amount of a substance in the body cannot be measured directly in humans and is not easily measured in laboratory animals. V_d is useful for determining the plasma concentration when a known amount of peptide is given or for determining the dose required to achieve a specific plasma level.

When a peptide is administered into the general circulation, it is uniformly and rapidly distributed into a single compartment, the plasma or central compartment, unless it is degraded or excreted instantaneously. The distribution of this substance will obviously affect its efficacy, duration of action, and rate of removal. To describe the quantity of peptide in the body (Q_b), the plasma concentration (C_p) is multiplied by the apparent volume of distribution (V_d). The equation is $Q_b = V_dC_p$. In solving this equation, the plasma concentration is used, since this is an easily obtained measurement. The entire body is considered to be a single compartment, with a homogeneous distribution at a concentration equal to that in the plasma. In most cases, the apparent volume of distribution is calculated by dividing the quantity of substance given by its concentration in plasma at time zero ($V_d = Q_b/C_p$).

Gut and pancreatic peptides are usually given intravenously or intraarterially. The oral route is not acceptable for peptides because most are destroyed by digestive enzymes. After injection, the peptide is distributed to various tissues. The rate and degree of distribution of the peptides are influenced by the following: the rate of blood flow; the extent of binding of the peptide to plasma proteins and to tissue; and the ability of the peptide to penetrate the various tissues. In most cases, the kidney and liver are the primary sites of excretion and metabolism, respectively.

The elimination of a peptide from the body can also be described quantitatively. After a peptide is infused intravenously or administered as a single bolus, the plasma levels of the peptide decline from an initially high concentration. This early rapid decline in plasma levels is called the distribution phase because the peptide is in the process of being distributed throughout the body. With time, further decreases in the plasma levels of the peptide reflect alterations in the concentration of the peptide in the body due to its elimination and/or inactivation.

Many substances are restricted to the plasma compartment, particularly large macromolecules similar in size to plasma proteins or substances that are avidly bound to circulating plasma proteins. If the substance is of low molecular weight (<1000) and not bound to plasma proteins, it will quickly diffuse into the extracellular water space.

The concept that a peptide is bound to a

plasma protein is important, since it is likely that only an unbound (free) peptide is able to exert its action, be metabolized, and be excreted. Thus, protein binding decreases the rate of these processes. If a substance is bound to plasma proteins, its half-life can be lengthened substantially.

The ability of a substance to enter the intracellular water depends on its ability to penetrate the cell membrane. Peptides that are insoluble in lipids penetrate across cell membranes only slightly if at all, and, therefore, tend to be excluded.

The absorption and excretion of a substance presumably proceed according to exponential or first-order kinetics. In other words, a constant fraction of the substance is removed for each unit of time. Since the excretion or elimination mechanisms are rarely saturated, the elimination of a substance is exponential. The rate of this elimination process can be expressed by its rate constant (k), which expresses the fractional change of this substance per unit of time, or by its half-life ($t_{1/2}$). Half-life is defined as the time needed to complete 50 percent of the elimination process. The values $t_{1/2}$ and k are independent of concentration and dose. When the decline in the plasma concentration of a peptide can be described by a single exponential term, the equation for this first-order rate constant and the half-time of the elimination process is

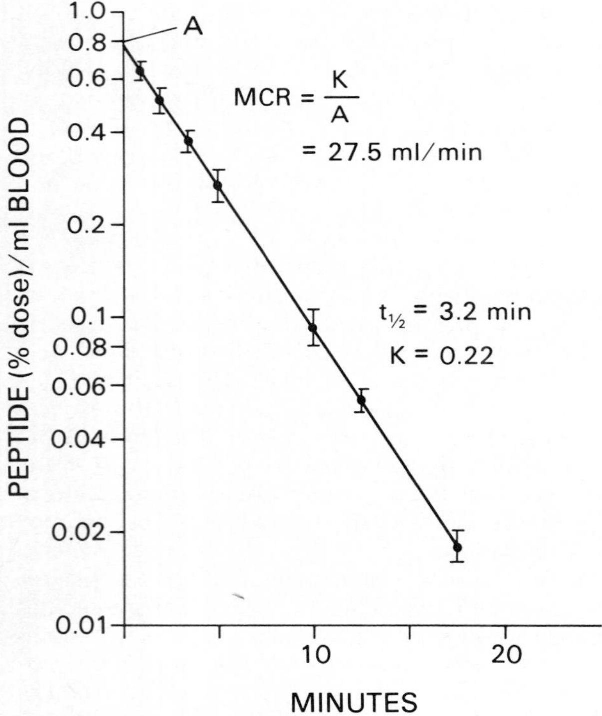

Figure 5-1. Disappearance of radioactive peptide from the blood after intravenous administration of iodinated peptide X (single pool model).

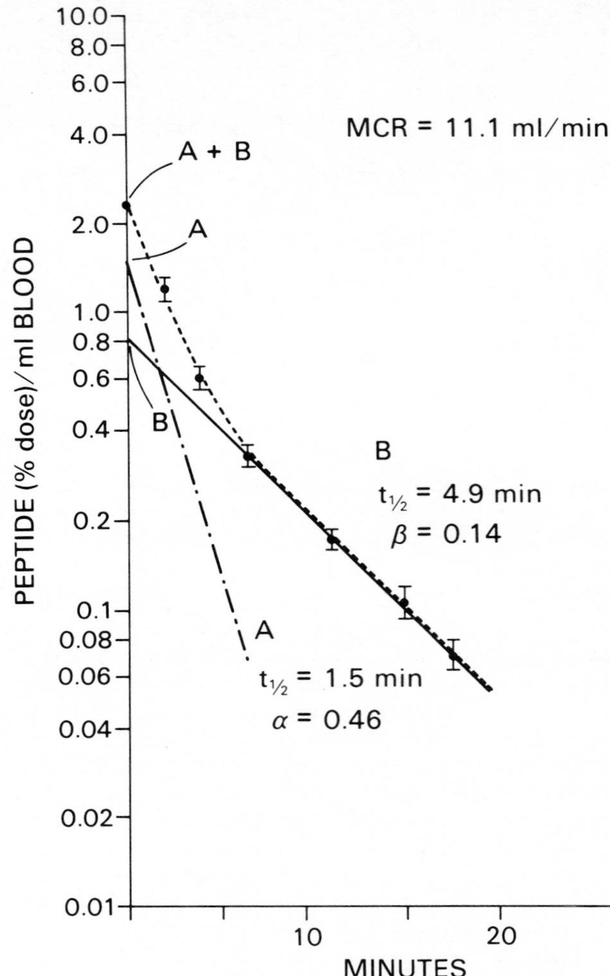

Figure 5-2. Disappearance of an iodinated peptide X from the plasma following the intravenous administration of iodinated peptide X (two-compartment model). The dotted-line curve is the actual disappearance of the peptide. α and β are the slopes of the corrected first and second exponentials. A and B are their intercepts. The formulas for calculation of the slope and MCR are: Slope (α or β) $= \frac{0.69}{t_{1/2}}$; MCR $= \frac{\alpha\beta}{A\beta + B\alpha}$. The values for A are generated by subtracting the values for B from the original value.

$$t_{1/2} = \frac{0.693}{k}$$

The equation for a single pool model can be described in a graphic fashion on semilog paper (Fig

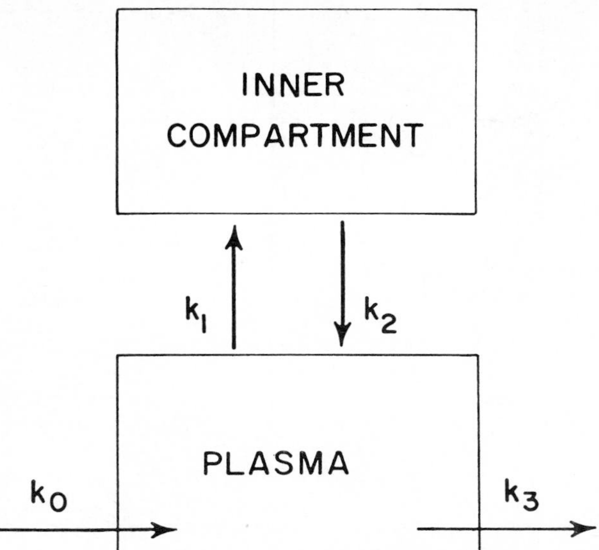

Figure 5-3. A two-compartment model for disappearance of exogenous gastrin from circulation. k_0 = rate of infusion; k_3 = rate of irreversible loss from plasma; k_1 and k_2 = rates of transfer between two compartments. (From Reeder et al [6], by permission of The American Physiological Society.)

5-1). The slope of the disappearance curve gives the rate constant, k.

Another important concept is clearance, usually expressed as the metabolic clearance rate (MCR). Clearance is a direct quantitation of the rate of elimination of a substance from the plasma, and it describes the volume of plasma completely cleared of the peptide per unit time. Its units are mL/min. The following formula gives derivation of the clearance value: clearance = dose administered (pg)/integrated area beneath the plasma concentration curve from time = 0 to time = infinity (pg/mL/min). In a single pool model, MCR can also be calculated: MCR = k (slope)/A (y-intercept) (Fig 5-1).

Many substances are absorbed and eliminated according to a two-compartment model (Fig 5-2). Initially, a substance is given into a central compartment (plasma pool), and then it is slowly absorbed and eliminated by a second compartment (Fig 5-3). As with the one-compartment model, the absorption and elimination processes behave according to first-order kinetics. In a plot of plasma concentration (ordinate) versus time (abscissa), it will be obvious that there are two distinct phases. The first or fast phase is characterized by a rapid elimination that is caused by the movement of the peptide from the systemic circulation (central compartment) to the second compartment. The second or slow phase is dominated by elimination processes of the kidney and liver. The rate constants for the distribution and elimination phases, which are called the distribution and elimination half-lives, can be calculated. The term ($t_{1/2\beta}$), elimination half-life, is generally termed the substance half-life.

In the two-compartment model, V_d is calculated using the area method (see Figure 5-2 for an explanation of the terms A and B):

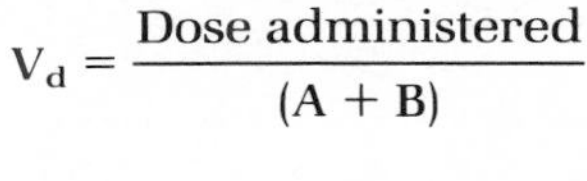

$$V_d = \frac{\text{Dose administered}}{(A + B)}$$

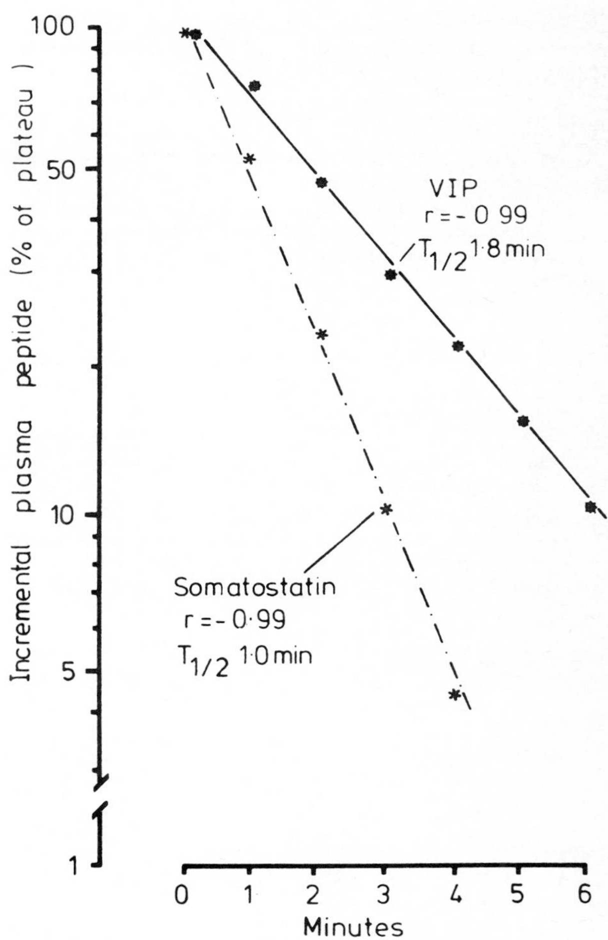

Figure 5-4. Regression lines of incremental VIP and somatostatin concentrations in peripheral plasma (expressed as percentage of plateau value) with time after stopping an infusion of actual 2-8 pmol/kg/min VIP or 8-2 pmol/kg/min somatostatin delivered during 40 minutes. Mean incremental plateau value taken as 100 percent at end of infusion (zero time). (From Chayvialle et al [17], by permission of British Medical Association.)

Clearance is a direct quantitation of the rate of elimination of the substance from the central compartment. The clearance formula (MCR) is shown below, when the pulse injection method is used:

$$MCR = \frac{\text{Dose}}{(A/\alpha + B/\beta)}$$

If the continuous infusion method is used, clearance is calculated as follows:

$$MCR = \frac{\text{infusion rate (pg/min)}}{\text{plasma concentration (pg/mL)}}$$

Studies from our laboratory have provided information on the pharmacokinetics of gastrin [6–8], secretin [9,10], cholecystokinin [11–16], vasoactive intestinal peptide [17], and somatostatin (Fig 5-4) [17].

REFERENCES

1. Gibaldi M, Perrier D: *Pharmacokinetics.* New York, Marcel Dekker Inc, 1982.
2. Mayer SE, Melmon KL, Gilman AG: Introduction; The dynamics of drug absorption, distribution, and elimination, in Gilman AG, Goodman LS, Gilman A (eds): *The Pharmacological Basis of Therapeutics.* 6th Ed. New York, Macmillan Publishing Co Inc, 1980, pp 1–27.
3. Riegelman S, Loo J, Rowland M: Concept of a volume of distribution and possible errors in evaluation of this parameter. J Pharm Sci 57:128, 1968.
4. Gibaldi M, Perrier D: Drug elimination and apparent volume of distribution in multicompartment systems. J Pharm Sci 61:952, 1972.
5. Jusko WJ, Gibaldi M: Effects of change in elimination on various parameters of the two-compartment open model. J Pharm Sci 61:1270, 1972.
6. Reeder DD, Jackson BM, Brandt EN Jr, et al: Rate and pattern of disappearance of exogenous gastrin in dogs. Am J Physiol 222:1571, 1972.
7. Villar HV, Reeder DD, Brandt EN Jr, et al: Disappearance half-time of autogenous antral gastrin in circulation. Physiologist 17:349, 1974.
8. Villar HV, Reeder DD, Rayford PL, et al: Rate of disappearance of circulating endogenous gastrin in dogs. Surgery 81:404, 1977.
9. Rayford PL, Curtis PJ, Fender HR, et al: Radioimmunoassay measurement of disappearance half-time of secretin. Surg Forum 26:385, 1975.
10. Curtis PJ, Fender HR, Rayford PL, et al: Disappearance half-time of endogenous and exogenous secretin in dogs. Gut 17:595, 1976.
11. Reeder DD, Villar HV, Brandt EN Jr, et al: Radioimmunoassay measurement of the disappearance half-time of exogenous cholecystokinin. Physiologist 17:319, 1974.
12. Rayford PL, Fender HR, Ramus NI, et al: Disappearance half-time of exogenous cholecystokinin from circulation in man and dogs. Gastroenterology 68:A-114/971, 1975.
13. Rayford PL, Fender HR, Ramus NI, et al: Release and half-life of CCK in man, in Thompson JC (ed): *Gastrointestinal Hormones.* Austin, University of Texas Press, 1975, pp 301–318.
14. Thompson JC, Fender HR, Ramus NI, et al: Cholecystokinin metabolism in man and dogs. Ann Surg 182:496, 1975.
15. Lilja P, Fagan C, Wiener I, et al: Disappearance half-time of CCK-99% correlated with gallbladder volume in man. Gastroenterology 80:1213, 1981.
16. Lilja P, Fagan CJ, Wiener I, et al: Infusion of pure cholecystokinin in humans. Correlation between plasma concentrations of cholecystokinin and gallbladder size. Gastroenterology 83:256, 1982.
17. Chayvialle J-A, Rayford PL, Thompson JC: Radioimmunoassay study of hepatic clearance and disappearance half-time of somatostatin and vasoactive intestinal peptide in dogs. Gut 22:732, 1981.

Chapter 6

Surgical Techniques

Courtney M. Townsend, Jr., M.D., and others

Careful observation is the foundation of physiologic study. Since Beaumont first peered into a gastrocutaneous fistula, many techniques have been developed for the study of gastrointestinal physiology. In this section, we describe surgical techniques that may be employed to study secretion, motility, and hormone release and metabolism.

Many of the techniques still bear the name of the investigator (Pavlov, Heidenhain, Herrera, and Shay, to name a few) who used them to make major contributions to our knowledge of gastrointestinal physiology. However, the techniques themselves are not an end, but simply a means to an end. This in no way detracts from the importance of surgical preparations. For example, the entire field of endocrinology began, in one sense, when Bayliss and Starling perfused an isolated segment of gut to discover the first hormone, secretin.

This is not a complete account of all surgical techniques that have been employed. We have used and are familiar with all the techniques described, and if these models are created as described, they will work. If future experience follows ours, however, they may not work the first time.

All of the following descriptions have been prepared by colleagues in our laboratory. I have been involved in the preparation of each segment, and all sections have been reviewed by Dr. Thompson and by me.

GASTRIC AND PANCREATIC FISTULAS

Isidoro Wiener, M.D., and William H. Nealon, M.D.

Gastric and pancreatic secretions may be collected by the creation of acute or chronic fistulas. Acute gastric fistulas use temporary catheters or cannulas; acute pancreatic fistulas may be constructed by placing a large Thomas cannula in the duodenum opposite the orifice of the pancreatic duct, which can then be cannulated, for short intervals (2–6 hours), at will.

Chronic fistulas involve insertion of more permanent cannulas. The methods are described below.

Gastric Fistulas (Fig 6-1)

Gastric secretions can be collected from an orogastric tube (difficult in most animals) or from temporary or permanent fistulas of the whole innervated stomach, or from isolated fundic pouches that may be innervated (Pavlov or Thomas) or denervated (Heidenhain). A simple fistula of the whole stomach is placed in the distal body of the stomach on the anterior surface near the greater curvature. A gastrotomy, 2 cm in length, is performed, and a Thomas-type metal or plastic cannula is placed in the stomach and secured with a purse-string suture. The cannula is exteriorized through a separate stab wound on the left side of the abdomen, well clear of the costal arch. This cannula may be used to study gastric secretion, although meal stimulation cannot be measured, and the possibility of reflux of duodenal bile or bicarbonate exists. The gastric fistula is useful for assessment of gastric acid output by the technique of intragastric titration [1] (Fig 6-2). For this reason, various gastric pouches have been devised whereby noncontaminated gastric secretions can be obtained and quantified.

Pavlov (Innervated Fundic) Pouch (see Fig 6-1)

In 1942, Thomas described a modification of the pouch that Pavlov popularized in 1902 [2]. This

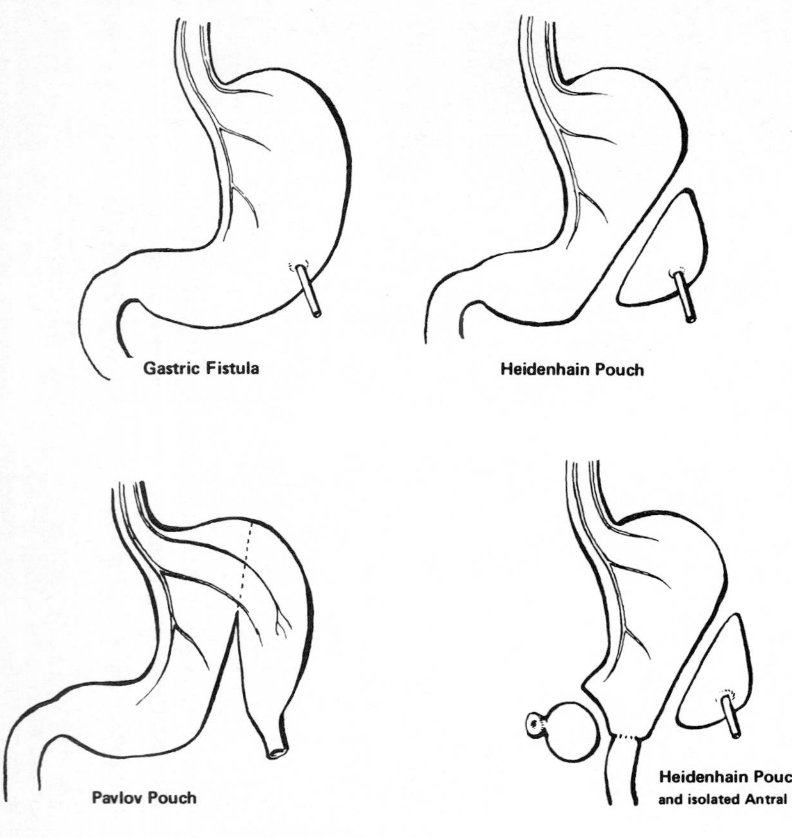

Figure 6-1. Experimental gastric pouches in common use (classic experimental preparations used in the study of gastric secretion). The gastric fistula is simply a cannula placed into the intact innervated stomach. The Heidenhain pouch is a denervated segment of fundic mucosa drained with a cannula. The Pavlov pouch is an innervated fundic pouch separated from the main stomach by an internal mucosal septum. Pouches of the antrum may be innervated or denervated. They allow study of the mechanisms for stimulation and suppression of gastrin release. The isolated antral pouch may be constructed in association with a Heidenhain pouch, as shown on the lower right, or with a Pavlov pouch or a gastric fistula. (From Thompson JC: Stomach and duodenum. In Sabiston DC Jr, ed): *Christopher's Textbook of Surgery.* 13th ed. Philadelphia, WB Saunders Co, 1985, pp 810–874.)

innervated pouch was first constructed after division of various muscular layers, and Thomas recommended a mucosal incision only.

In fasting mongrel dogs, a midline abdominal incision is made and an anterior gastrotomy, 2 cm long, is performed. Toothed clamps are used to grasp gastric mucosa at the proximal and distal limits of the intended pouch. The mucosa is drawn through the gastrotomy, and the resulting circle of everted mucosa is drawn into an elliptical configuration by placing traction on the two clamps. In the long axis of the ellipse, the two outer walls form ridges of mucosa divided by the two opposed mucosal layers, which communicate with the remainder of the stomach. A longitudinal mucosal incision is made along each ridge, and the two opposed layers of mucosa are closed in order to restore continuity of the main stomach. The free edges of mucosa on the two parallel ridges are then closed, thus establishing a barrier of two mucosal surfaces between the pouch and the stomach. The original gastrotomy is closed, and a Thomas-type cannula is placed, either in this gastrotomy or, in our experience, preferably through a separate stab wound at the most dependent area of the pouch. If desired, a second cannula can be placed in the remaining stomach for the purpose of administering gastric meals.

Heidenhain (Denervated Fundic) Pouch (see Fig 6-1)

The construction and use of a denervated fundic pouch was popularized by Heidenhain, and the pouch currently used has been modified by Gregory [3]. This pouch is especially useful for study of humoral stimulation of gastric secretion, but it has the disadvantage of insensitivity, since denervation removes vagal tone (acetylcholine) from the parietal cell mass. A gastric pouch is created by complete isolation of a segment of distal fundus along the greater curvature of the stomach. No antral mucosa should be in the pouch. Division of all layers of gastric wall results in a denervated area of gastric mucosa. Closure of the free edges of this segment produces a pouch into which a Gregory-type cannula can be placed. The defect in the main stomach is closed primarily. The cannula is passed through the abdominal wall and secured.

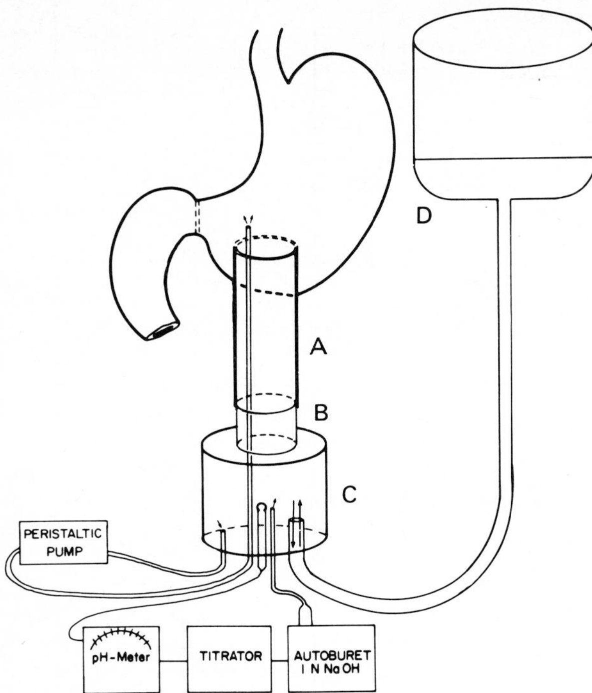

Figure 6-2. Schematic presentation of intragastric titration in dogs with gastric fistula: gastric cannula (A); hollow obturator (B); titration chamber (C); and barostat (D). (Modified from Konturek et al [1], with permission of the American Physiological Society.)

In a denervated pouch, gastric secretory responses to a meal or peptide stimulation can be measured.

Pancreatic Fistulas

The various methods that have been used to obtain pancreatic secretions from conscious animals have entailed either direct cannulation of the pancreatic duct or isolation of the small segment of duodenum into which the pancreatic duct is inserted. The fact that canine pancreatic and common bile ducts enter the duodenum in locations sufficiently distant from one another as to allow surgical isolation has made the latter method most popular [4]. Early efforts included the use of exteriorized duodenal loops [5], external rubber shunts from a duodenal pouch into the distal intestine [6], a duodenal pouch draining into a Roux-en-Y limb [7], and a series of cannulas that combined to allow collection of pancreatic secretion [8].

Herrera-type Pancreatic Fistula

A significant advance was made in 1968 with the description by Herrera et al [9] of a cannula that established chronic communication between the skin and the duodenum, with a side channel inserted into a small isolated pouch of duodenum containing the pancreatic papilla. This apparatus (Fig 6-3) permits normal drainage of pancreatic juice into the intestine and allows diversion of juices during studies.

After an overnight fast, mongrel dogs are anesthetized with sodium pentobarbital (Nembutal) anesthesia and given endotracheal intubation. One preoperative dose of penicillin G is administered intramuscularly and repeated daily for 3 days. A midline upper abdominal incision permits visualization of the pylorus and proximal half of the duodenum. Downward traction on the duodenum allows palpation of the common bile duct and the papilla, which are located at the end of the 0.5–2.0 cm course of the duct within the wall of the duodenum. The proximal limit of the duodenal pouch should be placed about 1 cm distal to the biliary papilla. Vascular connections between the duodenum and the pancreas are dissected, ligated, and divided, and the accessory pancreatic duct, in the posterior mesenteric leaflet, is ligated. After forming a 1 cm window in the mesentery, similar dissection is performed about 2.5 cm distal to the main pancreatic duct. The duodenum is then divided at these two locations and both free ends of the pouch are closed. An end-to-end duodeno-

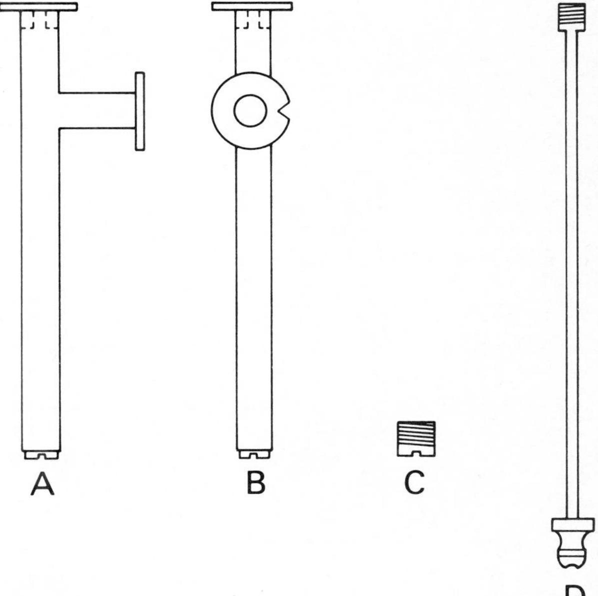

Figure 6-3. Herrera cannula (A,B) with screw-on plug (C) and obturator (D) for use during study.

duodenostomy is performed. An incision is made in the antimesenteric portion of the pouch and a purse-string suture is placed. The side channel of the cannula (see Fig 6-3) is placed in the pouch and secured. A duodenostomy is then created in the distal duodenum, and one free end of the cannula is placed in the duodenum and secured (Fig 6-4). The whole system is then generously wrapped in omentum, and the remaining free end of the cannula is exteriorized through a stab incision placed lateral to the rectus muscles. An external "bite block" stabilizes the cannula. The cannula is permitted to drain freely for 24 hours, after which the screw plug (see Fig 6-3C) is inserted. The dog is given Ringer's lactate by injection subcutaneously for 3 days, after which water and then food are resumed. With minimal care and adequate nutrition, dogs thus prepared can be maintained for 6–12 months.

ANTRAL POUCH AND ISOLATED ANTRAL VEINS

Isidoro Wiener, M.D., and William H. Nealon, M.D.

Antral Pouch (see Fig 6-1)

In the construction of antral pouches (innervated and denervated) in dogs, the stomach is divided immediately proximal to the pylorus in order to exclude duodenal mucosa [10–13]. The duodenum is divided just beyond the pylorus and the intervening tissue is discarded. The junction of the antrofundic mucosa of the opened stomach can be easily identified at operation by use of strips of pH testing paper applied after subcutaneous administration of 1 mg histamine base. The mucosa should be gently patted dry with a sponge immediately before the strips are laid transversely across the junction of antral and fundic mucosa.

Denervated

In preparing denervated antral pouches, the stomach is completely transected (along with vagal fibers of the nerves of Laterjet) at the level of the antrofundic junction [10]. Gastrointestinal continuity is restored with a gastroduodenostomy. The proximal end of the antral pouch is oversewn, and the distal end is brought through the body wall as an antrocutaneous fistula.

Innervated

Vagally innervated antral pouches are constructed by dividing the stomach at the level of the antrofundic junction with an incision beginning at the greater curvature just opposite the *incisura angularis.* This incision is carried to the lesser curvature, but the stomach is not completely divided. The gastric and antral lumina are separated with a double mucosal barrier, and gastrointestinal continuity is restored with a gastroduodenostomy [10].

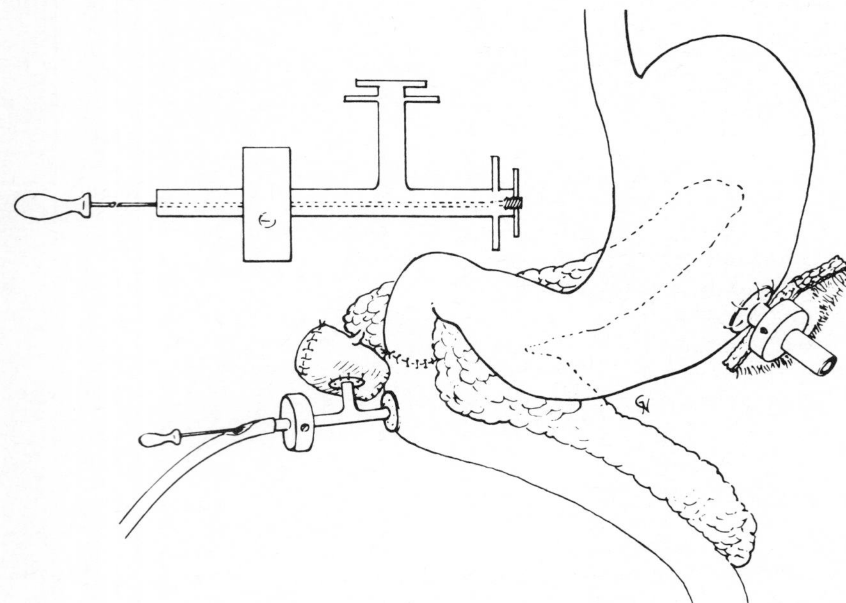

Figure 6-4. The final anatomic arrangements after Herrera cannula placement and gastric fistula with obturator in place to allow pancreatic juice diversion. (From Llanos et al, Surgery 81:661, 1977, with permission of The CV Mosby Co.)

Collection of Antral Venous Blood [13]

After an overnight fast, a healthy adult mongrel dog is anesthetized with thiopental sodium (Pentothal). The blood supply to the antrum is restricted to the right gastroepiploic vessels by carefully ligating the contributing branches from the fundic portion, the vessels along the lesser curvature, and the contributing vessels of the omentum. A splenic branch is then cannulated so that the flow of blood from the antrum can be diverted to make collections, by intermittent application of the choker (Fig 6-5).

SEGMENTAL PERFUSION OF THE INTESTINE

Masaki Fujimura, M.D., Felix Lluis, M.D., and Tsuguo Sakamoto, M.D.

We will describe several techniques for perfusion of isolated intestinal segments that we have used in acute and chronic studies in animals. We will also briefly describe the principles of intubation methods employed in humans.

The technique of isolated segmental perfusion of the intestine has been employed to study the transit or absorption of food in the gut. This technique has also been useful for study of release or action of gastrointestinal hormones by perfusion of various substances into a specific isolated segment.

Perfusion of Surgically Isolated Segments of Intestine in Dogs

In acute studies, a segment of the intestine can be isolated and perfused in the anesthetized animal. Experimental solutions can be administered with or without closure of the abdominal wall [14]. Acute models and studies have certain disadvantages; for example, operative trauma and anesthetic agents may produce systemic effects, which may affect motility or suppress hormone release.

Chronic isolation of segments of the small bowel yields stable experimental models. The most widely used preparation, originally designed to collect succus entericus, is the Thiry-Vella fistula or loop. A Thiry-Vella fistula is an experimental intestinal fistula that consists of an isolated intestinal segment with an intact blood supply. After the segment is isolated, intestinal continuity is restored by means of an end-to-end enteroenteros-

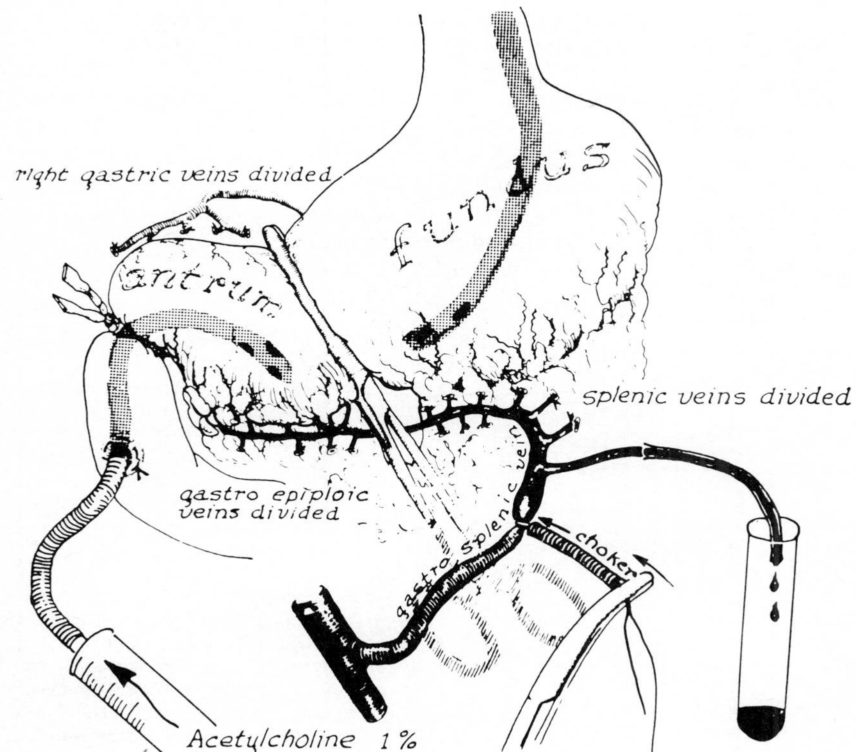

Figure 6-5. Technique for the selective sampling of antral venous blood. Acid secretion is collected via the fundic tube. If gastrin release is under study, acetylcholine can be instilled in the antral tube. When blood samples are not being collected, the choker is released and antral venous blood enters the systemic circulation. (From Charters et al [13], with permission of The CV Mosby Co.)

tomy. This isolated Thiry-Vella segment has been used to study intestinal absorption, secretion, or motility in response to intravenous or luminal stimulants.

As originally described by Thiry [15], one end of the segment was closed and the other was open as a mucocutaneous fistula. Later, Vella modified the original Thiry fistula to keep both ends of the segment open as fistulas [16,17]. With the modification, studies involving filling, emptying, and perfusion of the segment with test substances are more easily performed. The Thiry-Vella segment can be created at any site throughout the intestine and the length (usually 30–50 cm) can also vary, depending upon the purpose of the study. The fistulous opening can be created either by means of a mucocutaneous stoma or by installing Thomas-type metal cannulas into the lumen of the segment. Balloon catheters can be used to fill, empty, and subdivide the segments. Berger et al [18] observed no physiologic or histologic deterioration in Thiry-type fistulas in dogs studied repeatedly over 5 years.

Perfusion of Intestinal Segments by Intubation

Humans

When used correctly, human intestinal perfusion techniques may provide highly accurate and reproducible results [19,20]. Several technical devices have been used during the past 20 years. Accurate placement of the tube at the desired level of the intestine is facilitated by fluoroscopy and by measuring (from the incisors) the length of tube inserted.

The double-lumen perfusion system [21] has two main disadvantages that limit its usefulness for clinical studies [19]. The length of the intestinal segment under study is unknown but is longer than the distance between the two apertures, because of proximal reflux. Since no method of segment isolation is used, proximal endogenous secretions contaminate the test segment.

Most problems can be obviated by use of a triple-lumen perfusion system [22], which introduces the concept of "mixing" and "study" segments. The accuracy of the results is improved by providing a segment for mixing of fasting intestinal contents and test solution and by sampling the same bolus of intestinal contents at two different points of the study segment (Fig 6-6).

Polyvinyl tubing is used to construct multilumen tubes employed in the triple-lumen perfusion system. The subject swallows the tube with an attached rubber bag containing mercury, and normal peristaltic activity carries the tube to the desired level of the small intestine. The inclusion of a removable wire provides some stiffness and aids in rapid insertion [23]. A nonabsorbable marker (such as polyethylene glycol [24] or phenol red [25,26]) is used to examine the accuracy of segmental perfusion. The marker is infused along with the test solutions and should be recovered almost entirely at the point of sample withdrawal. When the marker is used to rule out the possibility of reflux, it should not be recovered from the sampling site. The marker provides information concerning the possible reflux of perfusate or its leakage around the distal collecting tube; the experiment should be excluded if either reflux or leakage is significant. Multilumen tubes have also been utilized in diverting chyme from the intestine while withdrawing intraluminal samples to evaluate the role of the intestinal phase of digestion in humans [20].

Balloons attached to the tubes are used when-

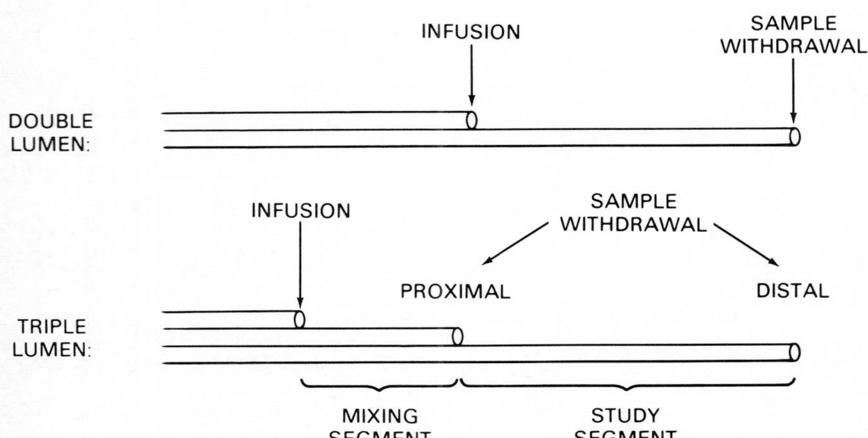

Figure 6-6. Comparison between the double- and triple-lumen systems used in studies of intestinal absorption or perfusion. In the double-lumen system, the length of the study segment is unknown because of proximal reflux. The triple-lumen perfusion system introduces the concept of "mixing" and "study" segments, and sampling of the same bolus of intestinal contents at two different points. When balloons are not used to isolate the study segment, the results are more accurate with the triple-lumen system because it provides a segment for mixing intestinal fasting contents and the test solution.

ever isolation of a given segment is an important part of the experimental design. Balloons are carefully inflated to a volume that causes awareness but not pain.

Experimental Animals

In awake animals, orogastric or nasogastric tubes are not easily placed or maintained in proper position. Segmental perfusion studies in animals became widely used after the introduction of gastric and intestinal cannulas by Thomas [27] in 1941 and duodenopancreatic cannulas by Herrera et al [9] in 1968 (see Figs 6-3 and 6-4).

Generally, cannulas are implanted at both ends of the intestinal segments to be perfused, so that administration of experimental solutions is by proximal cannulas and drainage is through the distal cannulas. Balloon catheters are inserted through the cannulas in order to occlude and perfuse the desired segment. A Dacron cuff may be wrapped around the bowel in order to splint the intestinal wall. When the balloon is inflated and the catheter pulled back, the cuff aids in holding the balloon in proper position and ensures a tight seal [28,29]. A triple-lumen catheter, described above, has been used successfully in dogs with chronic jejunal fistulas [30].

Preparation of Dogs with Gastric, Pancreatic, and Three Intestinal Cannulas

We have used this model in order to study the stimulatory and inhibitory roles of individual segments of small intestine (duodenum, jejunum, and ileum) on pancreatic exocrine secretion and on release of gastrointestinal hormones.

Construction of Cannulas

The gastric and intestinal cannulas (modifications of Thomas cannulas [27]) that are used in this preparation are illustrated in Figure 6-7.

Operative Procedures

Two operations are performed on each dog. Gastric and pancreatic fistulas are created as described at the beginning of this chapter and as illustrated in Figure 6-4.

The gastric and pancreatic cannulas are brought out through stab wounds in the abdominal wall, 2 cm or more below the costal margin, taking care that there is no tension on the cannula.

After complete recovery from the operation, usually 3 weeks, a second operation is carried out. The upper part of the abdomen, where gastric and pancreatic cannulas are located, is isolated from

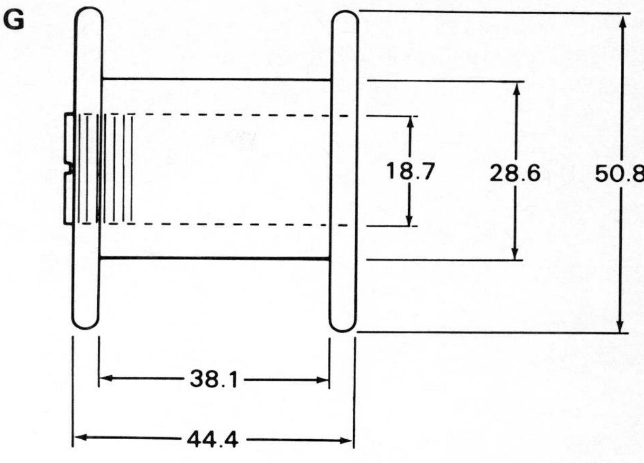

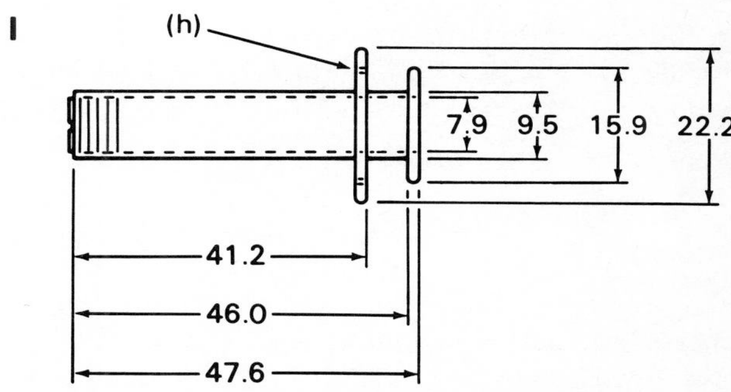

Figure 6-7. Construction illustration of cannulas used in this preparation (unit, mm). G. Gastric cannula made of plexiglass. I. Small intestinal cannula made of stainless steel. (h), 6 holes equally spaced to fix to the seromuscular layer of small intestine with string. A bite block made of nylon which stabilizes intestinal cannula against the skin and small intestine is not shown in the figure. Herrera cannula for pancreatic fistula is illustrated in Figure 6-3.

the operative field with sterile drapes, and the abdomen is opened through a lower midline abdominal incision. Intestinal cannulas are inserted into the small intestine at three separate sites (Fig 6-8, left): one just distal to the ligament of Treitz, one in the terminal ileum, and one half-way between the two (midintestine). The cannulas are fixed to the intestinal wall, and the upper jejunal and midintestinal cannulas are brought out on the right side and the ileal cannula on the left. Dogs are allowed to recover from the operation for at least 3 weeks before studies are performed.

Complications and Mortality

We initially inserted all cannulas (gastric, pancreatic, and three intestinal) at the same operation,

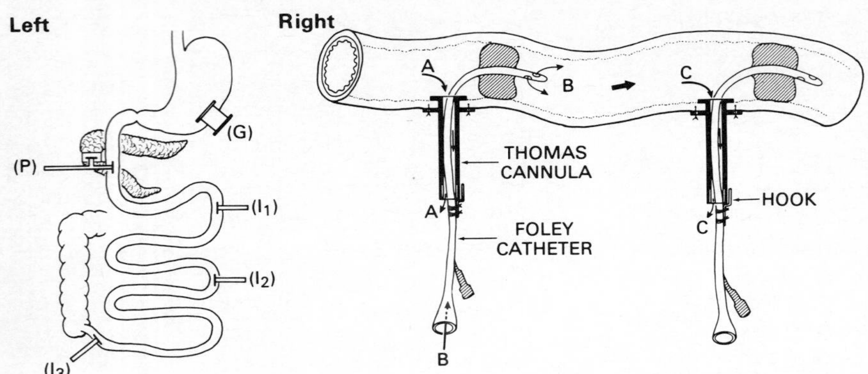

Figure 6-8. *Left:* Operative procedure. Placement of gastric (G) and pancreatic (P) cannulas during the first operation. In second operation, three intestinal cannulas (I_1, I_2, and I_3) are inserted (see text for explanation). *Right:* Isolation of a given segment of small intestine during every perfusion study. A, fasting intestinal contents escape. B, infusion of perfusate. C, recovery of perfusate.

but mortality was high (8 of 11). We had no deaths (zero of 7) with the two-stage procedure. Significant adhesions were found in only one of seven dogs. Of 21 intestinal cannulas implanted in the second operation, three were lost: two came out of the lumen, and one slipped through the abdominal wall.

Perfusion Experiments

Dogs were deprived of food but not water for 24 hours before each experiment. A Foley catheter (no. 12F) was inserted into the lumen of the intestine from each cannula located at both ends of the intestinal segment to be studied (Fig 6-8, right). To aid the catheter in migrating distally with the peristaltic contractions of the gut, the balloon was inflated with only 3 mL of water. Once the migration was accomplished, the catheter was pulled back to a position in which the balloon was located 5 cm distal to the entrance of the intestinal cannula, and 7 mL of air was added to effect complete occlusion of the lumen. Prevention of proximal or distal reflux of the perfusate and its contamination by succus entericus from above was thus effected. The fact that both cannulas are open during the experiment also serves these purposes. Before each study, 100 mL of saline containing phenol red (100 mg/L) was infused rapidly through both balloon catheters and fluid from both intestinal cannulas was collected. During the control (basal) period of the experiment, the phenol red solution was perfused (in the same manner and at the same flow rate as the luminal stimulant) for more than one hour. Fluid from the proximal cannulas and aspirate from distal balloon catheters were also collected. All fluid collected in this manner was observed by titrating it to pH 7–8 for the presence of red coloration in order to examine the accuracy of the segmental perfusion. For the duodenal perfusion, gastric juice was examined in the same manner. The catheters were fixed with a hook to the outside wall of the intestinal cannulas, so that the position of the balloon was maintained throughout the experiment.

Perfusion of jejunal or ileal segments is performed through the proximal catheter. Duodenal infusion is achieved through the duodenal limb of the pancreatic cannula, since we found that vomiting often occurs when a balloon is inflated in the first portion of the duodenum.

MEASUREMENT OF MOTILITY

Masaki Fujimura, M.D.

Early studies of gastrointestinal motility in conscious animals were achieved by direct observation through abdominal fistulas, segments of bowel transplanted under the skin, or a window (glass or celluloid) constructed in the anterior abdominal wall. Studies of motility were also accomplished in anesthetized animals during laparotomy. However, these techniques did not allow precise quantification of motility, and no permanent recordings of electrical activity could be made.

Radiographic techniques introduced by Cannon [31] made it possible to study the transit of radiopaque material along the gut in conscious animals. Recently, techniques have been developed that use cineradiography or isotope scintigraph image intensifiers and video tape recordings.

Current studies of gut motility are performed in vitro and in vivo. The development of techniques using segments or strips of the gut wall has been extremely useful. The prepared strips are attached to a strain-gauge transducer, and isometric contractions can be recorded. This technique has the advantage of allowing study of the gut directly without nervous or humoral influences. The results do not always relate to motility observed in vivo.

A balloon kymography technique, popularized by Bayliss and Starling [32], has been used for many years to record contractions of the circular muscle layer or intraluminal pressures. Balloons introduced in vitro or in vivo into the lumen of the gut segment to be studied are inflated and are connected to a pressure-sensing device or to a volume recorder. Changes in pressure or volume in the balloon can be recorded. Although it is much more direct and quantitative, there are several disadvantages of this technique; for example, the measurement obtained is that of intraballoon rather than intraluminal pressure, the balloon itself may stimulate motility, and the balloon, if too large, may evoke a reflex contraction. Even if the measurements go well, there may be difficulty establishing a relationship between the pressures measured and the activities of the gut muscle.

Open-tip catheters or catheter-tip transducers connected to strain-gauge transducers and recorders are more useful and reliable for measurement of intraluminal pressures. A disadvantage is that the recording from an open-tip catheter represents the activity at only one point in the lumen of the gut. A miniature balloon has been preferred for intraluminal measurements if bowel content is thick in order to prevent the blocking of catheter tips. The pressure recorded from the miniature balloon represents the mean pressure in any area of the gut [33]. There are difficulties in interpretation of the pressure changes obtained by these techniques because they record pressures only in whatever sealed cavity the catheters happen to lie. Moreover, the precise location of the tip of the catheter may not be clear.

Electrical Recording

Recently, with the improvement of electrical recorders, both myoelectrical [34,35] and mechanical [36,37], activities of the gut can be recorded. These techniques are currently the most accurate and sensitive for study of gut motility in experimental animals. Myoelectrical activities are recorded by either monopolar or bipolar electrodes implanted chronically on the serosal surface of the gut. Monopolar recording is used to record potential differences between an exploring electrode on the serosal surface of the gut and an indifferent electrode (on the leg, for example); bipolar recording is used to measure potential differences between adjacent electrodes. Bipolar recordings are preferred because artefacts produced by respiration or other motion are fewer.

Bellahsene et al [38] have recently developed an improved non-invasive method for recording and analyzing the electrical activity (electrogastrogram) of the human stomach obtained through transcutaneous recordings. The new method has a high signal-to-noise ratio and appears to be an attractive one in detecting gastric motor disturbances.

Mechanical activities may be recorded by means of strain-gauge transducers implanted chronically on the serosal surface of the gut [39]. The greatest advantage of this technique is that direct contractions of the gut wall may be recorded repeatedly in awake animals. Both electrodes and strain-gauge force transducers are small, so it is simple to implant several at one operation; they will allow for the simultaneous recording from multiple parts of the gut, without stimulation of mucosal receptors.

Insertion of Electrodes or Strain-Gauge Force Transducers

The gut is exposed by means of a midline laparotomy incision made with the animal under general anesthesia. Sterilized electrodes or strain-gauge transducers are secured with fine (5-0) monofilament sutures to the serosal surface of the gut. Strain-gauge force transducers are fixed in a circle in order to detect contraction of circular muscle. The lead wires exit from the abdominal cavity through a stab wound on the abdominal wall and are brought through a subcutaneous tunnel to exit between the scapulae. The wires are fixed to the skin with sutures, and the ends are soldered to an electrical connector, which is either fixed to the skin by sutures or placed in a pocket inside a canvas jacket. The protective jacket is placed on the dog to protect the external parts of the lead wires and connector from damage. The dogs are fasted for 3 days after surgery, and hydration is maintained by parenteral administration of Ringer's lactate solution (50 mL/kg/day). Recordings are performed by connecting the wires to a recorder.

INTRACEREBROVENTRICULAR AND CISTERNAL PUNCTURE

Masaki Fujimura, M.D., and
George H. Greeley, Jr., Ph.D.

Cannulation of the cerebral ventricles or the cisterna magna has been used for studies that involve the central neural action of regulatory agents, and for studies on the movement of these substances among cerebrospinal fluid, brain, and blood compartments. Two different techniques have been used: either a single cannula is inserted into one of the lateral ventricles or the cisterna magna for administration, or two cannulas are inserted simultaneously, one in a ventricle and one in the cisterna, for perfusion between the two [40–42]. Before cannulation is attempted, the investigator should be familiar with the stereotaxic coordinates of the experimental animal's brain [43–45].

We have often used dogs because of ease of cannulation, and we will describe the technique of cannulation. The dog is anesthetized with sodium pentobarbital (30 mg/kg, IV) and intubated with an inflatable endotracheal tube. The dog is then placed in a prone position with the head supported by a head holder or by an assistant, in such a manner that the calvarium is maintained in a horizontal plane. A midline scalp incision is begun at the external occipital protuberance and carried anteriorly for about 5 cm. The vault of the skull is exposed by incising the aponeurosis of the temporal muscle near its origin from the sagittal crest and by retracting the muscle to the side. A 2 mm drill hole is placed on a line connecting the two external auditory meati, 14 mm lateral to the median sagittal plane. The bone is opened with the drill at a right angle to the surface of the bone. This vertical plane through the skull facilitates tight fixation of chronic cannulas. Ashcroft et al [41] selected a point 0.8 mm lateral to the medial sagittal plane and 3.7 cm anterior to the external occipital protuberance and drilled the bone vertically. Fenstermacher [42] described placement of the hole 12 mm lateral to the midline and 5 mm posterior to the external auditory meatus. Regardless of which approach is chosen, it is important to remember that a constant landmark for entry into the lateral ventricle is a point situated midway on a line extending from the lateral canthus of the eye to the external occipital protuberance. After the drill penetrates the skull to the dura, it is removed and a 22-gauge spinal needle is inserted with gentle downward pressure for 15 mm below the surface of the skull. Every 1–2 mm, the stylet is removed and the lumen is observed for the presence of cerebrospinal fluid, which will slowly rise in the needle when the ventricle is entered. A slow flow without respiratory and pulse movements indicates communication with the subarachnoid space in a sulcus. In this case, the needle with the stylet must be pushed further inward. When the tip of the cannula is in the lateral ventricle, the flow will show respiratory and pulse fluctuations. The needle should then be attached to the head-holding device, or fixed directly to the skull with dental cement for acute studies.

A special cannula that can be tightly fixed to the skull is necessary for chronic studies [41,46,47]. Cannulation of the lateral ventricle can be done directly with the chronic cannula instead of a needle. We have used a standard procedure in order to avoid bleeding or damage to the brain caused by several trials with a chronic cannula (which is an 18-gauge needle). After puncture of the lateral ventricle with a 22-gauge spinal needle, the stylet of the needle is removed and a slender guide wire is inserted. The spinal needle is then removed, and the chronic cannula is inserted along the guide wire to the same depth as the needle puncture. A stainless steel plate is soldered around the cannula and is fixed directly to the skull with two screws, and the wound is closed. Penicillin (100,000 U, IM) is given daily for 3 days after surgery. Heparin (10,000 U/mL) solution is flushed through the cannula every few days to prevent formation of a membrane around the cannula tip. The dog can be used for experiments one week after surgery. Injections into the lateral ventricle should be performed aseptically, and after each experiment, antibiotics are given to prevent encephalitis.

Cannulation of the cisterna magna is performed with the dog similarly anesthetized. The head of the dog is held firmly by a head holder or an assistant at a right angle to the cervical spine. For an acute study, a 22-gauge spinal needle with stylet is inserted through the skin, at the point halfway between the occipital protuberance and the first cervical vertebra in the dorsal midline. The needle is directed perpendicularly to the spinal column, through the skin and musculature and into the atlantooccipital interspace. Then the needle is pushed strongly to penetrate the ligamentum flavum, under which the dura mater is found. The stylet of the needle is removed when the dura mater is penetrated, and a successful puncture is obvious when CSF flows up the shaft of the needle, pulsating with each heart beat. The head is slowly returned to the normal position, and the needle is fixed to the skin with skin sutures or to a head-holding device.

For chronic studies, a cannula that can be fixed tightly to the occipital bone is implanted surgically [41,48,49].

GASTRIC SECRETION IN THE RAT

Talaat Khalil, M.D.

Various methods have been devised for acute, semiacute, or chronic study of gastric acid secretion in rats. Studies may be performed with anesthetized or conscious rats; rats may be free to move about, or some restraint may be employed. (Unfortunately, we know of no comparative studies which examine the effects of these variables on acid secretion.) Regardless of whatever method is used, it is advisable to minimize the sources of variation that might affect gastric secretion in rats and to standardize the procedures. The most common techniques are described below. Any of the methods may be used to study stimulants or inhibitors of gastric secretion.

Shay Rat [50]

With the rat under light ether anesthesia, the abdomen is opened through a midline incision. The duodenum is identified and the junction between the pylorus and the duodenum is picked up gently with forceps. The stomach itself is not disturbed. A silk ligature is placed around the pylorus with care to avoid damage to blood vessels or excessive traction on the stomach. A no. 8 French catheter is then passed into the stomach from the mouth. The stomach is lavaged with 4 mL of saline, and the catheter is gradually withdrawn while suction is applied to recover any remaining fluid. The stomach is inspected to assure complete gastric emptying. (If the fluid cannot be withdrawn easily, or if the stomach contains food residue or feces, the animal is not used.) The abdominal wall is then closed. The animal is placed in its cage and receives nothing by mouth during the remainder of the experiment. Four hours later, the animal is again anesthetized with ether, the abdomen is opened, and a ligature placed at the esophagogastric junction. The stomach is removed, washed in saline, the greater curvature opened and the gastric juice drained into a graduated centrifuge tube through a funnel. The stomach is opened along the entire greater curvature, laid open, and the mucosa examined for ulcerations [50]. Ulcers are usually measured along their longest dimension, and the sum of these measurements (in mm) is the ulcer index for the rat.

Gastric Perfusion in Rats (Ghosh) [51]

We use a modification of the method of Ghosh and Schild [51]. A rat is anesthetized with sodium pentobarbital, a tracheostomy is performed, the abdomen is opened through a midline incision, and a polyethylene catheter is inserted through a duodenotomy into the stomach and doubly ligated in position; the proximal ligature is at the pylorus. A no. 6 French catheter is passed down the esophagus until the tip just reaches the rumen of the stomach. A ligature is placed around the esophagus in the neck. The stomach is mobilized by gentle traction on the rumen. Handling the glandular portion is avoided in order to prevent trauma to the secreting mucosa. The stomach is washed by a slow stream of tap water through the esophageal tube from a reservoir held 50 cm above the rat until the effluent is clear. The stomach is returned into the abdomen and a moistened sponge is placed against the rumen to keep it collapsed during the experiment. The stomach is perfused through the esophageal tube with 0.9 percent saline warmed to body temperature at a constant rate of 1 mL/min. The gastric effluent is collected in 10-minute samples and acid output is measured by titration with 0.01N NaOH (Figs 4-1 and 4-2).

Gastric Fistula in the Rat

This model was described first by Lane et al [52] in 1957. The abdomen is opened through a midline incision, and the stomach delivered through the incision to expose the rumen. An incision about 3 mm long is made 6 mm proximal to the junction of the rumen with the glandular stomach. The discoid end of the cannula is inserted and concentric purse string sutures are used to insure a leak-proof closure. The incision should be placed so that the disc in the stomach will be at its most dependent portion when gastric juice is being collected. The cannula is brought out through a small (3 mm) incision in the body wall about 1.5 cm to the left of the midline and 2 or 3 cm below the costal margin. Through the abdominal incision, a suture is passed through the peritoneal surface adjacent to the shaft of the cannula and then through the eye of the cannula and tied. This suture anchors the cannula to the inner abdominal wall.

When gastric secretion is to be collected, food is withdrawn and animals placed in Bollman cages at least 14 hours before study to avoid coprophagia. The animal is offered water ad libitum. Before starting the collection, the water is withdrawn. The plugs of the cannulas are removed and the stomach is washed with warm water and secretion is collected in test tubes.

GALLBLADDER FISTULAS

Tsuguo Sakamoto, M.D., Masaki Fujimura, M.D., and William H. Nealon, M.D.

In order to study the motor function of the gallbladder, pressure and motility recordings from gallbladder fistulas have been made in various laboratory animals, including the dog [53–63], cat [64,65], primate [66–69], and opossum [70]. Fried et al [61] from our laboratory have shown significant correlation between fat-stimulated elevations of plasma CCK concentrations and changes in the intraluminal pressure of the gallbladder in dogs with chronic gallbladder fistulas (see Fig 4-3).

A fasting dog weighing between 15 and 25 kg is anesthetized with IV sodium pentobarbital (Nembutal) (25 mg/kg). The abdomen is opened through an upper midline incision. The gallbladder volume is estimated by aspiration of bile through a fundic puncture. Then a silastic tube (I.D. 1.6 mm, O.D. 3.2 mm) is inserted 3 cm into the gallbladder through a small fundic cystostomy (Fig 6-9). The gallbladder catheter is secured in the fundus with a purse-string suture. The other end of the catheter is brought out from the abdomen through a small Thomas-type cannula where it is secured. The total length of the gallbladder catheter is approximately 30 cm, with ample length to avoid tension within the abdomen. The cystic duct is not ligated. A gastric fistula is also inserted so as to allow free drainage of acid gastric juice and thereby prevent release of endogenous secretin during experiments. An additional duodenal fistula or pancreatic fistula (Herrera type) may be placed to study the effect of luminal stimulants, such as fat and amino acids [61] and to correlate simultaneous gallbladder and pancreatic responses. After operation, the lumen of the gallbladder should be rinsed with sterile saline through the gallbladder catheter to remove any blood clots. The dog is given antibiotics for 4 days postoperatively and allowed to recover for at least 2 weeks. The gallbladder catheter should be sterile all the time. Periodic cleaning of the catheter, bacteriologic examinations of bile, and administration of antibiotics after each experiment are, we believe, helpful.

A pressure transducer (Statham P23Dc) is connected to the gallbladder catheter by means of a saline-filled polyethylene tube, and intragallbladder pressures are recorded on a polygraph (Grass or Beckman Instruments). The transducer is secured to the body of the dog with a jacket. The gallbladder is perfused constantly with isotonic saline at the rate of 1.0 mL/min by a Harvard infusion pump.

Experiments are begun after the gallbladder pressure has stabilized at a baseline. Test materials are given with an interval of at least 15 minutes between doses. This method of perfusion is suitable for comparison of multiple doses of test materials given by bolus injections or for short term infusion [63]. The contractile responses recorded by this method are easily reproducible on the same day, but they vary from day to day. If there is need for long term measurement of gallbladder

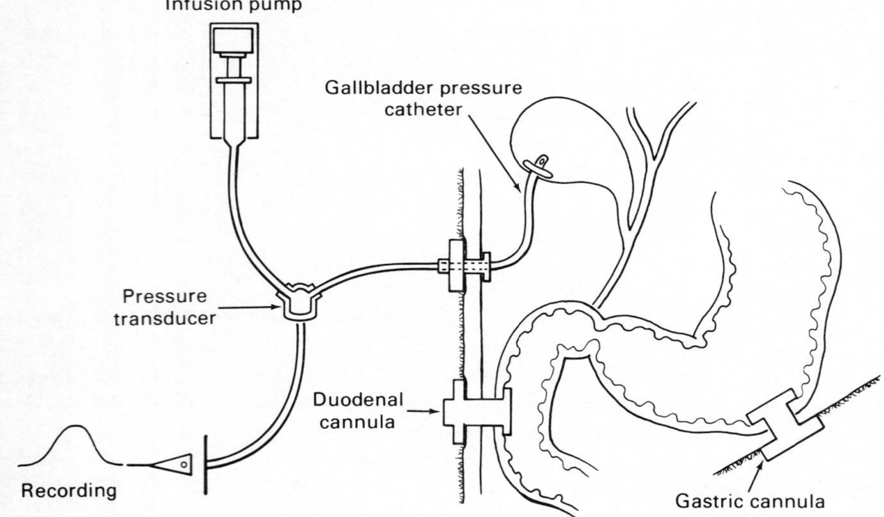

Figure 6-9. Infusion manometry system to measure the gallbladder pressure in dogs.

emptying or refilling (during either the postprandial state or the interdigestive state), the intraluminal pressure of the gallbladder is measured without perfusion [58,67]. When compared, contractile responses recorded with or without perfusion do not differ significantly after bolus injections, whereas results obtained by saline perfusion are higher than those of nonperfusion methods in response to continuous infusion of stimulants.

Changes in gallbladder volume can also be measured with this preparation. The gallbladder catheter is connected to the stopcock. Then gallbladder bile is aspirated slowly and completely by a syringe and then returned into the gallbladder slowly. Without giving stimulants, manipulation of withdrawal and refilling of bile does not affect the gallbladder volume, even though the volume is measured every 5 minutes (unpublished data).

Several variations of this method have been described. Ivy and Oldberg [53] originally created gallbladder fistulas with ligation of the cystic duct in an anesthetized dog. Vagne and Grossman [56] installed a Gregory-type metal cannula into the gallbladder and then ligated the cystic duct in a dog. The intragallbladder pressure was recorded in the conscious state. Jones et al [59] placed a balloon catheter into the gallbladder through a metal cannula which was secured in the fundus of the gallbladder. The cystic duct was left open and the balloon was connected to the transducer with a water-filled catheter. Williams and Huang [58] used a Teflon catheter (no. 7 F) to measure gallbladder pressure in conscious dogs. In conscious primates, O'Brien et al [66] observed gallbladder emptying by measuring intraduodenal appearance of radiolabeled insulin, which was injected into the gallbladder through the gallbladder catheter. Miranda et al [60] devised a gallbladder catheter with two side holes in the midpoint, which conducted pressure from the two separate points. This catheter was introduced through the fundus of the gallbladder into the duodenum. Measurements of pressure were accomplished by a slow pull-through during constant perfusion.

Schoetz et al [69] devised a double-catheter system in an anesthetized baboon. This system consisted of two separate catheters placed into the gallbladder. One of the catheters was connected to a pressure transducer and the other connected to the syringe, which cyclically infused or withdrew a present volume of bile at a constant rate. Thus, this system can record serial changes in the pressure-volume curve, and establish gallbladder compliance.

BILE SECRETION AND BILIARY MANOMETRY

Guillermo Gomez, M.D.

The first biliary fistula was reported by Schwann in 1844 [71] after he placed a catheter into the gallbladder. In 1923, Rous and McMaster [72] described a fistula of the common duct which has been used to study bile flow for many years with minor modifications. Their technique employs a double bile cannula that permits collection of bile from the proximal extrahepatic biliary tract and reinfusion of bile either directly into the duodenum or through the distal common duct. Cholestasis, infection, and catheter migration are frequent complications. Modifications in design with use of more inert materials have improved the long-term results of this preparation [73,74].

In order to obtain good results in chronic studies of bile secretion, the enterohepatic circulation and the integrity of the biliary tract must be preserved. These restrictions can be met in dogs by means of intermittent catheterization of the common bile duct through a duodenal cannula [27,75]. Comparison between chronic and intermittent catheterization of the biliary tract has revealed the advantages of the latter [76].

We have adopted intermittent catheterization in chronic studies of bile secretion in dogs. This method enables us to perform direct manometry of the sphincter of Oddi in conscious dogs. We reserve double cannulation of the common duct for acute experiments and the gallbladder fistula for measurements of gallbladder volume and pressure. (For the technique of gallbladder fistula for measurement of gallbladder pressure or volume, see the previous section of this chapter.)

Common Duct Fistula

These fistulas are used in studies of bile secretion (volume and composition) and of biliary tract pressure.

Acute Fistula

We [77] use a technique similar to the method described in anesthetized dogs by Wyatt in 1967 [55]. Under general anesthesia, laparotomy is performed and the common duct is dissected (Fig 6-10). The cystic duct is ligated, but the cystic artery is preserved. The pylorus is ligated and the stomach is drained through a Foley catheter. To collect hepatic bile, a plastic catheter is directed towards the liver through a small choledochotomy; a purse-string suture prevents bile leakage and prevents catheter displacement. For studies of sphincter of Oddi function, a side-hole plastic catheter is placed inside the distal common duct a few millimeters above the choledochal sphincter. A ligature that encircles the distal common bile duct fixes the catheter and isolates the sphincter from the remainder of the biliary tract. This system measures the resistance to flow that is produced by the sphincter. To measure duodenal motility, a second Foley catheter is introduced into the duodenum 5 cm distal to the sphincter of Oddi; the balloon filled with water reflects the duodenal pressure changes which are measured by a pressure transducer (Fig 6-10).

Chronic Fistulas

Laparotomy is performed with the dog under general anesthesia. The accessory pancreatic duct is ligated and a modified Thomas cannula is inserted into the duodenum and sutured in place opposite the papilla of Vater to allow its visualization [74]. A second Thomas cannula is placed in the most dependent portion of the stomach. Duodenal and gastric cannulas are exteriorized through right- and left-sided abdominal incisions, respectively. Cholecystectomy is usually performed. For studies, a strong beam of light is used to visualize the papilla through the duodenal cannula, and an olive-tipped (no. 6 French) ureteral catheter is inserted under direct vision and passed up the common duct. The catheter is secured in position by a rubber cork in the Thomas cannula. Bile is collected by gravity in graduated test tubes. This cork occludes the duodenal cannula and allows the placement of other catheters inside the duodenum for simultaneous luminal infusions or pressure measurements (Fig 6-11).

For studies of biliary and sphincter of Oddi pressure, we use a 16-gauge, 8-inch single lumen catheter in which an 0.8-mm lateral orifice is cut 15 mm from the sealed end. Up-downward displacement of the catheter allows sequential pressure measurement of duodenum, sphincter of Oddi and common duct, or vice versa.

Manometry System for Measurement of Gallbladder and Biliary Tract Pressure

Perfused pressure catheters (described above) are connected to wide-range pressure transducers (Statham series P23Dc), and the pressures are recorded on a polygraph (Grass or Beckman Instru-

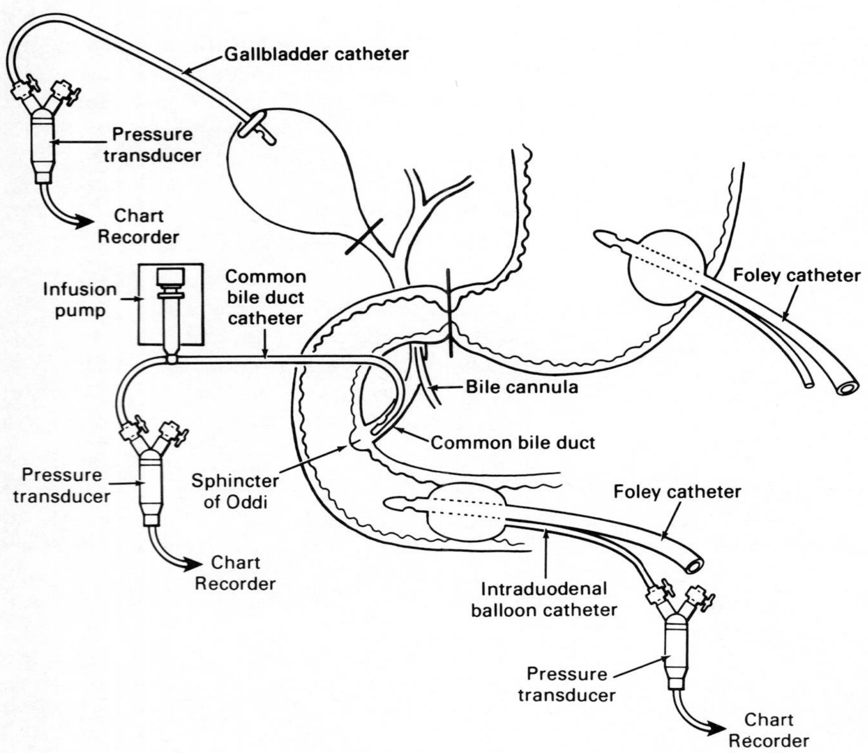

Figure 6-10. Acute preparation modified from Wyatt [55] for studies of sphincter of Oddi pressure in dogs.

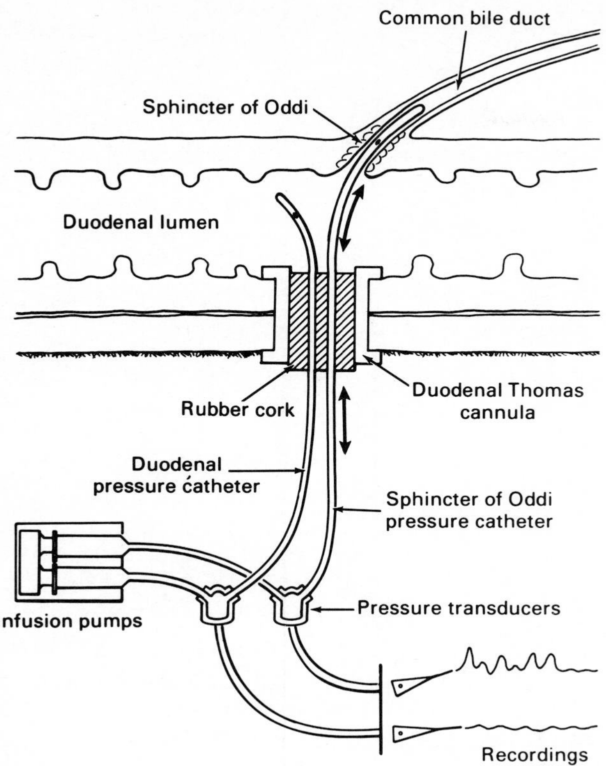

Figure 6-11. Infusion manometry system for biliary tract pressure measurement in conscious dogs. Duodenal pressure is simultaneously performed.

ments) that is calibrated before and at regular intervals during each experiment. Perfusion of the system is maintained by using a continuous syringe infusion pump (Harvard Apparatus Co.) at 0.7 to 1.25 mL/min flow rate of normal saline in order to obtain adequate sensitivity (a rise of at least 48 cmH_2O/sec when the catheter is occluded). Atmospheric and duodenal pressures are used as basal lines. Pressure values (peak, trough, height and frequency of waves) are read and calculated from the recording. Duodenal pressure is simultaneously recorded by means of a second catheter in order to identify the phase of the interdigestive migrating complex. This pressure is also determined by downward displacement of the main catheter and is subtracted in the calculations of sphincteric pressure [78] (Fig 6-12).

ISOLATED PERFUSED PANCREAS

William H. Nealon, M.D.

Exocrine pancreatic function can be studied readily in vitro by use of the isolated perfused pancreas. The technique may be applied to small animals, such as rabbits [79] or rats [80,81], as well as to larger animals, such as pigs [82] or dogs [83], and to humans [83a]. It is well suited for assessment of both exocrine and endocrine function.

In the rat, we use the modification of the method of Grodsky and Fanska [81], as described by Elahi et al. [80]. The pancreas is perfused through direct cannulation of the celiac and superior mesenteric arteries, and venous effluent is collected by cannulation of the portal vein. In addition, we perform a small duodenotomy on the antimesenteric surface opposite the entry of the pancreatic duct. We visualize the ampulla and pass a PE-50 polyethylene cannula into the duct. Ligation of the proximal common bile duct in the mesentery of the duodenum allows us to collect pure pancreatic secretion.

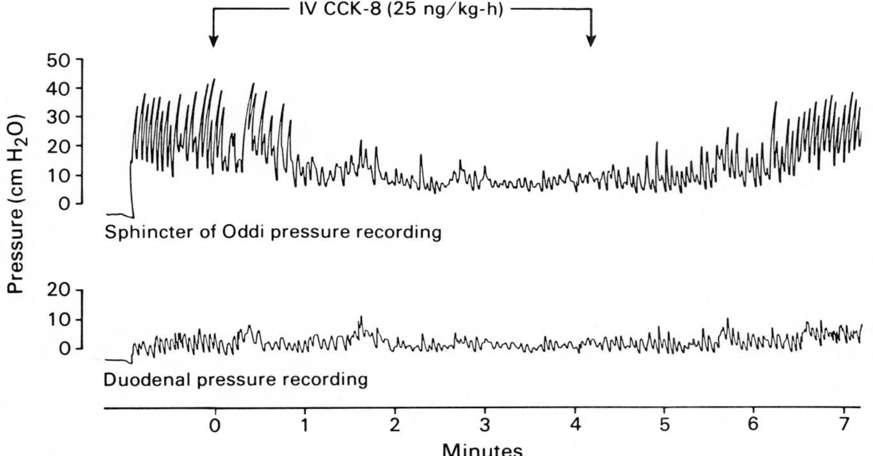

Figure 6-12. Relaxation of the sphincter of Oddi in conscious dogs induced by CCK-8 measured by means of perfused manometry technique. The intraduodenal pressure simultaneously registered is subtracted in the sphincteric pressure calculations. The first straight segment of both recordings corresponds to the atmospheric pressure.

Male Sprague-Dawley rats are anesthetized with ketamine and a wide T-shaped abdominal incision is performed. Peritoneal attachments between the pancreas and the colon, liver, diaphragm, and stomach are divided sharply. The pancreas is swept cephalad across the transverse mesocolon until the superior mesenteric vessels are visualized. The duodenum is divided after identifying and preserving the small branch from the superior mesenteric artery, which supplies the uncinate process. The stomach is mobilized and is used to manipulate the pancreas without direct trauma to the gland. The gastrohepatic ligament is incised and the left gastric vessels are identified, ligated, and divided. The esophagus and short gastric vessels are ligated and divided, and a splenectomy is performed. Using the mobilized stomach to facilitate manipulation of the pancreas, the peritoneum overlying the aorta is incised and all tissues are swept to the right. Finally, the plane between omental fat and pancreatic parenchyma is opened, and all vessels are ligated and divided from left to right up to the right gastroepiploic artery. The stomach is ligated and divided at the pylorus and discarded. Loop ties are placed around the proximal common bile duct, the portal vein, and the common hepatic artery in the porta hepatis, as well as around the celiac artery, the superior mesenteric artery, and the proximal and distal aorta.

Heparin (50 U/100 g body weight, 0.1 mL/100 g volume, using 500 U/mL solution) is administered through the inferior vena cava and ties are secured on the hepatic artery and the aorta. The aorta is divided at the proximal and distal ties and the posterior wall is incised longitudinally. Metal cannulas (22 gauge) are placed into the superior mesenteric and celiac arteries and tied and the perfusion pump is started at a rate of 1 cc/min and gradually advanced to 4 cc/min over the next 30 minutes. The antimesenteric border of the duodenum is incised and the ampulla of Vater is cannulated with PE-50 polyethylene tubing. The proximal common bile duct is ligated and divided. The portal vein is divided adjacent to the liver and a 19 gauge metal cannula is inserted so that the venous effluent is delivered into a fraction collector. All retroperitoneal attachments are divided and the gland is transported to a platform where weight of the preparation and temperature are monitored. An external heat lamp is used to avoid excess heat loss and paraffin is placed over the gland to retain hydration. All secretagogues may be administered via side arm in the perfusate delivery system. Perfusion pressure is monitored with a water manometer (Fig 6-13).

The perfusate is buffered Krebs-Ringer solution, containing 0.5 percent HSA and 4 percent T-40 dextran (Sigma), equilibrated against a mixture of O_2 (95 percent) and CO_2 (5 percent), with the pH adjusted to 7.4. The flow rate is adjusted to 4 mL/min and perfusion pressure to 60 cmH_2O. The preparation is allowed to equilibrate for 15 minutes before studies begin.

The portal vein effluent may be analyzed for glucose levels and for radioimmunoassay of the pancreatic hormones—insulin, glucagon, somatostatin, or pancreatic polypeptide. The pancreatic secretions may be assayed for bicarbonate and protein content.

The isolated perfused dog pancreas is prepared in much the same fashion, with the exception that the distal splenic artery may be used for placement of a pressure transducer catheter to facilitate perfusion pressure measurement. In each preparation, the duodenum may be removed surgically in order to eliminate this rich source of endogenous hormones.

PORTACAVAL TRANSPOSITION

Tsuguo Sakamoto, M.D.

This technique was developed and has been used to study hepatic metabolism and blood flow in conscious dogs [84,85]. The method can be extended by the use of additional surgical tech-

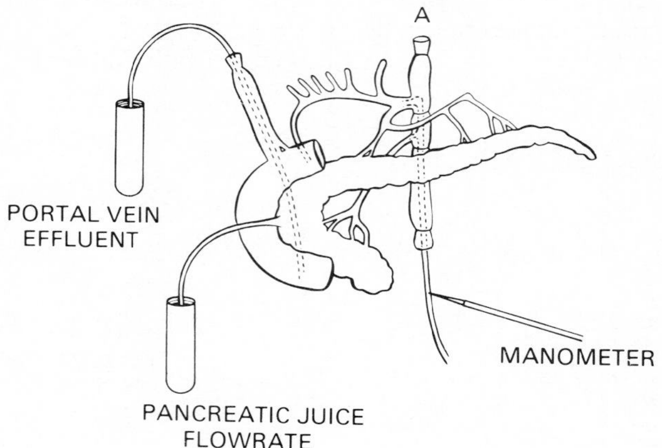

Figure 6-13. Perfusion of the pancreas, schematic representation. Perfusion is carried out through the catheter inserted into the ligated segments of both the celiac and superior mesenteric arteries at their origin in the aorta (A). Perfusion pressure is monitored with the manometer.

niques, such as gastric fistula, pancreatic fistula, and gallbladder fistula. Briefly, portacaval transposition is accomplished by mobilizing and dividing the inferior vena cava and the portal vein, and by anastomosing the proximal portal vein to the distal vena cava and the proximal vena cava to the distal portal vein. Thus, the liver is perfused with systemic venous blood and all portal venous blood flows directly into the systemic circulation. Administration of test materials into the intrahepatic portal venous system may thereby be accomplished by infusion into a hind leg vein, while administration of test agents into the systemic venous system is accomplished by infusion into a front leg vein (Fig 6-14).

After an overnight fast, the dog is anesthetized by intravenous injection of pentobarbital (25 mg/kg). The abdomen is opened through a midline incision. The inferior vena cava is dissected from the retroperitoneum. All tributaries into the vena cava between the confluence of the iliac veins and the liver, including the right adrenal vein and the lumbar veins, are divided and ligated. The entire portal vein is mobilized from its origin at the junction of the superior mesenteric and splenic veins to its bifurcation at the liver. All tributaries of the portal vein distal to its origin are divided and ligated. Next, the optimal point of division of the vena cava and the portal vein is chosen in order to avoid tension and twisting of the anastomosis. The

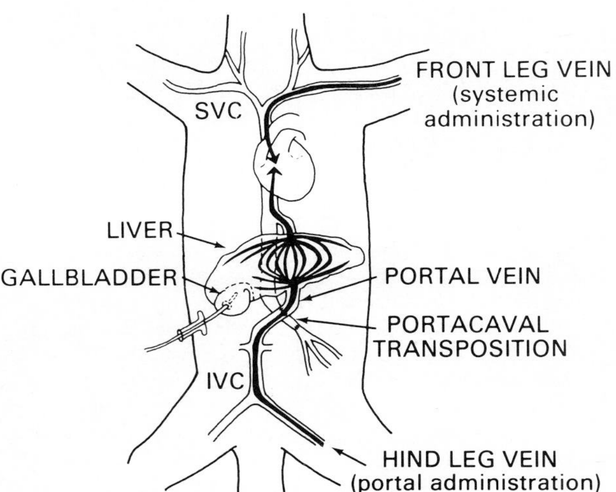

Figure 6-14. Diagram of operative preparation in dogs. Not shown are the modified Herrera pancreatic fistula (Herrera et al [9]) and the gastric fistula. IVC and SVC = superior and inferior vena cava, respectively. (From Sakamoto et al [63], by permission of The Rockefeller University Press.)

portal vein and the suprarenal inferior vena cava are each divided between vascular clamps. In order to minimize the period of mesenteric venous obstruction, the distal portal vein is first anastomosed end-to-end to the proximal vena cava. The distal vena cava is anastomosed end-to-end to the proximal portal vein. Both anastomoses are performed using two continuous sutures of 5-0 monofilament (Fig 6-14) [63]. We have not used hypothermia (as described by Starzl et al [85]) and we have not occluded the superior mesenteric artery (as described by Child et al [84]). The duration of the postoperative fast depends upon the experiments planned. If we construct a Herrera pouch, the dogs are not given food until the fourth postoperative day. If a gastric fistula is constructed, food is withheld for only one day. Until food intake is resumed, dogs receive parenteral fluids by clysis.

The dogs are usually not studied until one month postoperatively. We have performed indocyanine green clearance studies 3 months after portacaval transposition. Hepatic clearance of indocyanine green was significantly higher in comparison to normal controls [63]; this indicates that portacaval transposition does not impair hepatic function.

In this model, some of the substances that are infused into the hind leg vein may escape into the systemic circulation through collateral pelvic vessels. For example, we have observed that gastric acid output in response to pentagastrin (5 μg/kg/hr, which is supposed to be eliminated almost completely by the liver), given via the hind leg vein is reduced to 15 percent of acid secreted when pentagastrin is given via the front leg veins. This suggests a clearance of 85 percent, which is somewhat less than that reported after direct portal injection [86,87]. Systemic escape appears to increase with time.

REFERENCES

1. Konturek SJ, Rayford PL, Thompson JC: Effect of pH of gastric and intestinal meals on gastric acid and plasma gastrin and secretin responses in the dog. Am J Physiol 233:E537, 1977.
2. Thomas JE: A simplified procedure for preparing an improved Pavlov pouch. Proc Soc Exp Biol Med 50:58, 1942.
3. Gregory RA: Gastric secretory responses after portal venous ligation. J Physiol 144:123, 1958.
4. Thomas JE: Symposium: Exocrine pancreatic function. Methods for collecting pancreatic juice. Gastroenterology 36:362, 1959.
5. Sircus W: The effect of corticotrophin and corticosteroids on the external secretion of the pancreas in dogs. Gut 2:338, 1961.

6. Archambeau J, Greenlee H, Harper P: A modified total pancreatic fistula. Proc Soc Exp Biol Med 107:986, 1961.
7. Woods LP, Foster JH: Chronic pancreatic fistula—a new experimental technique. J Surg Res 3:9, 1963.
8. Preshaw RM, Grossman MI: Stimulation of pancreatic secretion by extracts of the pyloric gland area of the stomach. Gastroenterology 48:36, 1965.
9. Herrera F, Kemp DR, Tsukamoto M, et al: A new cannula for the study of pancreatic function. J Appl Physiol 25:207, 1968.
10. Thompson JC, Tramontana JA, Lerner HJ, et al: Physiologic scope of the antral inhibitory hormone. Ann Surg 156:550, 1962.
11. Peskin GW, Thompson JC: The gastric antrum. Am J Med Sci 239:231, 1960.
12. Thompson JC, Daves IA, Davidson WD, et al: Studies on the humoral control of gastric secretion in dogs with autogenous and homotransplanted antral and fundic pouches. Surgery 58:84, 1965.
13. Charters AC, Odell WD, Davidson WD, et al: Gastrin: Immunochemical properties and measurement by radioimmunoassay. Surgery 66:104, 1969.
14. Parsons DS: Methods for investigation of intestinal absorption, in Code CF (ed): *Handbook of Physiology. Sect. 6: Alimentary Canal. Vol. III. Intestinal Absorption.* Washington, D.C., American Physiological Society, 1968, pp 1177–1216.
15. Thiry L: Uber eine neue Methode, den Dunndarm zu isolieren. Sitzber Akad Wiss Wein Math-Naturw Kl I 50:77, 1864.
16. Vella L: Nuovo methodo per avere il succo enterico puro e stabilirne le proprieta fisiologiche. Med Acad Sci Inst Bologna, Ser 4, 2, Fasc. 3e:515, 1880.
17. Vella L: Neues verfahren zur gewinnung reinen darmsaftes und feststellung seiner physiologischen eigenschaften. Moleshott's Untersuch Naturl Mensch Thiere 13:40, 1888.
18. Berger EY, Kanzaki G, Homer MA, et al: Simultaneous flux of sodium into and out of the dog intestine. Am J Physiol 196:74, 1959.
19. Fordtran JS: Segmental perfusion techniques. Gastroenterology 56:987, 1969.
20. Clain JE, Go VLW, Malagelada J-R: Inhibitory role of the distal small intestine on the gastric secretory response to meals in man. Gastroenterology 74:704, 1978.
21. Fordtran JS, Levitan R, Bikerman V, et al: The kinetics of water absorption in the human intestine. Trans Assoc Am Physicians 74:195, 1961.
22. Whalen GE, Harris JA, Geenen JE, et al: Sodium and water absorption from the human small intestine. The accuracy of the perfusion method. Gastroenterology 51:975, 1966.
23. Schmitt MG Jr, Wood CM, Soergel KH: A method for rapid placing of small intestinal perfusion tubes. Gut 15:227, 1974.
24. Jacobson ED, Bondy DC, Broitman SA, et al: Validity of polyethylene glycol in estimating intestinal water volume. Gastroenterology 44:761, 1963.
25. Isenberg JI, Ippoliti AF, Maxwell VL: Perfusion of the proximal small intestine with peptone stimulates gastric acid secretion in man. Gastroenterology 73:746, 1977.
26. Preshaw RM, Cooke AR, Grossman MI: Quantitative aspects of response of canine pancreas to duodenal acidification. Am J Physiol 210:629, 1966.
27. Thomas JE: An improved cannula for gastric and intestinal fistulas. Proc Soc Exp Biol Med 46:260, 1941.
28. Meyer JH, Way LW, Grossman MI: Pancreatic bicarbonate response to various acids in duodenum of the dog. Am J Physiol 219:964, 1970.
29. Meyer JH, Kelly GA, Spingola LJ, et al: Canine gut receptors mediating pancreatic responses to luminal L-amino acids. Am J Physiol 231:669, 1976.
30. Barbezat GO: Triple-lumen perfusion of the canine jejunum. Gastroenterology 79:1243, 1980.
31. Cannon WB: The movements of the intestines studied by means of the rontgen rays. Am J Physiol 6:251, 1902.
32. Bayliss WM, Starling EH: The movements and innervation of the small intestine. J Physiol 24:99, 1899.
33. Connell AM: Methodology of investigations of alimentary motility, in Demling L, Ottenjann R (eds): *Gastrointestinal Motility. International Symposium on Motility of the G-I Tract.* Stuttgart, Georg Thieme Verlag, 1971, p 1.
34. Alvarez WC, Mahoney LJ: Action currents in stomach and intestine. Am J Physiol 58:476, 1922.
35. McCoy EJ, Bass P: Chronic electrical activity of gastroduodenal area: Effects of food and certain catecholamines. Am J Physiol 205:439, 1963.
36. Jacoby HI, Bass P, Bennett DR: In vivo extraluminal contractile force transducer for gastrointestinal muscle. J Appl Physiol 18:658, 1963.
37. Itoh Z, Takeuchi S, Aizawa I, et al: Characteristic motor activity of the gastrointestinal tract in fasted conscious dogs measured by implanted force transducers. Am J Dig Dis 23:229, 1978.
38. Bellahsene BE, Hamilton JW, Webster JG, et al: An improved method for recording and analyzing the electrical activity of the human stomach. IEEE Trans Biomed Engineering BME-32:911, 1985.
39. Bass P, Wiley JN: Contractile force transducer for recording muscle activity in unanesthetized animals. J Appl Physiol 32:567, 1972.
40. Bhawe WB: Experiments on the fate of histamine and acetylcholine after their injection into the cerebral ventricles. J Physiol 140:169, 1958.
41. Ashcroft GW, Dow RC, Moir ATB: The active transport of 5-hydroxyindol-3-ylacetic acid and 3-methoxy-4-hydroxyphenyl-acetic acid from a recirculatory perfusion system of the cerebral ventricles of the unanaesthetized dog. J Physiol 199:397, 1968.
42. Fenstermacher JD: Ventriculocisternal perfusion as a technique for studying transport and metabolism within the brain, in Marks N, Rodnight R (eds): *Research Methods in Neurochemistry.* New York, Plenum Press, 1972, pp 165–178.

43. Lim RKS, Liu C-N, Moffitt RL: *A Stereotaxic Atlas of the Dog's Brain.* Springfield, IL, Charles C Thomas, 1960.
44. Dua-Sharma S, Sharma KN, Jacobs HL: *The Canine Brain in Stereotaxic Coordinates.* Cambridge, The Massachusetts Institute of Technology, 1970.
45. Pellegrino LJ, Pellegrino AS, Cushman AJ: *A Stereotaxic Atlas of the Rat Brain.* New York, Plenum Press, 1979.
46. Haley TJ, Dickinson RW: A note on an indwelling cannula for intraventricular injection of drugs in the unanesthetized dog. J Am Pharmacol Assoc 45:432, 1956.
47. Myers RD: Blood-brain barrier: Techniques for the intracerebral administration of drugs, in Iversen LL, Iversen SD, Snyder SH (eds): *Handbook of Psychopharmacology.* New York, Plenum Press, 1975, pp 1–28.
48. Pappenheimer JR, Heisey SR, Jordan EF, et al: Perfusion of the cerebral ventricular system in unanesthetized goats. Am J Physiol 203:763, 1962.
49. Feldberg W, Myers RD, Veale WL: Perfusion from cerebral ventricle to cisterna magna in the unanaesthetized cat. Effect of calcium on body temperature. J Physiol 207:403, 1970.
50. Shay H, Sun DCH, Gruenstein M: A quantitative method for measuring spontaneous gastric secretion in the rat. Gastroenterology 26:906, 1954.
51. Ghosh MN, Schild HO: Continuous recording of acid gastric secretion in the rat. Br J Pharmacol 13:54, 1958.
52. Lane A, Ivy AC, Ivy EK: Response of the chronic gastric fistula rat to histamine. Am J Physiol 190:221, 1957.
53. Ivy AC, Oldberg E: A hormone mechanism for gallbladder contraction and evacuation. Am J Physiol 86:599, 1928.
54. Ivy AC, Janecek HM: Assay of Jorpes-Mutt secretin and cholecystokinin. Acta Physiol Scand 45:220, 1959.
55. Watt AP: The relationship of the sphincter of Oddi to the stomach, duodenum and gall-bladder. J Physiol 193:225, 1967.
56. Vagne M, Grossman MI: Cholecystokinetic potency of gastrointestinal hormones and related peptides. Am J Physiol 215:881, 1968.
57. Williams RD, Huang TT: New technique for experimental, repeated, long-term measurement of biliary pressure. Surgery 65:454, 1969.
58. Williams RD, Huang TT: The effect of vagotomy on biliary pressure. Surgery 66:353, 1969.
59. Jones DT, Isaza J, Woodward ER: A new method for long-term measurement of gallbladder contraction in the conscious dog. J Surg Res 11:187, 1971.
60. Miranda M, Espinoza M, Csendes A: Manometric characteristics of the extrahepatic biliary tract in dogs. Dig Dis Sci 26:417, 1981.
61. Fried GM, Ogden WD, Swierczek J, et al: Release of cholecystokinin in conscious dogs: Correlation with simultaneous measurements of gallbladder pressure and pancreatic protein secretion. Gastroenterology 85:1113, 1983.
62. Traynor OJ, Dozois RR, DiMagno EP: Canine interdigestive and postprandial gallbladder motility and emptying. Am J Physiol 246:G426, 1984.
63. Sakamoto T, Fujimura M, Newman J, et al: Comparison of hepatic elimination of different forms of cholecystokinin in dogs. Bioassay and radioimmunoassay comparisons of cholecystokinin-8-sulfate and -33-sulfate. J Clin Invest 75:280, 1985.
64. Jansson R, Svanvik J: Effects of intravenous secretin and cholecystokinin on gallbladder net water absorption and motility in the cat. Gastroenterology 72:639, 1977.
65. Behar J, Biancani P: Effect of cholecystokinin and the octapeptide of cholecystokinin on the feline sphincter of Oddi and gallbladder. J Clin Invest 66:1231, 1980.
66. O'Brien JJ, Shaffer EA, Williams LF Jr, et al: A physiological model to study gallbladder function in primates. Gastroenterology 67:119, 1974.
67. LaMorte WW, Gaca JM, Wise WE, et al: Choledochal sphincter relaxation in response to histamine in the primate. J Surg Res 28:373, 1980.
68. Schoetz DJ Jr, LaMorte WW, Wise WE, et al: Mechanical properties of primate gallbladder: Description by a dynamic method. Am J Physiol 241:G376, 1981.
69. Schoetz DJ Jr, Wise WE Jr, LaMorte WW, et al: Histamine receptors in primate gallbladder. Dig Dis Sci 28:353, 1983.
70. Ryan J, Cohen S: Gallbladder pressure-volume response to gastrointestinal hormones. Am J Physiol 230:1461, 1976.
71. Schwann T: Versuche, um auszumitteln, ob die Galle im Organismus eine fur das Leben wesentliche Rolle spielt. Arch Anat Physiol Wissensch Med, p 127, 1844.
72. Rous P, McMaster PD: A method for the permanent sterile drainage of intraabdominal ducts, as applied to the common duct. J Exp Med 37:11, 1923.
73. Jonson G: Permanent biliary fistulas in the dog. A new method. Acta Chir Scand Suppl 316:1, 1963.
74. Madrid JA, Salido GM, Mañas M, et al: Use of a bidirectional cannula to study biliary secretion in conscious dogs. Lab Anim 17:307, 1983.
75. Snape WJ, Thomas JE: A simple method for the study of biliary tract function in unanesthetized dogs. Fed Proc 4:66, 1945.
76. Snape WJ, Wirts CW, Cantarow A: Comparison of two types of permanent external bile-fistula dogs for studying liver function. Proc Soc Exp Biol Med 66:468, 1947.
77. Lonovics J, Fujimura M, Lluis F, et al: Cholecystokinin-induced relaxation of the sphincter of Oddi may partially be mediated by substance P. Gastroenterology 88:1480, 1985.
78. Carr-Locke DL, Gregg JA: Endoscopic manometry of pancreatic and biliary sphincter zones in man. Basal results in healthy volunteers. Dig Dis Sci 26:7, 1981.

79. Saito T: A technique for the perfusion of the isolated rabbit pancreas. Jpn J Pharmacol 34:43, 1984.
80. Elahi D, Muller DC, Andersen DK, et al: The effect of age and glucose concentration on insulin secretion by the isolated perfused rat pancreas. Endocrinology 116:11, 1985.
81. Grodsky GM, Fanska RE: The in vitro perfused pancreas. Methods Enzymol 39:364, 1975.
82. Lindkaer Jensen S, Kuhl C, Vagn Nielsen O, et al: Isolation and perfusion of the porcine pancreas. Scand J Gastroent Suppl 37:57, 1976.
83. Roy MW, Lee KC, Jones MS, et al: Neural control of pancreatic insulin and somatostatin secretion. Endocrinology 115:770, 1984.
83a. Brunicardi FC, Sun YS, Druck P, et al: Splanchnic neural regulation of glucagon release in the isolated perfused human pancreas. Am J Surg, in press.
84. Child CG III, Barr D, Holswade GR, et al: Liver regeneration following portacaval transposition in dogs. Ann Surg 138:600, 1953.
85. Starzl TE, Lazarus RE, Schlachter L, et al: A multiple catheter technique for studies of hepatic metabolism and blood flow in dogs with portacaval transposition. Surgery 52:654, 1962.
86. Thompson JC, Reeder DD, Davidson WD, et al: Effect of hepatic transit of gastrin, pentagastrin, and histamine measured by gastric secretion and by assay of hepatic vein blood. Ann Surg 170:493, 1969.
87. Strunz UT, Thompson MR, Elashoff J, et al: Hepatic inactivation of gastrins of various chain lengths in dogs. Gastroenterology 74:550, 1978.

Section Three

Models for Study

Chapter 7

Receptors for Gastrin and Cholecystokinin

Pomila Singh, Ph.D., and James C. Thompson, M.D.

Hormones initiate their effects by interacting with receptors on or within target cells; this interaction is followed by a chain of cellular events, culminating in a biologic response that is specific for the hormone. Gastrointestinal peptide hormones have been shown to interact with receptors on cell membranes [1–5]. The mechanism of action of the hormone involves high-affinity, low-capacity receptors, specific to the hormone on the target cell membranes, and a second intracellular messenger of action. These second messengers, such as calcium or the cyclic nucleotides, are triggered by the interaction of hormone and receptor, which in turn triggers other cellular events that result in measurable biologic effects. Thus, besides the concentration of the circulating hormone, other factors important to the biologic effectiveness of the hormone are 1) the actual concentration of the hormone available for binding at the target cell; 2) population of receptors available for binding at the cellular membrane; and 3) the availability of second messengers.

The study of membrane receptors for gut peptide hormones and of the physiologic effects of these hormones has become an important part of current research on gastrointestinal hormones. We should ask whether syndromes of gut dysfunction may be related to abnormalities of gut hormone receptors.

GASTRIN RECEPTORS

Studies in the mid-1970s indicated the presence of gastrin receptors (GR) on the plasma membrane of rat antral smooth muscle and rat fundic mucosa, but the binding of gastrin (G-17-I) was not correlated with any biologic end point. Extensive studies have since been carried out on the characterization of GR in different parts of the gastrointestinal tract, and certain biologic effects of gastrin have now been correlated with either the population or the presence or absence of specific gastrin-binding sites (receptors) on the plasma membranes of specific cell populations of the tissues.

Physicochemical Characterization

Using ^{125}I-labeled native gastrin I, specific GR in the crude membrane fraction (250–20,000 g) of rat oxyntic gland membranes were first described by Brown and Gallagher [6]. Since then, others have described specific, high-affinity, gastrin-binding sites (gastrin receptors) in mucosa from stomach, duodenum, and colon of rats [1,7], dogs [2,8,9], and rabbits [10] by using radiolabeled analogues of MG as the ligand in their binding studies. The radiolabeled analogues that have been used include 15-leucine synthetic human gastrin 17-I (LG) [1,7–9] and 11-norleucine synthetic human gastrin 13-I (NorLG) [10], in which Met in position 15 of the hormone has been replaced by Leu or Norleu. Since Met in the native hormone is sensitive to oxidation during iodination with chloramine T, these analogues of MG have been used preferentially in estimating GR [7,10].

Milder forms of iodination procedures, which do not substantially alter the biologic activity of polypeptide hormones, have become available recently, and we have examined several of these methods for iodination of both MG and LG. We have successfully iodinated the native gastrin molecule itself (with almost complete retention of biologic and receptor binding activity) by two methods, Iodo-Gen and EnzymoBead [11]. We have compared MG and LG for their ability to estimate the number of specific binding sites and observed no significant difference between the two compounds according to this criterion.

Using 15-Leu gastrin 17-I [1,7] or MG [11], a single class of specific, high-affinity binding sites (K_d, 0.3–0.4 nM) with a low capacity of approximately 4 fmol/mg crude membrane protein in the rat oxyntic gland (fundic) mucosa and duodenal mucosa (Table 7-1), and more than 40 fmol/mg purified plasma membrane from rat fundic mucosa has been described [11]. High-affinity binding sites for gastrin have also been described on isolated rabbit gastric mucosal cells [12] and canine parietal and nonparietal cells [2,8,9]. The receptors are protein in nature and hence denatured at higher temperatures [7]. In a recent study, the kinetics of binding of gastrin to gastrin receptors in crude membranes of oxyntic gland mucosa of rats was studied in some detail. The association rate constant (K_{+1}) of the binding was estimated to be $2 \times 10^6\ M^{-1}\ S^{-1}$ and the dissociation rate constant (K_{-1}) was estimated to be $1 \times 10^3\ S^{-1}$ [12].

The GR appear to have the highest affinity for gastrin 17-I, followed by cholecystokinin (CCK) > caerulein > pentagastrin [1,7,11]. These peptides display similarity in their COOH-terminal peptide chains, which explains the competitive inhibition afforded by each for binding to the gastrin receptors. Secretin, on the other hand, has been shown to demonstrate a noncompetitive inhibition to the binding of 15-Leu-G to GR [1].

It has been further shown that gastrin autoregulates the level of its own receptors [13]; the receptors are proportional to serum gastrin in a manner similar to that observed with estrogen regulation of the estrogen receptors. Thus, feeding the rat or performing a vagotomy results in increased gastrin levels, followed by increasing gastrin receptor levels, while the opposite results from fasting or feeding a liquid diet or after antrectomy [13]. This autoregulation explains the appearance of GR in the oxyntic gland mucosa of rats around the time and age (day 25) of weaning when a solid diet is introduced for the first time with the appearance of normal gastrin levels in the antrum [14]. Antral mucosa, liver, spleen, and kidneys do not contain gastrin receptors [1]. The autoregulation of GR in the rat gastric mucosa by gastrin has been shown to involve an initial down-regulation of GR on injection of gastrin 17, which is then restored to control levels within 3 hours. Therefore, the half-life of gastrin receptors appears to be approximately 3 hours. This is then followed by an up-regulation of the concentration of GR, which is cyclohexamide sensitive, indicating the involvement of a protein synthesis step in the further synthesis of GR under the influence of gastrin [15].

An interesting observation is that before the age of 40 days in the rat, corticosteroids appear to enhance GR levels on the gastric mucosa, by an

Table 7-1. **Gastrin receptors (GR) on crude membranes of gastrointestinal mucosa from rats**

Gastrointestinal mucosal tissue	*GR* (fmol/mg protein)*
Antrum	0.0 ± 0.0
Fundus	4.3 ± 0.8†
Proximal duodenum	0.0 ± 0.0
Distal duodenum	1.2 ± 0.4
Colorectal	3.9 ± 1.1

* GR was estimated from a Scatchard plot of MSA binding data using MG, iodinated by Iodo-Gen, as the radiolabeled ligand in the assay.
† Figures represent mean ± SEM values observed in three to five separate experiments.
(From Singh et al [11], by permission of The American Physiological Society.)

indirect or direct pathway, as yet unknown; however, after 40 days it has no effect [16,17]. There also is a slight sex difference in the GR population expressed per milligram crude membrane protein, which is lower in the 60-day-old female rat (2.5 fmol) than in the same age male rat (4.0 fmol). Before the age of 40 days, however, there is no sex difference in the GR population [18]. The lower GR levels in adult female rats appear to be due to lower serum gastrin levels, which can be increased by ovariectomy and further increased by ovariectomy plus adrenalectomy to resemble levels in adult male rats. This then up-regulates the GR population in the surgically operated female rats to male levels [18].

Trophic Effects of Gastrin in Relation to Gastrin Receptor Levels

The trophic effect of gastrin on gastric mucosa has been shown in a number of studies [19,20, inter alia]. Some of the direct trophic responses that have been recorded in male Sprague-Dawley rats include stimulation of mucosal hyperplasia of the oxyntic gland, mitosis, DNA, protein and RNA synthesis in vivo and in vitro, maintenance of epithelial cell lines by gastrin, and decrease in doubling time of the cells [19]. The stimulation of nucleic acid and protein synthesis by gastrin appears to require an intact pathway for polyamine synthesis, at least in the oxyntic gland and duodenum, since difluoromethylornithine (an irreversible inhibitor of ornithine decarboxylase) inhibits the trophic response to pentagastrin in the stomach and duodenum but not in the colon [21]. In dogs with Heidenhain pouch gastric fistulas, direct infusion of G-17-II at a D_{50} dose for acid secretion (160 μg/kg BW) for 4 hours significantly enhanced DNA synthesis by 500 percent in the pouch and 100 percent in the main stomach [19]. Indirect evidence for the involvement of gastrin and the trophic effects on gastric mucosa include parietal cell hyperplasia in patients with the Zollinger-Ellison (gastrinoma) syndrome in whom serum gastrin levels are greatly increased, and gastric mucosal atrophy after antrectomy in humans as a possible result of loss of circulating gastrin [19].

The effectiveness of different forms of gastrin in stimulating DNA synthesis and increasing total DNA content of gastric mucosa appears to be similar for the naturally occurring hormone, G-17-I, G-17-II, and G-34-II on a molar basis, while the synthetic pentagastrin is reportedly less potent [20]. Pentagastrin was observed to exert trophic effects on oxyntic gland mucosa, duodenum, and colon, but it had no effect on the esophagus, antrum, or diaphragm.

The possibility that the trophic effects of gastrin are mediated via the interaction of gastrin with its receptors was only recently shown in studies in which pentagastrin, given to young, 10-day-old rats, was ineffective in stimulating gastric mucosal DNA synthesis, possibly because of the absence of gastrin receptors in these rats. Pentagastrin, however, was very effective in inducing DNA synthesis in stomachs of 28-day-old rats, which contain the full adult complement of gastrin receptors [22].

Studies from our laboratory further demonstrated the presence of specific, high affinity (K_d, 0.5 nM) gastrin receptors in a mouse colon cancer cell line (MC-26) [23]. We have demonstrated that the growth rate in vivo of MC-26 cells is significantly increased in the presence of pentagastrin [24,25] and that there is a strong possibility that the trophic effect is mediated by gastrin receptors, which have been shown by us to be very sensitive to the circulating levels of pentagastrin [26,27]. We have also recently shown the inhibition of in vivo growth of MC-26 cells by proglumide [28], a specific receptor antagonist for gastrin and CCK [29]. On the other hand, tetragastrin was not found to have any promoting effect on chemically induced colonic tumors in Wistar rats [30], which could be due to the known reduced half-life of tetragastrin versus pentagastrin and the 1,000-fold smaller biologic activity of tetragastrin compared to gastrin (unpublished data from our laboratory). There is, thus, enough evidence to indicate that gastrin may indeed be trophic for both normal and cancerous gastrointestinal cells. This possibility derives further support from our finding of high-affinity gastrin receptors on a number of other gastrointestinal cancer cell lines [11] and in human cancers in vivo [31]. Of the 12 different gastrointestinal cancer cell lines we have screened for the presence of GR, we have so far identified one human stomach cancer cell line (AgS), as well as four of the seven different clones derived from this cell line, one human colon cancer cell line (LoVo), and one mouse colon cancer cell line (MC-26) to be highly positive. A human pancreatic (H2T) and a duodenal (HUTU) cancer cell line have also been observed to be slightly positive for GR. The affinity of these gastrin-binding sites for the cancer cell lines, interestingly, appears to be similar to that observed for normal cells from the fundic mucosa of rats.

At least one clone (AgS-12) of the seven AgS clones tested was negative for the presence of specific gastrin-binding sites, whereas the others were in various stages of retention of the gastrin receptors. Studies with estradiol receptors in human breast cancer tissues have shown that malignant mammary cells are similar in various stages of estradiol receptor loss, which greatly influences the responsiveness of the tumors to endocrine manipulation [32]. At present we are investigating the possibilities that gastrin is trophic for all the AgS clones to the same extent or that its action is dependent upon the absolute level of gastrin receptors present on the cell lines.

Besides gastrin, there are other factors and hormones that may be involved in the growth of the gastric mucosa. Glucagon may be one such hormone, since it was found to stimulate DNA synthesis in both the colon and oxyntic gland mucosa, though only to 40 percent of that caused by pentagastrin [33]. It remains to be seen whether the effect of glucagon is direct or is mediated in some way via gastrin receptors. Enteroglucagon is also a strong candidate as a gut growth hormone. Vasoactive intestinal peptide (VIP) did not stimulate DNA synthesis on its own but inhibited the effect of pentagastrin, an effect that is probably indirect, since VIP has not been shown to inhibit the binding of gastrin to gastrin receptors [7]. Another interesting feature reported is that gastrin infused directly into the intestinal lumen of rats is effective in stimulating intestinal mucosal growth, without any circulation of gastrin. However, contrary to this, luminal and topical effects in the intestine and growth in the oxyntic gland and duodenal mucosa require the endocrine presence of gastrin [34]. Thus, these studies indicate that cells facing the lumen in the intestine are probably responsive to gastrin, whereas responsive cells in the oxyntic gland and duodenum are at a deeper location.

Epidermal growth factor (EGF) is yet another substance that has been shown to significantly increase DNA synthesis, RNA, and protein content of oxyntic gland mucosa in male rats when administered chronically over 5 days. It also potentiates the trophic effect of pentagastrin when administered acutely, although it is ineffective by itself as an acute dose [35]. The effect appears to be specific to gastric mucosa, since neither EGF nor pentagastrin altered skin growth [35]. The mechanism of potentiation of the trophic effects of pentagastrin by EGF, however, is intriguing, since secretin, which has been shown to noncompetitively inhibit binding of pentagastrin to gastrin receptors, also inhibits the trophic effects of pentagastrin alone but not those of pentagastrin plus EGF. This indicates a mechanistic route, bypassing binding to gastrin receptors in the latter case, possibly a post receptor event. This appears even more likely based on the finding that while EGF potentiates the trophic effect of pentagastrin, it inhibits gastric acid secretion, an effect opposing that of pentagastrin. This finding indicates either a separate pathway for the two effects of growth and acid secretion by pentagastrin on the same cell or separate effects on two different cell populations, one being enhanced by EGF and the other being reduced by it. The trophic effects of EGF and gastrin on gastric mucosa could be related to recent findings that human G-17 underwent phosphorylation by the EGF-stimulated tyrosine kinase of A431 cell membranes [36]. The authors have suggested a physiologic role for gastrin phosphorylation by EGF in the effects of the two hormones on growth of gastrointestinal cells, since phosphorylation takes place on tyrosine molecules, known to be a key event in the control of cellular growth. As pointed out earlier, the mechanism of EGF stimulation of tyrosine kinase may, however, be quite different from that of inhibition of parietal cell acid secretion and may involve two different populations of gastric mucosal cells. The various factors that may be trophic to the gut have been reviewed by Johnson [19].

Parietal Cell, Acid Secretion, and Gastrin Receptors

The physiology of the parietal cell has been extensively investigated by Soll et al [2,8,37]. The major pathways for parietal cell stimulation for acid secretion, as summarized by Soll [38], are 1) neurocrine, via acetylcholine and similar chemical messengers through a synaptic route, 2) endocrine, via gastrin and other similar chemical messengers through the blood route, 3) paracrine, via histamine and other similar chemical messengers through an extracellular route, and 4) luminal, via amino acids and other similar chemical messengers from food through direct topical effects. The role of gastrin in acid secretion by parietal cells has been clearly demonstrated only recently. Studies with histamine antagonists that completely block histamine stimulation indicate that gastrin has an independent acid secretory effect, although this is much reduced in the absence of histamine. The concentrated effort of Soll and his group indicates that the isolated canine parietal cells are equipped with histamine, gastrin, and acetylcholine receptors, with potentiating interaction between the three groups of stimulants in addition to an independent effect relayed by the binding of the three groups of hormones to their own respective receptors. Whether gastrin can additionally initiate histamine release from either the enterochromaffin cells (ECF) (which in the case of rats have been shown to store histamine [39]), or the mast-like cells (which also store histamine in a number of species) by first interacting with specific gastrin receptors on these cells, remains to be studied.

As described recently [2,8,9], the characteristics of GR on the isolated canine parietal and nonparietal cells are reportedly different from those described for the GR on crude cell membrane preparations from rat gastric mucosa [1]. GR on canine parietal cells appear to have a slightly higher binding affinity for gastrin, 10^{11} M^{-1}. The main difference, however, appears to be that in the rat only one class of binding sites has been shown, reportedly with no positive or negative cooperativity [1], whereas in the dog a curvilinear Scatchard plot of the binding data has been obtained [2], which is indicative of either a heterogeneous population of binding sites or negative cooperativity between the binding sites. Negative cooperativity between membrane binding sites for peptide hormones is not uncommon, as has been reported for CCK [3] and insulin [40].

There appears to be a good relationship between the binding of gastrin to its receptors on canine parietal cells and the accumulation of aminopyrine, a biologic index of parietal cell function [2]. In the words of the authors, analogues of gastrin and CCK inhibit ^{125}I-gastrin binding in a dose-dependent fashion, and the rank order of potency for this competition is similar to that for stimulation of aminopyrine (AP) accumulation by parietal cells. Gastrin binding for parietal cells was not inhibited by unrelated hormones or by histamine, carbachol, or the inhibitors of these latter agents. These data indicate that the GR detected in the binding studies are linked to gastrin stimulation of aminopyrine accumulation by isolated canine parietal cells. Further support for this view comes from studies of cGMP analogues in which the dibutyryl but not 8-bromo analogues displaced ^{125}I-gastrin binding. Dibutyryl cGMP (Bt_2cGMP) also inhibited stimulation of AP accumulation by gastrin but not by histamine or cholinergic agents. A correlation was found between Bt_2cGMP inhibition of gastrin binding and gastrin stimulation of parietal cell function. Bt_2cGMP was first shown to inhibit CCK binding and action on pancreatic acini.

The rank order of affinity of gastrin and CCK analogues for parietal cell ^{125}I-gastrin binding differs from that found for CCK receptors or pancreatic acini [3], indicating the existence of closely related but distinct gastrin and CCK receptors in stomach and pancreas, respectively. GR on rabbit fundic mucosa dispersed cells have also been described [11,41]. The penultimate C-terminal amino acid, aspartic acid, has been shown to be important to binding of the gastrin molecule to its receptor on these cells and to its acid secretory function. Replacement by B-Asp acid or B-Ala negatively affects binding and function, while replacement with glutamic acid was less inhibitory [41]. Based on various structure-activity studies, Morley [42] has schematically represented the importance of C-terminal amino acids on the gastrin molecule for binding to the receptor on the substrate (Fig 7-1).

Gastrin Receptor Antagonists

As described above, Bt_2cGMP is an effective inhibitor of gastrin binding to its receptor, and of the biologic effects of gastrin [43]. Bt_2cGMP would then be described as a GR antagonist. If an antagonist blocks the receptor binding of the hormone and also inhibits its biologic effects (as is the case with Bt_2cGMP), it will definitely indicate the importance of binding of the hormone to its receptor for initiation of the biologic effect under investigation. Recently, another antagonist of gastrin action, proglumide, DL-4-benzamido-*N,N*-dipropyl glutaramic acid, the structure of which is only mildly similar to that of the C-terminal chain of gastrin, has been shown to be a competitive inhibitor of binding of gastrin to its receptor [29]. Gastrin-stimulated growth of parietal cells is inhibited by these antagonists, while histamine H_2-receptor antagonists are ineffective [44]. More recently, it has been demonstrated that proglumide, administered as a bolus injection or infusion, inhibits gastric acid secretion 13 to 62 percent compared to the histamine receptor antagonist cimetidine, which inhibits gastric acid secretion by 83 to 86 percent, though both were ineffective in lowering gastrin levels [45]. Proglumide is a weak inhibitor for gastric acid secretion compared to cimetidine, as shown in the finding that in patients with the Zollinger-Ellison syndrome, proglumide was much less effective compared with cimetidine, while in patients with duodenal ulcers, proglumide was as effective as cimetidine [45].

Gastrin Receptors in Aged Rats

In humans, both basal and stimulated gastric acid secretion has been shown to decrease with aging [46–48]. In our own laboratory, we have similarly observed a significant decrease in the basal and pentagastrin-stimulated gastric acid secretion of 24–32-month-old rats compared to 3-month-old

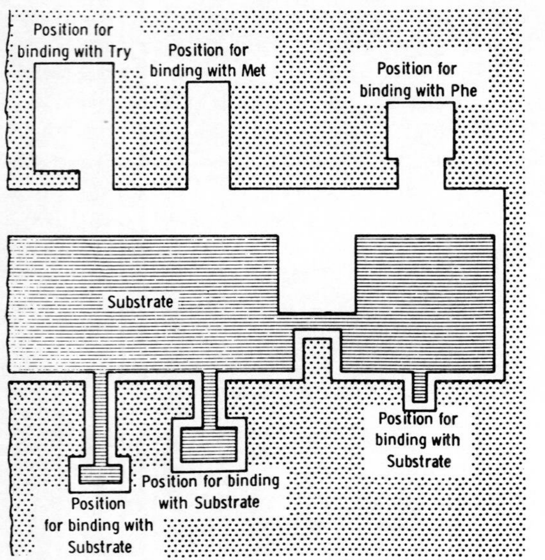

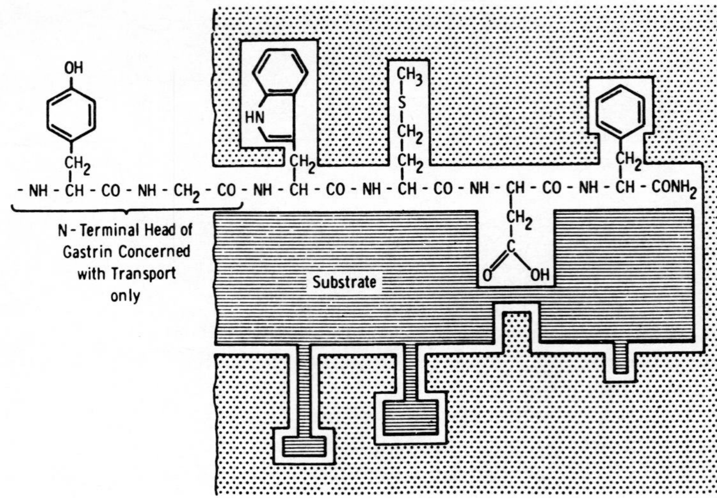

Figure 7-1. Schematic representation of the theory of hormonal action of the gastrins. Left: Cell receptor site equipped to receive a substrate but lacking an aspartyl group necessary for its function as an enzyme. Right: Missing carboxy group supplied by the C-terminal sequence of a gastrin molecule at exactly the required position. Receptor site can now function as an enzyme. (From Morley [38], by permission of The Royal Society.)

rats [49]. The fall in gastric acid secretion in older individuals probably results from a loss of parietal cells [50]. This possibility is corroborated by our studies [11,51], in which we observed a significantly lower number of specific gastric binding sites in the fundic mucosa of aged rats compared to that of young rats (Table 7-2). Serum gastrin levels have also been found by us to be significantly reduced in the aged rats [49], which agrees with the finding of involution of gastrin-cell population in old (27-month-old) rats [52]. Based on our studies, there is thus further strong evidence of age-associated changes in gastric physiology, which is reflected in similar changes in the effector (gastrin-binding) system.

CHOLECYSTOKININ RECEPTORS

Since the latter part of the 1970s, there has been great interest in receptors for cholecystokinin. The interaction of CCK with cell-surface receptors on the pancreatic acini, a target gland for a number of secretagogues including CCK and related peptides, was first studied in 1978 by using a ^{3}H-labeled probe with a very low specific activity [53]. Hence, the correlation between the biologic activity of the ligand and its binding to the receptor was poor, leading to inconclusive results. These studies were soon followed by more conclusive investigations using the iodinated probe and having a much higher specific activity. This made the binding assay studies sensitive enough for the detection of high-affinity binding sites, binding to which could then be correlated to activation of secretagogue in the pancreatic acini.

Physicochemical Characteristics of CCK Receptors

In early studies using the ^{3}H-caerulein probe, curvilinear Scatchard plots from the binding data were obtained, with an equilibrium affinity of 12 nM using isolated pancreatic cells and 18 nM using pancreatic total (crude) membranes from rats [4,53]. Recently, ^{125}I-labeled CCK-33 linked by the Bolton Hunter reagent (^{125}I-Bh-CCK-33) with a very high specific activity of 900–1300 Ci/mmol of ligand has been used [54], which has resulted in the detection of high-affinity binding sites in addition to the low-affinity binding sites described by the earlier studies.

The affinities of the two classes of binding sites, however, appear to be species-specific. Sankaran et al [55] reported affinity values of 26 pM and 2.2 nM for the high- and low-affinity sites on the mouse pancreatic acini, with binding capacities of approximately 1.9 fmol and 280 fmol/mg acinar protein, corresponding to 1,301 and 216,800

Table 7-2. **Total number and binding affinity of specific gastrin binding sites on the mucosal membranes of the gastrointestinal tract from young and old rats**

	Rat age in months					
	3		*6*		*24*	
Source	*GBS*[1]	K_d[2]	*GBS*	K_d	*GBS*	K_d
Fundus	5.1 ± 0.55 (n = 11)	0.21 ± 0.05 (n = 3)	2.9 ± 0.7 (n = 7)	0.30 ± 0.07 (n = 3)	0.4 ± 0.6* (n = 6)	0.41 ± 0.12 (n = 2)
Antrum	ND[3] (n = 6)	ND (n = 6)	ND (n = 6)	ND (n = 6)	4.7 ± 0.91 (n = 6)	3.7 ± 1.2 (n = 3)
Duodenum	3.0 ± 0.33 (n = 6)	0.27 ± 0.06 (n = 3)	1.1 ± 0.47 (n = 4)	0.37 ± 0.11 (n = 3)	1.3 ± 0.66 (n = 4)	0.43 ± 0.13 (n = 3)
Colon	4.2 ± 0.85 (n = 6)	0.44 ± 0.11 (n = 3)	2.1 ± 0.55 (n = 6)	0.4 ± 0.08 (n = 3)	2.3 ± 1.01 (n = 4)	0.55 ± 0.07 (n = 2)

1 = number of specific gastrin binding sites in fmol/mg crude membrane protein, estimated by SSA, using ^{125}I-MG, iodinated by Iodo-Gen.
2 = equilibrium dissociation constant values in nM, determined from a Scatchard plot of multi-point specific binding data.
n = number of observations per 2–3 separate experiments. For GBS measurement, tissues from three animals were pooled per observation point. For K_d determination, tissues from six rats were pooled per measurement.
3 = ND, not detectable.
* = statistically significant ($p < 0.05$) compared to both 3- and 6-month-old rat values.
(From Singh et al [11], by permission of The American Physiological Society.)

sites per cell, respectively. The same group reported 3- to 6-fold higher affinity values for binding of ^{125}I-CCK-33 to the two classes of CCK binding sites on rat pancreatic acini [54]. It is interesting that, on examining CCK binding with either total, particulate [5], or purified plasma membranes [56] from rat and mouse pancreas, the same group of workers have reported the presence of only one class of binding sites, with binding affinities of 1.8 nM and 1.35 nM and a capacity of 204 fmol and 20 pmol/mg membrane protein, respectively. Thus, the binding affinities reported for either the total or purified plasma membrane do not appear to be very different, but the capacity is about 20-fold higher in purified membrane preparation, which agrees with the concept of cell-surface receptors. The presence of cellular membrane CCK receptors on pancreatic acini has been further confirmed by autoradiographic localization of the radiolabeled probe [57]. The finding of only one class of binding sites on membrane preparations versus two classes of binding sites on whole cells of the pancreatic acini by the same group of workers is thus a curious finding which remains unexplained.

Two classes of binding sites have also been reported on guinea pig acini by Jensen et al [3]. A Scatchard plot of the ability of CCK-33 to inhibit binding of ^{125}I-CCK-33 obtained by these workers was curvilinear with an upward concavity; based on this result, the authors postulated that two classes of binding sites were probably present, the affinities and capacities of which cannot be clearly distinguished, and thus no specific calculation of affinity or capacity is yet possible. The total binding capacity of the two classes of binding sites has, however, been calculated to be 9,000 sites per acinar cell, which is much less than the combined values for the two classes of binding sites reported in rat or mouse pancreatic acini [55,56].

We have, in addition, recently reported the specific binding of CCK to normal and cancerous pancreatic membranes from humans [58]. The optimal binding conditions were similar for normal and cancerous pancreatic membranes. Maximum binding was observed at 30°C after 45 to 60 minutes of incubation, in the presence of 1.5 mM calcium and 5 mM magnesium. CCK-R in normal pancreatic membranes ranged from 11.9 to 200 fmol/mg protein, which probably reflects the degree of tissue deterioration before storage. Two classes of CCK-R were clearly definable with 10-fold differences in their binding affinities ($K_{d(1)}$, 0.04 nM and $K_{d(2)}$, 0.2–0.5 nM). Out of five cancerous pancreatic membranes, four were positive for CCK-R, with values ranging from 1.5–120 fmol/mg protein. This probably reflects differences in hormone dependence or dedifferentiation in situ. In only one cancerous pancreatic membrane was there retention of both types of normal binding sites, with similar binding affinities. In other cancerous pancreatic membranes, the types and binding affinity of CCK-R underwent significant changes. These changes indicate either dedifferentiation or hormone independence of cancerous pancreatic membranes and may be either the cause or the result of development of cancer.

On dog pancreatic membranes, we have also observed the presence of two classes of CCK receptors (unpublished data from this laboratory). Pancreatic tissues from the dogs were collected with or without in vivo perfusion of PO_4-buffered saline containing Trasylol and EDTA. The concentration of CCK-R measured on the perfused dog pancreatic membranes was found to be double that of nonperfused pancreatic membranes, indicating the importance of the method of collection of tissue on the final results of the receptor assay. A total of 105 ± 17 fmol of type I CCK-R (K_d, 0.04 ± 0.006 nM) and 101 ± 19 fmol of type II CCK-R (K_d, 0.51 ± 0.04 nM) was observed on the perfused dog pancreatic membranes.

Most of the other binding characteristics of CCK to pancreatic acini (cells or membranes) from the different animal species, however, have been reported to be similar by various groups of workers. A brief summary of the various findings on the binding of ^{125}I-CCK to its receptors follows: 1) it is reversible, 2) it is temperature-dependent (maximal at 37°C), 3) it is saturable, 4) it is specific to CCK and structurally related peptides (gastrin and caerulein), 5) it is inhibited by nonpeptide competitive antagonists such as Bt_2cGMP, 6) it is unaffected by other pancreatic secretagogues, such as secretin, VIP, glucagon, eledoisin, kassinin, substance P, carboxylcholine, litorin, pancreatic polypeptide, atropine, neurotensin, leucine enkephalin, methionine enkephalin, and somatostatin, 7) it shows accelerated dissociation of bound ^{125}I-CCK in the presence of agonists but not antagonists, indicating the presence of negative cooperativity between the binding sites, 8) it has a binding pH optimum of 5.5–6.5, and 9) it binds to trypsin-sensitive molecules, which indicate the proteinaceous nature of the CCK receptor [56]. Binding has been reported to be maximal in the presence of 5 mM magnesium and 1 mM EDTA and is inhibited in the presence of monovalent cations such as sodium and potassium [5]. We have, however, observed the binding of CCK to human pancreatic membranes to be maximal in the presence of the divalent cations (magnesium and calcium) and significantly reduced in the absence of calcium [58].

In spite of the reported presence of two classes of specific CCK-binding sites on the plasma membranes of pancreatic acini, the CCK-binding protein (linked covalently to ^{125}I-CCK-33 by disuccinimidyl suberate) was initially reported to separate as one homogeneous macromolecule on gel electrophoresis of the solubilized plasma membrane fraction (from mouse pancreatic acini) [56]. The molecular weight of CCK-binding protein thus separated was reported to be 80,000 in the presence or absence of dithiothreitol, indicating an absence of polymeric forms connected by disulfhydryl bonds [56]. In a later report, however, the same authors [59] reported the presence of a 120,000 molecular weight (M_r) CCK-binding protein in the absence of reducing agent and an 80,000 M_r unit in the presence of dithiothreitol, indicating a subunit structure of the binding protein in which a 76,000 M_r binding unit is linked to a 40,000 M_r nonbinding unit by a disulfide bond. Rosenzweig et al [60] have reported an 80,000 M_r monounit CCK receptor. The size of the receptor thus appears to be similar to that reported for glucagon [61], prolactin [62], and gonadotropin [63] but smaller than that for insulin [64], EGF [65], and IGF [66]. The binding kinetics of the purified CCK receptors are significantly altered with a reduced affinity for CCK [67].

CCK Receptors on Gallbladders

Specific CCK receptors have been demonstrated recently on cell membranes prepared from the muscularis layer of bovine gallbladders [68], but the mucosal and serosal membranes were reportedly devoid of CCK receptors. A single class of CCK binding sites, with a high affinity (K_d, approx. 0.6 nM) and capacity (100.5 ± 15.7 fmol/mg protein) was described [68]. We have, on the other hand, observed the presence of two classes of CCK binding sites on rabbit gallbladders (unpublished data from our laboratory). On membranes prepared from either the total gallbladder or only the muscular layer of gallbladder from rabbits, we were able to measure an equal distribution of approximately 200 fmol/mg protein of type I (K_d, 0.02 nM) and type II (K_d, 0.48 nM) sites, indicating a major distribution of CCK-R on the muscular layer of rabbit gallbladders. We have also determined the presence of specific CCK binding sites on the gallbladders and sphincter of Oddi of dogs by a single point assay which did not allow us to calculate the affinity or define the type of binding sites but gave us an approximate idea of the total number of binding sites; this was calculated to be 3.5 fmol for the gallbladder and 9.5 fmol for the sphincter of Oddi.

CCK-Analogue Structural Correlates of Receptor Binding and Biologic Response in the Pancreatic Acini

As pointed out earlier, it has been shown by almost all investigators that binding to CCK receptors on pancreatic acini is specific to CCK and related peptides. Analogue specificity of binding to CCK receptors has been unanimously reported to be in the following order in terms of concentration for half-maximal effect ($EC_{1/2}$): caerulein ($EC_{1/2}$, 0.3 nM) > CCK-8 ($EC_{1/2}$, 0.6 nM) > CCK-7 = CCK-33 ($EC_{1/2}$, 2 nM) > tyrosine-Hnl(SO_3H)-CCK-6 ($EC_{1/2}$, 17 nM) > des(SO_3H)-CCK-7 ($EC_{1/2}$, 1 μM) > gastrin I ($EC_{1/2}$, 2 μM) [3]. CCK-4 has even a lower binding affinity than gastrins I and II [56]. Additionally, an excellent correlation (K = 0.99) has been reported between the binding and biologic (amylase secretion) potencies of CCK and its analogues [54].

Nonpeptide-specific competitive antagonists, unlike CCK analogues, are unable to displace or increase the dissociation of ^{125}I-CCK-33 bound to pancreatic acini but do competitively inhibit the binding of ^{125}I-CCK-33 to the CCK receptors [3]. Interestingly, butyryl derivatives of cGMP, which were shown to be specific antagonists of the actions of CCK on pancreatic acinar cells [3], were observed to inhibit the binding of ^{125}I-CCK in close correlation to their ability to inhibit the increase in amylase release caused by an equimolar dose of CCK-33 [3]. The relative potencies of the cyclic nucleotides in inhibiting the two functions of binding and amylase release have been calculated to be Bt_2cGMP ($EC_{1/2}$, 0.1 mM) > $O^{2'}$ Bt_2cGMP ($EC_{1/2}$, 1 mM) > N^2Bt_2cGMP ($EC_{1/2}$, 10 mM) [3]. Unlike butyrylated cyclic GMP nucleotides, butyrylated cyclic AMP or nonbutyrylated cyclic GMP has not been observed to have any antagonist effects [5].

Recently a potent nonpeptide CCK antagonist has been described that was isolated from the fungus *Aspergillus alliaceus* and named asperlicin [69]. Its chemical designation is [2S-[2α,9β, 9(R*),9$\alpha\beta$]]-6,7-dihydro-7-[[2,3,9,9α-tetrahydro-9-hydroxy-2-(2-methylpropyl)-3-oxo-1H-imidazo-[1,2-α]indol-9-yl]methyl]-quinazolino[3,2-α][1,4]-benzodiazepine-5,13-dione. The compound reportedly has 300 to 400 times the affinity for pancreatic, ileal, and gallbladder CCK-R of proglumide, a standard antagonist of CCK actions used currently. More interestingly, unlike proglumide, asperlicin was found to be highly selective for peripheral CCK-R relative to brain CCK-R and gastrin receptors and was found to inhibit guinea pig gallbladder contraction in vivo. Asperlicin thus has immense potential for physiologic and pharmacologic studies.

Repeated observations have shown that not all the binding sites on pancreatic acini need to be occupied by CCK-33 in order to elicit the biologic response of amylase secretion. In the case of rat pancreatic acini Sankaran et al [55] have reported that concentrations of CCK 10 times lower (equal to 90 pM) than that needed for half-maximal inhibition of ^{125}I-CCK binding is necessary for half-maximal stimulation of amylase release. In other words, only 90 pM of CCK was required to half-maximally stimulate amylase release in rats, which is close to the K_d of high-affinity sites (64 pM in the case of this species); for this reason, the authors speculated that only the high-affinity sites for CCK need to be occupied for eliciting most of the amylase secretory response. Jensen et al [3] studied guinea pig pancreatic acini and similarly reported a need for occupancy of only 40 percent of the total (high- and low-affinity) binding sites by the six different CCK analogues tested in order to elicit the maximal amylase secretory response.

An unusual biphasic response of amylase secretion to CCK has been observed by a number of workers [3,55]. Lower doses of CCK increasingly stimulate the secretion of amylase, and high doses progressively reduce the stimulated levels to basal, which is an intriguing phenomenon and has been variously explained based on different models for binding. In the guinea pig acini, maximal stimulation of amylase release occurred with a concentration of 0.3 nM CCK-8, which was effective in inhibiting 40 percent of the binding by ^{125}I-CCK-33, while higher concentrations of CCK-8 caused a progressive decline in amylase secretion from the maximal levels in direct proportion to its ability to further inhibit ^{125}I-CCK binding. In other words, while 40 percent receptor occupation stimulated enzyme secretion, occupation of the rest of the 60 percent of the binding sites caused a progressive decrease in the stimulated amylase secretion [3]. Based on these findings, the authors have proposed that ^{125}I-CCK-33 binds to at least one class of interacting binding sites whose affinities are influenced by the extent to which they are occupied by agonists but not by antagonists.

In the case of insulin, De Meyts et al [70] have similarly proposed that curvilinear Scatchard plots are indicative of one rather than two classes of binding sites, which exhibit negative cooperativity at higher concentrations. Others, however, believe that accelerated dissociation of bound ligand, in the presence of unlabeled hormone, is reflective of two classes of binding sites on Scatchard analysis of the binding data [71,72]. Sankaran et al [55] subscribe to the latter interpretation based on their findings that unlabeled CCK enhanced only 2-fold dissociation, versus an 80-fold difference in K_d, between the proposed two binding sites.

Since in a standard model of negative cooperativity an equal number of low- and high-affinity binding sites has been proposed [73], the finding of an 100-fold difference in the binding capacity of low- and high-affinity sites by Sankaran et al [55] has been interpreted as indicative of the presence of two classes of binding sites in mouse pancreatic acini, in which one or both can exhibit site-site interaction. In mouse pancreatic acini, a biphasic effect of CCK has been demonstrated [55] similar to that reported for guinea pig acini [3] on amylase release, in which maximal secretion was evident in the presence of 150–200 pM of CCK-33, while at higher concentrations a progressive decrease in the secretion was observed, a reduction to only 15–20 percent of maximally stimulated levels in the presence of 30 nM CCK-33 (Fig 7-2). Perhaps each class of CCK receptors binds to two molecules of CCK. The first CCK molecule has a higher affinity constant than the second molecule, and the ratio of the two binding affinities is given as the cooperativity coefficient, C. For the observed biphasic effect of CCK on amylase release, two plausible explanations have been given. First, one CCK receptor that binds to two molecules of CCK regulates this function so that binding of one stimulates amylase and binding of the second inactivates the stimulation. However, since the authors could not fit their data into this model, a second explanation given by them is that both CCK receptors regulate amylase release; the high-affinity site stimulates the release, while the low-affinity site inactivates it. The data appeared to fit this model better, especially by incorporating a cooperativity function into the high-affinity receptors [55].

Other biologic effects of CCK that have been examined in relation to its binding include 1) stimulation of 2[^{3}H]deoxyglucose (DG) transport and inhibition of α[^{3}H]aminoisobutyric (AIB) acid in mouse pancreatic acini, and 2) increase in cellular cGMP and outflux of calcium in guinea pig pancreatic acini [3]. The effects on 2[^{3}H]glucose and amino acid transport were reportedly monophasic and were half-maximal at 0.85 and 0.44 nM, respectively [55]. Thus, it was postulated that glucose uptake and amino acid transport function could not be regulated by high-affinity sites (which with a K_d of 26 pM would be fully occupied at concentrations far less than that required to regulate the function). Low-affinity sites, with a K_d of 2.2 nM, would be fully occupied after these two functions are fully stimulated (Fig 7-3) [55]. Since these functions follow simple saturation kinetics, their regu-

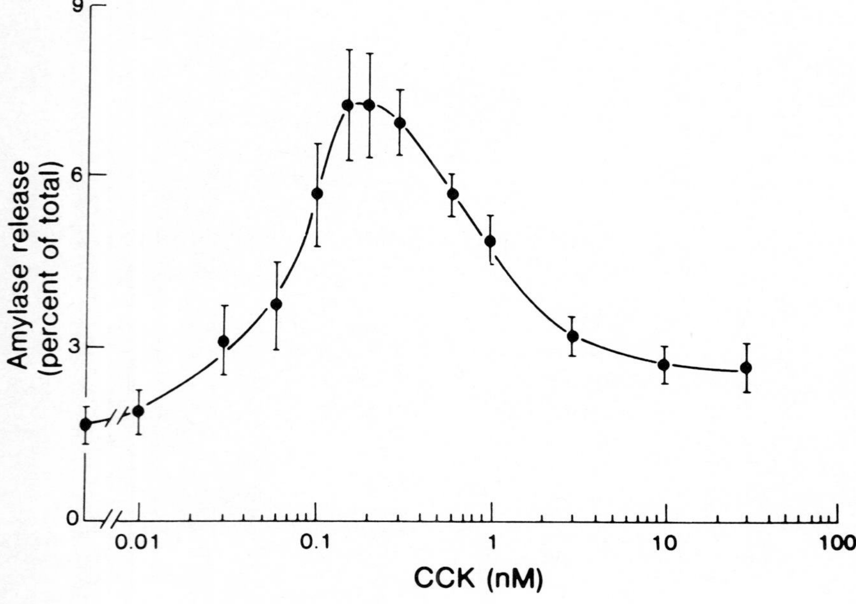

Figure 7-2. CCK-stimulated amylase release from isolated mouse pancreatic acini. Dose-response relationship of CCK-stimulated amylase release. Isolated acini were incubated with varying concentrations of CCK for 20 minutes. Values are means ± SE of four experiments. (From Sankaran et al [51], by permission of The American Physiological Society.)

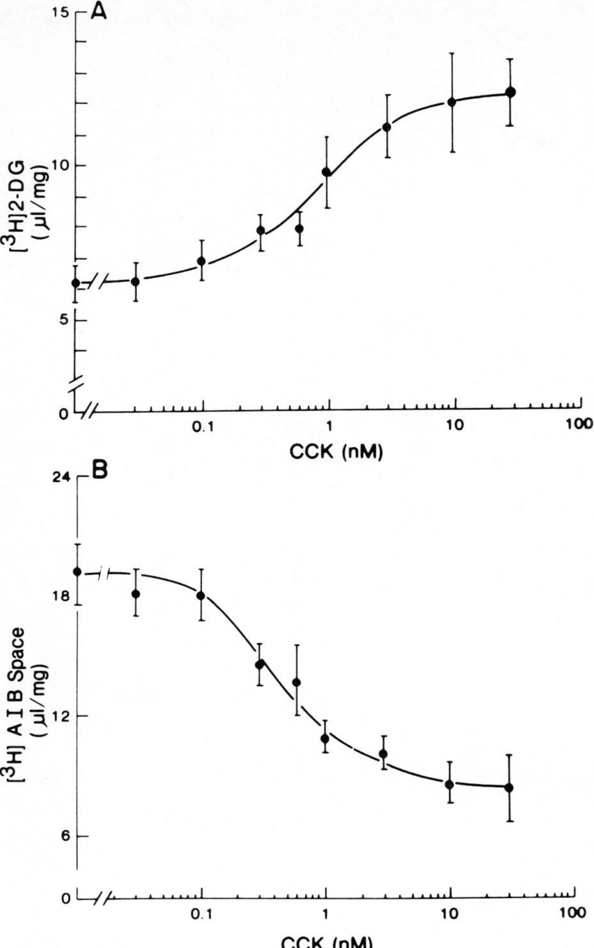

Figure 7-3. Effect of CCK on uptake of 2-$[^3H]$DG and $[^3H]$AIB by isolated mouse pancreatic acini. **A.** Dose-response relationship of CCK-stimulated 2-$[^3H]$DG uptake. Acini were incubated with varying concentrations of CCK for 10 minutes, followed by a 30-minute pulse with 100 nM 2-$[^3H]$DG. Values are means ± SE of four experiments. Line is best fit of data by Eq. 1 (see Methods), with $K_m = 0.85 \pm 0.22$ nM, $J_o = 6.15 \pm 0.20$ µL/mg, and $J_{max} = 5.92 \pm 0.44$ µL/mg. **B.** Dose-response relationship of CCK-induced inhibition of $[^3H]$AIB uptake. Acini were incubated with varying concentrations of CCK for 10 minutes, followed by a 40-minute pulse with 100 nM $[^3H]$AIB. Values are means ± SE of from experiments. Line is best fit of data by Eq. 2 (see Methods), with $K_m = 0.44 \pm 0.09$ nM, and J_{insens}, hormone-insensitive component = 8.39 ± 0.30 µL/mg. (From Sankaran et al [51], by permission of The American Physiological Society.)

lation is thought to be by one class of binding sites as against the proposed regulation of amylase release by the two classes of binding sites [55].

In a study of the ability of CCK-8 to alter cGMP and calcium function in guinea pig acini, CCK-8 was observed to cause a 5-fold increase in outflux of 45 calcium and a 17-fold increase in cGMP. A dose-response curve was monophasic and identical for these two functions [3]. The maximal stimulation of calcium outflux and cGMP generation occurred with a concentration of 3 nM CCK, corresponding to the dose of CCK reportedly effective in inhibiting 77 percent of the binding of ^{125}I-CCK-33 to the pancreatic acini. This indicates the need for only 77 percent occupation of binding sites to invoke maximal effects on the above two functions [3].

Amino Acid Constituents of CCK and Relation to Binding and Biologic Functions

Morley [42], in 1968, concluded that C-terminal gastrin-CCK tetrapeptide amide was the smallest C-terminal fragment that retained biologic activity and that the aspartic acid residue was essential for intrinsic hormone activity [42]. On the same lines, replacement of the penultimate aspartic acid residue with alanine has been shown to cause a 500-fold decrease in the potency towards calcium outflux [74] and a 30- to 150-fold decrease in the potency towards gallbladder contraction [75]. Replacement of the penultimate aspartic acid with β-alanine was found to cause a 300-fold decrease in the stimulation of enzyme secretion. Replacement by glutamic acid, resulting in an increase in the distance between the side-chain COOH-group and the peptide backbone, caused a 1,000-fold decrease in the potency [76]. These changes in the ability of the peptide to secrete amylase were repeatedly accompanied by corresponding changes in its ability to inhibit binding of ^{125}I-labeled CCK to guinea pig pancreatic acini [76]. The presence of an N-terminal "protecting group," such as B-butyloxycarbonyl (BOC), has been shown to modify the biologic activities of C-terminal fragments of CCK molecules [76]. In binding studies, blocking of N-terminal with BOC in the substituted 32 aspartic C-terminal heptapeptide with either β-alanine or glutamic acid was found to be 10 to 12 times more potent, respectively, when compared with peptides blocked with benzyloxycarbonyl [76]. The N-terminal deamino analogue of CCK heptapeptide was found to be 10 times less potent than the unaltered peptide in stimulating amylase secretion and 100 times less potent in increasing residual stimulation of enzyme secretion [76], indicating that the N-terminal amide selectively influences the rate at which the bound peptide dissociates from its receptors when the acini are washed.

The COOH-terminal phenylaninine residue of CCK has also been shown to be essential for biologic function, although not for binding [77]. This finding has led to the development of a new class of CCK antagonists that lack the C-terminal phenylalanine but have all the other components necessary for binding to the receptor, namely CCK-27-32 amide [77,78]. CCK-27-32-NH_2 molecule in fact appears to be the most potent receptor antagonist, being 30 times more potent than Bt_2cGMP [77].

Length of C-Terminal Peptide Chain and Tissue Specificity of Action

A characteristic feature of the action of CCK on its target tissues, which at the present time include pancreatic acini [3,55], cerebral cortex [79], stomach chief cells [80], and gallbladder [81], is that its dose-response curve (DRC) is broad, spanning up to a 10,000-fold range of concentration [82], and for a number of its biologic effects, such as stimulation of gallbladder contraction [81] and pancreatic enzyme secretion [3,55], the DRC has a biphasic contour. We find it interesting that biphasic dose-response curves of these effects can be elicited by caerulein, gastrin, and COOH-terminal fragments of CCK as small as tetrapeptide [83]. In the guinea pig pancreatic acini, however, the full spectrum of CCK activity appears to require the presence of at least the unsulfated COOH-terminal heptapeptide of CCK [82]. COOH-terminal fragments, with 4 to 6 amino acids, have been shown to possess only part of the full spectrum of CCK activity [82].

The relationship between the number of C-terminal amino acids and the effects on enzyme secretion and binding to the pancreatic acini is diagrammatically represented in Figure 7-4. The details are as follows: the COOH-terminal tetrapeptide amide produces maximal stimulation of enzyme secretion but causes only a small (10 percent) reduction in amylase secretion with supramaximal concentrations. Adding a NH_2-terminal glycine to CCK-4 does not alter the biologic activity of the peptide, suggesting that the glycine residue is inert and functions to produce proper spacing between the COOH-terminal tetrapeptide portions of CCK and the remaining biologically active NH_2-terminal portion of the peptide [82]. Adding an NH_2-terminal methionine to CCK-5 increases the potency with which the peptide causes maximal stimulation of enzyme secretion and increases the efficacy of the peptide for causing supramaximal inhibition of enzyme secretion. Thus, methionine does not simply serve a spacer function but increases both the potency and supramaximal efficacy of the peptide. Adding an NH_2-terminal tyrosine to CCK-6 increases the potency with which the peptide causes maximal stimulation of enzyme secretion and increases its efficacy for causing supramaximal inhibition of secretion. Both the maximal stimulation and the reduction in stimulation

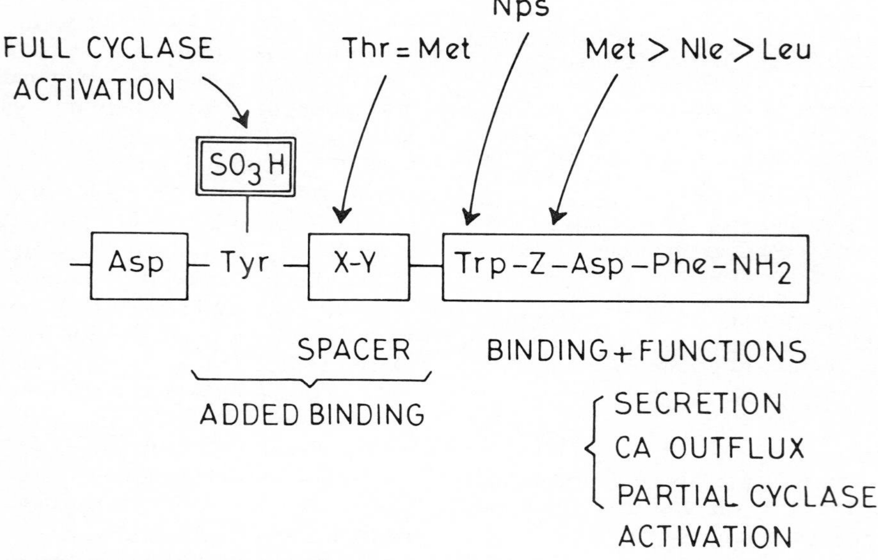

Figure 7-4. Structural requirements for the binding and biologic activities of pancreozymin-like peptides. (From Christophe et al [77], by permission of Raven Press.)

seen with supramaximal concentrations of unsulfated CCK-7 are identical to those seen with CCK, thus demonstrating that this peptide is the smallest COOH-terminal peptide that expresses the full spectrum of biologic activity of CCK.

Adding a sulfate ester to the tyrosine residue of des(SO_3H)-CCK-7 does not alter the configuration of the dose-response curve but does increase the potency of the peptide. Adding an NH_2-terminal aspartyl residue to CCK-7 causes a further 3- to 10-fold increase in potency, with no change in the concentration of the dose-response curve. Extending the NH_2-terminal of CCK-8 either does not change or reduces by as much as 10-fold [3] the potency with which the peptide stimulates enzyme secretion; however, it does not alter the configuration of the dose-response curve [3].

Extensive studies carried out by Jensen et al [82] have further demonstrated that increasing lengths of COOH-terminal fragments of CCK inhibit binding of ^{125}I-CCK and stimulate enzyme secretion with equal potency. These findings indicate that the limited abilities of CCK-6, CCK-5, and CCK-4 to cause supramaximal inhibition of enzyme secretion are not attributable to their binding to all of the CCK receptors. Further, each peptide tested had the same efficacy for increasing calcium outflux and cGMP as for maximal stimulation of enzyme secretion. Moreover, with each peptide tested, there is a fixed relationship between the dose-response curve for stimulation of calcium outflux and the up-stroke of the dose-response curves for stimulation of enzyme secretion. In contrast, the down-stroke of the dose-response curve for stimulating enzyme secretion is not accompanied by a change in the calcium outflux or cGMP. Thus, the mechanisms whereby supramaximal concentrations of CCK and COOH-terminal fragments cause a reduction in enzyme secretion are not mediated by changes in calcium outflux or cGMP. The mechanism that accounts for the supramaximal inhibition of enzyme secretion is as yet unknown. The limited ability of CCK-6, CCK-5, and CCK-4 to cause supramaximal inhibition appears to reflect binding of these peptides to CCK receptors combined with the limited ability to activate the unknown cellular processes that produce supramaximal inhibition (that is, they function as partial agonists).

Based on these findings, Jensen et al [83] have proposed a two-site model for the CCK receptors. The essential feature of this hypothesis is as follows: 1) each CCK receptor has two functionally distinct binding sites, I and II; 2) site I has a relatively high affinity for CCK and occupation of site I is a prerequisite for occupation of site II by CCK; 3) the dissociation of CCK from site I is relatively rapid; 4) the dissociation of CCK from site II is slow when site I is vacant but rapid when site I is occupied. Their findings indicate that the two different CCK binding sites have different structural requirements for activation by CCK. At site I, COOH-terminal fragments of CCK, having as few as four amino acids, are full agonists and cause outflux of cellular calcium as well as the up-stroke of the dose-response curve for enzyme secretion. At site II, COOH-terminal fragments of CCK having seven or more amino acids are full agonists and cause a down-stroke of the dose-response curve for enzyme secretion, whereas COOH-terminal fragments having fewer than seven amino acids are partial agonists with little or no intrinsic efficacy and cause little or no supramaximal inhibition of enzyme secretion. In contrast, the model proposed by Williams' group [55] invokes the binding of CCK first to the high-affinity receptors; when occupied by CCK these receptors stimulate amylase release by releasing one pool of calcium and this may also initiate other responses in acini, such as the stimulation of digestive enzymes. Next, the low-affinity receptors are occupied by CCK, inhibiting amylase release and regulating glucose and amino acid transport by acting through another pool of calcium. Furthermore, this low-affinity receptor may also be mediating the inhibition of the synthesis of pancreatic protein that is observed at high concentrations of CCK [84].

CCK Binding in the Brain

The most striking difference between CCK receptors in the pancreas and brain appears to be in the selectivity for CCK analogues and Bt_2cGMP. Pancreatic CCK receptors exhibit a very high degree of agonistic selectivity, while the brain CCK receptor is not as selective. The most and least potent CCK analogues (CCK-8, CCK-4) differ by only 10-fold in their binding to brain receptors [79]. Bt_2cGMP is also 40 times more potent as an inhibitor in pancreas versus brain [85], and 5′-GMP, which is 20 times less potent compared with Bt_2cGMP in pancreas, is equally as potent in the brain. The increased specificity of the pancreatic receptors may be important in the function of CCK as a hormone in the digestive system, since a receptor must distinguish CCK from other closely related molecules such as gastrin.

CCK Receptor Antagonists

Proglumide is a derivative of glutaramic acid that has been used for approximately 10 years in

Europe and Japan to treat patients with peptic ulcers. The claimed effectiveness of proglumide has been attributed to its ability to reduce secretion of gastric acid; recent studies show proglumide can inhibit binding of radiolabeled gastrin to a heterogeneous mixture of gastric mucosal cells as well as to a crude preparation of gastric mucosal membrane [86]. In pancreatic acini from guinea pig pancreas, proglumide and benzotript (*N-p*-chlorobenzoyl-L-tryptophan) caused a rightward shift in the dose-response curve for CCK-stimulated amylase secretion but did not alter the maximal increase in amylase secretion caused by CCK [86]. At relatively low concentrations, proglumide did not alter the stimulation of enzyme secretion caused by secretagogues whose effects are mediated by adenosine 3′-5′-monophosphate (e.g., VIP or secretin) and did not alter the stimulation of enzyme secretion caused by secretagogues that have a mode of action similar to that of CCK but act through different receptors (e.g., bombesin, physalaemin, eledoisin, and ionophore A23187). There was a close correlation between the ability of proglumide or benzotript to inhibit binding of ^{125}I-labeled CCK to its receptors on pancreatic acini and the abilities of this compound to inhibit the action of CCK on enzyme secretion and on calcium outflux. These results indicate that proglumide and benzotript are members of a different class of CCK receptor antagonists compared to Bt_2cGMP [87].

REFERENCES

1. Takeuchi K, Speir GR, Johnson LR: Mucosal gastrin receptor. I. Assay standardization and fulfillment of receptor criteria. Am J Physiol 237:E284, 1979.
2. Rutten MJ, Soll AH: Hormone regulation of parietal cell function: Gastrin interaction with a specific receptor. Ann NY Acad Sci 372:637, 1981.
3. Jensen RT, Lemp GF, Gardner JD: Interaction of cholecystokinin with specific membrane receptors on pancreatic acinar cells. Proc Natl Acad Sci USA 77:2079, 1980.
4. Deschodt-Lanckman M, Robberecht P, Camus J, et al: The interaction of caerulein with the rat pancreas. 1. Specific binding of [^{3}H]caerulein on plasma membranes and evidence for negative cooperativity. Eur J Biochem 91:21, 1978.
5. Steigerwalt RW, Williams JA: Characterization of cholecystokinin receptors on rat pancreatic membranes. Endocrinology 109:1746, 1981.
6. Brown J, Gallagher ND: A specific gastrin receptor site in the rat stomach. Biochem Biophys Acta 538:42, 1978.
7. Takeuchi K, Speir GR, Johnson LR: Mucosal gastrin receptor. II. Physical characteristics of binding. Am J Physiol 237:E295, 1979.
8. Soll AH, Amirian DA, Thomas LP, et al: Gastrin receptors on nonparietal cells isolated from canine fundic mucosa. Am J Physiol 247:G715, 1984.
9. Soll AH, Amirian DA, Thomas LP, et al: Gastrin receptors on isolated canine parietal cells. J Clin Invest 73:1434, 1984.
10. Magous R, Bali J-P: High-affinity binding sites for gastrin on isolated rabbit gastric mucosal cells. Eur J Pharmacol 82:47, 1982.
11. Singh P, Rae-Venter B, Townsend CM Jr, et al: Gastrin receptors in normal and malignant gastrointestinal mucosa. Age-associated changes. Am J Physiol 249:G761, 1985.
12. Speir GR, Takeuchi K, Johnson LR: Characterization of the interaction between gastrin and its receptor in rat oxyntic gland mucosa. Biochim Biophys Acta 716:308, 1982.
13. Takeuchi K, Speir GR, Johnson LR: Mucosal gastrin receptor. III. Regulation by gastrin. Am J Physiol 238:G135, 1980.
14. Takeuchi K, Peitsch W, Johnson LR: Mucosal gastrin receptor. V. Development in newborn rats. Am J Physiol 240:G163, 1981.
15. Speir GR, Takeuchi K, Peitsch W, et al: Mucosal gastrin receptor. VII. Up- and downregulation. Am J Physiol 242:G243, 1982.
16. Peitsch W, Takeuchi K, Johnson LR: Mucosal gastrin receptor. VI. Induction by corticosterone in newborn rats. Am J Physiol 240:G442, 1981.
17. Johnson LR: Regulation of the mucosal gastrin receptor. Proc Soc Exp Biol Med 173:167, 1983.
18. Johnson LR, Peitsch W, Takeuchi K: Mucosal gastrin receptor. VIII. Sex-related differences in binding. Am J Physiol 243:G469, 1982.
19. Johnson LR: The trophic action of gastrointestinal hormones. Gastroenterology 70:278, 1976.
20. Johnson LR: New aspects of the trophic action of gastrointestinal hormones. Gastroenterology 72:788, 1977.
21. Seidel ER, Tabata K, Dembinski AB, et al: Attenuation of trophic response to gastrin after inhibition of ornithine decarboxylase. Am J Physiol 249:G16, 1985.
22. Majumdar APN, Johnson LR: Gastric mucosal cell proliferation during development in rats and effects of pentagastrin. Am J Physiol 242:G135, 1982.
23. Singh P, Townsend CM Jr, Walker JP, et al: Gastrin receptors in a mouse colon cancer cell line responsive to trophic effects of gastrin. Surg Forum 35:205, 1984.
24. Winsett OE, Townsend CM Jr, Glass EJ, et al: Gastrin stimulates growth of colon cancer. Surg Forum 33:384, 1982.
25. Winsett OE, Townsend CM Jr, Glass EJ, et al: Gastrin stimulates growth of colon cancer. Surgery 99:302, 1986.
26. Singh P, Walker JP, Townsend CM Jr, et al: Mouse colon cancer and trophic effects of pentagastrin in relation to gastrin receptor levels in vivo. Dig Dis Sci 29:80S, 1984.
27. Singh P, Walker JP, Townsend CM Jr, et al: Role of gastrin and gastrin receptors on the growth of a

transplantable mouse colon carcinoma (MC-26), in Balb/c mice. Cancer Res, 46:1612, 1986.

28. Beauchamp RD, Townsend CM Jr, Singh P, et al: Proglumide, a gastrin receptor antagonist, inhibits growth of colon cancer and enhances survival in mice. Ann Surg 202:303, 1985.
29. Cifarelli A, Setnikar I, Vidal y Plana RR: Antagonism of proglumide with human gastrin at the receptor site. Hepatogastroenterology 27 (Suppl):124, 1980.
30. Tatsuta M, Yamamura H, Iishi H, et al: Gastrin has no promoting effect on chemically induced colonic tumors in Wistar rats. Eur J Cancer Clin Oncol 21:741, 1985.
31. Rae-Venter B, Townsend CM Jr, Thompson JC, et al: Gastrin receptors in human colon carcinoma. Gastroenterology 80:1256, 1981.
32. McGuire WL, de la Garza M, Chamness GC: Evaluation of estrogen receptor assays in human breast cancer tissue. Cancer Res 37:637, 1977.
33. Johnson LR: Effect of exogenous gut hormones on gastrointestinal mucosal growth. Scand J Gastroenterol (Suppl) 17:89, 1982.
34. Johnson LR, Guthrie PD, Dudrick SJ: Effects of luminal gastrin on the growth of rat intestinal mucosa. Gastroenterology 81:71, 1981.
35. Johnson LR, Guthrie PD: Stimulation of rat oxyntic gland mucosal growth by epidermal growth factor. Am J Physiol 238:G45, 1980.
36. Baldwin GS, Knesel J, Monckton JM: Phosphorylation of gastrin-17 by epidermal growth factor-stimulated tyrosine kinase. Nature 301:435, 1983.
37. Soll AH, Grossman MI: Cellular mechanisms in acid secretion. Ann Rev Med 29:495, 1978.
38. Soll AH: Potentiating interactions of gastric stimulants on [^{14}C] aminopyrine accumulation by isolated canine parietal cells. Gastroenterology 83:216, 1982.
39. Soll AH, Lewin KJ, Beaven MA: Isolation of histamine-containing cells from rat gastric mucosa: Biochemical and morphologic differences from mast cells. Gastroenterology 80:717, 1981.
40. De Meyts P, Bianco AR, Roth J: Site-site interactions among insulin receptors. Characterization of the negative cooperativity. J Biol Chem 251:1877, 1976.
41. Magous R, Martinez J, Lignon MF, et al: The role of the Asp-32 residue of cholecystokinin in gastric acid secretion and gastrin receptor recognition. Regul Pept 5:327, 1983.
42. Morley JS: Structure-function relationships in gastrin-like peptides. Proc R Soc Lond (Biol) 170:97, 1968.
43. Soll AH: Pharmacology of inhibitors of parietal cell function. J Clin Gastroenterol 3 (Suppl 2):85, 1981.
44. Rovati AL: Inhibition of gastric secretion by anti-gastrinic and H_2-blocking agents. Scand J Gastroenterol 11:113, 1976 (suppl 42).
45. Lamers CBHW, Jansen JBMJ: The effect of a gastrin-receptor antagonist on gastric acid secretion and serum gastrin in the Zollinger-Ellison syndrome. J Clin Gastroenterol 5:21, 1983.
46. Borgstrom S, Emas S, Lilja B, et al: Acid response to pentagastrin in relation to age and body stature in male and female ulcer patients. Scand J Gastroenterol 8:209, 1973.
47. Miyoshi A, Ohe K, Inagawa T, et al: A statistical study on the age distribution of gastric secretion in patients with peptic ulcer. Hiroshima J Med Sci 29:21, 1980.
48. Schuster MM: Disorders of the aging GI system. Hosp Prac Sept:95, 1976.
49. Khalil T, Fujimura M, Greeley GH Jr, et al: Effect of aging on serum gastrin and antral gastrin content in Sprague-Dawley rats. Gastroenterology 88:1445, 1985.
50. Portis SA, King JC: The gastrointestinal tract in the aged. JAMA 148:1073, 1952.
51. Singh P, Khalil T, Thompson JC: Effect of aging on gastrin receptors in the rat gut. Dig Dis Sci 29:80S, 1984.
52. Lehy T, Gres L, Ferreira de Castro E: Quantitation of gastrin and somatostatin cell populations in the antral mucosa of the rat. Cell Tissue Res 198:325, 1979.
53. Christophe J, DeNeef P, Deschodt-Lanckman M, et al: The interaction of caerulein with the rat pancreas. 2. Specific binding of [^{3}H]caerulein on dispersed acinar cells. Eur J Biochem 91:31, 1978.
54. Sankaran H, Goldfine ID, Deveney CW, et al: Binding of cholecystokinin to high affinity receptors on isolated rat pancreatic acini. J Biol Chem 255:1849, 1980.
55. Sankaran H, Goldfine ID, Bailey A, et al: Relationship of cholecystokinin receptor binding to regulation of biological functions in pancreatic acini. Am J Physiol 242:G250, 1982.
56. Sakamoto C, Williams JA, Wong KY, et al: The CCK receptor on pancreatic plasma membranes: Binding characteristics and covalent cross-linking. FEBS Lett 151:63, 1983.
57. Williams JA, Sankaran H, Roach E, et al: Quantitative electron microscope autoradiographs of ^{125}I-cholecystokinin in pancreatic acini. Am J Physiol 243:G291, 1982.
58. Singh P, Townsend CM Jr, Upp J, et al: Characterization of cholecystokinin receptors (CCK-R) in normal and cancerous human pancreas. Fed Proc 45:291, 1986.
59. Sakamoto C, Goldfine ID, Williams JA: Characterization of cholecystokinin receptor subunits on pancreatic plasma membranes. J Biol Chem 258:12707, 1983.
60. Rosenzweig SA, Miller LJ, Jamieson JD: Identification and localization of cholecystokinin-binding sites on rat pancreatic plasma membranes and acinar cells: A biochemical and autoradiographic study. J Cell Biol 96:1288, 1983.
61. Johnson GL, MacAndrew VI Jr, Pilch PF: Identification of the glucagon receptor in rat liver membranes by photoaffinity crosslinking. Proc Natl Acad Sci USA 78:875, 1981.
62. Borst DW, Sayare M: Photoactivated cross-linking of prolactin to hepatic membrane binding sites. Biochem Biophys Res Commun 105:194, 1982.
63. Rebois RV, Omedeo-Sale F, Brady RO, et al: Covalent

cross-linking of human chorionic gonadtropin to its receptor in rat testes. Proc Natl Acad Sci USA 78:2086, 1981.

64. Pilch PF, Czech MP: Interaction of cross-linking agents with the insulin effector system of isolated fat cells. Covalent linkage of ^{125}I-insulin to a plasma membrane receptor protein of 140,000 daltons. J Biol Chem 254:3375, 1979.
65. Hock RA, Nexø E, Hollenberg MD: Isolation of the human placenta receptor for epidermal growth factor—urogastrone. Nature 277:403, 1979.
66. Kasuga M, van Obberghen E, Nissley SP, et al: Structure of the insulin-like growth factor receptor in chicken embryo fibroblasts. Proc Natl Acad Sci USA 79:1864, 1982.
67. Szecowka J, Goldfine ID, Williams JA: Solubilization and characterization of CCK receptors from mouse pancreas. Regul Pept 10:71, 1985.
68. Steigerwalt RW, Goldfine ID, Williams JA: Characterization of cholecystokinin receptors on bovine gallbladder membranes. Am J Physiol 247:G709, 1984.
69. Chang RSL, Lotti VJ, Monaghan RL, et al: A potent nonpeptide cholecystokinin antagonist selective for peripheral tissues isolated from *Aspergillus alliaceus.* Science 230:177, 1985.
70. De Meyts P, Roth J, Neville DM Jr, et al: Insulin interactions with its receptors: Experimental evidence for negative cooperativity. Biochem Biophys Res Commun 55:154, 1973.
71. Kahn CR, Freychet P, Roth J: Quantitative aspects of the insulin-receptor interaction in liver plasma membranes. J Biol Chem 249:2249, 1974.
72. Pollet RJ, Standaert ML, Haase BA: Insulin binding to the human lymphocyte receptor. Evaluation of the negative cooperativity model. J Biol Chem 252:5828, 1977.
73. Rodbard D, Bertino RE: Theory of radioimmunoassays and hormone-receptor interactions: II. Simulation of antibody divalency, cooperativity and allosteric effects, in O'Malley BW, Means AR (eds): *Receptors for Reproductive Hormones.* New York, Plenum Press, 1973, pp 327–341.
74. Gardner JD, Conlon TP, Klaeveman HL, et al: Action of cholecystokinin and cholinergic agents on calcium transport in isolated pancreatic acinar cells. J Clin Invest 56:366, 1975.
75. Ondetti MA, Rubin B, Engel SL, et al: Cholecystokinin-pancreozymin: Recent developments. Am J Dig Dis 15:149, 1970.
76. Pan G-Z, Martinez J, Bodanszky M, et al: The importance of the amino acid in position 32 of cholecystokinin in determining its interaction with cholecystokinin receptors on pancreatic acini. Biochim Biophys Acta 678:352, 1981.
77. Spanarkel M, Martinez J, Briet C, et al: Cholecystokinin-27-32-amide. A member of a new class of cholecystokinin receptor antagonists. J Biol Chem 258:6746, 1983.
78. Jensen JR, Jones SW, Gardner JD: COOH-terminal fragments of cholecystokinin. A new class of cholecystokinin receptor antagonists. Biochim Biophys Acta 757:250, 1983.
79. Innis RB, Snyder SH: Distinct cholecystokinin receptors in brain and pancreas. Proc Natl Acad Sci USA 77:6917, 1980.
80. Kasbekar DK, Jensen RT, Gardner JD: Pepsinogen secretion from dispersed glands from rabbit stomach. Am J Physiol 244:G392, 1983.
81. Poitras P, Iacino D, Walsh JH: Dibutyryl cGMP: Inhibitor of the effect of cholecystokinin and gastrin on the guinea pig gallbladder *in vitro.* Biochem Biophys Res Commun 96:476, 1980.
82. Jensen RT, Lemp GF, Gardner JD: Interactions of COOH-terminal fragments of cholecystokinin with receptors on dispersed acini from guinea pig pancreas. J Biol Chem 257:5554, 1982.
83. Christophe J, Svoboda M, Calderon-Attas P, et al: Gastrointestinal hormone-receptor interactions in the pancreas, in Jerzy Glass GB (ed): *Gastrointestinal Hormones.* New York, Raven Press, 1980, pp 451–476.
84. Korc M, Bailey AC, Williams JA: Regulation of protein synthesis in normal and diabetic rat pancreas by cholecystokinin. Am J Physiol 241:G116, 1981.
85. Saito A, Goldfine ID, Williams JA: Characterization of receptors for cholecystokinin and related peptides in mouse cerebral cortex. J Neurochem 37:483, 1981.
86. Vidal y Plana RR, Cifarelli A, Bizzarri D: Effects of antigastrin drugs on the interaction of ^{125}I-human gastrin with rat gastric mucosa membranes. Hepato-Gastroenterol 27:41, 1980.
87. Hahne WF, Jensen RT, Lemp GF, et al: Proglumide and benzotript: Members of a different class of cholecystokinin receptor antagonists. Proc Natl Acad Sci USA 78:6304, 1981.

Chapter 8

Blood-Brain Barrier

George H. Greeley, Jr., Ph.D.

An extensive distribution of more than 25 different biologically active peptides in the gut and in the central nervous system (CNS) has been described for a wide variety of warm- and cold-blooded (vertebrates and invertebrates) species. Some of these peptides are secretin [1,2], cholecystokinin (CCK) [3–13], glucagon [14], VIP [2,14–19], somatostatin [14], peptide histidine isoleucine (PHI) [20], motilin [2], peptide YY (PYY) [21], neuropeptide Y (NPY) [22], pancreatic polypeptide (PP) [23–25], enkephalins [26], endorphins [27], thyrotropin-releasing hormone (TRH) [28], corticotropin-releasing factor (CRF) [29,30], bombesin [31], insulin [32], calcitonin gene-related peptide [33,34], growth hormone-releasing factor (GHRF) [35–37], and neurotensin [38]. Of these peptides, NPY and CCK-8 are the most abundant peptides in the CNS. For instance, the concentrations of NPY and CCK-8 in the anterior hypothalamus and cerebral cortex of the rat are approximately 1.0 nmol/g and 0.5 nmol/g, respectively.

Whether these brain-gut peptides can move freely between the blood and brain compartments across the blood-brain barrier and blood-cerebrospinal fluid (CSF) barrier has been asked ever since studies in which the peripheral administration of certain peptides resulted in central effects in humans and laboratory animals [39–42]. Although several of these brain-gut peptides have been detected in the CSF [43–50], whether these peptides gain access to the CSF from the general circulation or are released into the CSF and then into the peripheral circulation from the brain is unclear.

The systemic circulation is separated from the major compartments of the brain by the blood-brain barrier (BBB) and blood-CSF barrier. There are two possible routes for the transfer of blood-borne substances into the CNS: via the brain capillaries or via CSF. The BBB can be viewed as a screen that surrounds the brain and functions as a regulatory barrier between the systemic circulation and the brain. The brain capillary endothelial cell is the actual anatomic basis for the BBB, whereas the choroid plexus is the structural site of the blood-CSF barrier. The selective permeability of these barriers serves to control the composition and concentration of substances in the environment of the neurons, axons, and glial cells.

In order for water-soluble substances (a majority of peptides) to enter the brain, they must pass into the extracellular space of the brain or into the CSF. Although most substances can move freely between the extracellular space of the brain and the CSF (there is no barrier), they must penetrate the cerebral capillaries before they can enter the extracellular space of the brain from the systemic circulation. Cerebral capillaries, unlike extracerebral capillaries, are joined by tight junctions [51]. Tight junctions also exist between epithelial cells of the choroid plexus.

Although many essential nutrients necessary for CNS survival are transported into the CNS via specific, carrier-mediated transport systems, such systems for peptides across the BBB have not been documented. Nonetheless, many peptides appear capable of penetrating the interstitial space of the brain, especially at the circumventricular organs, which are less restrictive. The BBB may be nonexistent or weakly developed at the circumventricular organs (organum vasculosum lamina terminalis, median eminence, subfornical organ, pineal gland, area postrema), which are highly vascular beds of the brain [52]. In any case, there are numerous reports indicating that many peptides can cross the BBB [53–57].

As stated earlier, the epithelium of cerebral vessels has a low permeability to polar substances because of its intercellular junctions and an absence of pinocytosis; however, there are mechanisms for facilitated diffusion and active transport of certain solutes. Sex steroids, adrenal steroids, and thyroid hormones can diffuse through the BBB. Because peptides have a limited cerebrovascular permeability, they may enter the brain through the choroid plexus and CSF. In addition, polypeptides or peptides synthesized in the anterior pituitary may conceivably travel to the hypothalamus via the portal venous retrograde blood flow [58–60].

The observation that peptides in the systemic circulation do not penetrate the BBB with any effectiveness does not negate the possibility that peptides in the systemic circulation can affect the CNS. Many peptides appear to affect nerve terminals in the area of the circumventricular organs. Peptides can also gain access to the CSF by moving, albeit slowly, through nonspecific routes. Although the BBB is poorly permeable to large molecules, the blood-CSF barrier is more permeable to many small substances [61]. In most cases, the concentration of such substances in the blood is higher in comparison to their levels in the CSF, since they are actively transported from the CSF into the blood. The CSF-brain barrier is more permeable. Hence, substances with access to the CSF may affect tissue adjacent to the ventricular system. It is possible that a peptide or its fragment penetrates the BBB by first penetrating the CSF near the circumventricular organs. It is also possible for the BBB to be altered, at least temporarily, allowing entrance of various substances [62]. Both neural and humoral factors may temporarily modify the BBB [63]. The BBB of perinatal animals also seems less restrictive [64].

There are several methods one can use to determine whether a peptide found in the systemic circulation can be transferred from the blood into the brain. One approach is to monitor uptake of a radioactive peptide into the brain after its systemic administration. A second method is to use autoradiography, and a third is to monitor simultaneously the concentrations of the peptide in the CSF, brain, and systemic compartments by means of a specific radioimmunoassay. A fourth method uses a mathematical analysis of penetration of radioactive substances and determines permeability coefficients.

With each method, there are shortcomings. With the radioactive uptake method, one must verify whether the radioactive test substance found in the CSF or CNS is the authentic peptide that is being tested. Actually, this criticism applies to all of the methods mentioned. It is also conceivable that administration of the peptide may change the permeability of the BBB temporarily and this possibility must be examined [63].

Since most radioimmunoassays make use of an antiserum that relies on only a single or a couple of determinants of the peptide, one must verify that the radioimmunoassay is measuring the intact molecule and more importantly that one is measuring the biologically active portion of the molecule.

The method of Oldendorf [65,66] for measuring the uptake of peptides into the brain is another popular approach. Oldendorf's technique quantitates the passage of a substance from systemic blood into the brain. This technique relies on the simultaneous administration of two different isotopic substances, with a subsequent determination of their brain uptake index (BUI). The BUI uses the ratio of the radioactive substance in the CNS to that injected. Injection of a large amount of substance results in a lower ratio. This method seems to be applicable for amino acids, since their plasma levels are approximately their K_m; however, in the case of peptides, low concentrations of a peptide are needed to detect substantial transport (high BUI), and this is accomplished only by using peptides with extremely high specific activities. In addition, during a single pass, the net movement of a test substance into or out of the CNS can be difficult to predict, since its overall direction and magnitude are contingent upon its concentration in the brain and its injectate.

Rapoport et al [67] believe that the Oldendorf technique is inadequate to examine the uptake of substances whose permeability coefficients are less than 10^{-6} cm/sec. They suggest that use of the Oldendorf technique may result in the inability to detect brain uptake of certain peptides. In light of Rapoport's contention, it is worth mentioning that a bolus injection of peptide may result in little brain uptake if the peptide is degraded quickly in the liver or kidneys or if it is bound substantially to circulating proteins.

Greenberg et al [57] contend that peptides can readily penetrate the BBB. They use the intracarotid artery quick injection technique of Oldendorf [66] to determine the brain uptake index of radiolabeled peptides in comparison to ^3H_2O or ^{14}C-antipyrine as counterlabels. The normalized BUI values for ^{3}H-MIF-I, ^{3}H-2-MSH, and ^{14}C-AVP are 13.7, 9.6, and 113.0, respectively, at 15 seconds after injection, which is consistent with their having readily penetrated the BBB. The penetration of the BBB by these peptides also fits with the observation of their CNS effects.

Kruse-Larsen and Rehfeld [68] have monitored the gastrin levels in CSF and serum concurrently with a radioimmunoassay and found that the gastrin concentrations in CSF ranged from 2 to 8 pM (mean 5 pM), whereas in serum, the gastrin concentrations were 13 to 409 pM (mean 61 pM). This observation suggests that there is no correlation between serum and CSF gastrin levels and that gastrin appears to be restricted by the BBB. The same conclusion was reached independently by Cornford et al [65].

Straus et al [10] found that a number of intravenously administered peptides, including insulin, angiotensin, calcitonin, ACTH, and lactogen, undergo receptor-mediated uptake into brain tissue. However, the sites of uptake have been restricted to the circumventricular areas of the brain. Straus concluded that uptake of blood-borne peptides into cortical tissue where the blood-brain barrier is intact does not occur.

VIP, a 28 amino acid peptide, exists in both the gut and the brain. Ebeid et al [69] have studied the effect of portal systemic shunt and hepatic insufficiency on plasma levels of VIP and found a significant rise in plasma VIP during hepatic failure in humans and dogs. To ascertain whether brain VIP was similarly affected, they measured CSF levels of VIP by radioimmunoassay before and after an end-to-side portacaval shunt. The levels of VIP in the CSF did not increase significantly unless the animal became encephalopathic (grade III). They concluded that VIP does not cross the BBB. Additionally, they injected 1 μg of radiolabeled VIP intravenously into seven rats. These rats were killed 1 and 2 hours later, and their brains were compared with other organs. In contrast to a high concentration of radioactive material recovered from other organs (e.g., the lung), only background radioactivity was recovered from the brain [70], suggesting that VIP does not penetrate the BBB and that the elevated VIP levels in CSF in dogs and monkeys are of central origin.

In contrast, Kato et al [71] found that synthetic VIP, administered either intraventricularly or intravenously, caused a significant and dose-related increase in plasma prolactin levels in rats, suggesting that VIP might pass through the BBB and act on the central nervous system or that it acted directly on the anterior pituitary.

Kastin et al [55,72] found that [D-Ala^3]-delta sleep-inducing peptide can penetrate the BBB of rats. β-Endorphin can apparently penetrate the blood-cerebrospinal fluid barrier but is unable to cross into the brain [73,74] of rabbits.

Pardridge [75–81] performed numerous studies on the transport of various hormones and metabolic substrates through the BBB. In 1981, he concluded that there were two routes of penetration into the brain available for blood-borne substances: 1) lipid-mediation for lipid-soluble compounds such as steroid hormones, melatonin, or free fatty acids; and 2) carrier-mediation in the case of water-soluble compounds that have an affinity for one of nine specific transport systems located in the BBB. With regard to circulating peptides, the absence of peptide carriers in the BBB prevents the rapid distribution of peptides into the vast majority of brain interstitial or synaptic spaces. However, recent studies [82] indicate that some peptides (e.g., insulin) may bind specific receptors on the blood side of the BBB and thereby transmit messages to cells on the brain side of the BBB without the peptides' traversing the capillary wall. Moreover, direct in vitro evidence for insulin receptors on brain capillaries has recently been obtained [83].

Passaro et al [84] recently studied the appearance of ^{125}I-CCK-8 in the peripheral circulation of the rabbit after injection into the lateral ventricle and in the CSF after intravenous (IV) administration. They found that ^{125}I-CCK-8 diffused rapidly by a noncarrier-mediated mechanism into the peripheral blood after injection into the lateral bulk flow ventricle of a rabbit. In contrast, ^{125}I-CCK-8 was not observed in the CSF after IV injection. They speculated that this unidirectional transport mechanism from CSF to blood may apply to other neuropeptides as well. Peptides that are injected into the CSF can apparently pass quickly into the system circulation because of the rapid bulk flow of CSF [84]. They apparently escape the brain at the arachnoid villi. Hence, it is imperative to consider the notion that intracerebroventricular (ICV) injection is nearly equal to IV administration when examining the peripheral actions of centrally administered peptides.

Zhu et al [85] have studied the effects of IV and ICV infusion of CCK (CCK-8 SO_4 and CCK-33) and bombesin (which releases enteric CCK) on concentrations of CCK in plasma and CSF in dogs using the Fenstermacher ventriculocisternal perfusion technique [86]. They found that plasma CCK-33 concentrations increased after IV infusion of both CCK-33 and bombesin. However, the concentration of CCK-33 in the CSF increased only after direct ventricular infusion of CCK-33, but not after IV or ventricular administration of bombesin. These findings suggest that CCK-33 does not easily penetrate the BBB. In contrast to the findings of Passaro et al [84], Zhu et al also found that CCK-8 sulfate does not cross the BBB.

Lu et al [87] performed ICV infusion of CCK-8 and found a rapid elevation of peripheral pancreatic polypeptide, which was prevented by vagotomy or administration of atropine. Peripheral levels of CCK-8, CCK-33, and gastrin were unaffected. Although speculative, the disparities between the findings of Passaro et al [84] and those of Lu [87] and Zhu [85] and colleagues may be due to the fact that Passaro et al [84] used rabbits as an experimental animal, whereas Lu [87] and Zhu [85] and their colleagues used dogs. Furthermore, Passaro et al [84] used iodinated CCK-8, whereas Zhu [85] and Lu [87] and colleagues used authentic CCK-8 sulfate or CCK-33. It is conceivable that the character of CCK-8 is altered by iodination, which alters access across the CSF-blood barrier.

Morley et al [88] found that ICV administration of calcitonin potently inhibited gastric secretion in rats. Central administration of calcitonin was approximately 1000 times more potent than parenteral administration. They concluded that calcitonin exerts its effects by a direct action on the CNS. In addition, they studied the effect of ICV calcitonin on insulin and TRH-induced gastric acid secretion and found that gastric acid secretion returned to basal levels after ICV calcitonin administration. This is further evidence that calcitonin is a central inhibitor of gastric acid secretion. Morley et al [88] also found that ICV administration of calcitonin in rats inhibited the development of stress-induced ulcers.

REFERENCES

1. Charlton CG, O'Donohue TL, Miller RL, et al: Secretin in the rat hypothalamo-pituitary system: Localization, identification and characterization. Peptides 3:565, 1982.
2. Mutt V: VIP, motilin, and secretin, in Krieger DT, Brownstein MJ, Martin JB (eds): *Brain Peptides.* New York, John Wiley & Sons, 1983, pp 871–901.
3. Morley JE: Minireview. The ascent of cholecystokinin (CCK)—from gut to brain. Life Sci 30:479, 1982.
4. Loren I, Alumets J, Håkanson R, et al: Distribution of gastrin and CCK-like peptides in rat brain. Histochemistry 59:249, 1979.
5. Lamers CB, Morley JE, Poitras P, et al: Immunological and biological studies on cholecystokinin in rat brain. Am J Physiol 239:E232, 1980.
6. Dockray GJ: Immunochemical evidence of cholecystokinin-like peptides in brain. Nature 264:568, 1976.
7. Goltermann NR, Rehfeld JF, Roigaard-Petersen H: *In vivo* biosynthesis of cholecystokinin in rat cerebral cortex. J Biol Chem 255:6181, 1980.
8. Rehfeld JF, Kruse-Larsen C: Gastrin and cholecystokinin in human cerebrospinal fluid; immunochemical determination of concentrations and molecular heterogeneity. Brain Res 155:19, 1978.
9. Dockray GJ: Immunoreactive component resembling cholecystokinin octapeptide in intestine. Nature 270:359, 1977.
10. Straus E, Ryder SW, Eng J, et al: Immunochemical studies relating to cholecystokinin in brain and gut. Recent Prog Horm Res 37:447, 1981.
11. Dockray GJ: Cholecystokinin-like peptides in avian brain and gut. Experientia 35:628, 1979.
12. Beinfeld MC, Meyer DK, Eskay RL, et al: The distribution of cholecystokinin immunoreactivity in the central nervous system of the rat as determined by radioimmunoassay. Brain Res 212:51, 1981.
13. Simon-Assmann PM, Yazigi R, Greeley GH Jr, et al: Biologic and radioimmunologic activity of cholecystokinin in regions of mammalian brains. J Neurosci Res 10:165, 1983.
14. Shimatsu A, Kato Y, Matsushita N, et al: Effects of glucagon, neurotensin, and vasoactive intestinal polypeptide on somatostatin release from perifused rat hypothalamus. Endocrinology 110:2113, 1982.
15. Dockray GJ, Gregory RA: Relations between neuropeptides and gut hormones. Proc R Soc Lond 210:151, 1980.
16. Jirikowski G, Reisert I, Pilgrim C: Nerve cells immunoreactive for vasoactive intestinal polypeptide in dissociation cultures of rat hypothalamus and midbrain. Neurosci Lett 31:75, 1982.
17. Besson J, Rotsztejn W, Poussin B, et al: Release of vasoactive intestinal peptide from rat brain slices by various depolarizing agents. Neurosci Lett 28:281, 1982.
18. Triepel J: Vasoactive intestinal polypeptide (VIP) in the medulla oblongata of the guinea pig. Neurosci Lett 29:73, 1982.
19. Johansson BB, Fahrenkrug J, Wikkelsø C, et al: Vasoactive intestinal polypeptide in human cerebrospinal fluid. Front Horm Res 9:189, 1982.
20. Christofides ND, McGregor GP, Woodhams PL, et al: Ontogeny of PHI in the rat brain. Brain Res 264:359, 1983.
21. Greeley GH Jr, Partin M, Hill FLC, et al: Distribution of peptide YY in the canine alimentary canal. Gastroenterology 88:1403, 1985.
22. Allen YS, Adrian TE, Allen JM, et al: Neuropeptide Y distribution in the rat brain. Science 221:877, 1983.
23. Olschowka JA, O'Donohue TL, Jacobowitz DM: The distribution of bovine pancreatic polypeptide-like immunoreactive neurons in rat brain. Peptides 2:309, 1981.
24. Langslow DR, Kimmel JR, Pollock HG: Studies of the distribution of a new avian pancreatic polypeptide and insulin among birds, reptiles, amphibians and mammals. Endocrinology 93:558, 1973.
25. Adrian TE, Bloom SR, Bryant MG, et al: Distribution and release of human pancreatic polypeptide. Gut 17:940, 1976.
26. Polak JM, Bloom SR, Sullivan SN, et al: Enkephalin-

like immunoreactivity in the human gastrointestinal tract. Lancet 1:972, 1977.
27. Konturek SJ: Opiates and the gastrointestinal tract. Am J Gastroenterol 74:285, 1980.
28. Morley JE, Garvin TJ, Pekary AE, et al: Thyrotropin-releasing hormone in the gastrointestinal tract. Biochem Biophys Res Commun 79:314, 1977.
29. Petrusz P, Merchenthaler I, Maderdrut JL, et al: Corticotropin-releasing factor (CRF)-like immunoreactivity in the vertebrate endocrine pancreas. Proc Natl Acad Sci USA 80:1721, 1983.
30. Kruseman ACN, Linton EA, Rees LH, et al: Corticotropin-releasing factor immunoreactivity in human gastrointestinal tract. Lancet 2:1245, 1982.
31. Moody TW, O'Donohue TL, Jacobowitz DM: Biochemical localization and characterization of bombesin-like peptides in discrete regions of rat brain. Peptides 2:75, 1981.
32. Hendricks SA, Roth J, Rishi S, et al: Insulin in the nervous system, in Krieger DT, Brownstein MJ, Martin JB (eds): *Brain Peptides*. New York, John Wiley & Sons, 1983, pp 903–939.
33. Rosenfeld MG, Mermod J-J, Amara SG, et al: Production of a novel neuropeptide encoded by the calcitonin gene via tissue-specific RNA processing. Nature 304:129, 1983.
34. Gibson SJ, Polak JM, Bloom SR, et al: Calcitonin gene-related peptide immunoreactivity in the spinal cord of man and of eight other species. J Neurosci 4:3101, 1984.
35. Leidy JW Jr, Robbins RJ: Isolated rat hypothalamic cells produce authentic rat hypothalamic growth hormone releasing factors in vitro. Endocrinology 116 (Suppl):34, 1985.
36. Shibasaki T, Hotta M, Masuda A, et al: Secretion of growth hormone-releasing factor-like immunoreactivity from rat hypothalamus in vitro. Endocrinology 116 (Suppl):34, 1985.
37. Christofides ND, Stephanou A, Suzuki H, et al: Distribution of immunoreactive growth hormone-releasing hormone in the human brain and intestine and its production by tumors. J Clin Endocrinol Metab 59:747, 1984.
38. Aronin N, Carraway RE, Difiglia M, et al: Neurotensin, in Krieger DT, Brownstein MJ, Martin JB (eds): *Brain Peptides*. New York, John Wiley & Sons, 1983, p 753.
39. Olson RD, Kastin AJ, Montalbano-Smith D, et al: Neuropeptides and the blood-brain barrier in goldfish. Pharmacol Biochem Behav 9:521, 1978.
40. Kastin AJ, Olson RD, Schally AV, et al: CNS effects of peripherally administered brain peptides. Life Sci 25:401, 1979.
41. Miller LH, Groves GA, Bopp MJ, et al: A neuroheptapeptide influence on cognitive functioning in the elderly. Peptides 1:55, 1980.
42. Sandman CA, Walker BB, Lawton CA: An analog of MSH/ACTH 4-9 enhances interpersonal and environmental awareness in mentally retarded adults. Peptides 1:109, 1980.
43. Allen JP, Kendall JW, McGilvra R, et al: Immunoreactive ACTH in cerebrospinal fluid. J Clin Endocrinol Metab 38:586, 1974.
44. Yamada T, Takami MS, Gerner RH: Bombesin-like immunoreactivity in human cerebrospinal fluid. Brain Res 223:214, 1981.
45. Nutt JG, Mroz EA, Leeman SE, et al: Substance P in human cerebrospinal fluid: Reductions in peripheral neuropathy and autonomic dysfunction. Neurology 30:1280, 1980.
46. Patel YC, Rao K, Reichlin S: Somatostatin in human cerebrospinal fluid. N Engl J Med 296:529, 1977.
47. Oliver C, Charvet JP, Codaccioni JL, et al: T.R.H. in human C.S.F. Lancet 1:873, 1974.
48. Fahrenkrug J, Schaffalitzky de Muckadell OB, Fahrenkrug A: Vasoactive intestinal polypeptide (VIP) in human cerebrospinal fluid. Brain Res 124:581, 1977.
49. Nemeroff CB, Widerlov E, Bissette G, et al: Elevated concentrations of CSF corticotropin-releasing factor-like immunoreactivity in depressed patients. Science 226:1342, 1984.
50. Pavlinac DM, Lenhard LW, Parthemore JG, et al: Immunoreactive calcitonin in human cerebrospinal fluid. J Clin Endocrinol Metab 50:717, 1980.
51. Angevine JB Jr, Cotman CW: *Principles of Neuroanatomy*. New York, Oxford University Press, 1981, pp 365–366.
52. Weindl A: Neuroendocrine aspects of circumventricular organs, in Ganong WF, Martini L (eds): *Frontiers in Neuroendocrinology 1973*. New York, Oxford University Press, 1973, pp 3–25.
53. Volicer L, Loew CG: Penetration of angiotensin II into the brain. Neuropharmacology 10:631, 1971.
54. Kastin AJ, Nissen C, Schally AV, et al: Blood-brain barrier, half-time disappearance, and brain distribution for labeled enkephalin and a potent analog. Brain Res Bull 1:583, 1976.
55. Kastin AJ, Nissen C, Schally AV, et al: Additional evidence that small amounts of a peptide can cross the blood-brain barrier. Pharmacol Biochem Behav 11:717, 1979.
56. Hoffman PL, Walter R, Bulat M: An enzymatically stable peptide with activity in the central nervous system: Its penetration through the blood-CSF barrier. Brain Res 122:87, 1977.
57. Greenberg R, Whalley CE, Jourdikian F, et al: Peptides readily penetrate the blood-brain barrier: Uptake of peptides by synaptosomes is passive. Pharmacol Biochem Behav 5 (Suppl 1):151, 1976.
58. Bergland RM, Page RB: Pituitary-brain vascular relations: A new paradigm. Science 204:18, 1979.
59. Oliver C, Mical RS, Porter JC: Hypothalamic-pituitary vasculature: Evidence for retrograde blood flow in the pituitary stalk. Endocrinology 101:598, 1977.
60. Bergland RM, Davis SL, Page RB: Pituitary secretes to brain. Experiments in sheep. Lancet 2:276, 1977.
61. Brightman MW: The intracerebral movement of proteins injected into blood and cerebrospinal fluid of mice. Prog Brain Res 29:19, 1968.
62. Sankar R, Domer FR, Kastin AJ: Selective effects of

α-MSH and MIF-1 on the blood-brain barrier. Peptides 2:345, 1981.

63. Long JB, Holaday JW: Blood-brain barrier: Endogenous modulation by adrenal-cortical function. Science 227:1580, 1985.
64. Braun LD, Cornford EM, Oldendorf WH: Newborn rabbit blood-brain barrier is selectively permeable and differs substantially from the adult. J Neurochem 34:147, 1980.
65. Cornford EM, Braun LD, Crane PD, et al: Blood-brain barrier restriction of peptides and the low uptake of enkephalins. Endocrinology 103:1297, 1978.
66. Oldendorf WH: Brain uptake of radiolabeled amino acids, amines, and hexoses after arterial injection. Am J Physiol 221:1629, 1971.
67. Rapoport SI, Klee WA, Pettigrew KD, et al: Entry of opioid peptides into the central nervous system. Science 207:84, 1980.
68. Kruse-Larsen C, Rehfeld JF: Gastrin in human cerebrospinal fluid: Lack of correlation with serum concentrations. Brain Res 176:189, 1979.
69. Ebeid AM, Soeters PB, Fischer JE: The effect of portal systemic shunt and hepatic insufficiency on plasma levels of vasoactive intestinal peptide. Gastroenterology 70:A100/958, 1976.
70. Ebeid AM, Smith A, Escourrou J, et al: Increased immunoreactive vasoactive intestinal peptide in the cerebro-spinal fluid (CSF) of dogs and monkeys in hepatic failure. J Surg Res 25:538, 1978.
71. Kato Y, Iwasaki Y, Iwasaki J, et al: Prolactin release by vasoactive intestinal polypeptide in rats. Endocrinology 103:554, 1978.
72. Kastin AJ, Nissen C, Coy DH: Permeability of blood-brain barrier to DSIP peptides. Pharmacol Biochem Behav 15:955, 1981.
73. Merin M, Hollt V, Przewłocki R, et al: Low permeation of systemically administered human β-endorphin into rabbit brain measured by radioimmunoassays differentiating human and rabbit β-endorphin. Life Sci 27:281, 1980.
74. Houghten RA, Swann RW, Li CH: β-endorphin: Stability, clearance behavior, and entry into the central nervous system after intravenous injection of the tritiated peptide in rats and rabbits. Proc Natl Acad Sci USA 77:4588, 1980.
75. Pardridge WM, Mietus LJ: Transport of steroid hormones through the rat blood-brain barrier. J Clin Invest 64:145, 1979.
76. Pardridge WM, Mietus LJ: Transport of albumin-bound melatonin through the blood-brain barrier. J Neurochem 34:1761, 1980.
77. Pardridge WM, Mietus LJ: Palmitate and cholesterol transport through the blood-brain barrier. J Neurochem 34:463, 1980.
78. Pardridge WM, Oldendorf WH: Transport of metabolic substrates through the blood-brain barrier. J Neurochem 28:5, 1977.
79. Pardridge WM: Carrier-mediated transport of thyroid hormones through the rat blood-brain barrier: Primary role of albumin-bound hormone. Endocrinology 105:605, 1979.
80. Pardridge WM, Cornford EM, Braun LD, et al: Transport of choline and choline analogues through the blood-brain barrier, in Barbeau A, Growdon JH, Wurtman RJ (eds): *Nutrition and The Brain.* New York, Raven Press, 1979, pp 25–33.
81. Pardridge WM: Transport of nutrients and hormones through the blood-brain barrier. Diabetologia 20:246, 1981.
82. van Houten M, Posner BI: Insulin binds to brain blood vessels *in vivo.* Nature 282:623, 1979.
83. Haskell JF, Meezan E, Pillion DJ: Identification of the insulin receptor of cerebral microvessels. Am J Physiol 248:E115, 1985.
84. Passaro E Jr, Debas H, Oldendorf W, et al: Rapid appearance of intraventricularly administered neuropeptides in the peripheral circulation. Brain Res 241:335, 1982.
85. Zhu X-G, Greeley GH Jr, Lewis BG, et al: Blood-CSF barrier to CCK and effect of centrally-administered bombesin on release of brain CCK. J Neurosci Res 15:393, 1986.
86. Fenstermacher JD: Ventriculocisternal perfusion as a technique for studying transport and metabolism within the brain, in Marks N, Rodnight R (eds): *Research Methods in Neurochemistry.* New York, Plenum Press, 1972, pp 165–178.
87. Lu Q-H, Greeley GH Jr, Zhu X-G, et al: Intracerebroventricular administration of cholecystokinin-8 elevates plasma pancreatic polypeptide levels in awake dogs. Endocrinology 114:2415, 1984.
88. Morley JE, Levine AS, Silvis SE: Intraventricular calcitonin inhibits gastric acid secretion. Science 214:671, 1981.

Chapter 9

Actions of Gut Peptides

James C. Thompson, M.D., and others

The three chief endocrine effects of regulatory peptides of the gut involve secretion, motility, and growth. Peptides may stimulate or inhibit these actions. They may work together to achieve synergy in either stimulation or inhibition. Although gut hormones may affect secretion in the liver, small bowel, and colon, we have chosen as models for consideration the effect of gastrointestinal hormones on gastric and pancreatic secretion. Although motor actions outside the abdomen may be influenced by some gut peptides (VIP, for example, has strong actions on respiratory and vascular smooth muscle), we have limited our discussion on motility to the gut and biliary tree. A summary of the trophic actions of gastrointestinal hormones on the gut and pancreas concludes this segment.

GASTRIC SECRETION

R. Daniel Beauchamp, M.D., and James C. Thompson, M.D.

The normal flow and ebb of acid gastric secretion after a meal provide clear evidence of regulatory mechanisms that are designed to initiate and later curtail gastric secretion. These mechanisms involve the regulatory peptides of the gut. We will provide a summary of the morphologic and physiologic bases for gastric secretion as well as a summary of the role of gut peptides in the stimulation and inhibition of gastric secretion.

Structure and Function of Gastric Glandular Mucosa

Several cell types are found in the glandular mucosa of mammals. The surface of the glandular stomach is lined by a simple columnar epithelium of surface mucous cells. On the surface of the mucosa are found numerous tubular invaginations, the gastric pits (also called foveolas or crypts), which empty the gastric gland (Fig 9-1).

Surface mucous cells and mucous neck cells are found lining the gastric pits. The chief components of the gastric glands are parietal cells (oxyntic cells), which produce and secrete hydrochloric acid and intrinsic factor, and chief cells, which secrete pepsinogen. Less numerous in the gastric gland are enteroendocrine (or argentaffin) cells, which may be part of the so-called APUD system (if such a system exists). These cells contain various endocrine or paracrine polypeptides, and little is known of their true physiologic function (Fig 9-2). Mast cells are also found in the gastric glands [1]. These cells store heparin, histamine, and other vasoactive substances. In the antral glands are also found gastrin cells (G cells), which synthesize, store, and secrete gastrin.

The most remarkable aspect of gastric secretion is the ability of parietal cells to concentrate hydrogen ions more than one million times. Pure parietal cell secretion contains between 150–170 meq/L of H^+, between 165–170 meq/L of chloride, 7 meq/L of potassium, and is free of sodium [2,3].

Grossman has suggested that the parietal cells are probably directly stimulated by at least five chemical agents: acetylcholine, gastrin, entero-oxyntin (the proposed intestinal phase hormone), amino acids, and histamine [4,5]. Conversely, nonparietal gastric secretion is virtually identical to extracellular fluid. Acid concentration within the lumen of the stomach and duodenum is, therefore, dependent upon the admixture of parietal and nonparietal secretions [6].

On a molecular level, cAMP and calcium appear to have important roles in the stimulation of acid secretion by the parietal cells. Roth and Ivy [7] demonstrated in 1944 that caffeine increases gastric acid secretion in mammals. Theophylline is

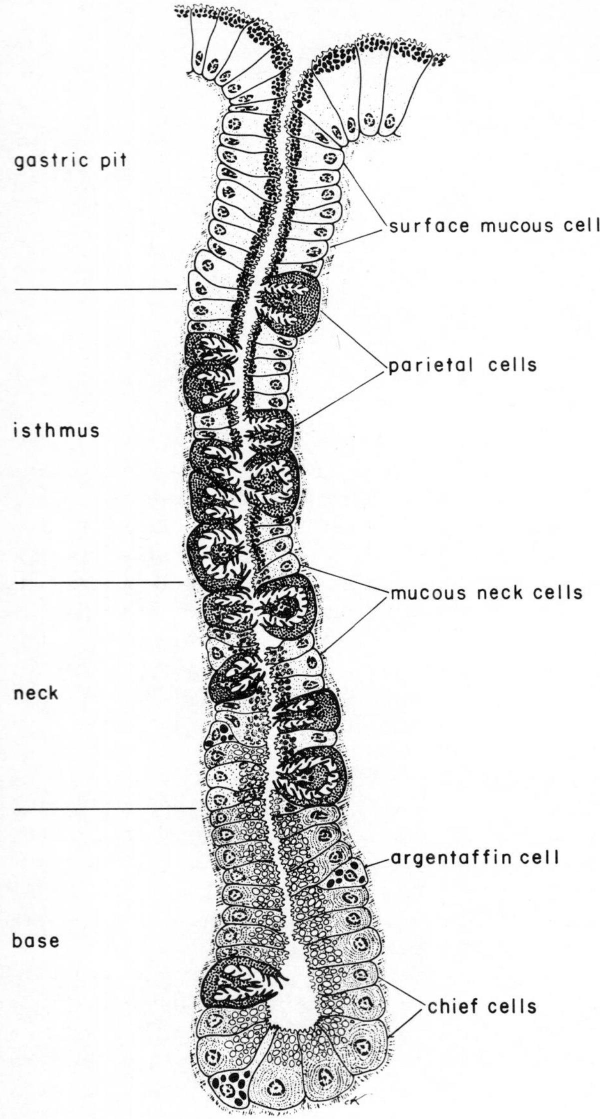

GASTRIC GLAND

Figure 9-1. Diagram of a gastric gland from fundic mucosa. (By permission of S Ito and RJ Winchester, J Cell Biol 16:541, 1983.)

another xanthine derivative that inhibits phosphodiesterase activity and therefore causes an increase in tissue cAMP. Fromm et al [8] have shown that cAMP, dibutyryl cAMP, and theophylline can all increase acid secretion from isolated rabbit fundic mucosa.

Cyclic AMP appears to act as a secondary messenger in histamine-stimulated acid secretion from frog gastric mucosa [9]. Histamine has also been found to stimulate cAMP production in isolated mammalian parietal cells [10]. The evidence for direct stimulation of the parietal cell by histamine includes changes in oxygen consumption, aminopyrine accumulation, and morphologic transformation [11,12].

There is clear evidence, however, that increases in cAMP are not always necessary for acid secretion. Ekblad et al [13] demonstrated that tissue concentrations of cAMP in isolated piglet gastric mucosa initially rose but then fell after 30 minutes in the presence of histamine, despite continued acid secretion. They concluded that cAMP may be necessary for the initiation of acid secretion but not for its continuation.

Cholinergic stimulation of acid secretion is not associated with a rise in cAMP levels in isolated parietal cells but is dependent on the presence of extracellular calcium [14]. Cholinergic stimulation modifies plasma membrane calcium permeability, and the resulting increase in cytosolic calcium enhances acid secretion. Dibutyryl cAMP-mediated acid secretion, however, is independent of medium calcium content [13].

Isolated frog gastric mucosa as well as isolated mammalian gastric glands are heavily dependent upon the presence of calcium in the serosal solution [15,16]. We have shown that exogenous calcium can stimulate gastrin release and gastric acid secretion in cats [17] and in humans [18]. Gastrin is also dependent upon extracellular calcium for its in vitro secretagogue effect but simultaneously has a requirement for either histamine or a phosphodiesterase inhibitor for its activity [19].

Components of Gastric Secretion

Acid Secretion

It has been known that gastric juice contains hydrochloric acid since Prout reported his findings in 1822 [quoted in 19]. These findings were greatly expanded by the classic studies of Beaumont [20] on the fur trapper Alexis St. Martin.

Gastric parietal cells secrete hydrogen ions in a concentration that is more than a million times that of serum. This parietal cell secretion is regulated by chemical messengers that are released in response to a variety of stimuli and are capable of acting directly upon the parietal cell to cause acid secretion.

Gastric secretion may be spontaneous (basal or interdigestive) or it may be stimulated (prandial). Basal secretion is a small fraction of maximal acid

CELLTYPE	LOCALIZATION	SECRETION GRANULES (size in nm)	AMINES	PEPTIDES
EC_n	Stomach (Small intestine)	200	Serotonin	?
ECL	Stomach	450	Histamine Serotonin ?	?
G	Stomach (Duodenum) (Pancreas)	300	Tryptamine? Dopamine?	Gastrin ACTH-and Lipotropin-related peptides ?
D	Stomach Small intestine Pancreas	350		Somatostatin Met-Enkephalin ? Gastrin (Pancreas) ?
D 1 (H)	Stomach Small intestine Large intestine Pancreas	160		VIP
A	Pancreas (Stomach) (Small intestine?)	250		Glucagon, Glicentin Pancreas Glucagon, GLI-1 CCK-PZ?(Endorphin)
X (AL)	Stomach (Small intestine) (Large intestine) (Pancreas)	300		?
PP (F)	Pancreas (Stomach) (Small intestine) (Large intestine)	180		Pancreatic Polypeptide Met-Enkephalin ?
P	Stomach Small intestine (Pancreas)	120	?	Bombesin ?

Figure 9-2. Enteroendocrine cells. (Compiled by Grube and Forssman, Horm Metab Res 11:603, 1979). Only those cell types found in the gastric mucosa (and elsewhere) have been selected. The cell type nomenclature is the currently accepted terminology. Secretion granule size and ultrastructural characteristics as well as their content of amines and peptides are also indicated.

output. It is about 10 percent of maximal capacity in humans [21] but less than 1 percent in dogs [5].

Stimulated gastric secretion is a complex occurrence that is conventionally divided into three phases: cephalic, gastric, and intestinal (Fig 9-3). Pavlov, in 1902, observed that food stimulation of gastric secretion could be brought about by sham feeding or by introduction of food into the stomach [22]. Later it was found that intestinal stimuli can also cause acid secretion, as will be discussed later in the chapter.

Grossman and Konturek [23] suggested that parietal cells do not secrete with maximal efficiency unless all receptors are occupied. It is thought that for maximal acid secretion to occur, all receptors must be occupied by their respective secretagogues; however, in the face of blockade of one receptor, some acid secretion may still occur. This theory, though unproven, is helpful in explaining why vagotomy and H_2-receptor antagonists (cimetidine and ranitidine) work. Vagotomy removes vagal acetylcholine and the receptor antagonists block histamine from its receptor. The histamine receptor is clearly the most important, because when it is blocked, acid output is nearly abolished (see Fig 9-3).

Cephalic Phase. The cephalic phase of gastric acid secretion is stimulated by the sight, smell, or chewing of palatable food. This action stimulates the vagal nuclei in the medulla, which initiate impulses via the peripheral vagi, some of which terminate in the gastric mucosa, causing acid release. The cephalic phase probably contributes one third to one half of the stimulatory response to a meal in humans [24]. Feldman and Richardson [25] have shown in normal humans that gastric acid secretion and serum gastrin levels are increased by merely discussing appetizing food. The sight or smell of food and the combination of sight and smell also stimulate gastric acid secretion and

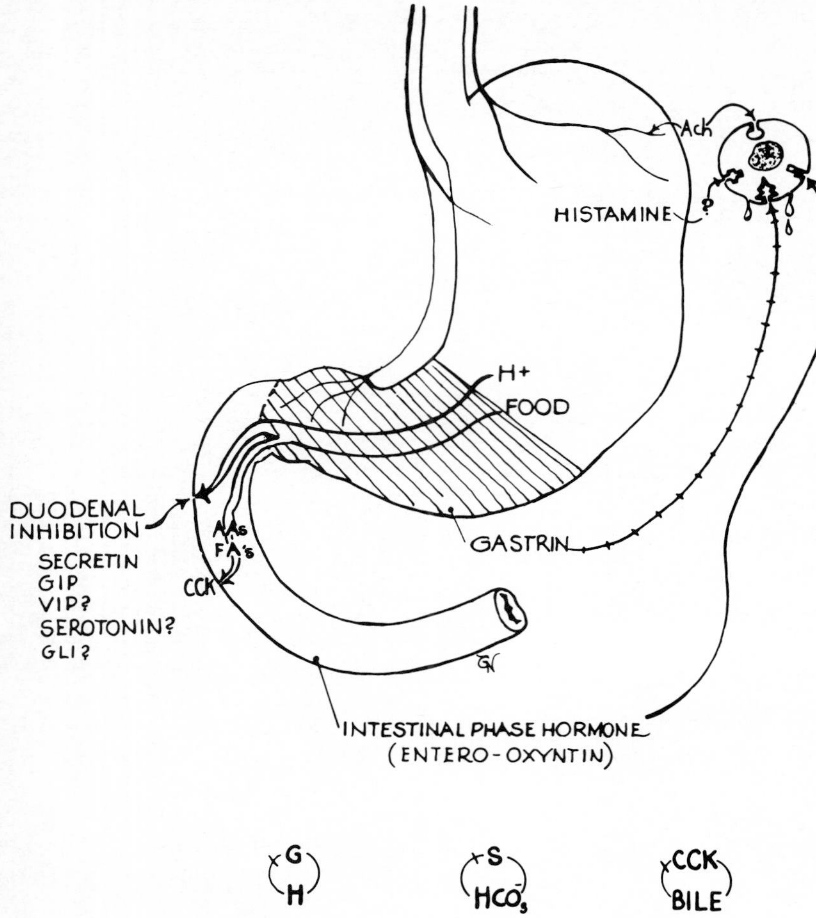

Figure 9-3. Schematic summary of some of the neurohumoral events that occur when a meal is eaten. Acetylcholine (ACh) is released from vagal nerve endings. Histamine is apparently released from stores within the mucosa. Gastrin is released by food (by a mechanism that is pH-sensitive) from antral mucosa (shaded area). Food in the small bowel stimulates release of the intestinal phase hormone. Each stimulant acts on the parietal cell (perhaps, as shown, each by means of a separate receptor on the cell membrane) to stimulate secretion of H^+. Delivery of acidified chyme into the duodenum evokes a series of events (some probably reflex, some humoral) that inhibit further gastric secretion. Some of the agents involved are listed. Amino acids (AAs) and fatty acids (FAs) (from partially digested food) cause release of CCK. Three feedback mechanisms, which act to halt hormone release, are shown diagramatically across the bottom as typical endocrine closed-loop relationships: acid (H^+) halts release of gastrin (G), HCO_3^- halts release of secretin (S), and intraduodenal bile appears to halt the release of CCK (Gomez G, et al: Bile inhibits release of cholecystokinin and neurotensin. Surgery, in press). (From Thompson [88], by permission of WB Saunders Co)

gastrin release. The acid secretion in response to discussing food was 66 percent of the response to modified sham feeding, and the responses to sight and smell were 23 to 46 percent of the response to sham feeding.

Sham feeding is a method for studying the cephalic phase of gastric secretion. In dogs with innervated antral pouches, the response of the main stomach to sham feeding was equal to the maximal response to exogenous gastrin [26]. Sham feeding in humans results in approximately 40 percent of the maximal acid response to exogenous pentagastrin [27]. Modified sham feeding or the "chew and spit" method has resulted in gastric acid secretion of 55–65 percent of the maximal response to pentagastrin [28,29].

The mechanism of vagally induced gastric secretion appears to be via direct stimulation of the parietal cell as well as possible stimulation of gastrin release [30]. The major mediator of the vagal stimulatory effect is acetylcholine. Specific muscarinic receptors have been detected on the parietal cell [31]. Atropine abolishes acid secretion in response to sham feeding in the dog [32]; however, in humans neither atropine nor pirenzepine (a peripheral muscarinic antagonist) can completely inhibit the gastric secretory response to modified sham feeding, even when given in large near-toxic doses [33].

What, then, are the additional mediators of acid secretion in response to modified sham feeding in humans? There is evidence that paracrine histamine release from gastric mucosal mast cells may be responsible for a portion of the cephalic phase of acid secretion. Histamine-(H_2) antagonists alone greatly reduce the acid response to modified sham feeding, and combined with pirenzepine, they completely abolish the acid secretion to modified sham feeding response [34]. Other candidates for comediators of the cephalic phase of gastric acid secretion are bombesin [35,36], enkephalin, substance P, and gastrin [37], all of which may have a concerted effect on physiologic acid secretion.

Gastric Phase. The gastric phase of gastric secretion is stimulated by food in the stomach. The degree of physical distention of the stomach and the chemical composition of the meal are the determinants of acid response to a meal. The major gastric stimulant of gastric secretion is gastrin (see Chapter 14). Gastrin is released by vagal stimulation, contact with food (especially amino acids), and calcium and alcohol. Release of gastrin is in dynamic equilibrium; it is released by these stimulants and release is later curtailed by antral acidification [38]. There is clear evidence that the vagus carries both stimulatory and inhibitory impulses for gastrin release. This evidence is summarized later in this chapter (Inhibition of Gastric Secretion).

Distention of the stomach with inert aqueous solutions causes acid secretion. In humans, gastric distention results in acid secretion that is approximately one third the maximal response to a meal [39–41]. In dogs, distention of the whole stomach stimulates moderate rates of acid secretion by mechanisms that do not primarily involve release of gastrin [6].

Fundic distention stimulates secretion through vagovagal and intramural cholinergic reflexes [42]. In dogs, graded distention of a vagally innervated antral pouch causes graded increases in gastrin levels and gastric acid secretion from an innervated gastric fistula. The release of gastrin can be completely abolished if distention is carried out with an acidified solution (100 mM HCl); however, the acid secretory response is only partially decreased. Vagal denervation of the antrum abolishes the acid secretory response caused by its distention. This has been called the pyloro-oxyntic reflex [43].

Separate distention of the fundic or antral portions of the stomach increases gastric acid secretion in humans [42,44]. A later study, however, found that antral distention decreases gastrin secretion in healthy subjects and concluded that gastrin does not participate in human distention-mediated effects [45].

There is evidence that a long (vagovagal) reflex as well as short (intramural) pathways are activated by gastric distention [1,5]. In humans, proximal gastric vagotomy reduces the acid response to fundic distention by 50 percent, whereas atropine inhibits the response to fundic [46] as well as total gastric distention by 80 percent [47]. In the dog, Grossman found that distention of the neurally intact antrectomized stomach causes an increase in acid secretion that is probably mediated by the vagovagal reflex [48]. Furthermore, vagally denervated Heidenhain pouch distention yields slight stimulation of acid secretion. When this was performed in the presence of exogenous histamine or gastrin, there was a marked augmentation of acid secretion. Grossman postulated that this was caused by a local intramural reflex [5] (Table 9-1).

Another component of the gastric phase of acid secretion may be released by chemical stimulation. Commonly ingested chemical substances known to stimulate acid secretion are caffeine, alcohol, calcium, and protein digestive products.

Caffeine and other xanthine derivatives, such as theophylline, can stimulate gastric acid secretion [7,8,49]. These compounds inhibit the phosphodiesterase-mediated breakdown of cAMP.

Daves et al [50] found that ethanol stimulates gastric acid secretion both by a direct effect on the

Table 9-1. **Distention-induced gastric reflexes for gastrin release and acid secretion in the dog**

Part distended	*Vagi*	*Path*	*Target*	*Product*	*Effect of vagotomy*
Oxyntic gland area	Intact	Vagovagal	Parietal cell	Acid	Decreased
				Gastrin	Abolished
			G cell		
	Cut	Intramural	Parietal cell	Acid	
			Parietal cell	Acid	Abolished
Pyloric gland area	Intact	Vagovagal	G cell	Gastrin	Decreased
	Cut	Intramural	G cell	Gastrin	

Data from Grossman MI [5].

parietal cells and by gastrin release. However, Cooke [51] found that intragastrically infused ethanol solutions of 8–16 percent caused no greater amount of acid secretion or gastrin release than water infusion in humans. More recently, a study was conducted in humans in which intragastrically infused solutions of 5, 10, and 20 percent ethanol were compared to equicaloric and equimolar control solutions. The 5 and 10 percent ethanol solutions stimulated significantly greater gastric acid secretion than control solutions or water. Serum gastrin levels were unchanged. In the same study, white wine or bourbon caused an increase in gastric acid secretion stimulated by a liquid protein meal, while white wine alone significantly increased gastrin levels [52].

In humans, oral calcium carbonate causes a significant increase in serum gastrin when compared to oral sodium bicarbonate [53], and it stimulates gastric acid secretion [54]. A recent study of healthy volunteers and duodenal ulcer patients confirmed that intragastric calcium increases secretion of gastric acid. The ulcer patients appeared to be more sensitive to this effect. Gastrin levels also increased; however, the correlation between acid secretion and circulating gastrin levels was weak [55].

Chemical properties of food contribute to gastric acid secretion. Protein breakdown products are responsible for the chemical stimulus of acid secretion [56]. Peptides and amino acids cause gastrin release and may also directly stimulate the oxyntic gland area [57].

Feldman et al [58] demonstrated in humans that the increase in plasma gastrin that occurs during intragastric amino acid administration can account for the observed increase in acid secretion. Exogenously administered gastrin G-17 at dosages that gave the same plasma levels obtained from an amino acid meal caused similar acid secretion. Strong correlation between incremental serum gastrin changes and gastric acid secretion in response to a peptone meal stimulation was shown by Lam et al [59] in another study in humans.

Tryptophan and phenylalanine are the two most potent individual amino acid stimulants of gastric acid secretion as well as of gastrin release in humans [60]. Amino acids can apparently stimulate parietal cells directly without mediation of gastrin. Debas and Grossman [57] and Konturek et al [61] have reported that application of amino acids directly to the fundic mucosa of the Heidenhain pouch in the dog causes an increase in acid secretion without a change in gastrin levels. Some doubt has been cast upon these studies because of the possibility that solutions at high pH may cause passage of CO_2 from the blood into the intragastric lumen. Much of the titratable acidity that accumulates in the Heidenhain pouch as a result of high pH protein solution is apparently carbonic acid [5,62].

Additional evidence that amino acids act independently of gastrin to cause acid secretion is available. Intravenous infusion of L-amino acids in both dogs and humans stimulates secretion of gastric acid without causing significant change in gastrin levels [63–66].

The presence of food in the stomach also appears to contribute to acid secretion by a buffering action. When the antral pH is elevated, gastrin release is facilitated by buffering the feedback inhibition of antral acidification.

Intestinal Phase. There is clear evidence that various stimuli applied within the small bowel can cause gastric acid secretion. Instillation of protein, amino acids, or acid into the proximal jejunum and distention of the jejunum can cause gastric acid secretion from the denervated gastric pouch of a dog [67].

Duodenal perfusion with peptide or amino acid solutions in humans or animals produces an increase in gastric acid secretion that is 30–40 percent of peak acid secretion [68–70]. There is strong evidence that absorbed amino acids account for much of the increase in acid secretion that results from intestinal exposure to peptide or amino acid solutions. Intravenous L-amino acids cause an increase in gastric acid secretion in the innervated as well as the denervated dog stomach [71]. In humans, intravenous infusion of phenylalanine and tryptophan significantly stimulated gastric acid secretion to about 50 percent of the response to intragastric peptone, whereas alanine and histidine had no effect. This effect was independent of gastrin elevation [72].

In dogs with portacaval transposition, intravenous L-amino acid mixtures caused a dose-dependent increase in gastric acid secretion from the innervated stomach. The response was greater when amino acids were given into the peripheral circulation than when given into the hepatic circulation. This is probably due to the hepatic uptake of the amino acids [64].

Orloff et al [73] have shown that identical increases in dog Heidenhain pouch gastric acid secretion occurred in response to mixed L-amino acids administered intrajejunally or via the portal vein. Elevations of plasma amino nitrogen were also similar. Again, peripherally administered IV amino acids caused the most secretion of acid. In dogs with portacaval shunts, intrajejunal amino acid infusion caused the same increase in acid secretion as occurred from peripheral IV infusion. Orloff et al [73,74] have shown that portacaval shunting results in increased gastric acid secretory response in humans and in dogs.

Distention of the small intestine also causes an increase in gastric acid secretion [70]. While a substantial portion of the intestinal phase of gastric acid secretion can be accounted for by absorbed amino acids, the response to distention should at least suggest that a hormone is involved. Grossman proposed the name "entero-oxyntin" for the intestinal phase hormonal secretagogue [75]. Evidence for and against a separate intestinal phase hormone is reviewed in Chapter 26.

Other Humoral Stimulants. Other hormones or hormone candidates have stimulatory effects on gastric acid secretion. Cholecystokinin (CCK) has a C-terminal pentapeptide identical to that of gastrin. CCK administered alone is a stimulant of gastric acid secretion. In the presence of gastrin, however, it acts as a competitive inhibitor of acid secretion [76].

Bombesin is a polypeptide isolated from the skin of frogs and is a potent stimulant of gastrin release and gastric acid secretion. Bombesin-like immunoreactivity has been demonstrated in the mammalian stomach and duodenum [77], where it is called gastrin-releasing peptide (GRP). The true physiologic role for GRP is not known at this time, but it does fulfill the function of a local releasing agent (or "on" switch) for most gut hormones.

Enkephalins are peptides with opiate-like actions that have been demonstrated to have a stimulatory effect on gastric acid secretion in dogs and an inhibitory effect in humans [78–80]. High concentrations of enkephalin-like immunoreactivity were found in the antral mucosa and lesser amounts in the proximal small intestine of humans [81]. Naloxone infusion reduces basal acid secretion and secretory response to a meal in humans but has no effect on serum gastrin levels [82].

Inhibition of Gastric Acid Secretion

Multiple inhibitory factors are also involved in the regulation of gastric acid secretion. The physiologic significance of most of these inhibitory substances is not yet clear. Most of the substances to be mentioned are covered in detail in other parts of this book (see Index). Once a meal has been eaten, cephalic stimulation is removed and therefore vagal activity is decreased. There is evidence, however, that the vagus itself has a mixed stimulatory and inhibitory effect upon gastrin-stimulated gastric acid secretion. In dogs with Heidenhain pouches, sham feeding causes an inhibition of gastrin-stimulated acid secretion [26]. This inhibition by sham feeding was abolished by either truncal vagotomy or resection of the antrum and duodenal bulb [83,84]. This appears to be a humorally mediated event, and the inhibitory substance has been referred to as vagogastrone by Grossman et al [75].

Debas [85] has postulated the presence of a powerful inhibitor of acid secretion and of gastrin release that originates from the mucosa of the proximal stomach. He has recently summarized the supporting evidence for this phenomenon. Release of this inhibitor appears to be dependent upon intact vagal innervation of the proximal stomach. We have shown that after a selective proximal vagotomy patients have an increased gastrin release during a standard meal, which suggests that the innervated fundic portion of the stomach normally inhibits gastrin release [86].

Rising concentrations of inhibitory factors as well as declining levels of stimulants are responsible for the decreasing gastric secretion after the first postprandial hour. Gastric phase stimulation decreases as gastric distention declines when gastric contents move into the intestine. Acidification of the antrum has been clearly demonstrated to suppress gastrin release [87]. Diminution of gastrin release may occur with an antral pH as high as 5, and at about pH 1.5 there is no release of gastrin [88].

Somatostatin is a 14 amino acid polypeptide found in the stomach that has inhibitory actions upon gastric secretions and may participate in the gastric as well as intestinally mediated inhibition of gastric acid secretion. Bloom et al [89] have shown that somatostatin inhibits fasting and stimulates levels of gastrin release and acid secretion.

Somatostatin appears to have a direct inhibitory effect on the parietal cell, as it has been shown to cause a sharp decrease in gastric acid output in response to a meal, to pentagastrin, or to histamine [90]. In conscious cats, somatostatin inhibits pentagastrin but not histamine-stimulated acid and pepsin secretion and delays the occurrence of tachyphylaxis to pentagastrin. Conversely, metiamide, an H_2-antagonist, did not delay tachyphylaxis but inhibited gastric acid secretion due to histamine and pentagastrin. This suggests that somatostatin occupies or modifies the gastrin receptors on parietal cells, thereby delaying tachyphylaxis [91].

Further evidence of direct inhibition of parietal cells by somatostatin was recently furnished by Short et al [92]. When antisomatostatin antibodies were infused with pentagastrin into the isolated perfused rat stomach, there was a 32 percent increase of acid secretion over pentagastrin stimulation alone, without an increase over basal gastrin release into the perfusate. Antisomatostatin antibodies perfused in the absence of pentagastrin significantly increased basal gastrin release but not acid output.

In humans, plasma somatostatin levels have been shown to increase in response to a meal and to duodenal acidification. The concentrations obtained are sufficient to cause inhibition of gastric acid secretion when somatostatin is given exogenously [93–95]. Recently, high affinity, specific somatostatin binding sites were described in the mucosa of the rabbit and human fundus [96]. As with GRP, the true physiologic role of somatostatin in gastric secretion is unknown, but it does fulfill the function of a local suppressor agent (or "off" switch) regarding the release of most gut hormones.

Prostaglandins may also have a role in the gastric phase of inhibition of acid secretion. Exogenous prostaglandins, PGE_1 and PGE_2, cause inhibition of gastric acid secretion [97,98] and prevent ulcer formation [97] in the rat stomach. Prostaglandins also inhibit acid secretion from the denervated Heidenhain pouch and from the innervated Pavlov pouch of dogs [99–101]. PGE_1 inhibits gastrin- and histamine-stimulated acid production but fails to inhibit cAMP-stimulated secretion in frog gastric mucosa [102]. Soll [103] found that PGE_2 and PGI also inhibit histamine-stimulated aminopyrine accumulation in isolated canine mucosa. Aspirin and indomethacin treatment enhance gastric acid secretion, possibly by reducing endogenous prostaglandins [104,105].

Konturek et al [106], however, found that the exogenous PGE_2 analogue (15-R-15-methyl PGE_2) caused a reduction in modified sham feeding-induced acid and pepsin secretion; however, aspirin treatment sufficient to reduce mucosal PGE_2 generation by 90 percent failed to alter the acid or pepsin response to modified sham feeding.

As food moves into the small intestine, additional inhibitory mechanisms come into play. Inhibition of gastric acid secretion has been demonstrated by the introduction of acid, fat [22], and hyperosmolar solutions [107] into the small intestine. Acid instilled into the duodenum causes dose-dependent increases in pancreatic bicarbonate secretion and dose-dependent inhibition of gastric acid secretion [108]. In dogs, instillation of hydrochloric acid into the distal duodenum causes a decrease in portal venous concentrations of gastrin [109] as well as inhibition of gastric acid secretion. Simultaneously, there is a marked increase in pancreatic volume and bicarbonate secretion. When the acid is confined to the duodenal bulb and not allowed to come into contact with the distal duodenum, gastric acid secretion is still inhibited; however, there is no change in pancreatic secretion [110–112]. These studies suggest two distinct inhibitory mechanisms. Secretin has been suggested as being partially responsible for the gastric acid inhibition and pancreatic stimulation observed with duodenal acidification beyond the duodenal bulb. The other agent has been named bulbogastrone by Andersson [112], but there is scant current evidence in support of it. The effect may be due to somatostatin or to more than one agent (see below).

Serotonin, or 5-hydroxytryptamine, is a vasoactive amine secreted into the portal circulation. This compound is released from the duodenal mucosa in response to acidification. Peripheral as well as portal concentrations of serotonin are raised after duodenal acidification. The rise in serotonin levels has been correlated with suppression of acid secretion from innervated but not denervated dog gastric pouches [113].

Mate et al [114] from our laboratory demonstrated that secretin and serotonin have additive inhibitory effects on pentagastrin-stimulated gastric acid secretion. Methysergide, a serotonin antagonist, abolished the inhibitory effect of secretin on gastric acid secretion, and it reversed the inhibitory action of intraduodenal acidification on pentagastrin-induced gastric acid secretion. Since duodenal acidification causes measurable release of both secretin [115–118] and serotonin [113], the interaction of these two agents could explain the bulbogastrone effect.

Pavlov, in the late 19th century [22], found that ingested fat inhibits gastric secretion. Kosaka and Lim [119] reported that IV or subcutaneous administration of extracts of segments of small and large intestinal mucosa that had been exposed to olive oil-inhibited meat-stimulated gastric acid secretion in dogs with Heidenhain pouches. Intraduodenal instillation of fat preparations has been shown to inhibit meal-stimulated gastric acid and enzyme secretion in humans [120]. Bile acids, along with lipase emulsification of the fats, were demonstrated to be important to the mechanism of gastric inhibition by fats in the rat [121]. Johnson and Grossman [122] found evidence for an enterogastrone distinct from secretin or CCK. The inhibitory effect of enterogastrone appears to be independent of vagal innervation in the dog [123].

Others have since confirmed that fat, in an absorbable form, introduced into the small intestine causes inhibition of gastric acid secretion [110,119]. The inhibition of acid secretion by fats seems to involve more than one humoral mechanism. Gastric inhibitory polypeptide (GIP) is a candidate for part of this effect. Circulating levels of GIP show a biphasic response to food with an initial peak stimulated by glucose and a late plateau that occurs in response to fat [124]. Exogenously administered GIP is a potent inhibitor of gastrin-stimulated acid secretion in the Heidenhain pouch [125], and it suppresses food-stimulated gastric acid secretion and gastrin release [126].

GIP is a relatively weak inhibitor of gastrin-stimulated acid secretion from an innervated gastric fistula [127,128]. The powerful inhibitory action exerted by GIP on the denervated Heidenhain pouch is abolished by a cholinergic background infusion with bethanechol [128]. Additionally, intestinal fat inhibits secretion from the innervated gastric fistula more effectively than from the Heidenhain pouch. This suggests that GIP is of secondary importance in the inhibition of gastric acid secretion in the intact animal [127].

Neurotensin is another possible mediator of the gastric inhibitory action of intraintestinal fat. Neurotensin is a 13 amino acid polypeptide found largely in the jejunum and ileum in rats [129] and dogs [130]. Fat ingestion is the most potent stimulus for neurotensin release in humans [131].

In humans, exogenously administered neurotensin at doses that give plasma levels comparable to those obtained from a fatty meal causes significant inhibition of acid secretion without a change in gastrin levels [132,133]. This inhibitory effect was reportedly abolished by vagotomy [134]. However, Mate et al (unpublished data) recently found that if the postvagotomy PG dose is adjusted so that it gives an acid secretion equivalent to that prior to vagotomy, then neurotensin still inhibits gastric acid secretion. They also found that indomethacin treatment abolished this inhibitory effect of neurotensin, indicating that it is mediated by prostaglandins.

Intravenously administered fat (Lipomul) inhibits amino acid stimulated gastric acid secretion in humans [135], and IV as well as intrajejunal intralipid causes significant inhibition of pentagastrin-stimulated gastric acid secretion [136]. Only intrajejunally administered intralipid, however, caused a rise in plasma neurotensin-like immunoreactivity. Baume et al [137] had previously found that IV fat emulsion caused a dose-related inhibition of gastric acid secretion in the rat. The gastric acid response caused by fat seems to involve intestinal as well as postabsorptive mechanisms in humans, but Walker et al [138] found no inhibition of amino acid-stimulated gastric acid secretion by IV fat in dogs.

Hyperosmolar solutions of sugar, salts, and peptone inhibit gastric acid secretion when introduced into the small intestine. Ingested food has been shown to reach the duodenum in a hyperosmolar state, and stimulation of duodenal osmoreceptors inhibits gastric acid secretion and gastrin release [107]. The mechanism appears to be humorally mediated, at least in part, because it still operates when extrinsic nerves between the intestine and stomach have been severed [110].

Other endogenous compounds, neurotransmitters, or polypeptide hormones have been shown to have inhibitory actions on gastric secretion when administered exogenously; their physiologic significance is even less clear. Catecholamines can inhibit gastric acid secretion by both α- and β-adrenergic mechanisms. Both $\beta 1$- and $\beta 2$-adrenoceptors seem to mediate inhibition of pentagastrin-induced secretion, while α-adrenoceptors reduce histamine-induced secretion [139]. Vasoactive intestinal peptide (VIP) is a potent inhibitor of histamine- and gastrin-stimulated acid secretion, but its physiologic role is not known [77]. Glucagon is a 29 amino acid polypeptide that inhibits both gastric acid secretion and gastrin release [140].

Peptide YY (PYY), first isolated in porcine intestine and found to be structurally related to pancreatic polypeptide (PP) [141,142], has been shown to be a potent inhibitor of pentagastrin-stimulated gastric acid secretion in dogs [143–145]; this action is independent of cholinergic pathways [146]. PYY also inhibits pentagastrin-stimulated gastric acid and pepsin secretion in humans at doses that had no effect on secretin- and CCK-8-stimulated pancreatic and biliary secretions. Those effects were seen at doses that caused elevations of plasma PYY similar to concentrations seen after food ingestion [147].

Calcitonin is a potent inhibitor of vagal- and pentagastrin-stimulated gastric secretion in normal human subjects [148] as well as in peptic ulcer patients [149] and in cats [17].

Calcitonin gene-related peptide (CGRP) is a 37 amino acid polypeptide that has been detected in neural fibers in the CNS as well as throughout the peripheral nervous system, including the gastrointestinal tract [150]. Exogenously administered CGRP has a potent inhibitory effect on stimulated gastric acid secretion in both the rat and the dog [151], and Kraenzlin et al [152] found that CGRP infusion in humans resulted in significant inhibition of basal acid and pepsin gastric secretion.

Urogastrone, a polypeptide found in human urine, is similar to epidermal growth factor (EGF), first obtained from the submaxillary glands of mice [153]. Urogastrone appears to be identical to human EGF [154]. This polypeptide is a potent inhibitor of gastric acid secretion and intrinsic factor secretion, whether stimulated by pentagastrin, histamine, or insulin, but it does not significantly alter gastrin levels [155]. A recent study has shown that EGF, when applied to the luminal side, acts directly on guinea pig gastric mucosa to inhibit histamine- and cAMP-stimulated acid secretion [156]. Nerve growth factor had no effect on this model.

Nerve growth factor (NGF) inhibits pentagastrin-stimulated acid secretion and food-stimulated gastrin release in dogs [157]. It also protects isolated gastric mucosa from taurocholate-induced injury [158].

The humoral influences (stimulatory and inhibitory) on gastric secretion have been reviewed [76] and are summarized in Figure 9-4.

Pepsinogen Secretion

Pepsin is the principal digestive enzyme of the stomach. It is formed by the proteolytic cleavage of the zymogen pepsinogen; this cleavage occurs in an acid environment below pH 5. Pepsinogen is produced in the chief cells of the gastric gland and is stored in zymogen granules.

Pepsinogen release appears to be under hormonal control similar to that for acid secretion. Histamine and pentagastrin both cause prolonged secretion of gastric acid and pepsinogen in dogs with Heidenhain pouches or gastric fistulas [159]. Vagal stimulation, cholinergic agents, and calcium also increase secretion of pepsinogen [160].

Pepsinogen secretion can be stimulated by duodenal infusion of acid at pH levels between 6.5 and 2.5, but acid concentrations below pH 2.5 cause an inhibition of pepsinogen response to food or insulin [161]. Secretin infusion also causes an

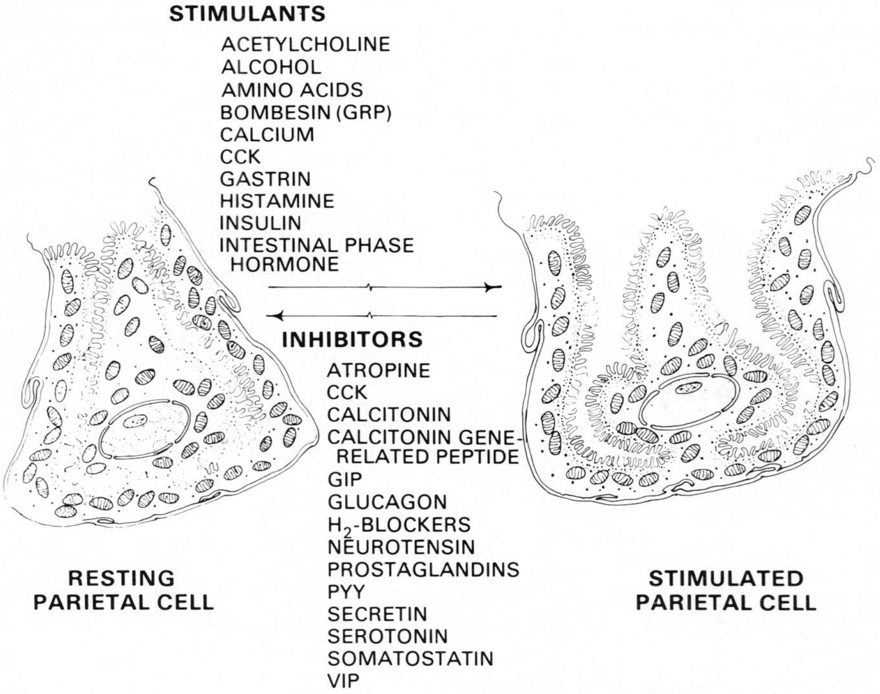

Figure 9-4. Agents that directly or indirectly stimulate or inhibit H^+ secretion from the parietal cell. CCK acting alone stimulates acid secretion; in the presence of gastrin (which is almost always the case under physiologic conditions), it is an inhibitor.

increase in pepsinogen secretion [162,163]. Entry of acid into the intestine is an important mechanism of stimulation of pepsinogen secretion. Infusion of pentagastrin at rates that produce maximal acid secretion causes no increase in pepsin secretion when the acid is prevented from entering the duodenum. Re-establishment of acid flow into the duodenum results in pepsin release [164].

Motilin, a polypeptide isolated from hog duodenal mucosa, stimulates pepsin output but not acid secretion [165]. Vagne et al [166] have reported a peptide fraction that has been isolated from hog intestine, is distinct from CCK, secretin, and motilin, and causes pepsin secretion with little effect on acid secretion.

Fat in the intestine inhibits gastric pepsin output in vagally intact and vagotomized dogs [167]. Other inhibitors of pepsinogen secretion include somatostatin [168] and prostaglandins and magnesium [160].

Bicarbonate Secretion

In 1948, Obrink [169] demonstrated the presence of bicarbonate in the gastric lumen when sodium thiocyanate was used to block acid secretion. He attributed this effect to leakage of bicarbonate across the gastric epithelial barrier. Subsequent studies have shown that blockage of acid secretion by sodium thiocyanate or by histamine H_2-receptor antagonists causes no leakage of bicarbonate into the gastric lumen and confirmed that there is, indeed, a small volume of alkaline secretion into the gastric lumen in vitro as well as in vivo in the guinea pig, dog, and human [170–174]. Immunocytochemical techniques have demonstrated high carbonic anhydrase activity in the guinea pig gastric mucosal parietal cells, surface mucous cells, and mucous neck cells [175]. The role of bicarbonate secretion is probably to protect the gastric mucosa against damage from hydrogen ions by forming an alkaline pH gradient across the mucous layer overlying the gastric epithelium [176].

Acetylcholine causes an increase in mucosal cGMP as well as alkaline secretion in the anesthetized dog fundic mucosa [177]. Isolated amphibian gastric mucosa demonstrated marked stimulation of alkaline secretion by carbachol and cGMP [170].

Prostaglandins appear to play an important role in bicarbonate secretion. Nonsteroidal anti-inflammatory drugs inhibit alkaline secretion in isolated amphibian mucosa and in mammalian mucosa in vivo [174,177–181]. Calcium also enhances bicarbonate secretion [182]. Alkaline secretion is not altered by cAMP, histamine, pentagastrin, CCK, secretin, or GIP [170,182,183]. The α-adrenergic agonist, norepinephrine, inhibits alkaline secretion, but isoprenaline, a β-agonist, had no effect [182].

The physiologic importance of gastric bicarbonate is not fully established. A recent study supports the concept that intraluminal bicarbonate serves a protective role [184]. Closed sacs of isolated frog gastric mucosa were readily ulcerated when exposed to exogenous hydrochloric acid and pepsin in Ringer's lactate solution without bicarbonate but were protected when bicarbonate was present in the Ringer's solution. Intracellular pH was higher when bicarbonate was present.

Mucus Secretion

Gastric mucus provides lubrication and also protection for the gastric epithelium. The organic components of mucous gel are glycoprotein (60–70 percent) and free protein (30 percent). These provide a mucous gel with a pH gradient for neutralization of gastric acid by bicarbonate secreted from the epithelium. This also inhibits pepsin acid digestion of the epithelium [185]. Further details of the structure of mucus are discussed elsewhere [186].

Zalewsky and Moody [187] observed that mucus is released by three mechanisms: exocytosis, apical expulsion, and cell exfoliation. Of these, exocytosis appears to be the most important. The thickness of the mucous gel layer depends upon the balance between the secretory rate and the rate of erosion by acid pepsin and intraluminal food.

Histamine also stimulates synthesis of mucus in the stomach of the cat [188,189], and cholinergic stimuli have been shown to increase mucus output [190].

Duodenal acidification increases gastric mucus production and is probably a secretin-mediated effect [188,191]. Secretin stimulates gastric mucus secretion in humans [192]. Exogenous somatostatin increases mucus output in humans [189]. CCK also stimulates mucus secretion and has additive effects with secretin [193].

Topical and parenteral PGE_2 stimulates mucus output in the rat, canine, and human stomachs [194]. An increase in the thickness of mucous gel is observed after topical treatment with 16,16-dimethyl-PGE_2 [195]. Interference with endogenous prostaglandin synthesis by aspirin decreases the thickness of the gel layer [196] and decreases the glycoprotein content of gastric juice [197]. Inhibition of protein synthesis in gastric mucosal tissues has been shown with aspirin [198].

Interference with the production of mucus,

along with alteration of acid and bicarbonate secretion, renders gastric mucosa more susceptible to ulceration.

Intrinsic Factor

Intrinsic factor is a polypeptide that binds and facilitates uptake of cyanocobalamin (vitamin B_{12}). Absence of intrinsic factor can lead to pernicious anemia. Intrinsic factor is secreted by parietal cells and like acid secretion is stimulated by histamine, pentagastrin, and cholinergic agents in vivo and inhibited by cimetidine [199]. A little understood aspect of intrinsic factor secretion is that it is secreted in amounts far in excess of that necessary to promote physiologic absorption of cyanocobalamin [199]. In rats, intrinsic factors seems to be produced and released from the chief cells. Carbachol is the most effective stimulant of intrinsic factor release in vitro from rat mucosal cells, a response that is inhibited by atropine and pirenzepine but not by prostaglandin E_2 or somatostatin [200]. Although release of intrinsic factor appears to be controlled by some of the regulatory mechanisms that mediate acid secretion, in other ways the regulation of its secretion appears to be distinct from that of pepsin and acid.

REFERENCES

1. Soll AH, Lewin K, Beaven MA: Isolation of histamine-containing cells from canine fundic mucosa. Gastroenterology 77:1283, 1979.
2. Hollander F: Gastric secretion of electrolytes. Fed Proc 11:706, 1952.
3. Hollander F: The significance of sodium and potassium in gastric secretion. A review of the problem. Gastroenterology 40:477, 1961.
4. Grossman MI: The chemicals that activate the "on" switches of the oxyntic cell. Mayo Clin Proc 50:515, 1975.
5. Grossman MI: Regulation of gastric acid secretion, in Johnson LR (ed): *Physiology of the Gastrointestinal Tract.* New York, Raven Press, 1981, pp 659–672.
6. Makhlouf GM, McManus JPA, Card WI: A quantitative statement of the two-component hypothesis of gastric secretion. Gastroenterology 51:149, 1966.
7. Roth JA, Ivy AC: The effect of caffeine upon gastric secretion in the dog, cat and man. Am J Physiol 141:1553, 1944.
8. Fromm D, Schwartz JH, Quijano R: Effects of cyclic adenosine 3′:5′-monophosphate and related agents on acid secretion by isolated rabbit gastric mucosa. Gastroenterology 69:453, 1975.
9. Harris JB, Nigon K, Alonso D: Adenosine-3,5′-monophosphate: Intracellular mediator for methyl xanthine stimulation of gastric secretion. Gastroenterology 57:377, 1969.
10. Wollin A, Soll AH, Samloff IM: Actions of histamine, secretin, and PGE_2 on cyclic AMP production by isolated canine fundic mucosal cells. Am J Physiol 237:E437, 1979.
11. Berglindh T, Helander HF, Obrink KJ: Effects of secretagogues on oxygen consumption, aminopyrine accumulation and morphology in isolated gastric glands. Acta Physiol Scand 97:401, 1976.
12. Soll AH: Physiology of isolated canine parietal cells: Receptors and effectors regulating function, in Johnson LR (ed): *Physiology of the Gastrointestinal Tract.* New York, Raven Press, 1981, pp 673–691.
13. Ekblad EBM, Machen TE, Licko V, et al: Histamine, cyclic AMP and the secretory response of piglet gastric mucosa. Acta Physiol Scand Suppl:69, 1978.
14. Berglindh T, Sachs G, Takeguchi N: Ca^{2+}-dependent secretagogue stimulation in isolated rabbit gastric glands. Am J Physiol 239:G90, 1980.
15. Jacobson A, Schwartz M, Rehm WS: Effects of removal of calcium from bathing media on frog stomach. Am J Physiol 209:134, 1965.
16. Berglindh T: Absolute dependence on chloride for acid secretion in isolated gastric glands. Gastroenterology 73:874, 1977.
17. Becker HD, Konturek SJ, Reeder DD, et al: Effect of calcium and calcitonin on gastrin and gastric secretion in cats. Am J Physiol 225:277, 1973.
18. Reeder DD, Becker HD, Thompson JC: Effect of intravenously administered calcium on serum gastrin and gastric secretion in man. Surg Gynecol Obstet 138:847, 1974.
19. Dick JA: The control of gastric secretion. Br J Hosp Med July:28, 1983.
20. Beaumont W: *Experiments and Observations on the Gastric Juice and the Physiology of Digestion.* Plattsburgh, NY, 1833.
21. Wormsley KG, Grossman MI: Maximal histalog test in control subjects and patients with peptic ulcer. Gut 6:427, 1965.
22. Pavlov JP: *The Work of The Digestive Glands.* Translated into English by WH Thompson. London, Charles Griffin & Co Ltd, 1902.
23. Grossman MI, Konturek SJ: Inhibition of acid secretion in dog by metiamide, a histamine antagonist acting on H_2 receptors. Gastroenterology 66:517, 1974.
24. Malagelada J-R: Gastric, pancreatic and biliary responses to a meal, in Johnson LR (ed): *Physiology of the Gastrointestinal Tract.* New York, Raven Press, 1981, pp 893–924.
25. Feldman M, Richardson CT: Role of thought, sight, smell, and taste of food in the cephalic phase of gastric acid secretion in humans. Gastroenterology 90:428, 1986.
26. Preshaw RM: Gastric acid output after sham feeding and during release or infusion of gastrin. Am J Physiol 219:1409, 1970.
27. Feldman M, Richardson CT, Fordtran JS: Effect of sham feeding on gastric acid secretion in healthy subjects and duodenal ulcer patients: Evidence for increased basal vagal tone in some ulcer patients. Gastroenterology 79:796, 1980.
28. Knutson U, Olbe L, Ganguli PC: Gastric acid and

plasma gastrin responses to sham feeding in duodenal ulcer patients before and after resection of antrum and duodenal bulb. Scand J Gastroenterol 9:351, 1974.

29. Konturek SJ, Kwiecien N, Obtulowicz W, et al: Cephalic phase of gastric secretion in healthy subjects and duodenal ulcer patients: Role of vagal innervation. Gut 20:875, 1978.
30. Smith CL, Kewenter J, Connell AM, et al: Control factors in the release of gastrin by direct electrical stimulation of the vagus. Am J Dig Dis 20:13, 1975.
31. Ecknauer R, Thompson WJ, Johnson LR, et al: Isolated parietal cells: [^{3}H]QNB binding to putative cholinergic receptors. Am J Physiol 239:G204, 1980.
32. Nilsson G, Simon J, Yalow RS, et al: Plasma gastrin and gastric acid responses to sham feeding and feeding in dogs. Gastroenterology 63:51, 1972.
33. Konturek SJ, Obtulowicz W, Kwiecien N, et al: Effects of pirenzepine and atropine on gastric secretory and plasma hormonal responses to sham-feeding in patients with duodenal ulcer. Scand J Gastroenterol 15 (Suppl 66):63, 1980.
34. Konturek SJ, Obtulowicz W, Kwiecien N, et al: Comparison of ranitidine and cimetidine in the inhibition of histamine, sham-feeding, and meal-induced gastric secretion in duodenal ulcer patients. Gut 21:181, 1980.
35. Grossman MI: Vagal stimulation and inhibition of acid secretion and gastrin release: Which aspects are cholinergic? in Rehfeld JF, Amdrup E (eds): *Gastrin and Vagus*. New York, Academic Press, 1979, pp 105–113.
36. Polak JM, Hobbs S, Bloom SR, et al: Distribution of a bombesin-like peptide in human gastrointestinal tract. Lancet 1:1109, 1976.
37. Konturek SJ: Cholinergic control of gastric acid secretion in man. Scand J Gastroenterol (Suppl) 72:1, 1982.
38. Jackson BM, Reeder DD, Thompson JC: Dynamic characteristics of gastrin release. Am J Surg 123:137, 1972.
39. Hunt JN, MacDonald I: The relation between the volume of a test-meal and the gastric secretory response. J Physiol 117:289, 1952.
40. Cooke AR: Potentiation of acid output in man by a distention stimulus. Gastroenterology 58:633, 1970.
41. Richardson CT, Walsh JH, Cooper KA, et al: Studies on the role of cephalic-vagal stimulation in the acid secretory response to eating in normal human subjects. J Clin Invest 60:435, 1977.
42. Grotzinger U, Bergegardh S, Olbe L: Effect of fundic distension on gastric acid secretion in man. Gut 18:105, 1977.
43. Debas HT, Konturek SJ, Walsh JH, et al: Proof of a pyloro-oxyntic reflex for stimulation of acid secretion. Gastroenterology 66:526, 1974.
44. Bergegardh S, Olbe L: Gastric acid response to antrum distension in man. Scand J Gastroenterol 10:171, 1975.
45. Schoon I-M, Bergegardh S, Grotzinger U, et al: Evidence for a defective inhibition of pentagastrin-stimulated gastric acid secretion by antral distension in the duodenal ulcer patient. Gastroenterology 75:363, 1978.
46. Schoon IM, Olbe L: Inhibitory effect of cimetidine on gastric acid secretion vagally activated by physiological means in duodenal ulcer patients. Gut 19:27, 1978.
47. Schiller LR, Walsh JH, Feldman M: Distention-induced gastrin release. Effects of luminal acidification and intravenous atropine. Gastroenterology 78:912, 1976.
48. Grossman MI: Secretion of acid and pepsin in response to distention of vagally innervated fundic gland area in dogs. Gastroenterology 42:718, 1962.
49. Cano R, Isenberg JI, Grossman MI: Cimetidine inhibits caffeine-stimulated gastric acid secretion in man. Gastroenterology 70:1055, 1976.
50. Daves IA, Miller JH, Lemmi CAE, et al: Mechanism and inhibition of alcohol-stimulated gastric secretion. Surg Forum 16:305, 1965.
51. Cooke AR: Ethanol and gastric function. Gastroenterology 62:501, 1972 (Letter).
52. Lenz HJ, Ferrari-Taylor J, Isenberg JI: Wine and five percent ethanol are potent stimulants of gastric acid secretion in humans. Gastroenterology 85:1082, 1983.
53. Reeder D, Conlee JL, Thompson JC: Changes in gastric secretion and serum gastrin concentration in duodenal ulcer patients after oral calcium antacid, in Demling L (ed): *Gastrointestinal Hormones*. Stuttgart, Georg Thieme Verlag, 1972, pp 19–22.
54. Levant JA, Walsh JH, Isenberg JI: Stimulation of gastric secretion and gastrin release by single oral doses of calcium carbonate in man. N Engl J Med 289:555, 1973.
55. Barclay G, Maxwell V, Grossman MI, et al: Effects of graded amounts of intragastric calcium on acid secretion, gastrin release, and gastric emptying in normal and duodenal ulcer subjects. Dig Dis Sci 28:385, 1983.
56. Richardson CT, Walsh JH, Hicks MI, et al: Studies on the mechanisms of food-stimulated gastric acid secretion in normal human subjects. J Clin Invest 58:623, 1976.
57. Debas HT, Grossman MI: Chemicals bathing the oxyntic gland area stimulate acid secretion in dog. Gastroenterology 69:654, 1975.
58. Feldman M, Walsh JH, Wong HC, et al: Role of gastrin heptadecapeptide in the acid secretory response to amino acids in man. J Clin Invest 61:308, 1978.
59. Lam SK, Isenberg JI, Grossman MI, et al: Gastric acid secretion is abnormally sensitive to endogenous gastrin released after peptone test meals in duodenal ulcer patients. J Clin Invest 65:555, 1980.
60. Byrne WJ, Christie DL, Ament ME, et al: Acid secretory response in man to 18 individual amino acids. Clin Res 25:108A, 1977.
61. Konturek SJ, Tasler J, Obtulowicz W, et al: Comparison of amino acids bathing the oxyntic gland area

in the stimulation of gastric secretion. Gastroenterology 70:66, 1976.
62. Spenney JG: Physical chemical and technical limitations to intragastric titration. Gastroenterology 76:1025, 1979.
63. Schafmayer A, Teichmann RK, Rayford PL, et al: Effect of parenteral L-amino acids on gastric secretion and serum gastrin in normal dogs and dogs with portacaval transposition. Surgery 85:191, 1979.
64. Landor JH, Ipapo VS: Gastric secretory effect of amino acids given enterally and parenterally in dogs. Gastroenterology 73:781, 1977.
65. Chatamra K, Pigott HWS, MacNaughton JI, et al: The effect of intravenous Aminoplex 5 on serum gastrin and gastric secretion. Postgrad Med J 51:1, 1975.
66. Isenberg JI, Maxwell V: Intravenous infusion of amino acids stimulates gastric acid secretion in man. N Engl J Med 298:27, 1978.
67. Thompson JC, Peskin GW: The intestinal phase of gastric secretion. Am J Med Sci 241:159, 1961.
68. Isenberg JI, Ippoliti AF, Maxwell VL: Perfusion of the proximal small intestine with peptone stimulates gastric acid secretion in man. Gastroenterology 73:746, 1977.
69. Konturek SJ, Kwiecien N, Obtulowicz W, et al: Intestinal phase of gastric secretion in patients with duodenal ulcer. Gut 19:321, 1978.
70. Konturek SJ, Radecki T, Kwiecien N: Stimuli for intestinal phase of gastric secretion in dogs. Am J Physiol 234:E64, 1978.
71. Mariano EC, Landor JH: Gastric secretory response to intravenous amino acids in eviscerated dogs. Arch Surg 113:611, 1978.
72. McArthur KE, Isenberg JI, Hogan DL, et al: Intravenous infusion of L-isomers of phenylalanine and tryptophan stimulate gastric acid secretion at physiologic plasma concentrations in normal subjects and after parietal cell vagotomy. J Clin Invest 71:1254, 1983.
73. Orloff MJ, Villar-Valdes H, Rosen H, et al: Humoral mediation of the intestinal phase of gastric secretion and of acid hypersecretion associated with portacaval shunts. Surgery 66:118, 1969.
74. Orloff MJ, Abbott AG, Rosen H: Nature of the humoral agent responsible for portacaval shunt-related gastric hypersecretion in man. Am J Surg 120:237, 1970.
75. Grossman MI, and others: Candidate hormones of the gut. Gastroenterology 67:730, 1974.
76. Thompson JC: Hormonal influences on gastric secretion, in Rob C (ed): *Advances in Surgery*. Chicago, Year Book Medical Publishers, 1978, pp 53–83.
77. Rayford PL, Miller TA, Thompson JC: Secretin, cholecystokinin and newer gastrointestinal hormones. N Engl J Med 294:1093, 1157, 1976.
78. Konturek SJ, Tasler J, Cieszkowski M, et al: Comparison of methionine-enkephalin and morphine in the stimulation of gastric acid secretion in the dog. Gastroenterology 78:294, 1980.
79. Konturek SJ, Pawlik W, Walus KM, et al: Methionine-enkephalin stimulates gastric secretion and gastric mucosal blood flow. Proc Soc Exp Biol Med 158:156, 1978.
80. Konturek SJ, Kwiecien N, Obtulowicz W, et al: Effect of enkephalin and naloxone on gastric acid and serum gastrin and pancreatic polypeptide concentrations in humans. Gut 24:740, 1983.
81. Polak JM, Bloom SR, Sullivan SN, et al: Enkephalin-like immunoreactivity in the human gastrointestinal tract. Lancet 1:972, 1977.
82. Feldman M, Walsh JH, Taylor IL: Effect of naloxone and morphine on gastric acid secretion and on serum gastrin and pancreatic polypeptide concentrations in humans. Gastroenterology 79:294, 1980.
83. Sjodin L: Inhibition of gastrin-stimulated canine acid secretion by sham feeding. Scand J Gastroenterol 10:73, 1975.
84. Sjodin L, Andersson S: Effect of resection of antrum and duodenal bulb on sham-feeding-induced inhibition of canine gastric secretion. Scand J Gastroenterol 12:43, 1977.
85. Debas HT: Proximal gastric vagotomy interferes with a fundic inhibitory mechanism. A hypothesis for the high recurrence rate of peptic ulceration. Am J Surg 146:51, 1983.
86. Thompson JC, Lowder WS, Peurifoy JT, et al: Effect of selective proximal vagotomy and truncal vagotomy on gastric acid and serum gastrin responses to a meal in duodenal ulcer patients. Ann Surg 188:431, 1978.
87. Woodward ER: The role of the gastric antrum in the regulation of gastric secretion. Gastroenterology 38:7, 1960.
88. Thompson JC: The stomach and duodenum, in Sabiston DC Jr (ed): *Christopher's Textbook of Surgery* (13 Ed). Philadelphia, WB Saunders Co, 1986, pp 810–874.
89. Bloom SR, Mortimer CH, Thorner MO, et al: Inhibition of gastrin and gastric-acid secretion by growth-hormone release-inhibiting hormone. Lancet 2:1106, 1974.
90. Barros D'Sa AA, Bloom SR, Baron JH: Direct inhibition of gastric acid by growth-hormone release-inhibiting hormone in dogs. Lancet 1:886, 1975.
91. Albinus M, Blair EL, Hirst BH, et al: The effects of somatostatin and metiamide on tachyphylaxis of pentagastrin stimulated gastric acid and pepsin secretion in the conscious cat. J Physiol 266:801, 1977.
92. Short GM, Doyle JW, Wolfe MM: Effect of antibodies to somatostatin on acid secretion and gastrin release by the isolated perfused rat stomach. Gastroenterology 88:984, 1985.
93. Colturi TJ, Unger RH, Peters M, et al: Physiologic role for circulating somatostatin in gastric secretion in man. Gastroenterology 84:1129, 1983.
94. Bottcher W, Yamada T, Kauffman GL: Somatostatin is an enterogastrone. Gastroenterology 84:1112, 1983.

95. Colturi TJ, Unger RH, Feldman M: Role of circulating somatostatin in regulation of gastric acid secretion, gastrin release, and islet cell function. Studies in healthy subjects and duodenal ulcer patients. J Clin Invest 74:417, 1984.
96. Guijarro LG, Arilla E, Lopez-Ruiz MP, et al: Somatostatin binding sites in cytosolic fraction isolated from rabbit antral and fundic gastric mucosa. Regul Pept 10:207, 1985.
97. Robert A, Nezamis JE, Phillips JP: Effect of prostaglandin E_1 on gastric secretion and ulcer formation in the rat. Gastroenterology 55:481, 1968.
98. Ramwell PW, Shaw JE: Prostaglandin inhibition of gastric secretion. J Physiol 195:34, 1968.
99. Becker HD, Reeder DD, Thompson JC: The effect of prostaglandin E_1 on the release of gastrin and gastric secretion on dogs. Endocrinology 93:1148, 1973.
100. Robert A, Nezamis JE, Phillips JP: Inhibition of gastric secretion by prostaglandins. Am J Dig Dis 12:1073, 1967.
101. Conolly ME, Bieck PR, Payne NA, et al: Effect of the prostaglandin precursor, arachidonic acid, on histamine stimulated gastric secretion in the conscious dog, and observations on the effect of inhibiting endogenous prostaglandin synthesis. Gut 18:429, 1977.
102. Way L, Durbin RP: Inhibition of gastric acid secretion *in vitro* by prostaglandin E_1. Nature 221:874, 1969.
103. Soll AH: Specific inhibition by prostaglandins E_2 and I_2 of histamine-stimulated [^{14}C] aminopyrine accumulation and cyclic adenosine monophosphate generation by isolated canine parietal cells. J Clin Invest 65:1222, 1980.
104. Levine RA, Schwartzel EH: Effect of indomethacin on basal and histamine stimulated human gastric acid secretion. Gut 25:718, 1984.
105. Hunt JN, Smith JL, Jiang CL, et al: Effect of synthetic prostaglandin E_1 analog on aspirin-induced gastric bleeding and secretion. Dig Dis Sci 28:897, 1983.
106. Konturek SJ, Kwiecien N, Obtulowicz W, et al: Prostaglandins and vagal stimulation of gastric secretion in duodenal ulcer patients. Scand J Gastroenterol 18:43, 1983.
107. Teichmann RK, Swierczek JS, Rayford PL, et al: Effect of duodenal osmolality on gastrin and secretin release and on gastric and pancreatic secretion. World J Surg 3:623, 1979.
108. Johnson LR, Grossman MI: Characteristics of inhibition of gastric secretion by secretin. Am J Physiol 217:1401, 1969.
109. Becker HD, Reeder DD, Thompson JC: Physiologic mechanisms of duodenal feedback inhibition of gastric secretion. Surg Forum 25:412, 1974.
110. Andersson S: Gastric and duodenal mechanisms inhibiting gastric secretion of acid, in Code CF (ed): *Handbook of Physiology*. Baltimore, Williams & Wilkins Co, 1967, pp 865–878.
111. Windsor CWO, Cockel R, Lee MJR: Inhibition of gastric secretion in man by intestinal fat infusion. Gut 10:135, 1969.
112. Andersson S: Bulbogastrone, in Thompson JC (ed): *Gastrointestinal Hormones*. Austin, University of Texas Press, 1975, pp 555–562.
113. Jaffe BM, Kopen DF, Lazan DW: Endogenous serotonin in the control of gastric acid secretion. Surgery 82:156, 1977.
114. Mate L, Sakamoto T, Greeley GH Jr, et al: Regulation of gastric acid secretion by secretin and serotonin. Am J Surg 149:40, 1985.
115. Miyata M, Rayford PL, Thompson JC: Hormonal (gastrin, secretin, cholecystokinin) and secretory effects of bombesin and duodenal acidification in dogs. Surgery 89:209, 1980.
116. Chey WY, Kim MS, Lee KY, et al: Secretin is an enterogastrone in the dog. Am J Physiol 240:G239, 1981.
117. Fahrenkrug J, Schaffalitzky de Muckadell OB: Plasma secretin concentration in man: Effect of intraduodenal glucose, fat, amino acids, ethanol, HCl, or ingestion of a meal. Eur J Clin Invest 7:201, 1977.
118. O'Connor FA, Buchanan KD, Connon JJ, et al: Secretin and insulin: Response to intraduodenal acid. Diabetologia 12:145, 1976.
119. Kosaka T, Lim RKS: Demonstration of the humoral agent in fat inhibition of gastric secretion. Proc Soc Exp Biol Med 27:890, 1930.
120. Shay H, Gershon-Cohen J, Fels SS: The role of the upper small intestine in the control of gastric secretion; the effect of neutral fat, fatty acid, and soaps; the phase of gastric secretion influenced and the relative importance of the psychic and chemical phases. Ann Intern Med 13:294, 1939.
121. Menguy R: Studies on the role of pancreatic and biliary secretions in the mechanism of gastric inhibition by fat. Surgery 48:195, 1960.
122. Johnson LR, Grossman MI: Effects of fat, secretin, and cholecystokinin on histamine-stimulated gastric secretion. Am J Physiol 216:1176, 1969.
123. Halvorson HC, Middleton MD, Bibler DD Jr, et al: Influence of the vagus nerve on the inhibitory effect of fat in the duodenum. Am J Dig Dis 11:911, 1966.
124. Brown JC, Dryburgh JR, Moccia P, et al: The current status of GIP, in Thompson JC (ed): *Gastrointestinal Hormones*. Austin, University of Texas Press, 1975, pp 537–547.
125. Pederson RA, Brown JC: Inhibition of histamine-, pentagastrin-, and insulin-stimulated canine gastric secretion by pure "gastric inhibitory polypeptide." Gastroenterology 62:393, 1972.
126. Villar HV, Fender HR, Rayford PL, et al: Suppression of gastrin release and gastric secretion by gastric inhibitory polypeptide (GIP) and vasoactive intestinal polypeptide (VIP). Ann Surg 184:97, 1976.
127. Debas HT, Yamagishi T: Gastric inhibitory polypeptide (GIP) is not the primary mediator of the enterogastrone action of fat. Gastroenterology 74:1118, 1978.
128. Soon-Shiong P, Debas HT, Brown JC: Bethanechol

prevents inhibition of gastric acid secretion by gastric inhibitory polypeptide. Am J Physiol 247:G171, 1984.

129. Carraway R, Leeman SE: Characterization of radioimmunoassayable neurotensin in the rat. Its differential distribution in the central nervous system, small intestine, and stomach. J Biol Chem 251:7045, 1976.

130. Doyle H, Greeley GH Jr, Mate L, et al: Distribution of neurotensin in the canine gastrointestinal tract. Surgery 97:337, 1985.

131. Rosell S, Rokaeus A: The effect of ingestion of amino acids, glucose and fat on circulating neurotensin-like immunoreactivity (NTLI) in man. Acta Physiol Scand 107:263, 1979.

132. Blackburn AM, Bloom SR, Long RG, et al: Effect of neurotensin on gastric function in man. Lancet 1:987, 1980.

133. Skov Olsen P, Holst Pedersen J, Kirkegaard P, et al: Neurotensin inhibits meal-stimulated gastric acid secretion in man. Scand J Gastroenterol 18:1073, 1983.

134. Olsen PS, Pedersen JH, Kirkegaard P, et al: Neurotensin-induced inhibition of gastric acid secretion in duodenal ulcer patients before and after parietal cell vagotomy. Gut 25:481, 1984.

135. Varner AA, Isenberg JI, Elashoff JD, et al: Effect of intravenous lipid on gastric acid secretion stimulated by intravenous amino acids. Gastroenterology 79:873, 1980.

136. Petersen B, Christiansen J, Rokaeus A, et al: Effect of intravenous and intrajejunal fat infusion on gastric acid secretion and plasma neurotensin-like immunoreactivity in man. Scand J Gastroenterol 19:48, 1984.

137. Baume PE, Meng HC, Law DH: Intravenous fat emulsion and gastric secretion in the rat. Am J Dig Dis 11:1, 1966.

138. Walker JP, King L, Silva M, et al: Effect of different intravenous nutrients on release of gastrointestinal hormones and secretion of gastric acid. Gastroenterology 88:1626, 1985.

139. Daly MJ: The classification of adrenoceptors and their effects on gastric acid secretion. Scand J Gastroenterol 19 (Suppl 89):3, 1984.

140. Becker HD, Reeder DD, Thompson JC: Effect of glucagon on circulating gastrin. Gastroenterology 65:28, 1973.

141. Tatemoto K, Mutt V: Isolation of two novel candidate hormones using a chemical method for finding naturally occurring polypeptides. Nature 285:417, 1980.

142. Tanaka I, Tatemoto K, Taylor IL: Distribution of PYY in the canine gastrointestinal tract. Gastroenterology 86:1276, 1984.

143. Pappas TN, Debas HT, Goto Y, et al: Peptide YY inhibits meal-stimulated pancreatic and gastric secretion. Am J Physiol 248:G118, 1985.

144. Lluis F, Fujimura M, Guo Y-S, et al: Regulation of gastric acid secretion by peptide YY, secretin, and neurotensin. Gastroenterology 88:1478, 1985.

145. Guo Y-S, Fujimura M, Lluis F, et al: Peptide YY: A physiologic role in the regulation of gastric secretion. Gastroenterology 88:1408, 1985.

146. Lluis F, Fujimura M, Guo Y-S, et al: Peptide YY pancreatic action is independent of cholinergic pathways. Gastroenterology 88:1478, 1985.

147. Adrian TE, Savage AP, Sagor GR, et al: Effect of peptide YY on gastric, pancreatic, and biliary function in humans. Gastroenterology 89:494, 1985.

148. Hesch R-D, Hufner M, Schmidt H, et al: Gastrointestinal effects of calcitonin in man, in Demling L (ed): *Gastrointestinal Hormones*. Stuttgart, Georg Thieme Verlag, 1972, pp 94–103.

149. Becker HD, Reeder DD, Scurry MT, et al: Inhibition of gastrin release and gastric secretion by calcitonin in patients with peptic ulcer. Am J Surg 127:71, 1974.

150. Rosenfeld MG, Mermod J-J, Amara SG, et al: Production of a novel neuropeptide encoded by the calcitonin gene via tissue-specific RNA processing. Nature 304:129, 1983.

151. Tache Y, Pappas T, Lauffenburger M, et al: Calcitonin gene-related peptide: Potent peripheral inhibitor of gastric acid secretion in rats and dogs. Gastroenterology 87:344, 1984.

152. Kraenzlin ME, Ch'ng JLC, Mulderry PK, et al: Infusion of a novel peptide, calcitonin gene-related peptide (CGRP) in man. Pharmacokinetics and effects on gastric acid secretion and on gastrointestinal hormones. Regul Pept 10:189, 1985.

153. Gregory H: Isolation and structure of urogastrone and its relationship to epidermal growth factor. Nature 257:325, 1975.

154. Hirata Y, Orth DN: Epidermal growth factor (urogastrone) in human fluids: Size heterogeneity. J Clin Endocrinol Metab 48:673, 1979.

155. Elder JB, Ganguli PC, Gillespie IE, et al: Effect of urogastrone on gastric secretion and plasma gastrin levels in normal subjects. Gut 16:887, 1975.

156. Finke U, Rutten M, Murphy RA, et al: Effects of epidermal growth factor on acid secretion from guinea pig gastric mucosa: In vitro analysis. Gastroenterology 88:1175, 1985.

157. Townsend CM Jr, Watson LC, Perez-Polo JR, et al: Nerve growth factor (NGF) inhibits release of gastrin (G) and secretion of gastric acid (H^+). Fed Proc 41:1499, 1982.

158. Swierczek J, Sakamoto T, Perez-Polo JR, et al: Nerve growth factor is cytoprotective for bile salt-induced gastric mucosal damage. Surg Forum 34:162, 1983.

159. Thompson JC, Davidson WD, Patton JJ, et al: Histamine stimulation of gastric pepsin secretion in the dog. Arch Surg 97:805, 1968.

160. Samloff IM: Pepsinogens, pepsins, and pepsin inhibitors. Gastroenterology 60:586, 1971.

161. Friedman MHF, Pincus IJ, Thomas JE, et al: Stimulation of pepsin secretion by means of acid in the intestine. Am J Physiol 140:708, 1944.

162. Brooks AM, Isenberg J, Grossman MI: The effect of secretin, glucagon, and duodenal acidification on

pepsin secretion in man. Gastroenterology 57:159, 1969.

163. Braganza JM, Gibbs ACC, Howat HT: The influence of secretin on the secretion of pepsin in response to acid stimulants in the anaesthetized cat. J Physiol 252:791, 1975.
164. Braganza JM, Herman K, Hine P, et al: The effect of pentagastrin (I.C.I. 50, 123) on peptic secretion in man. J Physiol 289:9, 1979.
165. Brown JC, Mutt V, Dryburgh JR: The further purification of motilin, a gastric motor activity stimulating polypeptide from the mucosa of the small intestine of hogs. Can J Physiol Pharmacol 49:399, 1971.
166. Vagne M, Mutt V, Perret G, et al: A fraction isolated from porcine upper small intestine stimulating pepsin secretion in the cat. Digestion 14:89, 1976.
167. Grossman MI, Greengard H, Woolley JR, et al: Pepsin secretion and enterogastrone. Am J Physiol 141:281, 1944.
168. Hirschowitz BI: Pepsinogen. Postgrad Med J 60:743, 1984.
169. Obrink KJ: Studies on the kinetics of the parietal secretion of the stomach. Acta Physiol Scand 15 (Suppl 51):1, 1948.
170. Flemstrom G: Active alkalinization by amphibian gastric fundic mucosa in vitro. Am J Physiol 233:E1, 1977.
171. Flemstrom G, Sachs G: Ion transport by amphibian antrum in vitro. I. General characteristics. Am J Physiol 228:1188, 1975.
172. Garner A, Flemstrom G: Gastric HCO_3^- secretion in the guinea pig. Am J Physiol 234:E535, 1978.
173. Kauffman GL Jr, Reeve JJ Jr, Grossman MI: Gastric bicarbonate secretion: Effect of topical and intravenous 16,16-dimethyl prostaglandin E_2. Am J Physiol 239:G44, 1980.
174. Johansson C, Aly A, Nilsson E, et al: Stimulation of gastric bicarbonate secretion by E_2 prostaglandins in man, in Samuelsson B, Paoletti R, Ramwell P (eds): *Advances in Prostaglandin, Thromboxane, and Leukotriene Research.* New York, Raven Press, 1983, pp 395–401.
175. Lonnerholm G: Carbonic anhydrase in the intestinal tract of the guinea-pig. Acta Physiol Scand 99:53, 1977.
176. Williams SE, Turnberg LA: Demonstration of a pH gradient across mucus adherent to rabbit gastric mucosa: Evidence for a 'mucus-bicarbonate' barrier. Gut 22:94, 1981.
177. Cheung LY, Newton WT: Cyclic guanosine monophosphate response to acetylcholine stimulation of gastric alkaline secretion. Surgery 86:156, 1979.
178. Garner A: Effects of acetylsalicylate on alkalinization, acid secretion and electrogenic properties in the isolated gastric mucosa. Acta Physiol Scand 99:281, 1977.
179. Garner A: Mechanisms of action of aspirin on the gastric mucosa of the guinea pig. Acta Physiol Scand (Suppl):101, 1978.
180. Garner A, Heylings JR: Stimulation of alkaline secretion in amphibian-isolated gastric mucosa by 16,16-dimethyl PGE_2 and $PGF_{2\alpha}$. A proposed explanation for some of the cytoprotective actions of prostaglandins. Gastroenterology 76:497, 1979.
181. Garner A, Flemstrom G, Heylings JR: Effects of antiinflammatory agents and prostaglandins on acid and bicarbonate secretions in the amphibian-isolated gastric mucosa. Gastroenterology 77:451, 1979.
182. Flemstrom G: Effect of catecholamines, Ca^{++} and gastrin on gastric HCO_3^- secretion. Acta Physiol Scand (Suppl):81, 1978.
183. Flemstrom G: Gastric secretion of bicarbonate, in Johnson LR (ed): *Physiology of the Gastrointestinal Tract.* New York, Raven Press, 1981, pp 603–616.
184. Kivilaakso E: Contribution of ambient HCO_3^- to mucosal protection and intracellular pH in isolated amphibian gastric mucosa. Gastroenterology 85:1284, 1983.
185. Allen A: Structure of gastrointestinal mucus glycoproteins and the viscous and gel-forming properties of mucus. Br Med Bull 34:28, 1978.
186. Allen A: Structure and function of gastrointestinal mucus, in Johnson LR (ed): *Physiology of the Gastrointestinal Tract.* New York, Raven Press, 1981, pp 617–639.
187. Zalewsky CA, Moody FG: Mechanisms of mucus release in exposed canine gastric mucosa. Gastroenterology 77:719, 1979.
188. Vagne M, Perret G: Effect of duodenal acidification on gastric mucus and acid secretion in conscious cats. Digestion 14:332, 1976.
189. Vagne M, Perret G: Regulation of gastric mucus secretion. Scand J Gastroenterol 11 (Suppl 42):63, 1976.
190. Jerzy Glass GB, Boyd LJ: The influence of vagotropic and sympathicotropic stimuli on the secretion of gastric mucin and its fractions in man. Am J Dig Dis 17:355, 1950.
191. Vagne M: Dose-response curve to secretin on gastric mucus secretion in conscious cats. Digestion 10:402, 1974.
192. Andre C, Lambert R, Descos F: Stimulation of gastric mucous secretions in man by secretin. Digestion 7:284, 1972.
193. Rees WDW, Turnberg LA: Biochemical aspects of gastric secretion. Clinics Gastroenterol 10:521, 1981.
194. Johansson C, Aly A: Stimulation of gastric mucus output by somatostatin in man. Eur J Clin Invest 12:37, 1982.
195. Bickel M, Kauffman GL Jr: Gastric gel mucus thickness: Effect of distention, 16,16-dimethyl prostaglandin E_2, and carbenoxolone. Gastroenterology 80:770, 1981.
196. Johansson H, Lindquest B: Anti-inflammatory drugs and gastric mucus. Scand J Gastroenterol 6:49, 1971.
197. Menguy R, Masters YF: Effects of aspirin on gastric mucous secretion. Surg Gynecol Obstet 120:92, 1965.

198. Spohn M, McColl I: In vitro studies on the effect of salicylates on the synthesis of proteins by guinea pig gastric mucosal tissue. Biochim Biophys Acta 608:409, 1980.
199. Donaldson RM Jr: Intrinsic factor and the transport of cobalamin, in Johnson LR (ed): *Physiology of the Gastrointestinal Tract.* New York, Raven Press, 1981, pp 641–658.
200. Schepp W, Ruoff H-J, Miederer SE: Cellular origin and release of intrinsic factor from isolated rat gastric mucosal cells. Biochim Biophys Acta 763:426, 1983.

PANCREATIC SECRETION

William Nealon, M.D., and
James C. Thompson, M.D.

For descriptive purposes, pancreatic exocrine function has been classified into three secretory phases—cephalic, gastric, and intestinal—according to the site from which stimulatory impulses emanate. There is, however, no evidence to suggest that these phases are in any way isolated during the digestive process; rather they represent an orchestration of the responses to various stimuli that collectively compose the pancreatic exocrine response.

Pavlov [1] first demonstrated the cephalic phase of pancreatic secretion by sham feeding dogs with esophageal fistulas and Heidenhain stomach pouches. The cephalic phase stimuli (the sight, smell, chewing, or swallowing of food) activate central neural mechanisms. Afferent vagal impulses terminate in the vagal nuclei in the medulla; the nuclei initiate efferent stimuli, which traverse the peripheral vagal fibers and enter the pancreatic parenchyma, where acetylcholine is released from vagal nerve endings. Specific cholinergic receptors on the acinar cell membrane bind to acetylcholine, a cascade of intracellular events is initiated, and pancreatic enzymes are secreted.

The gastric phase is initiated when food enters the stomach and gastric distention activates vagovagal impulses, which further stimulate cholinergic fibers in the pancreas. At the same time, partial digestion products of proteins and cephalic phase cholinergic stimuli cause release of gastrin, which itself evokes stimulation of pancreatic enzymes. Thus, before food reaches the small bowel, both peptidergic and neurocrine impulses have reached the pancreas.

Acidified gastric chyme entering the duodenum is the signal for the initiation of the intestinal phase. The bolus of food has been mixed, liquefied and osmotically altered when it reaches the duodenum, but as yet minimal digestion has occurred. Pancreatic juice with the three major enzyme groups (amylytic, lipolytic, and proteolytic) flows into the duodenum, where activated enzymes begin the process of digestion. The accumulated products of fat and protein digestion promote further enzyme secretion. An alkaline, aqueous solution, rich in bicarbonate, is also released and is primarily responsible for the volume of juice secreted. A combination of cholinergic stimulation, initiated by the entry of nutrients into the small bowel, and humoral stimulation, dominated by release of secretin and cholecystokinin (CCK), causes the secretion of large amounts of enzyme-rich alkaline juice. The bicarbonate-rich fluid neutralizes gastric acid delivered to the duodenum in order to provide the proper pH for optimal enzyme function. Each of the three major enzyme groups is able to digest one of the three basic food components—carbohydrates, fats, or proteins. Oligosaccharides, fatty acids, and amino acids, which result from this digestive process, are absorbed by the intestinal mucosa. As bicarbonate flows into the duodenum, the pH is raised, halting further release of secretin, which in turn causes an end to water and bicarbonate secretion. The feedback signal to stop release of pancreatic enzymes has not been demonstrated. It should, teleologically, depend upon enzymes or their split products in the duodenal lumen. So far, the story has not been clearly told.

History

The physiology of pancreatic exocrine function developed from the work of Bernard and Heidenhain in the 19th century and flourished under Pavlov, who recognized the stimulatory influence of acid and nutrients in the duodenum on pancreatic secretion. Pavlov [1] divided vagus and splanchnic nerves and evoked a pancreatic exocrine response after nerve stimulation. The concept of a humoral stimulus in the digestive process was unrecognized until Bayliss and Starling [2] reported their historic work on the demonstration of secretin activity from the acidified duodenum. They correlated the pancreatic response to intestinal acid after vagotomy with the response to IV injections of the extract.

In 1925, Mellanby [3] attributed pancreatic response to a dual hormonal and nervous stimulation. According to his hypothesis, secretin was solely responsible for bicarbonate and water secretion, while vagus nerves caused enzyme release. This interpretation was widely accepted for nearly 20 years. Interestingly, only 3 years after Mellanby's report, Ivy and Oldberg [4] infused fat into the proximal gut of dogs and attributed the rapid contraction of the gallbladder to a putative humoral agent. They theorized that the hormone was present in duodenal extracts, and they named the substance cholecystokinin, for its effect on the gallbladder muscle. Fifteen years later, Harper and Raper [5] dispelled the notion of a purely nervous source of enzyme stimulation when they described a substance obtained from alcohol-extracted cat small intestinal mucosa that evoked a profound pancreatic protein secretion. They named this agent pancreozymin. Purification of these two agents, cholecystokinin and pancreozymin, by Mutt and Jorpes [6] in 1968 resulted in the startling discovery that they were identical 33 amino acid peptides. Because the cholecystokinetic function was the first described, the term cholecystokinin was chosen to apply to this peptide (see Chapter 15).

Further delineation of the relative extent to which each of the two mechanisms (nervous and hormonal) contributes to the regulation of pancreatic exocrine function came from Wang and Grossman in 1951 [7]; they examined autotransplanted canine pancreatic secretion after stimulation by various dietary components. The use of a denervated gland provided evidence for humoral regulation of both aqueous bicarbonate-rich and enzyme-rich pancreatic secretion during digestion.

The technologic advances that have made possible the isolation, sequencing, and synthesis of peptides, along with the development of radioimmunoassay, have permitted great progress in the work with the classic pancreatic peptides—secretin and CCK—while new peptides are added to the list of pancreatic secretagogues regularly.

In addition to the recognized physiologic stimulants, secretin and CCK, it is known that exogenous administration of gastrin, vasoactive intestinal peptide (VIP), bombesin, gastrin-releasing peptide (GRP), motilin, peptide histidine isoleucine [8], neurotensin, substance P, and growth hormone-releasing factor will stimulate pancreatic exocrine secretion [9]. Attempts using radioimmunoassay techniques have failed to correlate the postprandial plasma levels of these substances with plasma levels achieved during exogenous delivery of stimulatory doses of the agent. For this reason, only secretin and CCK serve an acknowledged physiologic role in pancreatic secretion [10].

Recent attention has been directed toward peptides that inhibit pancreatic secretion: glucagon, calcitonin [9], pancreatic polypeptide (PP) [11], calcitonin gene-related peptide (CGRP) [12], somatostatin [13], peptide YY (PYY) [14], neuropeptide Y (NPY) [11], and growth hormone-release inhibiting hormone [15]. Once again, a clear physiologic role for these agents has not yet been demonstrated, and the challenge of detecting minor inhibitory influences in the face of the overriding stimulation of the postprandial pancreas is a considerable one. The fact that a much greater maximally stimulated secretory volume and enzyme release can be achieved by exogenously administered peptides than that measured after a meal suggests that inhibitory impulses may play a role.

Cellular Kinetics of Secretion

As methods to make direct observations on cellular events have been developed, four broad categories of investigation have evolved: those directed at structure-function relationships, at protein synthesis and transport, at receptors, and at stimulus-secretion coupling. Studies on structure-function relationships are heavily dependent upon electron microscopy and have been used to establish that the cells lining pancreatic ductules primarily secrete water and bicarbonate, while acinar cells largely secrete digestive enzymes [16]. Studies of protein synthesis and transport have attempted to define the sequence of biochemical events that occur during the process in which the precursors of pancreatic enzymes present in zymogen granules in the basal regions of the cell transverse the intracellular cytosol for release into ductules. These studies have also explored the relative proportions of each enzyme released; various theories of the patterns of release have been proposed.

The questions of how a peptide hormone passes its signal to a cell and what events are activated within the cell have resulted in the development of the receptor theory and of the process that has been called stimulus-secretion coupling. The specific binding of a peptide or a neurotransmitter to the cell membrane can now be demonstrated by quantifying the binding of a labeled peptide and by measuring the kinetics of binding in the presence of varied amounts of unlabeled ligand. The consequent activation of a number of intracellular pathways has been called the stimulus-secretion coupling and, although ongoing investigations have demonstrated an increasingly complex process, hormone-stimulated secretion occurs through either calcium-dependent or adenylate cyclase (cyclic AMP)-mediated pathways.

In addition to discussing the above categories

that relate to acinar function, a series of studies on ductular secretion of bicarbonate and electrolytes will be summarized.

Structure-Function Relationship

Each different cell type within the pancreas can generally be related to individual products of secretion: acinar cells secrete digestive enzymes and a fluid rich in chloride and low in bicarbonate; duct cells secrete bicarbonate and water; and the islets of Langerhans synthesize and secrete peptide hormones [17–20]. The latter are composed of α cells (which produce glucagon), β cells (insulin), D cells (somatostatin and VIP), and F cells (PP) [17–19]. The ductal cell and its analogue, the centroacinar cell, combine with the acinar cell to compose the exocrine pancreas.

Acinar cells typically represent between 80 and 90 percent of the gland by volume, while ductular cells form about 4 percent and endocrine cells 2 percent; the balance of the gland is occupied by all extracellular matrix [21]. Six to eight acinar cells form a functional unit called the acinus, which is the basic subunit of the exocrine pancreas. This cluster of cells surrounds a lumen that emerges from the acinus in the form of a small ductlet, called the intercalated duct [21]. The acini are connected with excretory ducts by long intercalary and intralobular ducts whose walls are formed by cells that do not contain zymogen granules. Those cells contain carbonic anhydrase and secrete the aqueous component of the juice. Cells of the ducts frequently project into the acinus itself, where they are known as centroacinar cells [22] (Fig 9-5). The centroacinar cell functions as a ductal cell, producing a water and a bicarbonate-rich electrolyte secretion [23]. Both the acinar and centroacinar cells have microvillous processes. These serve to greatly increase the surface area of the individual cells [24]. Many acini, together with their intercalated and intralobular ducts, constitute a lobule, which is linked by interlobular ducts to the main duct that finally enters the duodenum [21].

Islets and acini are served by separate arterioles. Those to the islets break up into large sinusoids and drain into smaller capillaries that surround adjacent acini. Thus, blood flows from the islets to the acini, carrying high concentrations of hormones to cells that synthesize and secrete the enzymes of external secretion of the pancreas.

The acinar cell has traditionally been described as pyramidal in shape, with the apical portion directed toward the acinar lumen, and the basal limit, with its basement membrane, directed toward the capillary network. Blood-borne humoral peptide (or neurotransmitter) agonists may interact and bind to specific receptors along the cell basement membrane [25]. Acinar cells are held together by junctional complexes in the lateral membranes. The junctional complex consists of three morphologically defined structures: adher-

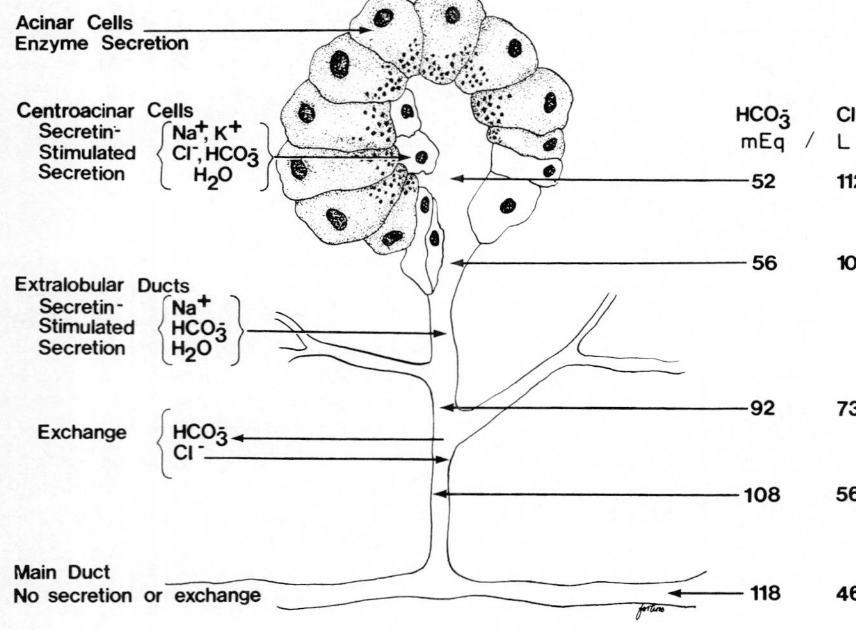

Figure 9-5. Secretion by centroacinar cells and by cells of the extralobular ducts of the pancreas. Chloride concentrations (right) were determined on fluid collected by micropuncture, and the bicarbonate concentrations were inferred from the fact that the fluid is isotonic. These data are for the cat pancreas, but other species seem to be similar. (Adapted from Lightwood and Reber, Gastroenterology 72:61, 1977.)

ing zonules, desmosomes, and terminal bars or "tight junctions" [26,27]. The terminal bars are able to restrict passage of secretory proteins as well as to affect tissue permeability to ions and small molecules [28,29]. The apical region of the acinar cell is characteristically rich with zymogen granules. Each of these saccular structures contains the full spectrum of digestive enzymes produced by the gland [30,31].

Digestive Protein Synthesis and Transport

Electron microscope studies of the various morphologic intracellular components of the acinar cells have coincided with efforts to define the processes of synthesis, segregation, storage, and final exocytotic expulsion of the various digestive enzyme species from the pancreatic acinar cell using cell fractionation procedures. Although controversies exist, the consensus is that this mechanism progresses in an orderly fashion from the basal to the apical pole of the acinar cell [32]. As early as 1955, the relationship between the rough endoplasmic reticulum and protein synthesis was drawn [33]. Scheele et al [34] later observed that pancreatic secretory proteins are synthesized initially with an amino acid terminal extension. Blobel and Dobberstein [35] proposed a signal peptide hypothesis, which simply theorized that this terminal amino acid fragment guides the growing protein chain by allowing for attachment of the polysome to the membrane. These nascent proteins, with an intact signal extension, have been termed preproproteins, and after cleavage of the terminal sequence they are called proproteins. The majority of pancreatic acinar secretory proteins are secreted in this form and are activated extracellularly by proteolytic cleavage (for example, conversion of trypsinogen to trypsin by enterokinase in the duodenum) [21].

The events that occur between the elaboration of the digestive enzyme precursor and its release into the duct depend upon packaging the peptides in secretory granules. After synthesis and sequestration within the endoplasmic reticulum, the protein migrates toward the Golgi apparatus, and it is in this region that the protein enzymes are enveloped in zymogen granules (Fig 9-6). The secretory proteins accumulate in storage granules that move to the apical regions of the acinar cell, where neurohumoral stimuli trigger exocytosis [21].

Palade [32], in his 1975 Nobel Prize address, summarized the components of his exocytosis theory of enzyme secretion. The process of exocytosis theoretically involves fusion of the granule membrane with the plasmalemma, allowing granule contents to escape into the lumen (Fig 9-7). This hypothetical model is intimately linked to the question of parallel versus nonparallel digestive protein secretion. According to the former con-

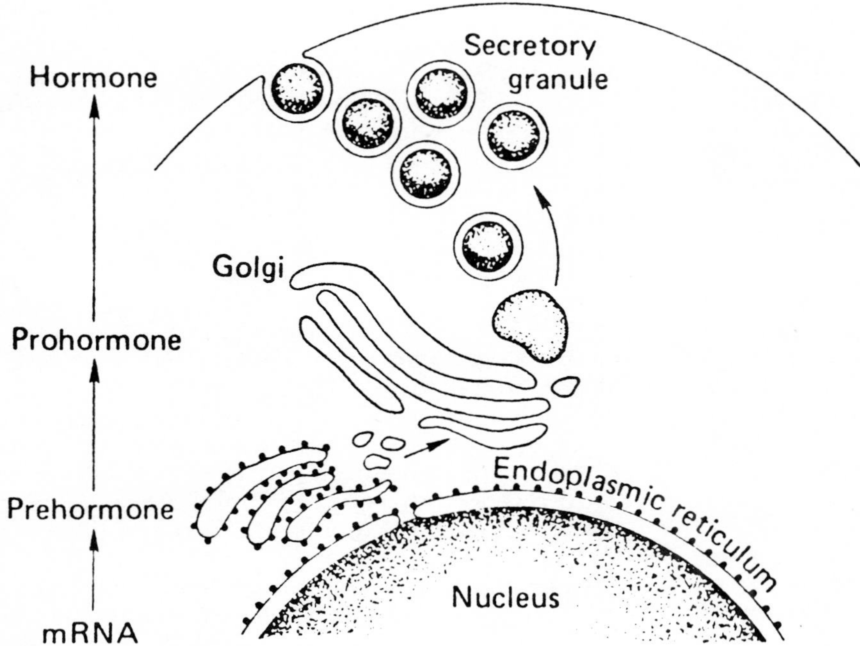

Figure 9-6. Intracellular transport of protein from the endoplasmic reticulum to the Golgi complex, packaging of newly synthesized polypeptide hormone into secretory granules, and release of hormone by exocytosis. At left are listed the molecular forms of the hormone (or information coding for the hormone) present in that portion of the cell. (From Williams JA, in Greenspan, G.L. (ed): *Basic and Clinical Endocrinology*. Los Altos, CA, Lange Medical Publishing Co, 1983, p. 1.)

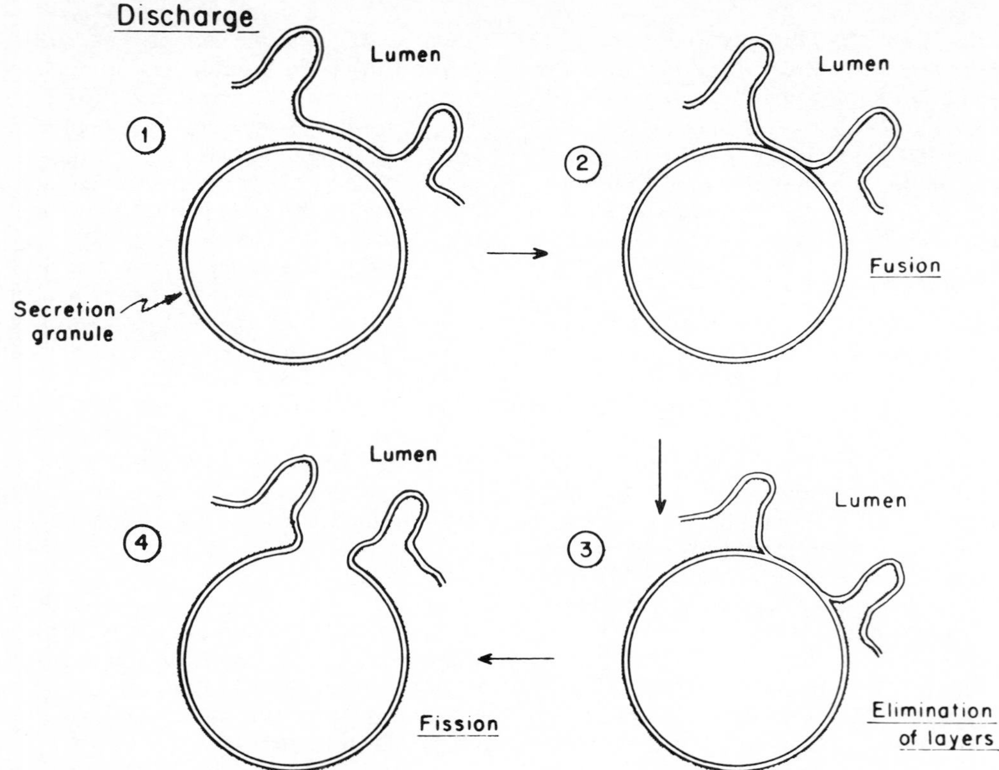

Figure 9-7. Diagram of membrane interactions during secretory discharge. (From Palade [32], with permission of the American Association for the Advancement of Science.)

cept, all enzyme secretion occurs through release of constant proportions of each individual enzyme, a theory that would be well supported by the exocytosis model. The implication in the alternative nonparallel concept is that individual cells may possess the ability to respond to secretory stimuli in a very specialized manner.

Scheele and Palade [31] and Steer and Glazer [36], using incubated pancreatic acinar preparations, measured constant proportions of enzymes released into the incubation medium after a variety of stimulants, a finding consistent with the theory of parallel secretion or mass transport.

Rothman [37] challenged both the exocytosis model and the parallel secretion model by pointing to evidence that suggested that digestive enzymes are secreted by transport across apical plasma membranes of the acinar cell from the cytoplasm as a result of equilibrium processes [37]. He based his hypothesis upon the conflicting observation that concentrations of various enzymes can be altered in collected secretions [36,37]. Rothman [37] theorized a release of enzymes by zymogen granules within the cells, allowing independent secretion of each component. The rate of enzyme synthesis may explain the preponderance of one or another enzyme in pancreatic juice [38], and evidence has been provided that suggests that synthetic rates may be altered by feeding [39,40], by starvation [40], and by variations in dietary composition. A preponderance of one dietary component results in a rise in the appropriate digestive enzyme [41–44]. Each study has evaluated these changes after a prolonged period of altered dietary conditions, which suggests that the mixture of digestive enzymes secreted in response to a single meal is stereotyped or preordained by previously induced synthetic patterns.

A recent study of enzyme responses in rabbit pancreas found a highly linked secretory pattern that supports both nonparallel secretion and exocytosis and theorizes the presence of acini throughout the gland with heterogeneous enzyme contents [45]. According to this hypothesis, varied proportions of secreted digestive enzymes may result from stimulation of alternate clusters of acini.

Since extrapancreatic sources of the conventional digestive enzymes, such as lipase, amylase, and certain peptidases, have been established, current interest has focused on those enzymes that appear to play a minor role in the process of digestion but that are of specific pancreatic origin [46]. The value of examining the function of enzymes such as these depends upon the degree to which precise determinations of pancreatic exocrine function may be made without a need to correct for extrapancreatic enzyme sources.

Receptors

The initial step in the mechanism of action of secretagogues on the release of pancreatic enzymes is the reversible binding of the secretagogue to receptors located on the surface of the plasma membrane of the pancreatic acinar cell. The apparent affinity of a secretagogue for its receptor is reflected in the range of concentrations over which it exhibits activity by competing with a known radiolabeled ligand for receptor binding sites [47,48]. Varied doses of nonlabeled peptides are incubated with the labeled ligand, and membrane binding is measured.

The known receptor sites on pancreatic acinar cells include CCK, high-affinity secretin, high-affinity VIP, bombesin, physalaemin/elediosin, and acetylcholine, along with putative binding by insulin, glucagon, and cholera toxins, among others [47]. Steigerwalt and Williams et al [49,50] have characterized specific CCK receptors on pancreatic membranes and brain [51] as well as on bovine gallbladder membranes [52]. Similar acinar CCK receptors have been detected by Jensen et al [53], who calculated a population of approximately 9,000 binding sites on each acinar cell.

Stimulus-Secretion Coupling

Secretagogue-receptor interaction is known to result in elevations of intracellular free calcium, cyclic AMP, and cyclic GMP in pancreatic acinar cells. This is thought to represent two functionally distinct sequences of biochemical events [54]. Some agonists interact with specific receptors to cause release of cellular calcium, accompanied by cGMP release. Others respond to specific receptors by stimulating activation of adenylate cyclase, increasing cellular cAMP. These two mechanisms, which couple the hormone stimulus to enzyme secretion, have distinct initial pathways but appear to interact at some intermediate phase within the cell. This interaction is considered to be the basis for the potentiation of enzyme secretion [55,56]. Potentiation occurs when a secretagogue that operates via cAMP and a hormone that increases calcium release combine to promote secretion of an enzyme that is substantially greater than the sum of the effects of each individual agent acting alone. The substances that act through calcium mobilization include CCK and its analogues, cholinergic agents, gastrin, and bombesin, while secretagogues that increase intracellular cAMP include secretin, VIP, and the cholera toxin [57] (Table 9-2).

The actions of secretagogues, such as CCK or cholinergic agents, were first thought to result from their ability to mobilize and transport extracellular calcium into pancreatic acinar cells [58]. This conclusion was reached after the demonstration of diminution or cessation of pancreatic enzyme secretion in incubation solutions that were free of calcium [59,60]. Studies with radiolabeled calcium have documented the absence of calcium influx after secretagogue stimulation [61]. The source of the free calcium release appears to be from intracellular pools. Hormone-receptor interaction leads to a breakdown of phosphatidylinositol in cell membranes [62]. Calcium bound to this substance is released into the cytosol. Stolze and Schulz [62] have shown an adenosine triphosphate-dependent calcium pump and a sodium-dependent calcium transport that contribute to the release of free calcium from the cytosol. As stimulation is sustained, the permeability of the plasma membrane increases, and calcium influx occurs [63]. With cessation of stimulation, there is a resynthesis of phosphatidylinositol and its calcium-binding properties, resulting in reconstitution

Table 9-2. **Division of regulatory peptides that stimulate acinar cells, according to intracellular messengers**

cAMP	*Calcium*	*Unknown*
β-Adrenergic catecholamines	α-Adrenergic catecholamines	Insulin
CGRP	Acetylcholine	Nerve growth factor
Secretin	Bombesin	Somatostatin
VIP	CCK	
Growth hormone-releasing factor	Gastrin	
Cholera toxin	GRP	

(Adapted from [57].)

of the "trigger pool" of membrane-bound calcium [64].

Those pancreatic secretagogues that cause release of calcium also increase cellular guanosine 3:5′-monophosphate (cyclic GMP) [65,66]. Although this release appears to be closely related to intracellular free calcium release, there seems to be no role for this substance as a mediator of stimulus-secretion coupling [67], that is, studies in which release of cGMP is depressed have not changed the secretory response.

VIP, secretin, and cholera toxin will increase pancreatic enzyme secretion in some species [68,69]. Their action is dependent upon cAMP and adenylate cyclase activation. The mediator of secretin and VIP stimulation of adenylate cyclase is guanosine triphosphate [57]. This is in contrast to cholera toxin, which itself acts as an enzyme to inhibit the degradation of guanosine triphosphate, resulting in a persistently activated state [70].

Both cyclic nucleotides and calcium-dependent processes appear to regulate Na^+-K^+-ATPase (Na^+-K^+ pump) activity in acinar cells for stimulated amylase release [71,72]. These pumps play a role in electrolyte secretion in the acini by channeling Na^+ out of the cell and into the acinar lumen.

Bicarbonate and Electrolyte Secretion

Isolation of duct cells and intact ducts from glands of copper-deficient rats in which acinar cells are selectively destroyed has provided information concerning secretin-stimulated electrolyte and fluid secretion [73,74]. As in the acinar cell, secretin stimulation of duct cells results in release of intracellular cAMP. The acinar cell adenylate cyclase is activated by both secretin and CCK, while duct cell adenylate cyclase responds only and quite specifically to secretin and its analogue, VIP [73]. The actual mechanism of cAMP mediation is not certain.

The concentrations of Na^+ and K^+ in pancreatic juice are independent of the rate of secretion and very nearly equal to the concentrations in plasma. If plasma composition remains constant, both the sum of the cations and the sum of the anions in pancreatic juice are independent of the rate of secretion. The osmotic pressure of pancreatic juice is identical to that of plasma.

The formation of intracellular HCO_3^- is dependent upon carbonic anhydrase to process both extracellular and intracellular HCO_3^-. Thus, inhibitors of carbonic anhydrase inhibit pancreatic secretion of bicarbonate-containing juice [75]. The majority of secreted HCO_3^- arises from extracellular HCO_3^-, which enters the cell as CO_2 and is reprocessed to HCO_3^- before extrusion. The presence of extracellular bicarbonate is required for duct cell function [76].

Nervous Control of Pancreatic Function

The pancreas contains a network of postganglionic cholinergic neurons that stimulate secretion of enzymes. These postganglionic neurons are activated by preganglionic parasympathetic fibers of the vagi. In addition, there are nervous connections between pancreatic postganglionic nerves and the intrinsic ganglia of the intestinal wall. These connections appear to mediate an enteropancreatic reflex. Preganglionic sympathetic fibers synapse with postganglionic cells in the celiac and associated ganglia, and the postganglionic fibers are distributed to pancreatic blood vessels.

All efforts have failed to clarify whether nervous or humoral influences predominate in the physiologic functioning of the exocrine pancreas. Certainly a physiologic role is apparent for cholinergic, adrenergic, and paracrine pathways [77]. Anatomic studies have documented the presence of both a vagal and a sympathetic nervous supply in the pancreas of humans and dogs [78]. Physiologic studies have demonstrated differences between species as well as unaccountable inconsistencies when the endogenous or exogenous stimulant is varied. Electrical stimulation of proximal vagal trunks does result in a small but definite rise in pancreatic exocrine function [79–81]; a background secretin infusion accentuates the effect [80]. In the pig and cat, systemic atropine reduces secretion of enzymes but not of bicarbonate [79–81], while in dogs, all exocrine function is blocked by atropine [80]. Debas and Yamagishi [82] have suggested a reflex arc between the antrum of the stomach and the pancreas. They observed that antral distention with acid or alkali caused protein and bicarbonate release in the canine pancreas. Both vagotomy and atropine inhibited the effect [82]. Their evidence appears sound.

Nutrient stimulation of exocrine pancreatic function, either by the products of fat or protein digestion or by hydrochloric acid, is dramatically depressed by both truncal and extragastric vagotomy [83–89]. Exogenous CCK-stimulated pancreatic secretion is unaffected by atropine or vagotomy [83,84,87,89,90], yet basal enzyme secretion is diminished [86,87,89]. Vagotomy typically does not influence the pancreatic bicarbonate response to exogenous secretin, but atropine does inhibit bicarbonate secretion in response to moderate doses of secretin [87,89]. This phenomenon has been examined by Singer et al [91]. The differential effect of atropine and vagotomy was interpreted by them as evidence that secretin stimulation is dependent upon intrapancreatic vagovagal interaction and is independent of intact vagal innervation via vagal trunks. CCK-secretin potentiation is unchanged by atropine, but secretin potentiation by intestinal l-phenylalanine is blocked [92]. A transplanted, denervated pancreas will respond to intestinal stimulants with enzyme and bicarbonate secretion, which is independent of vagal influences [87,93]. Recent work has stressed the notion of a cholinergic reflex which would explain the rapidity of response to intestinal stimuli [92]. We have found that vagotomy causes a significant decrease in pancreatic enzyme output stimulated by intraduodenal fat but causes no change in enzyme output in response to bombesin or exogenous CCK. Vagotomy caused no change in fat-stimulated release of CCK. We concluded that CCK release is independent of the vagus, and that the vagus stimulates pancreatic protein output by enteropancreatic reflexes that are independent of CCK [94]. Finally, support for parasympathetic pathways in pancreatic function is provided in studies of dispersed acini that have demonstrated specific muscarinic receptors that respond to acetylcholine [95].

The sympathetic nervous system has attracted much less interest, but norepinephrine is known to cause a decrease in caerulein-induced secretion of protein and fluid [96]. Hemodynamic studies have suggested that vasoconstriction does occur and may cause inhibition [97], while a study with isolated perfused cat pancreas suggests a specific norepinephrine-mediated inhibition [98].

More recently, Pearson et al [99] demonstrated that after blockade of the large cholinergic component of pancreatic response by atropine, electrical stimulation of an isolated rat pancreas resulted in release of amylase, which was abolished by β-adrenergic inhibitors. This minor adrenergic stimulation is consistent with the observation that dopamine stimulates pancreatic secretion in dogs [100].

The concept of peptidergic nerves arose from the observation that in vitro electrical stimulation of the guinea pig pancreas caused a release of amylase without calcium flux [101]. Transmitters in this system appear to be stored primarily in nerve terminals [102,103]. Most of these peptides are protease-sensitive and probably exert their influence locally. Among the peptides purported to have peptidergic behavior are somatostatin, enkephalin, VIP, and CGRP [21].

Stimulation of Regulatory Peptides

The classic hormones that influence pancreatic secretion are secretin and CCK. A treasure store of information concerning them has accumulated. They are the only two peptides that have a clear physiologic role in pancreatic exocrine secretion.

Secretin (see **Chapter 16**)

Bayliss and Starling [2], in 1902, showed that infusion of hydrochloric acid into a denervated loop of small intestine stimulated secretion from the pancreas. The responsible putative humoral substance was named secretin. Endogenous secretin is induced primarily by gastric acid delivery to the proximal duodenum [104–106]. Reduction of gastric acidity, either through histamine H_2-receptor blockade or through antacids or aspiration of gastric secretion, is associated with diminished secretin levels [105,106]. Studies have confirmed that a pH of 4.5 is the threshold for both secretin release and bicarbonate secretion; however, no additional augmentations of response occur with pH levels below 3.0 [107]. Both the length of acidified small bowel and the total hydrogen ion load have been correlated with plasma secretin levels [108,109].

VIP shares nine identical amino acids with secretin, activates intracellular adenylate cyclase, and mimics the actions of secretin; however, it is considerably less potent [110]. Its physiologic role is unclear, although it has been implicated in certain disease states [111,112].

CCK (see **Chapter 15**)

CCK was originally isolated and purified from hog proximal small intestine [6]. Like all peptides that stimulate pancreatic enzyme secretion, its C-terminal amino acid residue is amidated [57]. Exogenous administration results in a dose-dependent secretion of enzyme and water from the pancreas through specific receptor binding and calcium-dependent intracellular mechanisms, as previously described. CCK release has classically been attributed to intestinal perfusion with the products of fat digestion, peptones, and L-isomers of amino acids obtained from protein digestion. As radioimmunoassay methods have improved, meal- and specific nutrient-stimulated CCK levels have been obtained [112–115] and, in our own laboratory, correlated with the bioassay of gallbladder contractility in humans [114,116] and with both gallbladder function and pancreatic secretion in dogs [117].

The fact that both vagotomy and atropine inhibit meal-stimulated pancreatic enzyme secretion and gallbladder contraction led to the assumption that CCK release must also be vagus-dependent. Recent studies, however, have shown that meal- or nutrient-stimulated plasma CCK levels have been unaffected by vagotomy in dogs [90] and have actually been elevated in humans [118]. Pancreatic exocrine response to exogenous CCK administration is unaltered by vagotomy or systemic atropine [83,87,89].

Other Gut Peptides

Gastrin shares a common C-terminal pentapeptide-amide sequence with CCK and possesses a similar sulfated tyrosine residue. Gastrin stimulates pancreatic enzyme secretion in a fashion similar to that of CCK, but with only about one third the potency in dogs and even less in humans [119]. Gastrin is assumed to be the humoral agent in the gastric phase of pancreatic secretion [119,120]. Caerulein is a decapeptide analogue of CCK that is present in the skin of the blue frog, *Hyla caerulea* [121], truly only God knows why. It has both structural and functional similarities to CCK [121] (see molecular forms of CCK in Appendix).

A growing list of peptides that share no structural similarities with CCK but that evoke a pancreatic exocrine response through pathways identical to those described by CCK has emerged. One group is composed of peptides obtained from the skin of frogs and includes bombesin, alytesin, ranatensin, and litorin [122,123]. Gastrin-releasing peptide (GRP) has been termed mammalian bombesin and has a similar potent stimulatory effect on pancreatic secretion [124]. Although these agents stimulate CCK release, they are known from in vitro studies to have their own independent secretagogue function [125]. A second group of peptides that stimulate pancreatic protein secretion by release of intracellular calcium includes the mammalian putative hormones substance P and neurotensin [126,127]. Neurotensin has been shown to stimulate pancreatic enzyme secretion in a fashion that was additive with respect to CCK stimulation, suggesting a common biochemical pathway for both hormones [128].

Several gut hormones inhibit pancreatic exocrine function, including somatostatin [15], which is very potent, PP [129,130], whose physiologic role is uncertain, pancreatic glucagon [131], pancreatone [132], peptide YY [14], NPY [11], certain prostaglandins [133], calcitonin [134], and CGRP [12]. Somatostatin inhibits secretion of both bicarbonate and enzyme [26] and exerts a profound inhibition of release on all known gastrointestinal hormones tested [135]. PP has been shown to rise in plasma after meal stimulation in dogs [130] and humans [129]. PP release is vagally mediated [135]. Relatively little attention has been directed toward the various inhibitors of exocrine function. PP has attracted some interest because postprandial levels are comparable to effective exogenous levels [135]. The fact that the digestive response after a meal may reflect a balance of stimulatory and inhibitory impulses is easily conceivable and even likely, and yet efforts to document such an interaction have failed.

Exogenous administration of CCK or secretin is known to cause a much greater pancreatic response than that achieved after a meal, and this has been used as evidence for meal-stimulated release of inhibitors. Our laboratory has recently concentrated its efforts on certain inhibitors of pancreatic secretion. We have found that CGRP inhibits canine pancreatic secretion in conscious dogs, stimulated by either CCK, secretin, or duodenal perfusion with amino acids or with hydrochloric acid. The response is dose-dependent and reversible [12, unpublished data from this laboratory]. We have also [136] been engaged in investigations with peptide YY. Again, this peptide, which is in the same family as PP and NPY, provides a potent inhibitory effect on both endogenous and exogenous stimulation of pancreatic exocrine function.

The interaction of two or more peptides has been studied somewhat among stimulants of pancreatic secretion, particularly CCK and secretin. The term potentiation has been used to describe a unique form of interaction in which two stimulants combine to achieve a much greater response than is expected on the basis of individual effects alone. The term has also been applied when a second substance is able to accentuate exocrine response to the maximal dose for a second peptide. Gardner [54] has theorized that this process occurs when substances are combined that follow separate intracellular pathways. In addition to the classic interactions of CCK and secretin and the analogous response to secretin and a meal or to CCK and a meal, our laboratory has observed a potentiated response between neurotensin and secretin and between growth hormone-releasing factor and CCK [unpublished data].

Interactions such as these have not been explored in the inhibitors of pancreatic secretion. For this reason, our laboratory has undertaken a project in which various inhibitors have been infused alone and then together in order to detect any potentiation. We have tested PP, PYY, somatostatin, calcitonin, and CGRP [137] and found each to have an additive effect on the other without any potentiation. We did, however, make the observation that combining two peptides at doses that were ineffective alone actually resulted in a significant inhibition [137, unpublished data]. The implications of this finding may have an impact on the concept of a physiologic role for these peptides.

Traditionally, a physiologic role for a gut peptide is accepted only if plasma levels measured during effective exogenous doses of a peptide coincide with levels achieved after a meal. If we consider the fact that a meal characteristically results in an orchestrated release of a spectrum of gut hormones with both stimulatory and inhibitory functions and that many of these peptides will interact, then very low plasma levels may achieve biologic activity. Our finding of ineffective doses combining to achieve a potent inhibitory response certainly supports this hypothesis. We speculate that such interactions may be functional during digestion and that they have physiologic significance. The ability to achieve a response to several peptides combined at doses consistent with levels after a meal may be a more appropriate measure of the "physiologic" state.

Various theories might be proposed to explain the very rare success in defining a physiologic role for gut hormones. Certainly, the concept of potentiation accounts for a secretory response to low levels of individual peptides. A second alternative is the so-called paracrine system, which releases regulatory substances, often in high local concentrations, which are not reflected in peripheral plasma measurements.

Meal Stimulation

As in gastric physiology, the pancreatic exocrine response to meal stimulation has been divided into three phases: cephalic, gastric, and intestinal.

Cephalic Phase

The cephalic phase of pancreatic secretion has been examined in the dog [138] and in humans [139,140] by exposure to sight and smell of food or by sham feeding. Water and bicarbonate release is minimal, and therefore the enzyme-rich juice has been more readily quantified by performing studies with a background infusion of secretin [140]. The enzyme response was measured to be 50 percent of maximal secretion to exogenous CCK-8 [140]. Studies with atropine give conflicting messages [139,140], but the consensus is that vagal fibers carry this signal. The mechanism most commonly postulated for the cephalic phase of pancreatic secretion is gastrin release [138], although studies in humans have failed to reveal gastrin elevations during sham feeding [141]. This finding is consistent with the demonstration that antral acidification has no effect on the cephalic phase of pancreatic secretion but does abolish gastrin release [82,139]. This phase is usually regarded as simply a preparatory stage in which enzymes are passed into ducts awaiting water and bicarbonate secretion to deliver the digestive enzymes to the duodenum.

Gastric Phase

The obvious primary role of the stomach in pancreatic secretion is to serve as a conduit through which delivery of nutrient to the duodenum can be regulated. In addition, the intestinal response results from exposure to digestive products of protein and fat, suggesting a role for gastric pepsin and preliminary nutrient processing. Greater attention, however, has been directed toward the impact of gastrin release on pancreatic exocrine function and of presumed gastropancreatic reflexes under vagal control. Pancreatic exocrine response to antral distention is blocked by atropine [82] and is independent of gastrin release [82]. It is associated with a quantity of protein secretion too small to be considered an important contribution to overall pancreatic response to a meal. Exogenous gastrin analogue will result in a pancreatic exocrine response from an isolated perfused pancreas preparation [120] and in humans [142] (but only with doses known to be greater than maximal for gastric acid secretion) [142].

Intestinal Phase

When chyme reaches the proximal small bowel, the intestinal phase of pancreatic secretion is initiated. This is quantitatively the most important phase. The physiology of the phase primarily concerns itself with specific nutrient perfusion, especially peptides and fats, and the pancreatic responses.

Peptides. The products of protein digestion, amino acids and oligopeptides, will stimulate pancreatic exocrine secretion when perfused into the duodenum [143]. Some controversy has arisen regarding which amino acid evokes the strongest responses. In early work with humans, methionine, valine, and phenylalanine were found to be the only amino acids capable of stimulating pancreatic exocrine secretion alone [144]. Studies in dogs suggest that intestinal perfusion of amino acids individually will stimulate pancreatic secretion only when tryptophan or phenylalanine is used [143]. Nondigested proteins evoke no response from the pancreas [145]. Interestingly, the opposite conditions are found in the rat, where intact proteins in the intestine are stimulatory, while protein digests do not promote secretion [146]. The response to intestinal perfusion of amino acids is significantly less than maximal stimulation with CCK-8 [147]. The dynamics of stimulation appear to resemble those seen in gastric acid stimulation of bicarbonate secretion in that the secretory response is independent of concentration and is greatly determined by total area of exposed mucosa [145].

Fatty Acids and Monoglycerides. As with proteins, it is the products of early fat digestion that stimulate pancreatic exocrine response. Intact triglycerides do not stimulate, but fatty acids and monoglycerides evoke a pronounced response when exposed to the intestinal lumen. Chain lengths of C_8–C_{18} are all effective stimulants, and their potencies are inversely proportional to chain length [148]. The magnitude of fatty acid-stimulated pancreatic secretion has been compared with maximal exogenous CCK stimulation, with results varying from distinctly submaximal [147] to approximately equal to maximal [93]. Sodium oleate stimulation will result in water and electrolyte secretion slightly more than half the maximal exogenous secretion level [147].

Gastric Acid. The most potent stimulus to bicarbonate and volume secretion is gastric acid. In humans in the basal state, small amounts of acid may be delivered continuously to the duodenum [149], but the overall pancreatic response is low because the dynamics are unrelated to acid concentration but quite sensitive to total acid load [150]. The sensitivity of duodenal mucosa to acid pH has been shown to have a pH threshold of 4.5, above which no fluid or bicarbonate response occurs [150]. When pancreatic juice was diverted in dogs, the fluid and bicarbonate response to unbuffered gastric acid was comparable to maximal exogenous secretin stimulation [147]. In spite of this weight of information favoring a profound influence of gastric acid on pancreatic secretion, Rune [151] has shown that only a very short segment of duodenum is ever sufficiently acidified to stimulate pancreatic secretion. Some explanation for the observed pancreatic fluid and bicarbonate response to meals is the potentiation of effect by protein [152] and fat [153] digestive products. No such potentiation of enzyme secretion is known.

Feedback

Finally, a large amount of work has focused on a feedback mechanism for enzyme secretion by diverting pancreatic flow in the rat [154]. Both trypsin inhibitor and diversion of pancreatic juice result in pancreatic exocrine stimulation. This effect has not been reproduced in the dog [155] and only equivocally in the pig [156]. Efforts at reproduction in humans have failed. Inoue et al [157] were able to show an increased release of CCK in response to food after pancreatic duct ligation in dogs. The known feedback for bicarbonate secretion by alkaline pH makes a hypothesis of a similar mechanism for enzyme secretion an attractive one.

REFERENCES

1. Pavlov IP: *The Work of the Digestive Glands.* Translated by WT Thomas. London, Griffin, 1902.
2. Bayliss WM, Starling EH: The mechanism of pancreatic secretion. J Physiol (Lond) 28:325, 1902.
3. Mellanby J: The mechanism of pancreatic digestion on the function of secretin. J Physiol (Lond) 60:85, 1925.
4. Ivy AC, Oldberg E: A hormone mechanism for gallbladder contraction and evacuation. Am J Physiol 86:599, 1928.
5. Harper AA, Raper HS: Pancreozymin, a stimulant of the secretion of pancreatic enzymes in extracts of the small intestine. J Physiol 102:115, 1943.
6. Mutt V, Jorpes JE: Structure of porcine cholecystokinin-pancreozymin. 1. Cleavage with thrombin and with trypsin. Eur J Biochem 6:156, 1968.
7. Wang CC, Grossman MI: Physiological determination of release of secretin and pancreozymin from intestine of dogs with transplanted pancreas. Am J Physiol 164:527, 1951.
8. Dimaline R, Dockray GJ: Actions of a new peptide from porcine intestine (PHI) on pancreatic secretion in the rat and turkey. Life Sci 27:1947, 1980.
9. Thompson JC, Marx MM: Gastrointestinal hormones. Curr Prob Surg 21:1, 1984.
10. Tache Y: Nature and biological actions of gastrointestinal peptides: Current status. Clin Biochem 17:77, 1984.
11. Louie DS, Williams JA, Owyang C: Action of pancreatic polypeptide on rat pancreatic secretion: In vivo and in vitro. Am J Physiol 249:G489, 1985.
12. Nealon WH, Beauchamp D, Townsend CM Jr, et al:

Comparative potencies of calcitonin gene-related peptide and calcitonin in the regulation of canine pancreatic exocrine function. Surg Forum 36:142, 1985.
13. Boden G, Sivitz MC, Owen OE, et al: Somatostatin suppresses secretin and pancreatic exocrine secretion. Science 190:163, 1975.
14. Tatemoto K: Isolation and characterization of peptide YY (PYY), a candidate gut hormone that inhibits pancreatic exocrine secretion. Proc Natl Acad Sci USA 79:2514, 1982.
15. Konturek SJ, Tasler J, Obtulowicz W, et al: Effect of growth hormone-release inhibiting hormone on hormones stimulating exocrine pancreatic secretion. J Clin Invest 58:1, 1976.
16. Harper AA: Hormonal control of pancreatic secretion, in Code CF (ed): *Handbook of Physiology*. Baltimore, Williams & Wilkins, 1967, pp 969–995.
17. Bloom SR, Polak JM: The new peptide hormones of the gut, in Jerzy Glass GB (ed): *Progress in Gastroenterology*. New York, Grune & Stratton, 1977, pp 109–151.
18. Barros D'Sa AAJ, Bloom SR, Polak JM, et al: Inhibition of gastric acid secretion and G-cell release of gastrin by growth-hormone release-inhibiting hormone (GH-RIH). Clin Sci 49:26p, 1975.
19. Schusdziarra V, Ipp E, Harris V, et al: Studies of the physiology and pathophysiology of the pancreatic D cell. Metabolism 27 (Suppl 1):1227, 1978.
20. Sewell WA, Young JA: Secretion of electrolytes by the pancreas of the anaesthetized rat. J Physiol 252:379, 1975.
21. Gorelick FS, Jamieson JD: Structure-function relationships of the pancreas, in Johnson LR (ed): *Physiology of the Gastrointestinal Tract*. New York, Raven Press, 1981, pp 773–794.
22. Davenport HW: Pancreatic secretion. *Physiology of the Digestive Tract*. 5th Ed. Chicago, Year Book Medical Publishers, 1982, pp 143–154.
23. Churg A, Richter WR: Histochemical distribution of carbonic anhydrase after ligation of the pancreatic duct. Am J Pathol 68:23, 1972.
24. Ekholm R, Zelander T, Edlund Y: The ultrastructural organization of the rat exocrine pancreas. I. Acinar cells. J Ultrastruc Res 7:61, 1962.
25. Geuze JJ, Poort C: Cell membrane resorption in the rat exocrine pancreas cell after in vivo stimulation of the secretion, as studied by in vitro incubation with extracellular space markers. J Cell Biol 57:159, 1973.
26. Farquhar MG, Palade GE: Cell junctions in amphibian skin. J Cell Biol 26:263, 1965.
27. Schulz I: Electrolyte and fluid secretion in the exocrine pancreas, in Johnson LR (ed): *Physiology of the Gastrointestinal Tract*. New York, Raven Press, 1981, pp 795–819.
28. Claude P, Goodenough DA: Fracture faces of zonulae occludentes from "tight" and "leaky" epithelia. J Cell Biol 58:390, 1973.
29. Bolender RP: Stereological analysis of the guinea pig pancreas. I. Analytical model and quantitative description of nonstimulated pancreatic exocrine cells. J Cell Biol 61:269, 1974.
30. Kraehenbuhl JP, Racine L, Jamieson JD: Immunocytochemical localization of secretory proteins in bovine pancreatic exocrine cells. J Cell Biol 72:406, 1977.
31. Scheele GA, Palade GE: Studies on the guinea pig pancreas. J Biol Chem 250:2660, 1975.
32. Palade G: Intracellular aspects of the process of protein synthesis. Science 189:347, 1975.
33. Palade GE: A small particulate component of the cytoplasm. J Biophys Biochem Cytol 1:59, 1955.
34. Scheele G, Dobberstein B, Blobel G: Transfer of proteins across membranes. Biosynthesis *in vitro* of pretrypsinogen and trypsinogen by cell fractions of canine pancreas. Eur J Biochem 82:593, 1978.
35. Blobel G, Dobberstein B: Transfer of proteins across membranes. Presence of proteolytically processed and unprocessed nascent immunoglobulin light chains on membrane-bound ribosomes of murine myeloma. J Cell Biol 67:835, 1975.
36. Steer ML, Glazer G: Parallel secretion of digestive enzymes by the in vitro rabbit pancreas. Am J Physiol 231:1860, 1976.
37. Rothman SS: The digestive enzymes of the pancreas: A mixture of inconstant proportions. Annu Rev Physiol 39:373, 1977.
38. Solomon TE: Regulation of exocrine pancreatic cell proliferation and enzyme synthesis, in Johnson LR (ed): *Physiology of the Gastrointestinal Tract*. New York, Raven Press, 1981, pp 873–892.
39. Slot JW, Strous GJAM, Geuze JJ: Effect of fasting and feeding on synthesis and intracellular transport of proteins in the frog exocrine pancreas. J Cell Biol 80:708, 1979.
40. Webster PD, Singh M, Tucker PC, et al: Effects of fasting and feeding on the pancreas. Gastroenterology 62:600, 1972.
41. Grossman MI, Greengard H, Ivy AC: The effect of dietary composition on pancreatic enzymes. Am J Physiol 138:676, 1943.
42. Heisler S, Brondek G: Absence of effects of dibutyryl cyclic guanosine 3′,5′-monophosphate on release of α-amylase, ^{45}Ca efflux, and protein synthesis in rat pancreas in vitro. Experientia 31:936, 1973.
43. Robberecht P, Deschodt-Lanckman M, Camus J, et al: Rat pancreatic hydrolases from birth to weaning and dietary adaptation after weaning. Am J Physiol 221:376, 1971.
44. Snook JT: Dietary regulation of pancreatic enzymes in the rat with emphasis on carbohydrate. Am J Physiol 221:1383, 1971.
45. Adelson JW, Miller PE: Pancreatic secretion by nonparallel exocytosis: Potential resolution of a long controversy. Science 228:993, 1985.
46. Huijghebaert SM, Hofmann AF: Pancreatic carboxypeptidase hydrolysis of bile acid-amino acid conjugates: Selective resistance of glycine and taurine amidates. Gastroenterology 90:306, 1986.
47. Gardner JD: Receptors and gastrointestinal hormones, in Sleisenger MH, Fordtran JF (eds): *Gastro-*

intestinal Disease. Philadelphia, WB Saunders, 1978, pp 179–195.

48. Gardner JD: Receptors for gastrointestinal hormones. Gastroenterology 76:202, 1979.
49. Steigerwalt RW, Williams JA: Characterization of cholecystokinin receptors on rat pancreatic membranes. Endocrinology 109:1746, 1981.
50. Szecowka J, Goldfine ID, Williams JA: Solubilization and characterization of CCK receptors from mouse pancreas. Regul Pept 10:71, 1985.
51. Vigna SR, Steigerwalt RW, Williams JA: Characterization of cholecystokinin receptors in bullfrog (*Rana catesbeiana*) brain and pancreas. Regul Pept 9:199, 1984.
52. Steigerwalt RW, Goldfine ID, Williams JA: Characterization of cholecystokinin receptors on bovine gallbladder membranes. Am J Physiol 247:G709, 1984.
53. Jensen RT, Lemp GF, Gardner JD: Interaction of cholecystokinin with specific membrane receptors on pancreatic acinar cells. Proc Natl Acad Sci USA 77:2079, 1980.
54. Gardner JD: Regulation of pancreatic exocrine function in vitro: Initial steps in the actions of secretagogues. Ann Rev Physiol 41:55, 1979.
55. Gardner JD, Jackson MJ, Batzri S, et al: Potential mechanisms of interaction among secretagogues. Gastroenterology 74:348, 1978.
56. Peikin SR, Rottman AJ, Batzri S, et al: Kinetics of amylase release by dispersed acini prepared from guinea pig pancreas. Am J Physiol 235:E743, 1978.
57. Gardner JD, Jensen RT: Regulation of pancreatic enzyme secretion *in vitro*, in Johnson LR (ed): *Physiology of the Gastrointestinal Tract*. New York, Raven Press, 1981, pp 831–871.
58. Douglas WW: Stimulus-secretion coupling: The concept and clues from chromaffin and other cells. Br J Pharmacol 34:451, 1968.
59. Case RM, Clausen T: The relationship between calcium exchange and enzyme secretion in the isolated rat pancreas. J Physiol 235:75, 1973.
60. Williams JA, Chandler D: Ca^{++} and pancreatic amylase release. Am J Physiol 228:1729, 1975.
61. Gardner JD, Conlon TP, Klaeveman HL, et al: Action of cholecystokinin and cholinergic agents on calcium transport in isolated pancreatic acinar cells. J Clin Invest 56:366, 1975.
62. Stolze H, Schulz I: Effect of atropine, ouabain, antimycin A, and A23187 on "trigger Ca^{2+} pool" in exocrine pancreas. Am J Physiol 238:G338, 1980.
63. Schulz I, Wakasugi H, Stolze H, et al: Analysis of Ca^{2+} fluxes and their relation to enzyme secretion in dispersed pancreatic acinar cells. Fed Proc 40:2503, 1981.
64. Singh M, Webster PD III: Pancreatic exocrine secretion. Clinics Gastroenterol 10:555, 1981.
65. Kapoor CL, Krishna G: Hormone-induced cyclic guanosine monophosphate secretion from guinea pig pancreatic lobules. Science 196:1003, 1977.
66. Gunther GR, Jamieson JD: Increased intracellular cyclic GMP does not correlate with protein discharge from pancreatic acinar cells. Nature 280:318, 1979.
67. Gardner JD, Rottman AJ: Evidence against cyclic GMP as a mediator of the actions of secretagogues on amylase release from guinea-pig pancreas. Biochim Biophys Acta 627:230, 1980.
68. Gardner JD, Rottman AJ: Action of cholera toxin on dispersed acini from guinea pig pancreas. Biochim Biophys Acta 585:250, 1979.
69. Peikin SR, Costenbader CL, Gardner JD: Actions of derivatives of cyclic nucleotides on dispersed acini from guinea pig pancreas. Discovery of a competitive antagonist of the action of cholecystokinin. J Biol Chem 254:5321, 1979.
70. Cassel D, Selinger Z: Mechanism of adenylate cyclase activation by cholera toxin: Inhibition of GTP hydrolysis at the regulatory site. Proc Natl Acad Sci USA 74:3307, 1977.
71. Hootman SR, Ochs DL, Williams JA: Intracellular mediators of Na^+-K^+ pump activity in guinea pig pancreatic acinar cells. Am J Physiol 249:G470, 1985.
72. Maruyama Y, Petersen OH: Control of K^+ conductance by cholecystokinin and Ca^{2+} in single pancreatic acinar cells studied by the patch-clamp technique. J Membr Biol 79:293, 1984.
73. Schulz I: Bicarbonate transport in the exocrine pancreas. Ann NY Acad Sci 341:191, 1980.
74. Folsch UR, Creutzfeldt W: Pancreatic duct cells in rats: Secretory studies in response to secretin, cholecystokinin-pancreozymin, and gastrin in vivo. Gastroenterology 73:1053, 1977.
75. Rothman SS, Brooks FP: Pancreatic secretion in vitro in "Cl^--free," "CO_2-free," and low-Na^+ environment. Am J Physiol 209:790, 1965.
76. Schulz I, Strover F, Ullrich KJ: Lipid soluble weak organic acid buffers as "substrate" for pancreatic secretion. Pflugers Arch 323:121, 1971.
77. Singh M, Webster PD III: Neurohormonal control of pancreatic secretion. A review. Gastroenterology 74:294–309, 1978.
78. Tiscornia OM, Martinez JL, Sarles H: Some aspects of human and canine macroscopic pancreas innervation. Am J Gastroenterol 66:353, 1976.
79. Brown JC, Harper AA, Scratcherd T: Potentiation of secretin stimulation of the pancreas. J Physiol 190:519, 1967.
80. Hickson JCD: The secretory and vascular response to nervous and hormonal stimulation in the pancreas of the pig. J Physiol 206:299, 1970.
81. Holst JJ, Schaffalitzky de Muckadell OB, Fahrenkrug J: Nervous control of pancreatic exocrine secretion in pigs. Acta Physiol Scand 105:33, 1979.
82. Debas HT, Yamagishi T: Evidence for pyloropancreatic reflex for pancreatic exocrine secretion. Am J Physiol 234:E468, 1978.
83. Konturek SJ, Becker HD, Thompson JC: Effect of vagotomy on hormones stimulating pancreatic secretion. Arch Surg 108:704, 1974.
84. Konturek SJ, Tasler J, Obtulowicz W: Effect of atro-

pine on pancreatic responses to endogenous and exogenous cholecystokinin. Am J Dig Dis 17:911, 1972.

85. Konturek SJ, Radecki T, Biernat J, et al: Effect of vagotomy on pancreatic secretion evoked by endogenous and exogenous cholecystokinin and caerulein. Gastroenterology 63:273, 1972.
86. Moreland HJ, Johnson LR: Effect of vagotomy on pancreatic secretion stimulated by endogenous and exogenous secretin. Gastroenterology 60:425, 1971.
87. Singer MV, Solomon TE, Rammert H, et al: Effect of atropine on pancreatic response to HCl and secretin. Am J Physiol 240:G376, 1981.
88. Singer MV, Niebel W, Hoffmeister D, et al: Dose response effects of atropine on pancreatic response to low doses of secretin. Regul Rept (Suppl) 2:S108, 1983.
89. Debas HT, Konturek SJ, Grossman MI: Effect of extragastric and truncal vagotomy on pancreatic secretion in the dog. Am J Physiol 228:1172, 1975.
90. Fried GM, Ogden WD, Greeley G, et al: Correlation of release and actions of cholecystokinin in dogs before and after vagotomy. Surgery 93:786, 1983.
91. Singer MV, Niebel W, Uhde KH, et al: Dose-response effects of atropine on pancreatic response to secretin before and after truncal vagotomy. Am J Physiol 248:G532, 1985.
92. Beglinger C, Grossman MI, Solomon TE: Interaction between stimulants of exocrine pancreatic secretion in dogs. Am J Physiol 246:G173, 1984.
93. Solomon T, Grossman MI: Effect of atropine and vagotomy on response of transplanted pancreas. Am J Physiol 236:E186, 1979.
94. Fried GM, Ogden WD, Sakamoto T, et al: Experimental evidence for a vagally mediated and cholecystokinin-independent enteropancreatic reflex. Ann Surg 202:69, 1985.
95. Amsterdam A, Jamieson JD: Structural and functional characterization of isolated pancreatic exocrine cells. Proc Natl Acad Sci USA 69:3028, 1972.
96. Vaysse N, Bastie MJ, Pascal JP, et al: Effects of catecholamines and their inhibitors on the isolated canine pancreas. I. Noradrenaline and isoprenaline. Gastroenterology 72:711, 1977.
97. Thomas JE: Neural regulation of pancreatic secretion, in Code CF (ed): *Handbook of Physiology*. Baltimore, Williams & Wilkins, 1967, pp 955–968.
98. Elisha EE, Hutson D, Scratcherd T: The direct inhibition of pancreatic electrolyte secretion by noradrenaline in the isolated perfused cat pancreas. J Physiol 351:77, 1984.
99. Pearson GT, Singh J, Petersen OH: Adrenergic nervous control of cAMP-mediated amylase secretion in the rat pancreas. Am J Physiol 246:G563, 1984.
100. Iwatsuki K, Chiba S: Comparative study of the secretory response to dopamine and seven amino acid conjugated derivatives of the blood-perfused canine pancreas. Jpn J Pharmacol 30:621, 1980.
101. Pearson GT, Davison JS, Collins RC, et al: Control of enzyme secretion by non-cholinergic, non-adrenergic nerves in guinea pig pancreas. Nature 290:259, 1981.
102. Furness JB, Costa M: Types of nerves in the enteric nervous system. Neuroscience 5:1, 1980.
103. Snyder SH, Innis RB: Peptide neurotransmitters. Annu Rev Biochem 48:755, 1979.
104. Chey WY, Lee YH, Hendricks JG, et al: Plasma secretin concentrations in fasting and postprandial state in man. Am J Dig Dis 23:981, 1978.
105. Kim MS, Lee KY, Chey WY: Plasma secretin concentrations in fasting and postprandial states in dog. Am J Physiol 236:E539, 1979.
106. Schaffalitzky de Muckadell OB, Fahrenkrug J: Secretion pattern of secretin in man: Regulation by gastric acid. Gut 19:812, 1978.
107. Fahrenkrug J, Schaffalitzky de Muckadell OB, Rune SJ: pH threshold for release of secretin in normal subjects and in patients with duodenal ulcer and patients with chronic pancreatitis. Scand J Gastroenterol 13:177, 1978.
108. Thomas JE, Crider JO: A quantitative study of acid in the intestine as a stimulus for the pancreas. Am J Physiol 131:349, 1940.
109. Schaffalitzky de Muckadell OB, Fahrenkrug J, Nielsen J, et al: Meal-stimulated secretin release in man: Effect of acid and bile. Scand J Gastroenterol 16:981, 1981.
110. Makhlouf GM, Said SI: The effect of vasoactive intestinal peptide (VIP) on digestive and hormonal function, in Thompson JC (ed): *Gastrointestinal Hormones*. Austin, University of Texas Press, 1975, pp 599–610.
111. Modlin IM, Bloom SR, Mitchell SJ: Experimental evidence for vasoactive intestinal peptide as the cause of the watery diarrhea syndrome. Gastroenterology 75:1051, 1978.
112. Walsh JH, Lamers CB, Valenzuela JE: Cholecystokinin-octapeptidelike immunoreactivity in human plasma. Gastroenterology 82:438, 1982.
113. Jansen JBMJ, Lamers CBHW: Radioimmunoassay of cholecystokinin in human tissue and plasma. Clin Chim Acta 131:305, 1983.
114. Wiener I, Inoue K, Fagan CJ, et al: Release of cholecystokinin in man. Correlation of blood levels with gallbladder contraction. Ann Surg 194:321, 1981.
115. Lilja P, Wiener I, Inoue K, et al: Release of cholecystokinin in response to food and intraduodenal fat in pigs, dogs and man. Surg Gynecol Obstet 159:557, 1984.
116. Thompson JC, Fried GM, Ogden WD, et al: Correlation between release of cholecystokinin and contraction of the gallbladder in patients with gallstones. Ann Surg 195:670, 1982.
117. Fried GM, Ogden WD, Swierczek J, et al: Release of cholecystokinin in conscious dogs: Correlation with simultaneous measurements of gallbladder pressure and pancreatic protein secretion. Gastroenterology 85:1113, 1983.
118. Hopman WPM, Jansen JBMJ, Lamers CBHW: Plasma cholecystokinin response to a liquid fat

meal in vagotomized patients. Ann Surg 200:693, 1984.
119. Stening GF, Grossman MI: Gastrin-related peptides as stimulants of pancreatic and gastric secretion. Am J Physiol 217:262, 1969.
120. Lindkaer Jensen S, Rehfeld JF, Holst JJ, et al: Secretory effects of gastrins on isolated perfused porcine pancreas. Am J Physiol 238:E186, 1980.
121. Anastasi A, Erspamer V, Endean R: Isolation and amino acid sequence of caerulein, the active decapeptide of the skin of *Hyla caerulea*. Arch Biochem Biophys 125:57, 1968.
122. Erspamer V, Falconieri Erspamer G, Inselvini M, et al: Occurrence of bombesin and alytesin in extracts of the skin of three European discoglossid frogs and pharmacological actions of bombesin on extravascular smooth muscle. Br J Pharmacol 45:333, 1972.
123. May RJ, Conlon TP, Erspamer V, et al: Actions of peptides isolated from amphibian skin on pancreatic acinar cells. Am J Physiol 235:E112, 1978.
124. Inoue K, McKay D, Yajima H, et al: Effect of gastrin releasing peptide on the release of gastrointestinal hormones in dogs. Physiologist 25:218, 1982.
125. Deschodt-Lanckman M, Robberecht P, De Neef P, et al: In vitro action of bombesin and bombesin-like peptides on amylase secretion, calcium efflux, and adenylate cyclase activity in the rat pancreas. A comparison with other secretagogues. J Clin Invest 58:891, 1976.
126. von Euler US, Gaddum JH: An unidentified depressor substance in certain tissue extracts. J Physiol 72:74, 1931.
127. Carraway R, Leeman SE: The isolation of a new hypotensive peptide, neurotensin, from bovine hypothalami. J Biol Chem 248:6854, 1973.
128. Sakamoto T, Newman J, Fujimura M, et al: Role of neurotensin in pancreatic secretion. Surgery 96:146, 1984.
129. Schwartz TW: Pancreatic polypeptide: A hormone under vagal control. Gastroenterology 85:1411, 1983.
130. Taylor IL, Solomon TE, Walsh JH, et al: Studies on the metabolism and biologic activity of pancreatic polypeptide. Scand J Gastroenterol 13:182, 1978.
131. Dyck WP, Texter EC Jr, Lasater JM, et al: Influence of glucagon on pancreatic exocrine secretion in man. Gastroenterology 58:532, 1970.
132. Harper AA, Hood AJC, Mushens J, et al: Pancreotone, an inhibitor of pancreatic secretion in extracts of ileal and colonic mucosa. J Physiol 292:455, 1979.
133. Konturek SJ, Radecki T, Pucher A: Comparison of natural and synthetic prostaglandins on gastric and pancreatic secretions and peptic ulcer formation in conscious cats. Digestion 14:44, 1976.
134. Konturek SJ, Radecki T, Konturek D, et al: Effect of calcitonin on gastric and pancreatic secretion and peptic ulcer formation in cats. Am J Dig Dis 19:235, 1974.
135. Schwartz TW, Stadil F, Chance RE, et al: Pancreatic-polypeptide response to food in duodenal-ulcer patients before and after vagotomy. Lancet 1:1102, 1976.
136. Lluis F, Fujimura M, Guo Y-S, et al: Peptide YY is an important regulator of pancreatic exocrine secretion. Surg Forum 36:170, 1985.
137. Nealon WH, Beauchamp RD, Townsend CM Jr, et al: Additive interactions of calcitonin gene-related pancreatic peptide and calcitonin on pancreatic exocrine function in conscious dogs. Dig Dis Sci 30:984, 1985.
138. Preshaw RM, Cooke AR, Grossman MI: Sham feeding and pancreatic secretion in the dog. Gastroenterology 50:171, 1966.
139. Sarles H, Dani R, Prezelin G, et al: Cephalic phase of pancreatic secretion in man. Gut 9:214, 1968.
140. Defilippi C, Solomon TE, Valenzuela JE: Pancreatic secretory response to sham feeding in humans. Digestion 23:217, 1982.
141. Feldman M, Walsh JH: Acid inhibition of sham feeding-stimulated gastrin release and gastric acid secretion: Effect of atropine. Gastroenterology 78:772, 1980.
142. Valenzuela JE, Walsh JH, Isenberg JI: Effect of gastrin on pancreatic enzyme secretion and gallbladder emptying in man. Gastroenterology 71:409, 1976.
143. Meyer JH, Kelly GA, Jones RS: Canine pancreatic response to intestinally perfused oligopeptides. Am J Physiol 231:678, 1976.
144. Go VLW, Hofmann AF, Summerskill WHJ: Pancreozymin bioassay in man based on pancreatic enzyme secretion: Potency of specific amino acids and other digestive products. J Clin Invest 49:1558, 1970.
145. Meyer JH, Kelly GA, Spingola LJ, et al: Canine gut receptors mediating pancreatic responses to luminal L-amino acids. Am J Physiol 231:669, 1976.
146. Green GM, Olds BA, Matthews G, et al: Protein, as a regulator of pancreatic enzyme secretion in the rat. Proc Soc Exp Biol Med 142:1162, 1973.
147. Debas HT, Grossman MI: Pure cholecystokinin: Pancreatic protein and bicarbonate response. Digestion 9:469, 1973.
148. Malagelada J-R, DiMagno EP, Summerskill WHJ, et al: Regulation of pancreatic and gallbladder functions by intraluminal fatty acids and bile acids in man. J Clin Invest 58:493, 1976.
149. Lam SK, Isenberg JI, Grossman MI, et al: Gastric acid secretion is abnormally sensitive to endogenous gastrin released after peptone test meals in duodenal ulcer patients. J Clin Invest 65:555, 1980.
150. Meyer JH, Way LW, Grossman MI: Pancreatic bicarbonate response to various acids in duodenum of the dog. Am J Physiol 219:964, 1970.
151. Rune SJ: pH in the human duodenum. Digestion 8:261, 1973.
152. Fink AS, Miller JC, Jehn DW, et al: Digests of protein augment acid-induced canine pancreatic secretion. Am J Physiol 242:G634, 1982.
153. Fink AS, Meyer JH: Intraduodenal emulsions of

oleic acid augment acid-induced canine pancreatic secretion. Am J Physiol 245:G85, 1983.
154. Miyasaka K, Green GM: Effect of atropine on rat basal pancreatic secretion during return or diversion of bile-pancreatic juice. Proc Soc Exp Biol Med 174:187, 1983.
155. Magee DF, Naruse S: Effect of pancreatic juice on basal pancreatic and gastric secretion in dogs. J Physiol 330:489, 1982.
156. Lilja P, Greeley G, Thompson JC: Intraduodenal trypsin does not inhibit release of cholecystokinin in pig. Gastroenterology 82:1118, 1982.
157. Inoue K, Yazigi R, Watson LC, et al: Increased release of cholecystokinin after pancreatic duct ligation. Surgery 91:467, 1982.

MOTILITY: GUT AND BILIARY

Tsuguo Sakamoto, M.D., Yan-Shi Guo, M.D., and James C. Thompson, M.D.

Gastrointestinal motility can be regulated by three different mechanisms: the nervous system, intrinsic electrical activity, and humoral agents. The effect of gastrointestinal hormones on gut motility may be produced by concentrations of hormones that are truly physiologic in some instances or it may result only after administration of larger, "pharmacologic" concentrations. Physiologic concentrations are those achieved by natural release mechanisms—in the case of gut hormones, this usually means those concentrations of a peptide present in the blood after a meal. The concept is not always simple, however, since motility is often stimulated by an interplay of endocrine, paracrine, or neurocrine peptides as well as by local myogenic and neurogenic controls.

Recent advances in immunohistochemistry have provided some information about the localization of peptides as paracrine or neurocrine. However, it remains difficult to determine the relationship between local levels of peptide in the vicinity of receptors and gastrointestinal motility. We have no methods yet available to evaluate the physiologic role of regulatory peptides when they act in a paracrine or neurocrine manner. Therefore, we can assess the physiologic role of peptides on gastrointestinal motility only by the following criteria provided by Grossman [1], who stated that such agents should 1) be present in endocrine cells, 2) be released by feeding or other stimuli, thereby increasing plasma concentration and producing characteristic biologic actions, and 3) produce effects that could be reproduced by infusion of the exogenous peptide in amounts that yield plasma concentrations observed with endogenous release.

Two different kinds of motor activity are present throughout the gastrointestinal tract, namely, a digestive pattern of motility and an interdigestive pattern. Szurszewski [2] demonstrated a typical interdigestive motor complex in the dog intestine. This myoelectric complex is initiated in the duodenum and migrates down the intestine until it reaches the terminal ileum. The migrating motor complex (MMC) continuously recycles every 2 hours and shows four phases, namely, phase I, a relative absence of action potential activity; phase II, persistent but random action potential activity; phase III, sudden onset and continuous occurrence of bursts of large action potentials; and phase IV, rapid decrease in the incidence of action potentials.

These phasic changes of MMC were also found in the lower esophageal sphincter, the stomach, and the gallbladder [3,4]. The control mechanisms of the MMC are unclear. Both humoral and neural control may be involved.

The results of studies on the effects of gastrointestinal hormones on gastrointestinal motility are summarized in Table 9-3.

Gastrin

Gastrin causes contraction of the lower esophageal sphincter, and this effect is not antagonized by atropine [5]. Intravenous infusion of gastrin-17 has been reported to significantly increase the lower esophageal sphincter pressure at doses that yield serum concentrations of gastrin similar to those seen after a meal [6]. However, in other reports, the contraction of the lower esophageal sphincter can be seen only at pharmacologic doses of gastrin [7]. No correlation was found between concentrations of serum gastrin and lower esophageal sphincter pressure in clinical conditions associated either with hypergastrinemia or with decreased sphincter pressure [8]. We agree with the general conclusion that gastrin appears to have no physiologic role in the regulation of lower esophageal sphincter pressure.

Gastrin causes relaxation of the gastric fundus and contraction of the antrum in humans and various animals [9–13]. This action has been suggested as a physiologic role of gastrin [9,12]. Pharmacologic doses of gastrin delay gastric emptying of fluid in humans [14] and in the dog [15,16] and of solid food in humans [17]. The delay of gastric emptying can be explained, in part, by relaxation of the proximal stomach. Gastrin can cause con-

Table 9-3. **Summary of studies (with references) on the effects of different gastrointestinal hormones on gut motility**

Peptides	LES*	Stomach: Proximal	Stomach: Distal	Pylorus	Gastric emptying
Gastrin	+[5–8]	−[9]	+°[10–13]	−[d][49]	−[14–17]
CCK	−[45–48]	−°[48]	+−[50, 121]	+[49, 51]	−[15, 51, 52]
Secretin	−[a][61, 62]	−[48]	−[48, 63]	+[49]	−[52, 64]
VIP	−[a][95, 96]	−[97]	−[98]	−[99]	+[99]
GIP	−[a][122]	−[123]	−[123]		
Glucagon	−[a][124]	−[125]	−[125]	+−[126]	−[127]
Motilin	+°[75, 76]	+°[72, 80]	+°[72, 74, 77]	+[128]	+[91]
Substance P	+[102]	+[103]		+[103]	
Neurotensin	−[108]	+−[110, 111, 113]	−[110]		−[109]
Somatostatin		−[129]	−[129]		+−[130]
Bombesin			−[131]	+[132]	−[133]
Enkephalins			−[134]	+[134]	
PP	+[135]		+[136]		+[136]
PYY		−[137]	−[137]		

Peptides	Small intestine	Colon	Gallbladder	SO**
Gastrin	+[b][18, 21–23]	+[24, 25]	+[19, 20]	−[26]
CCK	+[b][53–55]	+[24, 58, 67, 25]	+°[19, 26–33, 42]	−°[26, 39–44, 138]
Secretin	−[b][65, 66]	−[67, 68]	+−[35, 36, 70, 71]	−[26]
VIP	+−[100, 101]	−[139]	−[36–38, 140]	
GIP				
Glucagon	+−[b][127, 141–143]	−[68, 127, 144]	−[26, 42, 145]	−[26]
Motilin	+°[c][72, 73, 78, 79, 81–88]		+°[4, 76]	
Substance P	+[104]	+[105]	+[106]	
Neurotensin	+[111, 112]	+[112, 117]	+[117]	−[UP]
Somatostatin	+−[c][146, 147]		−[129, 148, 149]	
Bombesin	+−[131]		+[131, 150]	
Enkephalins	+−[c][151, 152]	+[151]		
PP	+[153]	+[136]	−°[154, 155]	+[155]
PYY	−[156]	−[156]	x[157]	
PSP	−[119]			

* = lower esophageal sphincter; + = increase in motility; − = decrease in motility; [a] = antagonist to gastrin; ° = possible physiologic role; [b] = induction of fed pattern from fasted pattern; [c] = induction of migrating motor complexes; [d] = antagonist to CCK and secretin; ** = sphincter of Oddi; UP = unpublished data from our laboratory; x = no effect.

traction of the jejunum, ileum, and colon [13,18] and gallbladder [19,20] in various animals only at pharmacologic doses. Interdigestive MMCs of the stomach and intestine are disrupted by large doses of pentagastrin in dogs [21,22]. However, Erckenbrecht et al. [23] recently reported that pentagastrin (in a dose that stimulates gastric acid secretion to the same extent as the postprandial rise of gastrin) converted the normal interdigestive motility pattern to the digestive motility pattern in the upper gut in humans, whereas proglumide (a gastrin receptor antagonist) restored the periodic fasting pattern. This indicates that stimulation of upper intestinal motility might be one of the physiologic roles of gastrin in humans.

Physiologic doses of gastrin I increase the incidence of rectal and rectosigmoidal action potentials and the amplitude of intraluminal pressure in humans [24,25]. However, a postprandial slow increase in serum gastrin concentration does not correlate with rapid response of colonic motor activity to a meal [25].

Cholecystokinin

Cholecystokinin (CCK) causes contraction of the gallbladder and relaxation of the sphincter of Oddi [19,26]. The cholecystokinetic activity of CCK has been established in a number of different species using both in vivo and in vitro preparations

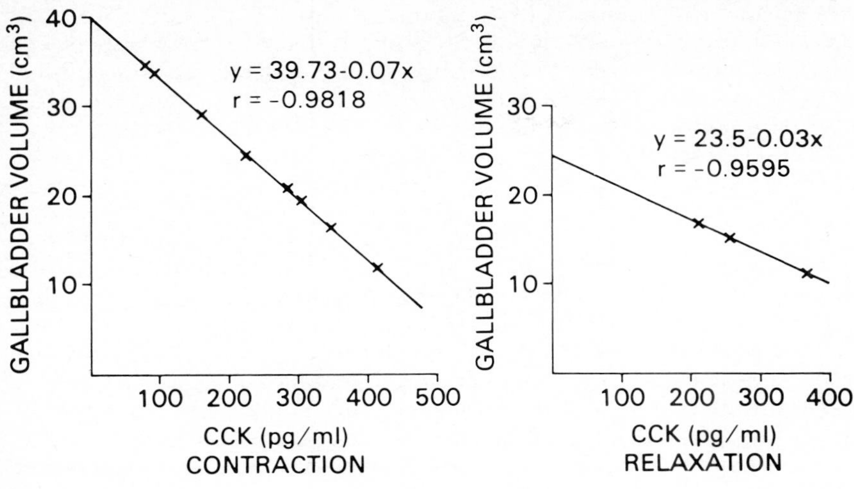

Figure 9-8. Linear regression analysis of CCK levels and gallbladder volume during contraction phase (0–16 min) and relaxation phase (18–60 min) in eight-volunteers after intraduodenal instillation of Lipomul. (From Wiener et al [31], by permission of the JB Lippincott Co.)

[26–30]. In humans, intravenous infusion of physiologic doses of CCK-33 causes gallbladder contraction [30]. Gallbladder kinetics in response to fat ingestion were found to correlate significantly with plasma concentrations of CCK-33 in normal individuals [31] (Fig 9-8), and in patients with gallstones [32] (Fig 9-9). These findings provide strong evidence that endogenous CCK plays a major role in the physiologic stimulation of gallbladder contraction. This action is not affected by either cholinergic or adrenergic blockades [27,28,33]. CCK can act directly on gallbladder muscle and possibly exerts its effect through receptor-operated calcium channels [34]. The cholecystokinetic activity of CCK is potentiated by secretin, whereas exogenous secretin itself has no effect on gallbladder contraction [35,36]. In contrast to secretin, vasoactive intestinal peptide (VIP) antagonizes CCK-induced gallbladder contraction both in vivo and in vitro [36–38]. The physiologic significance of these hormone-hormone interactions on gallbladder contraction is, however, unclear.

The effect of CCK on the sphincter of Oddi is controversial. The discrepancies in previous reports may be due to the impurity of peptides, differences in methods, and differences in species. CCK has been shown to increase common duct pressure and to decrease bile duct flow in dogs and rabbits [39,40]. In the opossum, CCK also increases contractile activity of the biliary sphincter and decreases common bile duct flow [41]. On the other hand, there is accumulating evidence that CCK causes relaxation of the sphincter of Oddi. Lin and Spray have demonstrated that CCK relaxed the sphincter of Oddi in conscious dogs [42] and that threshold doses of CCK for relaxation of the sphincter of Oddi are smaller than those required for gallbladder contraction [26]. Persson and Ekman [43] demonstrated that the sphincter muscle of Oddi can respond to CCK independently of duodenal smooth muscle. The effect of CCK on the sphincter of Oddi is unaffected by both cholinergic and adrenergic blockades [42,44]. CCK may act di-

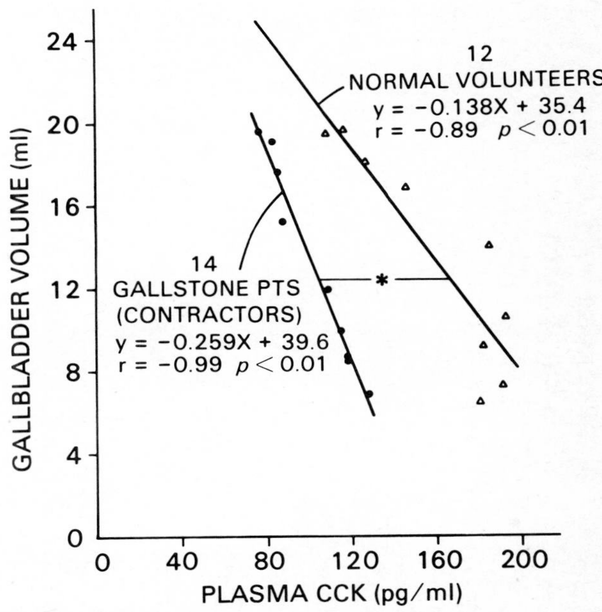

Figure 9-9. Linear regression analysis of gallbladder volume versus plasma concentrations of CCK 0–30 minutes after Lipomul administration. * = significant difference between slopes of regression. (From Thompson et al [32], by permission of the JB Lippincott Co.)

rectly on the sphincter of Oddi. We have unpublished studies in dogs that support its role in relaxation of the sphincter of Oddi in dogs. Thus, motor activity of the gallbladder and the sphincter of Oddi in response to food can be attributed mainly to the physiologic role of CCK. The relaxing effect of CCK on sphincter of Oddi is also enhanced by secretin or intraduodenal acid [26,42,44].

CCK causes relaxation of the human lower esophageal sphincter [45,46]. This effect may be mediated by stimulation of postganglionic, nonadrenergic, noncholinergic inhibitory neurons [47]. In dogs, the submaximal dose of CCK for pancreatic secretion and gallbladder contraction inhibits gastric emptying of fluid in a dose-dependent manner [15]. The inhibitory effect of CCK on gastric emptying may be caused by the decrease in intragastric pressure and increase in pyloric pressure [48–51]. In contrast, gastric emptying in humans is unaffected by physiologic doses of CCK [52].

During the interdigestive state, CCK given at a physiologic dose (ED_{50} for pancreatic secretion) increases duodenal and jejunal spike potentials and decreases the duration of phase II of MMCs. At a higher dose of CCK, phase III of MMCs is interrupted [53,54] (Fig 9-10). CCK greatly decreases the transit time for contrast material through the human small intestine [55] and increases human and cat colonic motility in vivo [24,56,57] and in vitro [58]. Recently, central administration of CCK-8 was reported to decrease the frequency of the MMCs in rats [59] (Fig 9-11), but intraluminal infusion of CCK-8 increased the myoelectric activity in the intestine of rabbits [60].

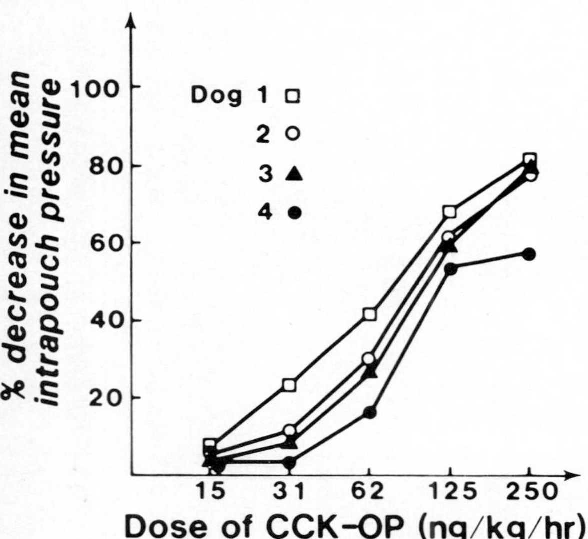

Figure 9-10. Effect of intravenous CCK-8 pressure within the gastric pouch during phase III motility after IV infusion of CCK-8. (From Schang and Kelly [53], by permission of the American Physiological Society.)

Secretin

Secretin itself has no effect on the lower esophageal sphincter in humans [61] or in the opossum [62], but it antagonizes gastrin-induced contraction of the lower esophageal sphincter [62]. The ED_{50} of secretin for pancreatic secretion can cause significant inhibition of intragastric pressure in conscious dogs [48], suggesting a physiologic role of secretin in relaxation of the stomach. In vitro, secretin decreases spontaneous phasic contraction of muscle strips from human fundus and antrum [63]. Physiologic doses of secretin cause significant delay of gastric emptying of liquid in humans [52,64]. This action may be due to inhibitory effects on intragastric pressure. Intraduodenal acidification inhibits MMCs in dogs. However, the inhibitory effects of secretin on MMCs can be seen only at pharmacologic doses [65]. In humans, pharmacologic doses of secretin can also inhibit basal motor activity of the duodenum and jejunum and antagonize the stimulatory effect of CCK [66]. The effect of secretin on intestinal motility appears to occur only with pharmacologic doses.

The effect of secretin on rectosigmoidal motility is chiefly inhibitory [67,68] and is found only with pharmacologic doses. Intraduodenal acidification has been reported to cause gallbladder contraction, presumably mediated by hormonal substances [69], possibly by secretin and CCK. In conscious dogs with chronic gallbladder fistulas, even when secretin is given alone intravenously at pharmacologic doses, the gallbladder does not respond [35,70], but the cholecystokinetic effects of CCK are augmented by exogenous or endogenously released secretin [35]. On the other hand, Lin and Spray [26,28] observed gallbladder contraction in response to secretin at a dose range of 1 to 4 U/kg/hr and found augmentation of cholecystokinetic effects between CCK and secretin. However, the doses of secretin used for augmentation of CCK on gallbladder contraction were much higher than ED_{50} of secretin for pancreatic secretion. Therefore, secretin is probably not a physiologic regulator of gallbladder contraction. Intraduodenal administration of acid also decreases choledochal resistance [44]. Exogenous secretin administered at doses that are lower than needed

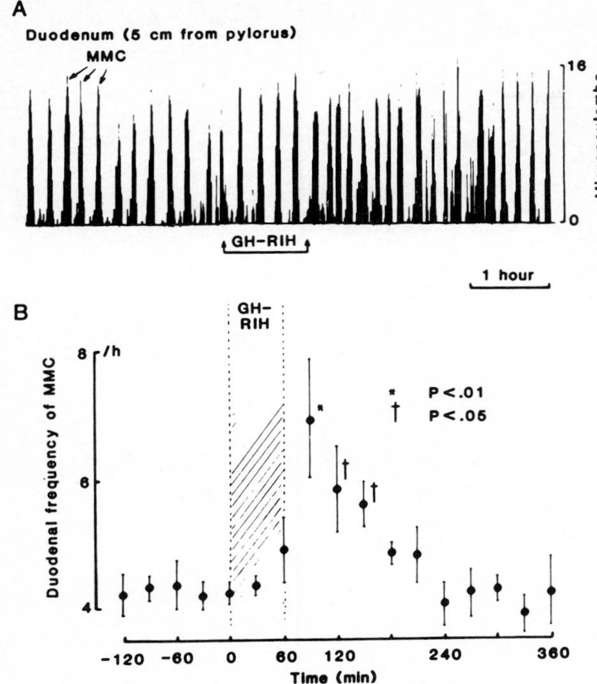

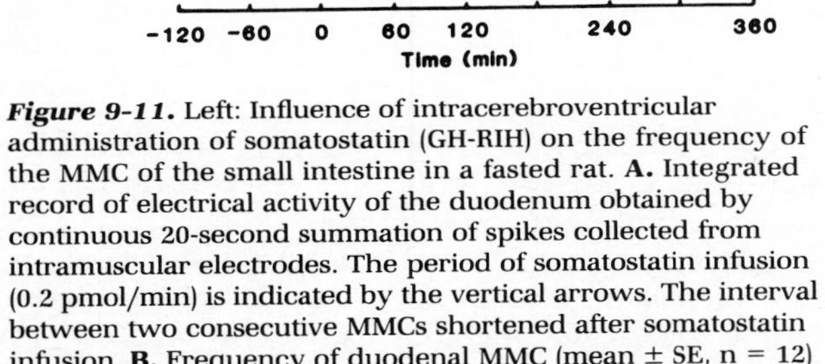

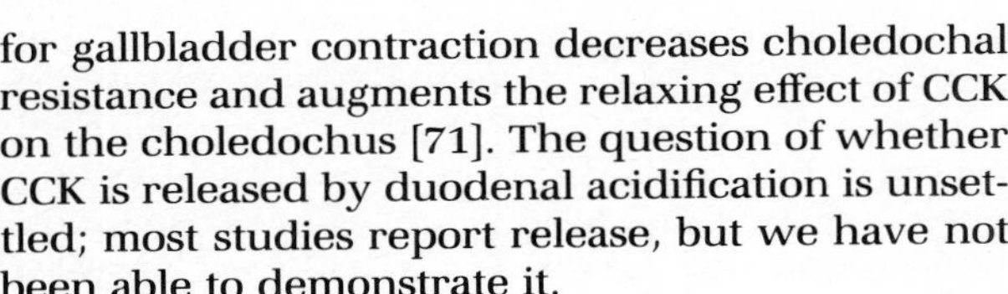

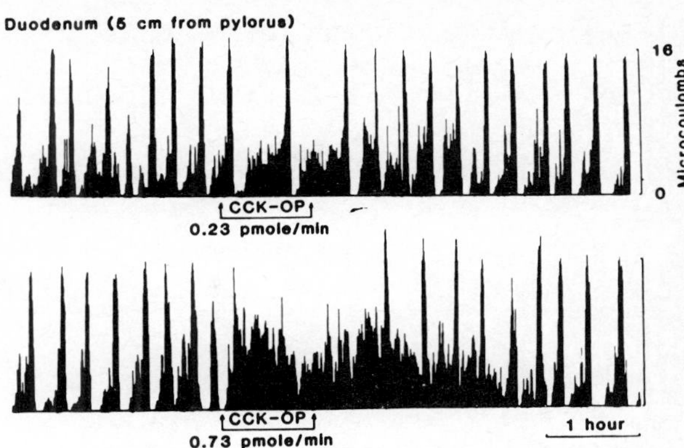

Figure 9-11. Left: Influence of intracerebroventricular administration of somatostatin (GH-RIH) on the frequency of the MMC of the small intestine in a fasted rat. **A.** Integrated record of electrical activity of the duodenum obtained by continuous 20-second summation of spikes collected from intramuscular electrodes. The period of somatostatin infusion (0.2 pmol/min) is indicated by the vertical arrows. The interval between two consecutive MMCs shortened after somatostatin infusion. **B.** Frequency of duodenal MMC (mean ± SE, n = 12) measured during consecutive 30-minute periods. Somatostatin infusion (0.2 pmol/min) significantly increased the frequency of MMC. Right: Comparative effects of two doses of CCK-OP administered intracerebroventricularly on the pattern of MMC of the small intestine in a fasted rat. The duration of the MMC cycle increased at the lower rate of infusion, while at the higher rate (0.73 pmol/min) the MMC was disrupted in a manner similar to that seen after a meal. (From Bueno and Ferre [59], by permission of the American Association for the Advancement of Science.)

for gallbladder contraction decreases choledochal resistance and augments the relaxing effect of CCK on the choledochus [71]. The question of whether CCK is released by duodenal acidification is unsettled; most studies report release, but we have not been able to demonstrate it.

Motilin

Motilin has significant effects on gastrointestinal smooth muscle. During the interdigestive state, the plasma levels of motilin fluctuate cyclically in humans and dogs, and peak levels are closely associated with the onset of phase III of the interdigestive myoelectrical activity of the stomach and duodenum [72,73] (Fig 9-12). The gallbladder and the lower esophageal sphincter also contract cyclically in synchrony with MMCs in the stomach and duodenum [3,4] (Figs 9-13 and 9-14). During the interdigestive state, intravenous physiologic doses of motilin can initiate MMCs in the gastroduodenal area [73,74] and cause synchronous contractions of the gallbladder and the lower esophageal sphincter [75,76]. Motilin in vitro has been shown to stimulate contractile activity of the canine stomach and duodenum [77] and rabbit small intestine [78].

Itoh et al [79] have shown that the induction of MMCs by exogenous motilin can be found only in the interdigestive state. Exogenous motilin has little effect on the digestive pattern of intestinal motor activity. In a study on an autotransplanted canine gastric pouch, exogenous motilin was found to synchronously induce an activity front (phase III) in the pouch, in the main stomach, and in the duodenum [80]. When antimotilin antibodies were given intravenously, the spontaneous occurrence of MMCs was interrupted temporarily,

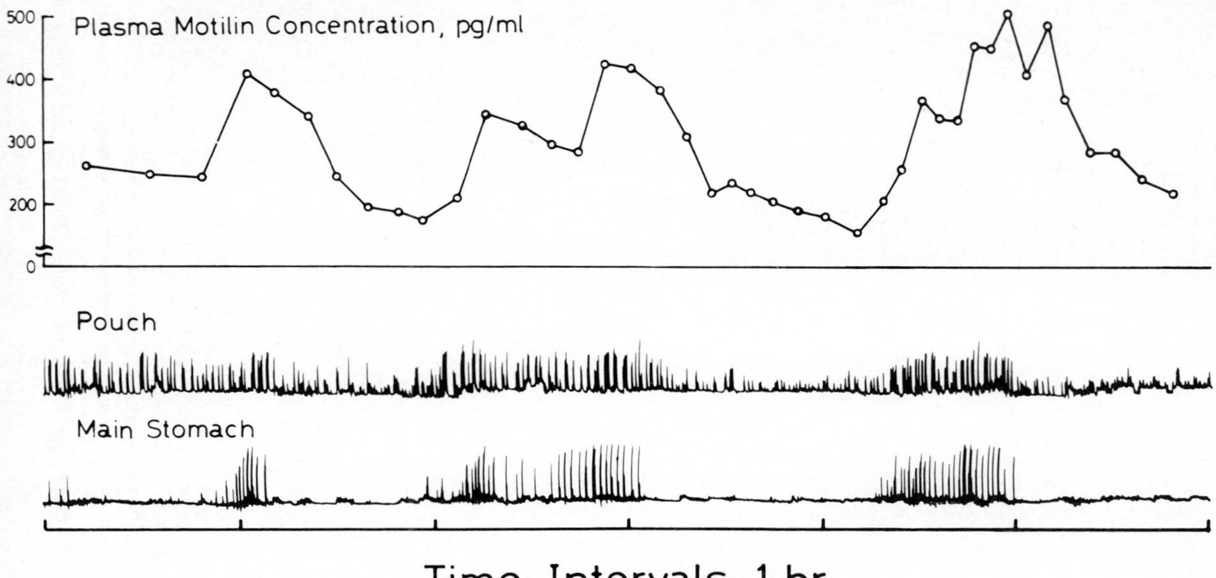

Figure 9-12. Comparison of changes in plasma immunoreactive motilin concentration and in contractile activity in the main stomach and the extrinsically denervated pouch in a dog. Contractile changes in the pouch are more closely correlated to plasma IRM concentration than those in the main stomach. (From Itoh et al [72], by permission of Plenum Publishing Corp.)

and plasma motilin concentrations were temporarily decreased in the conscious dog [81]. As plasma motilin levels rise again to the levels of the pre-antimotilin peak, regular MMCs reappear in the antrum and migrate abnormally. Thus, these studies strongly suggest a physiologic role for motilin in the initiation of MMCs of the stomach and duodenum. However, the MMCs can occur without a concomitant increase in plasma motilin levels [82]. Conversely, a peak plasma concentration of motilin does not always induce MMCs [83]. Exogenous gastrin, CCK, and secretin convert interdigestive patterns to digestive patterns without affecting cyclic changes in plasma motilin levels [84]. Therefore, the regulation of MMCs cannot be fully attributed to motilin.

Although exogenous somatostatin, at physiologic doses, decreases plasma levels of motilin and pancreatic polypeptide (PP), somatostatin induces an activity front (phase III) in the duodenum and jejunum. In addition, cyclic increases in plasma somatostatin levels are also observed simultaneously with the appearance of the activity front in the upper duodenum. Somatostatin, therefore, appears to be another candidate for the regulation of the MMCs [85]. Ectopic MMCs can be observed in the jejunum, while plasma motilin levels are depressed by infusion of somatostatin or PP. MMCs in the jejunum, therefore, seem to be motilin-independent, whereas MMCs in the gastroduodenal area are motilin-dependent [86,87].

Atropine suppresses both MMCs and fluctuation of plasma motilin concentrations in humans [88]. Cholinergic mechanisms may be involved, at least in part, in the regulation of MMCs. Plasma levels of motilin have been shown to increase after a mixed meal or after fat and water. Physiologic doses of exogenous motilin in humans accelerate gastric emptying of a mixed breakfast and of glucose, but not of fat [89–91]. In contrast, other studies have shown that ingestion of a mixed meal not only abolished the cyclic changes in plasma motilin levels but also resulted in a significant decrease in plasma motilin levels that was accompanied by induction of digestive myoelectric patterns in the stomach and duodenum [84,92].

VIP

VIP has been shown by immunocytochemical techniques to be localized in vagal neurons and in the myenteric and submucous plexus of the bowel in humans and many other mammalian species. VIP appears to play an important role in the enteric nervous system [93].

VIP is a putative neurotransmitter of the non-

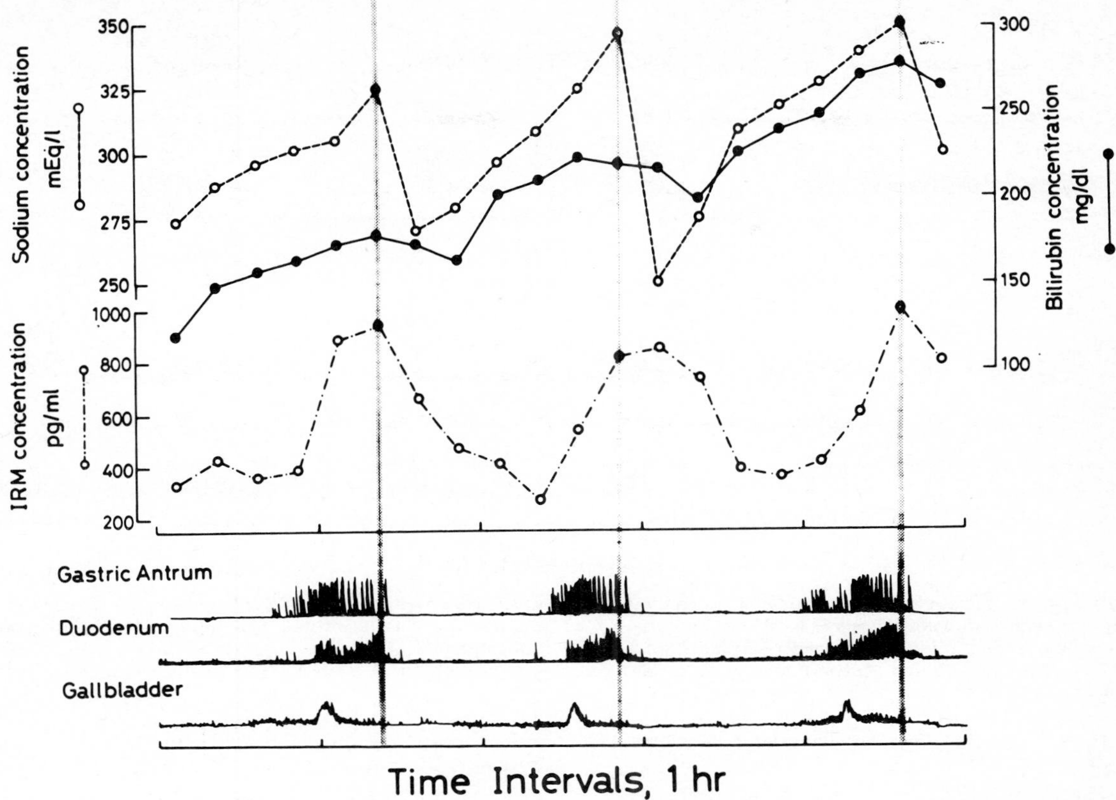

Figure 9-13. Interdigestive 5-hour changes in gallbladder bilirubin and sodium concentration (top), plasma immunoreactive motilin concentration (middle), and contractile activity in the gastric antrum, the duodenum, and the gallbladder (bottom) in a conscious dog. Three shaded vertical lines indicate simultaneous occurrence of concentration and motor events. (From Itoh et al [4], by permission of The American Gastroenterological Association.)

adrenergic, noncholinergic inhibitory system [94]. The effects of VIP on gastrointestinal motility are mostly inhibitory. VIP causes a dose-related relaxation of the lower esophageal sphincter in the anesthetized opossum. The effect of VIP is not blocked by tetrodotoxin or β-adrenergic antagonists [95]. In humans, VIP alone does not cause relaxation of the lower esophageal sphincter, but it antagonizes pentagastrin-induced contraction [96]. In the cat, VIP causes relaxation of the upper stomach [97]. In studies on canine antral smooth muscle, VIP decreased the force of both spontaneous and acetylcholine (ED_{50})-induced contractions [98]. Pentagastrin-induced muscle contractions are also antagonized by VIP [98]. Pyloric relaxation and a subsequent increase in a transpyloric flow were observed during injection of VIP [99]. In the preparation of ex vivo perfused isolated canine jejunal loop, VIP caused biphasic effects that consisted of initial relaxation and a later increase of the basal muscular tone [100]. VIP increased the number of migrating action potential complexes in the rabbit small intestine [101].

VIP alone produces dose-related decreases in resting gallbladder tension and antagonizes CCK-8-induced contractile activity of guinea pig gallbladder smooth muscle strip [38]. However, VIP has no effect on acetylcholine-induced contractions [38]. Although these effects require pharmacologic doses of VIP, they suggest the possible physiologic significance of VIP as a neurotransmitter.

Substance P

Substance P has potent stimulatory effects in vivo and in vitro on gastrointestinal motility in various species. It causes contraction of the lower esophageal sphincter of the opossum [102], contraction of the feline pylorus and stomach [103], contraction of rabbit large intestine and guinea pig ileum, an increase in myoelectric activity of the

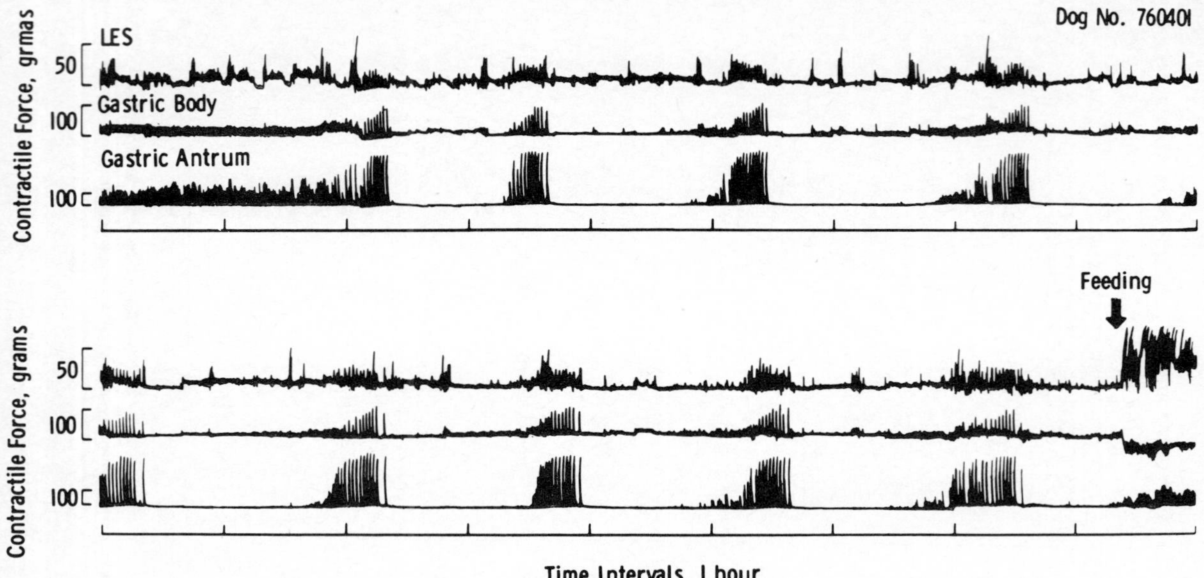

Figure 9-14. Eighteen-hour changes of contractile activity in the lower esophageal sphincter (LES) and stomach. The arrow indicates feeding. Note significant differences in contractile pattern before and after feeding. In the interdigestive state, simultaneous occurrence of contractile episodes is observed at regular intervals. (From Itoh et al [3], by permission of Plenum Publishing Corp.)

dog small bowel [104], and an increase in colonic motility in rats [105].

The contractile effects of substance P on the lower esophageal sphincter, stomach, pylorus, and small intestine can be blocked by atropine, which suggests that it may act on gastrointestinal smooth muscle via cholinergic pathways, at least in part. Substance P can induce gallbladder contraction in vivo and in vitro [106]. These effects are not influenced by either cholinergic or adrenergic blockades or tetrodotoxin in vitro. Substance P also relaxed the sphincter of Oddi in anesthetized dogs [107].

Neurotensin

Neurotensin causes relaxation of the human lower esophageal sphincter at a dose that yields plasma concentrations similar to those found after a meal [108] (Fig 9-15). Neurotensin, at physiologic doses, delays gastric emptying of oral glucose in healthy humans [109]. In the canine innervated antral pouch, motor activity is inhibited by physiologic doses of neurotensin. On the other hand, a denervated fundic pouch requires pharmacologic doses of neurotensin for inhibition of motility [110]. Neurotensin contracts the fundus and relaxes the small intestine in rats. These effects of neurotensin are not affected by antagonists to acetylcholine, histamine, and serotonin [111–113]. Therefore, neurotensin may act directly on smooth muscle via specific receptors, at least in the rat. However, neurotensin affects the contractility of guinea pig intestinal smooth muscle either in an excitatory or an inhibitory manner [112]. The mechanisms by which neurotensin acts on guinea pig smooth muscle consist of presynaptic and postsynaptic effects [112]. Pharmacologic doses of neurotensin increase colonic activity in cats [114], dogs [115], and humans [116], and this effect may be mediated through prostaglandins [115]. Neurotensin causes gallbladder contraction in conscious dogs [117]. Its effect on the gallbladder is atropine-sensitive [118]. However, in a study on in vitro rabbit gallbladder muscle strips, neurotensin had no effect on the contractile tension (unpublished data from our laboratory). Therefore, neurotensin may act on the gallbladder via cholinergic pathways.

Other Peptides

There are several other candidate hormones that may be involved in gastrointestinal motility, including somatostatin, bombesin, glucagon, gastric inhibitory polypeptide (GIP), enkephalins, PP, peptide YY (PYY), and pancreatic spasmolytic polypeptide (PSP) [119]. However, the physiologic

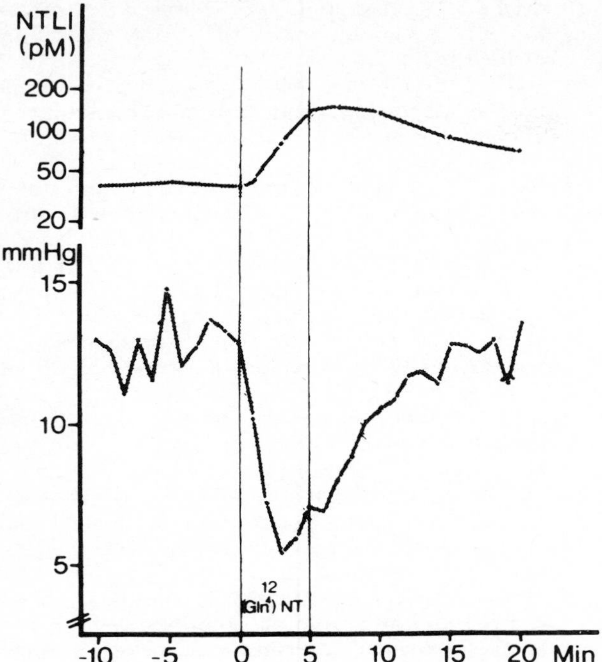

Figure 9-15. Plasma concentration of NTLI (upper curve) and LES pressure in response to IV infusion of 12 pmol $\times$ kg^{-1} $\times$ min^{-1} for 5 minutes (n = 6). Vertical lines indicate the infusion period. (From Rosell et al [108], by permission of Acta Physiologica Scandinavica.)

roles of these peptides in gastrointestinal motility are still far from clear (see Table 9-3).

As mentioned before, gastrointestinal motility is presumed to be regulated by an interplay of various gastrointestinal hormones as well as by local myogenic and neurogenic controls. Moreover, under physiologic conditions, several gastrointestinal hormones can be released in combination after a meal, in addition to the increase in neural tone, and intraluminal pressure caused by food. Therefore, gastrointestinal motility cannot be attributed to the effect of a single peptide.

Careful study of multiple experiments on the effects of gastrointestinal hormones on gut motility shows that conflicting results abound. Many of these discrepancies can be attributed to the following: 1) differences in species; 2) differences in doses of peptides; 3) differences in experimental models (e.g., in vivo or in vitro); 4) differences in methods of administration of peptides; 5) differences in recording techniques; and 6) differences in the effects of the anesthesia [120]. Also, we must face the sobering fact that some of the discrepancies result from error.

REFERENCES

1. Grossman MI: Physiological effects of gastrointestinal hormones. Fed Proc 36:1930, 1977.
2. Szurszewski JH: A migrating electric complex of the canine small intestine. Am J Physiol 217:1757, 1969.
3. Itoh Z, Honda R, Aizawa I, et al: Interdigestive motor activity of the lower esophageal sphincter in the conscious dog. Am J Dig Dis 23:239, 1978.
4. Itoh Z, Takahashi I, Nakaya M, et al: Interdigestive gallbladder bile concentration in relation to periodic contraction of gallbladder in the dog. Gastroenterology 83:645, 1982.
5. Jensen DM, McCallum R, Walsh JH: Failure of atropine to inhibit gastrin-17 stimulation of the lower esophageal sphincter in man. Gastroenterology 75:825, 1978.
6. Freeland GR, Higgs RH, Castell DO, et al: Lower esophageal sphincter and gastric acid response to intravenous infusions of synthetic human gastrin heptadecapeptide. Gastroenterology 71:570, 1976.
7. Walker CO, Frank SA, Manton J, et al: Effect of continuous infusion of pentagastrin on lower esophageal sphincter pressure and gastric acid secretion in normal subjects. J Clin Invest 56:218, 1975.
8. McCallum RW, Walsh JH: Relationship between lower esophageal sphincter pressure and serum gastrin concentration in Zollinger-Ellison syndrome and other clinical settings. Gastroenterology 76:76, 1979.
9. Okike N, Kelly KA: Vagotomy impairs pentagastrin-induced relaxation of canine gastric fundus. Am J Physiol 232:E504, 1977.
10. Strunz UT, Code CF, Grossman MI: Effect of gastrin on electrical activity of antrum and duodenum of dogs. Proc Soc Exp Biol Med 161:25, 1979.
11. Morgan KG, Schmalz PF, Go VLW, et al: Effects of pentagastrin, G_{17}, and G_{34} on the electrical and mechanical activities of canine antral smooth muscle. Gastroenterology 75:405, 1978.
12. Strunz UT, Grossman MI: Antral motility stimulated by gastrin: A physiological action affected by cholinergic activity, in Brooks FP, Evers PW (eds): *Nerves and the Gut.* Thorofare, NJ, Charles B Slack Inc, 1977, pp 233–239.
13. Smith AN, Hogg D: Effect of gastrin II on the motility of the gastrointestinal tract. Lancet 1:403, 1966.
14. Hunt JN, Ramsbottom N: Effect of gastrin II on gastric emptying and secretion during a test meal. Br Med J 4:386, 1967.
15. Debas HT, Farooq O, Grossman MI: Inhibition of gastric emptying is a physiological action of cholecystokinin. Gastroenterology 68:1211, 1975.
16. Strunz UT, Grossman MI: Effect of intragastric pressure on gastric emptying and secretion. Am J Physiol 235:E552, 1978.
17. Hamilton SG, Sheiner HJ, Quinlan MF: Continuous monitoring of the effect of pentagastrin on gastric emptying of solid food in man. Gut 17:273, 1976.

18. Mikos E, Vane JR: Effects of gastrin and its analogues on isolated smooth muscles. Nature 214:105, 1967.
19. Ryan JP: Motility of the gallbladder and biliary tree, in Johnson LR (ed): *Physiology of the Gastrointestinal Tract*. New York, Raven Press, 1981, pp 473–493.
20. Vagne M, Grossman MI: Cholecystokinetic potency of gastrointestinal hormones and related peptides. Am J Physiol 215:881, 1968.
21. Marik F, Code CF: Control of the interdigestive myoelectric activity in dogs by the vagus nerves and pentagastrin. Gastroenterology 69:387, 1975.
22. Wiesbrodt NW, Copeland EM, Kearley RW, et al: Effects of pentagastrin on electrical activity of small intestine of the dog. Am J Physiol 227:425, 1974.
23. Erckenbrecht JF, Caspari J, Wienbeck M: Pentagastrin induced motility pattern in the human upper gastrointestinal tract is reversed by proglumide. Gut 25:953, 1984.
24. Snape WJ Jr, Carlson GM, Cohen S: Human colonic myoelectric activity in response to Prostigmin and the gastrointestinal hormones. Am J Dig Dis 22:881, 1977.
25. Snape WJ Jr, Matarazzo SA, Cohen S: Effect of eating and gastrointestinal hormones on human colonic myoelectrical and motor activity. Gastroenterology 75:373, 1978.
26. Lin T-M: Actions of gastrointestinal hormones and related peptides on the motor function of the biliary tract. Gastroenterology 69:1006, 1975.
27. Hedner P: Effect of the C-terminal octapeptide of cholecystokinin on guinea pig ileum and gall-bladder in vitro. Acta Physiol Scand 78:232, 1970.
28. Amer MS, Becvar WE: A sensitive in-vitro method for the assay of cholecystokinin. J Endocrinol 43:637, 1969.
29. Sturdevant RA, Stern DH, Resin H, et al: Effect of graded doses of octapeptide of cholecystokinin on gallbladder size in man. Gastroenterology 64:452, 1973.
30. Lilja P, Fagan CJ, Wiener I, et al: Infusion of pure cholecystokinin in humans. Correlation between plasma concentrations of cholecystokinin and gallbladder size. Gastroenterology 83:256, 1982.
31. Wiener I, Inoue K, Fagan CJ, et al: Release of cholecystokinin in man. Correlation of blood levels with gallbladder contraction. Ann Surg 194:321, 1981.
32. Thompson JC, Fried GM, Ogden WD, et al: Correlation between release of cholecystokinin and contraction of the gallbladder in patients with gallstones. Ann Surg 195:670, 1982.
33. Amer MS: Studies with cholecystokinin *in vitro*. III. Mechanism of the effect on the isolated rabbit gallbladder strips. J Pharmacol Exp Ther 183:527, 1972.
34. Lonovics J, Varro V, Thompson JC: The role of calcium and cAMP in cholecystokinin(CCK)-stimulated rabbit gallbladder contraction. Gastroenterology 88:1480, 1985.
35. Stening GF, Grossman MI: Potentiation of cholecystokinetic action of cholecystokinin (CCK) by secretin. Clin Res 17:528, 1969.
36. Vagne M, Troitskaja V: Effect of secretin, glucagon and VIP on gallbladder contraction. Digestion 14:62, 1976.
37. Ryan J, Cohen S: Effect of vasoactive intestinal polypeptide on basal and cholecystokinin-induced gallbladder pressure. Gastroenterology 73:870, 1977.
38. Ryan JP, Ryave S: Effect of vasoactive intestinal polypeptide on gallbladder smooth muscle in vitro. Am J Physiol 234:E44, 1978.
39. Sarles JC, Bidart JM, Devaux MA, et al: Action of cholecystokinin and caerulein on the rabbit sphincter of Oddi. Digestion 14:415, 1976.
40. Watts J McK, Dunphy JE: The role of the common bile duct in biliary dynamics. Surg Gynecol Obstet 122:1207, 1966.
41. Becker JM, Moody FG: The dose/response effects of gastrointestinal hormones on the opossum biliary sphincter. Curr Surg 37:60, 1980.
42. Lin TM, Spray GF: Effect of pentagastrin, cholecystokinin, caerulein and glucagon on the choledochal resistance and bile flow of conscious dogs. Gastroenterology 56:1178, 1969.
43. Persson CGA, Ekman M: Effect of morphine, cholecystokinin and sympathomimetics on the sphincter of Oddi and intramural pressure in cat duodenum. Scand J Gastroenterol 7:345, 1972.
44. Hallenbeck GA: Biliary and pancreatic intraductal pressures, in Code CF (ed): *Handbook of Physiology. Section 6: Alimentary Canal.* Vol II. American Physiological Society, Washington, D.C., 1967, pp 1007–1025.
45. Resin H, Stern DH, Sturdevant RAL, et al: Effect of the C-terminal octapeptide of cholecystokinin on lower esophageal sphincter pressure in man. Gastroenterology 64:946, 1973.
46. Fisher RS, DiMarino AJ, Cohen S: Mechanism of cholecystokinin inhibition of lower esophageal sphincter pressure. Am J Physiol 228:1469, 1975.
47. Behar J, Biancani P: Effect of cholecystokinin-octapeptide on lower esophageal sphincter. Gastroenterology 73:57, 1977.
48. Valenzuela JE: Effect of intestinal hormones and peptides on intragastric pressure in dogs. Gastroenterology 71:766, 1976.
49. Fisher RS, Lipshutz W, Cohen S: The hormonal regulation of pyloric sphincter function. J Clin Invest 52:1289, 1973.
50. Sugawara K, Isaza J, Curt J, et al: Effect of secretin and cholecystokinin on gastric motility. Am J Physiol 217:1633, 1969.
51. Yamagishi T, Debas HT: Cholecystokinin inhibits gastric emptying by acting on both proximal stomach and pylorus. Am J Physiol 234:E375, 1978.
52. Valenzuela JE, Defilippi C: Inhibition of gastric emptying in humans by secretin, the octapeptide of cholecystokinin, and intraduodenal fat. Gastroenterology 81:898, 1981.
53. Schang J-C, Kelly KA: Inhibition of canine interdigestive proximal gastric motility by cholecystokinin octapeptide. Am J Physiol 240:G217, 1981.

54. Mukhopadhyay AK, Thor PJ, Copeland EM, et al: Effect of cholecystokinin on myoelectric activity of small bowel of the dog. Am J Physiol 232:E44, 1977.
55. Levant JA, Kun TL, Jachna J, et al: The effects of graded doses of C-terminal octapeptide of cholecystokinin on small intestinal transit time in man. Am J Dig Dis 19:207, 1974.
56. Mangel AW: Potentiation of colonic contractility to cholecystokinin and other peptides. Eur J Pharmacol 100:285, 1984.
57. Snape WJ Jr: Interaction of the octapeptide of cholecystokinin and gastrin I with bethanechol in the stimulation of feline colonic smooth muscle. Gastroenterology 84:58, 1983.
58. Egberts E-H, Johnson AG: The effect of cholecystokinin on human *Taenia coli*. Digestion 15:217, 1977.
59. Bueno L, Ferre J-P: Central regulation of intestinal motility by somatostatin and cholecystokinin octapeptide. Science 216:1427, 1982.
60. Sninsky CA, Wolfe MM, McGuigan JE, et al: Alterations in motor function of the small intestine from intravenous and intraluminal cholecystokinin. Am J Physiol 247:G724, 1984.
61. Cohen S, Lipshutz W: Hormonal regulation of human lower esophageal sphincter competence: Interaction of gastrin and secretin. J Clin Invest 50:449, 1971.
62. Lipshutz W, Cohen S: Interaction of gastrin I and secretin on gastrointestinal circular muscle. Am J Physiol 222:775, 1972.
63. Cameron AJ, Phillips SF, Summerskill WHJ: Comparison of effects of gastrin, cholecystokinin-pancreozymin, secretin, and glucagon on human stomach muscle in vitro. Gastroenterology 59:539, 1970.
64. Vagne M, Andre C: The effect of secretin on gastric emptying in man. Gastroenterology 60:421, 1971.
65. Mukhopadhyay AK, Johnson LR, Copeland EM, et al: Effect of secretin on electrical activity of small intestine. Am J Physiol 229:484, 1975.
66. Gutierrez JG, Chey WY, Dinoso VP: Actions of cholecystokinin and secretin on the motor activity of the small intestine in man. Gastroenterology 67:35, 1974.
67. Dinoso VP Jr, Meshkinpour H, Lorber SH, et al: Motor responses of the sigmoid colon and rectum to exogenous cholecystokinin and secretin. Gastroenterology 65:438, 1973.
68. Chowdhury AR, Lorber SH: Effects of glucagon and secretin on food- or morphine-induced motor activity of the distal colon, rectum, and anal sphincter. Am J Dig Dis 22:775, 1977.
69. Ivy AC, Oldberg E: A hormone mechanism for gallbladder contraction and evacuation. Am J Physiol 86:599, 1928.
70. Jansson R, Steen G, Svanvik J: A comparison of glucagon, gastric inhibitory peptide, and secretin on gallbladder function, formation of bile, and pancreatic secretion in the cat. Scand J Gastroenterol 13:919, 1978.
71. Lin T-M, Spray GF: Choledochal, hepatic and cholecystokinetic actions of secretin (S); potentiation by cholecystokinin (CCK). Gastroenterology 60:783, 1971.
72. Itoh Z, Nakaya M, Suzuki T: Neurohormonal control of gastrointestinal motor activity in conscious dogs. Peptides 2 (Suppl 2):223, 1981.
73. Vantrappen G, Janssens JJ, Peeters TL, et al: Motilin and the interdigestive migrating motor complex in man. Dig Dis Sci 24:497, 1979.
74. Lee KY, Chey WY, Tai H-H, et al: Radioimmunoassay of motilin. Validation and studies on the relationship between plasma motilin and interdigestive myoelectric activity of the duodenum of dog. Am J Dig Dis 23:789, 1978.
75. Itoh Z, Aizawa I, Honda R, et al: Control of lower-esophageal-sphincter contractile activity by motilin in conscious dogs. Am J Dig Dis 23:341, 1978.
76. Takahashi I, Suzuki T, Aizawa I, et al: Comparison of gallbladder contractions induced by motilin and cholecystokinin in dogs. Gastroenterology 82:419, 1982.
77. Green WER, Ruppin H, Wingate DL, et al: Effects of 13-nle-motilin on the electrical and mechanical activity of the isolated perfused canine stomach and duodenum. Gut 17:362, 1976.
78. Adachi H, Toda N, Hayashi S, et al: Mechanism of the excitatory action of motilin on isolated rabbit intestine. Gastroenterology 80:783, 1981.
79. Itoh Z, Honda R, Hiwatashi K, et al: Motilin-induced mechanical activity in the canine alimentary tract. Scand J Gastroenterol 11 (Suppl 39):93, 1976.
80. Thomas PA, Kelly KA: Hormonal control of interdigestive motor cycles of canine proximal stomach. Am J Physiol 237:E192, 1979.
81. Lee KY, Chang T-M, Chey WY: Effect of rabbit antimotilin serum on myoelectric activity and plasma motilin concentration in fasting dog. Am J Physiol 245:G547, 1983.
82. Fox JET, Track NS, Daniel EE: Relationship of plasma motilin concentration to fat ingestion, duodenal acidification and alkalinization, and migrating motor complexes in dogs. Can J Physiol Pharmacol 59:180, 1981.
83. Itoh Z, Aizawa I, Honda R, et al: Regular and irregular cycles of interdigestive contractions in the stomach. Am J Physiol 238:G85, 1980.
84. Lee KY, Kim MS, Chey WY: Effects of a meal and gut hormones on plasma motilin and duodenal motility in dog. Am J Physiol 238:G280, 1980.
85. Peeters TL, Janssens J, Vantrappen GR: Somatostatin and the interdigestive migrating motor complex in man. Regul Pept 5:209, 1983.
86. Janssens J, Vantrappen G, Peeters TL: The activity front of the migrating motor complex of the human stomach but not of the small intestine is motilin-dependent. Regul Pept 6:363, 1983.
87. Poitras P, Steinbach JH, VanDeventer G, et al: Motilin-independent ectopic fronts of the interdigestive myoelectric complex in dogs. Am J Physiol 239:G215, 1980.
88. You CH, Chey WY, Lee KY: Studies on plasma motilin concentration and interdigestive motility of

the duodenum in humans. Gastroenterology 79:62, 1980.
89. Christofides ND, Bloom SR, Besterman HS, et al: Release of motilin by oral and intravenous nutrients in man. Gut 20:102, 1979.
90. Christofides ND, Sarson DL, Albuquerque RH, et al: Release of gastrointestinal hormones following an oral water load. Experientia 35:1521, 1979.
91. Christofides ND, Long RG, Fitzpatrick ML, et al: Effect of motilin on the gastric emptying of glucose and fat in humans. Gastroenterology 80:456, 1981.
92. Itoh Z, Takeuchi S, Aizawa I, et al: Changes in plasma motilin concentration and gastrointestinal contractile activity in conscious dogs. Am J Dig Dis 23:929, 1978.
93. Said SI (ed): *Vasoactive Intestinal Peptide.* New York, Raven Press, 1982.
94. Fahrenkrug J: Vasoactive intestinal polypeptide: Measurement, distribution and putative neurotransmitter function. Digestion 19:149, 1979.
95. Rattan S, Said SI, Goyal RK: Effect of vasoactive intestinal polypeptide (VIP) on the lower esophageal sphincter pressure (LESP). Proc Soc Exp Biol Med 155:40, 1977.
96. Domschke W, Lux G, Domschke S, et al: Effects of vasoactive intestinal peptide on resting and pentagastrin-stimulated lower esophageal sphincter pressure. Gastroenterology 75:9, 1978.
97. Fahrenkrug J, Haglund U, Jodal M, et al: Nervous release of vasoactive intestinal polypeptide in the gastrointestinal tract of cats: Possible physiological implications. J Physiol 284:291, 1978.
98. Morgan KG, Schmalz PF, Szurszewski JH: The inhibitory effects of vasoactive intestinal polypeptide on the mechanical and electrical activity of canine antral smooth muscle. J Physiol 282:437, 1978.
99. Edin R, Lundberg JM, Ahlman H, et al: On the VIP-ergic innervation of the feline pylorus. Acta Physiol Scand 107:185, 1979.
100. Kachelhoffer J, Mendel C, Dauchel J, et al: The effects of VIP on intestinal motility. Study on *ex vivo* perfused isolated canine jejunal loops. Am J Dig Dis 21:957, 1976.
101. Sninsky CA, Wolfe MM, Martin JL, et al: Myoelectric effects of vasoactive intestinal peptide on rabbit small intestine. Am J Physiol 244:G46, 1983.
102. Mukhopadhyay AK: Effect of substance P on the lower esophageal sphincter of the opossum. Gastroenterology 75:278, 1978.
103. Lidberg P, Dahlstrom A, Lundberg JM, et al: Different modes of action of substance P in the motor control of the feline stomach and pylorus. Regul Pept 7:41, 1983.
104. Thor PJ, Sendur R, Konturek SJ: Influence of substance P on myoelectric activity of the small bowel. Am J Physiol 243:G493, 1982.
105. Krier J, Szurszewski JH: Effect of substance P on colonic mechanoreceptors, motility, and sympathetic neurons. Am J Physiol 243:G259, 1982.
106. Mate LJ, Sakamoto T, Thompson JC: The effect of substance P on gallbladder motility *in vivo* and *in vitro*. Proc Soc Exp Biol Med 175:257, 1984.
107. Lonovics J, Fujimura M, Lluis F, et al: Cholecystokinin-induced relaxation of the sphincter of Oddi may partially be mediated by substance P. Gastroenterology 88:1480, 1985.
108. Rosell S, Thor K, Rokaeus A, et al: Plasma concentration of neurotensin-like immunoreactivity (NTLI) and lower esophageal sphincter (LES) pressure in man following infusion of (Gln^4)-neurotensin. Acta Physiol Scand 109:369, 1980.
109. Blackburn AM, Bloom SR, Long RG, et al: Effect of neurotensin on gastric function in man. Lancet 1:987, 1980.
110. Andersson S, Rosell S, Hjelmquist U, et al: Inhibition of gastric and intestinal motor activity in dogs by (Gln^4) neurotensin. Acta Physiol Scand 100:231, 1977.
111. Rokaeus A, Burcher E, Chang D, et al: Actions of neurotensin and (Gln^4)-neurotensin on isolated tissues. Acta Pharmacol Toxicol 41:141, 1977.
112. Kitabgi P: Effects of neurotensin on intestinal smooth muscle: Application to the study of structure-activity relationships. Ann NY Acad Sci 400:37, 1982.
113. Huidobro-Toro JP, Kullak A: Excitatory neurotensin receptors on the smooth muscle of the rat fundus: Possible implications in gastric motility. Br J Pharmacol 84:897, 1985.
114. Hellstrom PM, Rosell S: Effects of neurotensin, substance P and methionine-enkephalin on colonic motility. Acta Physiol Scand 113:147, 1981.
115. Bardon T, Ruckebusch Y: Neurotensin-induced colonic motor responses in dogs: A mediation by prostaglandins. Regul Pept 10:107, 1985.
116. Calam J, Unwin R, Peart WS: Neurotensin stimulates defaecation. Lancet 1:737, 1983.
117. Sakamoto T, Mate L, Greeley GH Jr, et al: Effect of neurotensin on gallbladder contraction in dogs. Gastroenterology 86:1229, 1984.
118. Fujimura M, Sakamoto T, Khalil T, et al: Physiologic role of neurotensin in gallbladder contraction in the dog. Surg Forum 35:192, 1984.
119. Jørgensen KD, Diamant B, Jørgensen KH, et al: Pancreatic spasmolytic polypeptide (PSP): III. Pharmacology of a new porcine pancreatic polypeptide with spasmolytic and gastric acid secretion inhibitory effects. Regul Pept 3:231, 1982.
120. Lilja P, Wiener I, Inoue K, et al: Influence of different anesthetic agents on the release of cholecystokinin in dogs. Surgery 97:415, 1985.
121. Morgan KG, Schmalz PF, Go VLW, et al: Electrical and mechanical effects of molecular variants of CCK on antral smooth muscle. Am J Physiol 235:E324, 1978.
122. Sinar DR, O'Dorisio TM, Mazzaferri EL, et al: Effect of gastric inhibitory polypeptide on lower esophageal sphincter pressure in cats. Gastroenterology 75:263, 1978.
123. Brown JC, Dryburgh JR, Frost JL, et al: Properties

and actions of GIP, in Bloom SR (ed): *Gut Hormones.* New York, Churchill Livingstone, 1978, pp 277–282.
124. Jennewein HM, Waldeck F, Siewert R, et al: The interaction of glucagon and pentagastrin on the lower oesophageal sphincter in man and dog. Gut 14:861, 1973.
125. Stunkard AJ, van Itallie TB, Reis BB: The mechanism of satiety: Effect of glucagon on gastric hunger contractions in man. Proc Soc Exp Biol Med 89:258, 1955.
126. Phaosawasdi K, Boden G, Kolts B, et al: Hormonal effects on pyloric sphincter pressure (PSP): Are they of physiologic importance? Clin Res 27:270A, 1979.
127. Lin T-M: Effects of insulin and glucagon on secretory and motor function of the gastrointestinal tract, in Jerzy Glass GB (ed): *Gastrointestinal Hormones.* New York, Raven Press, 1980, pp 639–691.
128. Strunz U, Domschke W, Domschke S, et al: Potentiation between 13-nle-motilin and acetylcholine on rabbit pyloric muscle in vitro. Scand J Gastroenterol 11 (Suppl 39):29, 1976.
129. Tansy MF, Martin JS, Landin WE, et al: The differential action of somatostatin on the motor effector system of the canine gastrointestinal tract. Metabolism 27 (Suppl 1):1353, 1978.
130. Bloom SR, Ralphs DN, Besser GM, et al: Effect of somatostatin on motilin levels and gastric emptying. Gut 16:834, 1975.
131. Melchiorri P: Bombesin and bombesin-like peptides of amphibian skin, in Bloom SR (ed): *Gut Hormones.* New York, Churchill Livingstone, 1978, pp 534–540.
132. Bertaccini G, Impicciatore M: Action of bombesin on the motility of the stomach. Naunyn-Schmiedeberg's Arch Pharmacol 289:149, 1975.
133. Scarpignato C, Micali B, Vitulo F, et al: Inhibition of gastric empyting by bombesin in man. Digestion 23:128, 1982.
134. Edin R, Lundberg J, Terenius L, et al: Evidence for vagal enkephalinergic neural control of the feline pylorus and stomach. Gastroenterology 78:492, 1980.
135. Rattan S, Goyal RK: Effect of bovine pancreatic polypeptide on the opossum lower esophageal sphincter. Gastroenterology 77:672, 1979.
136. Lin T-M, Chance RE: Spectrum of gastrointestinal actions of bovine PP, in Bloom SR (ed): *Gut Hormones.* New York, Churchill Livingstone, 1978, pp 242–246.
137. Suzuki T, Nakaya M, Itoh Z, et al: Inhibition of interdigestive contractile activity in the stomach by peptide YY in Heidenhain pouch dogs. Gastroenterology 85:114, 1983.
138. Behar J, Biancani P: Effect of cholecystokinin and the octapeptide of cholecystokinin on the feline sphincter of Oddi and gallbladder. J Clin Invest 66:1231, 1980.
139. Piper PJ, Said SI, Vane JR: Effects on smooth muscle preparations of unidentified vasoactive peptides from intestine and lung. Nature 225:1144, 1970.
140. Jansson R, Steen G, Svanvik J: Effects of intravenous vasoactive intestinal peptide (VIP) on gallbladder function in the cat. Gastroenterology 75:47, 1978.
141. Wingate DL, Pearce EA, Thomas PA, et al: Glucagon stimulates intestinal myoelectric activity. Gastroenterology 74:1152, 1978.
142. Wingate DL, Pearce E: The physiological role of glucagon in the gastrointestinal tract, in Picazo J (ed): *Glucagon in Gastroenterology.* Baltimore, University Park Press, 1979, pp 19–38.
143. Chernish SM, Miller RE, Rosenak BD, et al: Hypotonic duodenography with the use of glucagon. Gastroenterology 63:392, 1972.
144. Taylor I, Duthie HL, Cumberland DC, et al: Glucagon and the colon. Gut 16:973, 1975.
145. Lin TM: Action of secretin (S), glucagon (G), cholecystokinin (CCK) and endogenously released S and CCK on gallbladder (GB), choledochus (C) and bile (B) flow in dogs. Fed Proc 33:391, 1974.
146. Ormsbee HS III, Koehler SL Jr, Telford GL: Somatostatin inhibits motilin-induced interdigestive contractile activity in the dog. Am J Dig Dis 23:781, 1978.
147. Thor P, Krol R, Konturek SJ, et al: Effect of somatostatin on myoelectrical activity of small bowel. Am J Physiol 235:E249, 1978.
148. Lin T-M, Spray GF, Tust RH: Action of somatostatin (SS) on choledochal sphincter (CS), gallbladder (GB) and bile flow (BF) in dogs. Fed Proc 36:557, 1977.
149. Creutzfeldt W, Lankisch PG, Folsch UR: Hemmung der sekretin- und cholezystokinin-pankreozymin-induzierten saft- und enzym-sekretion des pankreas und der gallenblasenkontraktion beim menschen durch somatostatin. Dtsch Med Wochenschr 100:1135, 1975.
150. Corazziari E, Torsoli A, Melchiorri P, et al: Effect of bombesin on human gallbladder emptying. Rendic Gastroenterol 6:52, 1974.
151. Korner MM, Berges W, Scholten T, et al: Differential effects of enkephalin analogue on the motility of the small and large intestine, in Wienbeck M (ed): *Motility of the Digestive Tract.* New York, Raven Press, 1982, pp 131–136.
152. Konturek SJ, Pawlik W, Tasler J, et al: Effects of enkephalin on the gastrointestinal tract, in Bloom SR (ed): *Gut Hormones.* New York, Churchill Livingstone, 1978, pp 507–512.
153. Bueno L, Fioramonti J, Rayner V, et al: Effects of motilin, somatostatin, and pancreatic polypeptide on the migrating myoelectric complex in pig and dog. Gastroenterology 82:1395, 1982.
154. Adrian TE, Mitchenere P, Sagor G, et al: Effect of pancreatic polypeptide on gallbladder pressure and hepatic bile secretion. Am J Physiol 243:G204, 1982.
155. Lin T-M, Chance RE: VI. Bovine pancreatic polypeptide (BPP) and avian pancreatic polypeptide (APP). Gastroenterology 67:737, 1974.

156. Lundberg JM, Tatemoto K, Terenius L, et al: Localization of peptide YY (PYY) in gastrointestinal endocrine cells and effects on intestinal blood flow and motility. Proc Natl Acad Sci USA 79:4471, 1982.
157. Lluis F, Fujimura M, Guo Y-S, et al: Peptide YY and gallbladder contraction. Gastroenterology 88:1479, 1985.

REGULATION OF GROWTH OF GUT AND PANCREAS

J. Patrick Walker, M.D., R. Daniel Beauchamp, M.D., and Courtney M. Townsend, Jr., M.D.

In establishing an understanding of the trophic actions of gastrointestinal hormones, we must look at extremes of circumstances to propose mechanisms of action in normal tissues. Although we suppose that normal levels of hormones are necessary for maintenance of normal structure and function, it is only in pharmacologic doses or in pathologic states that evidence is available for stimulation and maintenance of gut growth by gastrointestinal hormones. In patients with prolonged fasts, either self-imposed or produced by disease or circumstance, there is atrophy of organs and of portions of organs of the gut. Conversely, in patients or animals with hyperphagia, there is growth of the stomach, pancreas, and intestine. One of the proposed means for maintenance of normal organ structure and function is the release of physiologic concentrations of hormones (gastrin, cholecystokinin, and others) by food stimulus. This stimulus exerts control over the target organ by putative mechanisms, which we shall discuss. This biologic concept is represented pathologically in patients with the Zollinger-Ellison (ZE) syndrome, in whom a gastrin-producing islet tumor causes an increase, often massive, in both the size and number of parietal cells [1].

We should clarify initially the relationship between hypertrophy and hyperplasia: hypertrophy is growth in the size of an organ by increase in the size of cells, and hyperplasia is growth in the size of an organ by increase in cell number. Both phenomena may occur at the same time, in the same organ. In a simplistic manner, hypertrophy may be said to be associated with an increase in the tissue content of RNA and hyperplasia with an increase in DNA. We will summarize some experimental studies that have been carried out to investigate the trophic effects of gastrointestinal hormones on the organs of the gastrointestinal tract and pancreas.

Stomach

A discussion of trophic effects of gastrointestinal hormones on the stomach must begin with gastrin (see Chapter 14). Dragstedt et al [2] observed in 1951 that isolation of the antrum resulted in hyperfunction of acid-secreting cells. They proposed that the mechanism of action was through gastrin. Although parietal cell hyperplasia had been described in patients with the Zollinger-Ellison syndrome [1,3], the initial experimental studies on the growth-promoting effects of increased gastrin stores were not performed until the late 1960s by Crean et al [4,5] at Edinburgh. They produced duodenal obstruction in rats, which resulted in overgrowth of gastric mucosa and hypergastrinemia. This led to proportional increases in parietal and chief cell populations [4]. This finding is similar to the increase in mucosal volumes found during pregnancy and lactation (states of hyperphagia), in which parietal and peptic cell populations increase proportionally [5]. The opposite condition occurs with decreased gastrin stores, that is, after gastrectomy there is atrophy of the mass of parietal cells [6,7].

In 1967, Crean et al [8] reported a classic study in which they gave 2 mg of pentagastrin twice daily to Wistar rats for 21 days and found marked hyperplasia of the parietal cell population without other major changes in the gastric mucosa [9]. The amount of acid produced per parietal cell was also increased. The hyperplasia was different from that produced by duodenal obstruction and pregnancy in that it was selective for parietal cells and resulted in a change in the ratio of parietal to chief cells. Chronic administration of histamine also increased acid production (although not as much as pentagastrin) but did not produce parietal cell hyperplasia. These findings seemed to indicate a mechanism for hyperplasia beyond that of the classic hypothesis that work demands growth of producing tissues.

At about the same time, Johnson et al [10,11] induced increased incorporation of amino acids into proteins of the mucosa of the gastrointestinal tract by administration of gastrin to rats. In these studies, pentagastrin (but not histamine) increased incorporation of ^{14}C-labeled leucine in gastric and duodenal mucosa in a dose-related fashion. There was no effect on liver tissue.

Since secretin was known to inhibit gastrin-stimulated acid secretion, Stanley et al [12] tested the hypothesis that secretin would also inhibit trophic effects of pentagastrin in rat gastric mucosa.

They showed that secretin diminished the effects of chronic pentagastrin administration on both the parietal cell population and on acid secretory capacity.

In a follow-up study, Johnson and Guthrie [13] examined trophic responses of pentagastrin, secretin, histamine, and metiamide (an early H_2-receptor blocker) alone and in combination. They showed the expected finding that secretin inhibited both acid production and DNA synthesis stimulated by gastrin (Fig 9-16). They also found that when gastrin-induced production of acid was inhibited by metiamide, the trophic effect (as measured by DNA synthesis) persisted. The lack of trophic effect of histamine was again confirmed. The increased rate of DNA synthesis was found to correlate with time after pentagastrin administration [14].

The effects of cholinergic innervation on pentagastrin-stimulated synthesis of DNA in gastric mucosa were studied in Sprague-Dawley rats, tested with atropine and vagotomy, alone and in combination with pentagastrin [15]. Although atropine given alone and vagotomy increased DNA synthesis, as did pentagastrin, neither atropine nor vagotomy affected pentagastrin stimulation of DNA synthesis. The stimulation of DNA synthesis brought about by cholinergic ablation is thought to depend upon endogenous hypergastrinemia. Hollinshead et al [16] have recently shown that truncal vagotomy in dogs caused basal and postprandial hypergastrinemia within 24 to 48 hours.

Does gastrin act directly to stimulate growth? Evidence for a direct effect is provided by studies in which rat and human gastric mucosal cells in tissue culture were treated with pentagastrin [17]. Growth of the pentagastrin-treated cells was double that of the cells of the saline-treated controls. Willems et al [18] studied the kinetics of cell proliferation in canine fundic mucosa in response to food and gastrin; they concluded that endogenously released gastrin, but not histamine, is important for normal maintenance of growth of gastric mucosa. Antrectomy in rats caused a 65 percent decrease in RNA and a 75 percent decrease in DNA [19]; exogenous pentagastrin restored gastric mucosal RNA to 90 percent of controls but had no effect on DNA. Since pentagastrin was given for only 24 hours before sacrifice of animals, the lack of change in DNA content was assumed to be the length of turnover time for gastric mucosa (approximately 8 days in the rat).

Enochs and Johnson [20] studied the influence of pituitary and adrenal hormones on the trophic effects of pentagastrin and concluded that 1) hypophysectomy alone produced an increase in DNA synthesis in the gastric antrum and fundus but not in the duodenum; 2) adrenalectomy alone had no effect on fundus, antrum, or duodenum; 3) hypophysectomy with adrenalectomy increased antral and duodenal DNA synthesis but reduced DNA synthesis in the fundus by 30 percent (compared to hypophysectomized controls); 4) the trophic effects of pentagastrin were independent of adrenal hormones; 5) pentagastrin inhibited antral DNA synthesis in intact and in adrenalectomized and hypophysectomized animals. Hypophysectomy had previously been shown to reduce the volume of gastric mucosa and the parietal population [21,22].

In 1968, Steiner et al [23] showed that a 6-day fast diminished the weight of the small intestine (52 percent) proportionally more than the weight loss of the whole body (32 percent). Since most of

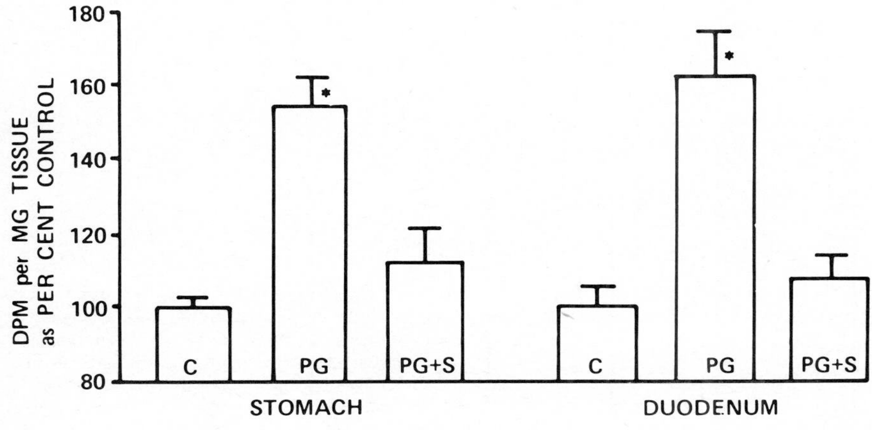

Figure 9-16. Disintegrations per minute (DPM) of [^{3}H]thymidine incorporated into gastric and duodenal DNA per milligram of wet weight of tissue expressed as 100 percent of the saline control animals. C = control animals; PG = pentagastrin, 250 μg/kg; PG + S = PG + secretin, 75 U/kg. Means and standard errors of the means of 16 observations in each group. * = $p < 0.001$. (From Johnson and Guthrie [13], with permission of Williams & Wilkins.)

the previous studies on the trophic effects of pentagastrin were done with fasted animals, Muller et al [24] treated fed guinea pigs with a short-term course of pentagastrin (3 days) and demonstrated a rate of synthesis of DNA and RNA that was greater than that of controls. This showed that the trophic effects could extend beyond those effects produced by the normal endogenous gastrin response to a meal. Dembinski et al [25] found that 48-hour administration of prostaglandins from the E and F series (or their analogues) stimulated increased uptake of tritiated thymidine in rat pancreas and gastroduodenal mucosa. Prolonged treatment for 10 days led to increased organ weights. Prostaglandin E_2 caused a dose-dependent increase in DNA and RNA content of the pancreas as well as of the gastric and duodenal mucosa. Prostacyclin (PGI_2) had no effect on growth of mucosa or pancreas. PGI_2 did inhibit gastric acidity by 50 percent and significantly increased serum gastrin levels, as did the E and F series of prostaglandins. The conclusion was that the growth-related effects were independent of gastrin levels.

Other gastrointestinal hormones affect the trophic actions of gastrin on the mucosa of the stomach, and some have trophic effects of their own. CCK, although structurally similar to gastrin, has no effect on gastric mucosa alone and does not alter the trophic effects produced by pentagastrin [26]. As previously mentioned, secretin reduces the trophic effects of pentagastrin [12,13]. Glucagon alone stimulates thymidine uptake in DNA from oxyntic mucosa but does not alter pentagastrin-induced stimulation [27]. Vasoactive inhibitory peptide (VIP) inhibited the trophic effects of pentagastrin but had no effect of its own [27].

An 8-hour infusion of somatostatin transiently reduced nuclear uptake of tritiated thymidine and the rate of cell division. When given with gastrin, the trophic effects of gastrin were inhibited [28]. In rats with chronic endogenous hypergastrinemia (produced by transposition of the antrum to the colon), a 3-week administration of somatostatin lowered parietal and peptic cell densities [29].

Johnson and Guthrie [30] recently reported that proglumide (thought to be a specific receptor-blocker for gastrin and CCK) inhibited the pentagastrin-stimulated increase of uptake of tritiated thymidine in gastric mucosa. Upp et al [31] have recently found that proglumide causes an increased uptake of tritiated thymidine at 48 hours and increased DNA content after 7 days of treatment in the rat. We have recently shown [32] that proglumide inhibits the growth of MC-26 mouse colon cancer and prolongs survival in tumor-bearing mice. This colon cancer has been shown to be stimulated by exogenous gastrin in vivo [33]. The DNA content of colon tumors and of normal fundic mucosa was significantly less in the proglumide-treated mice (Fig 9-17). Mice receiving proglumide for 3 weeks had a diminished colon weight as well as a significantly smaller colonic content of RNA and protein, but there was no effect on colonic DNA content compared with controls. We have no

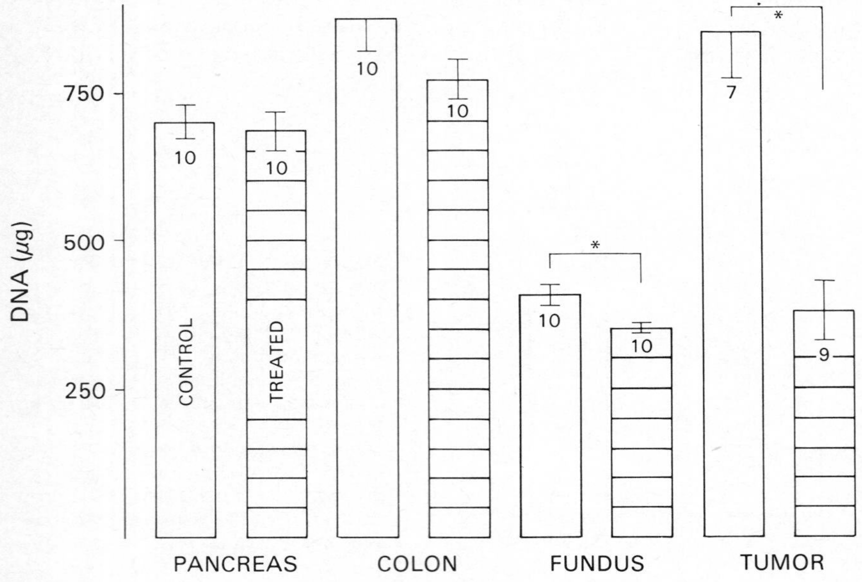

Figure 9-17. Balb/c mice receiving 3 weeks of proglumide, a CCK/gastrin antagonist. Tumor is a subcutaneous MC-26 mouse colon adenocarcinoma. Treatment was begun on the day of tumor cell injection, and mice were sacrificed 23 days later.

exogenous gastrin in this experiment and therefore were able to conclude that the proglumide effect was due to inhibition of the growth effects of endogenous gastrin or CCK on the colonic tumor.

The mode of action of the trophic effects of gastrin is still unknown. However, Seidel et al [34] have recently shown that treatment of rats with difluoromethylornithine (DFMO), concurrently with pentagastrin, inhibited the trophic effects of the hormone. DFMO is a selective, irreversible inhibitor of ornithine decarboxylase, the rate-limiting enzyme for the synthesis of polyamines (spermine, putrescine, and spermidine), which are necessary for tissue growth. DFMO alone had no effect on mucosal growth.

Epidermal growth factor (EGF) has been reported to increase DNA synthesis in the oxyntic mucosa but not in the duodenum and colon of the rat [35]. This increase was not inhibited by secretin, as is the hypertrophic effect by gastrin. EGF increased ornithine decarboxylase activity in the stomach and duodenum of young mice but not in the midgut or colon [36]. A 14-day treatment with bethanechol, a cholinergic agonist, produced a slight increase (9 percent) in oxyntic gland weight but did not affect DNA, pepsinogen, or protein content in treated rats [37].

Sircar et al [38] have shown that feeding rats chemically defined synthetic diets, such as Vivonex, reduced serum gastrin levels within one day and the concentration of gastrin in antral mucosa by 4 to 5 days; the mucosal change was correlated with decreased mucosal synthesis of DNA [39]. Neither antral gastrin nor mucosal DNA synthesis was lowered in chow-fed rats. Both starvation and total parenteral nutrition reduced gastric mucosal mass as well as antral gastrin in the rat [40,41]. These mucosal changes were reversed by administration of exogenous gastrin [42]. Normal diet appears to contain a factor that maintains gastrin levels and thereby the gastric mucosa. Fat, protein, minerals (including iron), and bulk supplements did not restore gastrin levels or the DNA synthetic response [39].

Besides starvation hypogastrinemia, and the Zollinger-Ellison (ZE) syndrome (hypergastrinemia), other clinical situations may prominently display the trophic effects of hormones. These situations are found in patients after intestinal resection and in those with renal failure. Extensive resection of the small bowel produces hyperplasia of the mucosa of the small intestine and of the gastric mucosa [42–45]. Resection is rapidly followed by elevated levels of circulating gastrin and gastric acid hypersecretion [46–49]. Gastric hypoplasia produced by antrectomy can be reversed by small intestinal resection, with resultant elevation of circulating gastrin [50]. Although the functional significance of hypertrophy of gastric mucosa remains to be determined [51], other trophic actions of gastrin, such as colonic mucosal hypertrophy, may play an important role.

We find it interesting (and challenging) that postresectional hyperplasia of the jejunum and ileum does not—at least in rats—appear to be related to endogenous gastrin levels [50,52]. Deveney et al [53] studied the effects of increased acid secretory capacity and gastrin levels on intestinal morphology and pancreatic function in rats. Colonic and pancreatic weights were increased in all rats with hypergastrinemia (caused by antral transposition to the colon), and hypertrophy of the small bowel was found in rats with hypergastrinemia only when the acid secretory capacity of the stomach was maintained. Why the presence of acid should be necessary for small bowel hypertrophy, regardless of gastrin levels, but not be required (at least in the presence of hypergastrinemia) for hypertrophy of the colon and pancreas is unexplained. We have recently confirmed that fundusectomy in rats produces a prolonged and profound increase in serum gastrin levels, and found that rats sacrificed from 2–6 weeks after fundusectomy had hypertrophy of the pancreas and the colon [54]. This effect did not, however, persist, and animals sacrificed 5–7 months later showed no difference in pancreatic or colonic weights.

Hypergastrinemia in renal failure patients is well known [55], and in some few patients there may be an increase in gastric acid output as well [56]. Although the etiology of the hypergastrinemia is unknown, decreased renal catabolism and chronic antacid use are implicated; there is also some evidence of fundic hyperplasia [57]. Although bleeding from peptic ulcers is a well-recognized complication of renal transplant surgery, bleeding is generally (and correctly) attributed to immunosuppression (particularly by steroids), to stress, and in some cases to anticoagulation.

Paradoxically, Takeuchi and Johnson [58] have shown that pentagastrin stimulation of gastric mucosal proliferation protects against stress ulceration in rats. However, this study was conducted in rats with low endogenous stores of gastrin produced by feeding of liquid diets.

The trophic actions of gastrointestinal hormones may be responsible for some aspects of gut development (see Chapter 11). Gastrin has been linked ontogenetically with development of the rat gastrointestinal tract [59]. Hypergastrinemia has long been linked with congenital hypertrophic pyloric stenosis. Dodge and Karim [60,61] were able to induce pyloric stenosis in pups by administration of exogenous gastrin to pregnant bitches. However, a woman with proven ZE syndrome and greatly elevated levels of serum gastrin gave birth to a normal child with no evidence of pyloric stenosis [62]. The cord blood serum gastrin level was elevated, indicating placental transport of the hormone. Although the experimental evidence is tantalizing, the etiology and possible pathogenetic role of gastrin in the development of congenital hypertrophic pyloric stenosis remain obscure. Secretin (which produces contraction of the pylorus) does not appear to play a role in pyloric stenosis [63].

Pancreas

The first report of a trophic effect of gastrointestinal hormones on the pancreas was by Rothman and Wells [64], who reported in 1967 that pancreatic weights were significantly increased in rats given CCK but not secretin or methacholine. An increase in pancreatic weight, protein, and DNA content, as well as an increased incorporation of labeled thymidine into DNA in rats, was reported in 1973 in rats treated with CCK [65]; confirmation was provided later that year [66]. Proglumide (a specific competitive inhibitor of gastrin and CCK receptors) blocks the CCK-8-stimulated increase in tritiated thymidine uptake in rats after 48 hours of treatment. Proglumide alone, given for 6 days, was also found to stimulate pancreatic growth in the rat [67]. Upp et al [31] have confirmed these findings.

The interactions of caerulein (a decapeptide analogue of CCK from frog skin [68,69]) and secretin have been studied in rats [70]. Caerulein plus secretin has a synergistic action on the pancreas, that is, pancreatic weight, protein, DNA, and trypsinogen content were enhanced to a greater extent when the peptides were given together than when given individually. The trophic effects of caerulein and secretin are not limited to rats. We have shown trophic effects of caerulein and secretin alone (as well as in combination) on the pancreas of Syrian golden hamsters [71]. In these studies, secretin alone produced increased DNA content of the pancreas. Trophic effects on the hamster pancreas have also been demonstrated with CCK-8 [72].

Dembinski and Johnson [73] showed secretin stimulation of DNA content, and Solomon et al [74] have described the kinetics and site of cellular DNA synthesis after stimulation with caerulein and secretin. Solomon et al [74] found that uptake of tritiated thymidine reached a peak after 2 days of treatment, whereas DNA content increased after 3 days and peaked at 5 days of treatment (Fig 9-18). Autoradiography revealed increased synthesis of DNA; potentiation was seen when caerulein and secretin were given together.

The hypertrophic response to CCK causes an increase in amylase content, but dose-response curves of protein secretion in relation to CCK in the hypertrophic pancreas are the same as in control animals [75]. This pancreatic hypertrophy apparently does not alter the number of affinity of CCK receptors.

Release of endogenous secretin by intraduodenal acid and of endogenous CCK by intraduodenal amino acids has been shown to be trophic

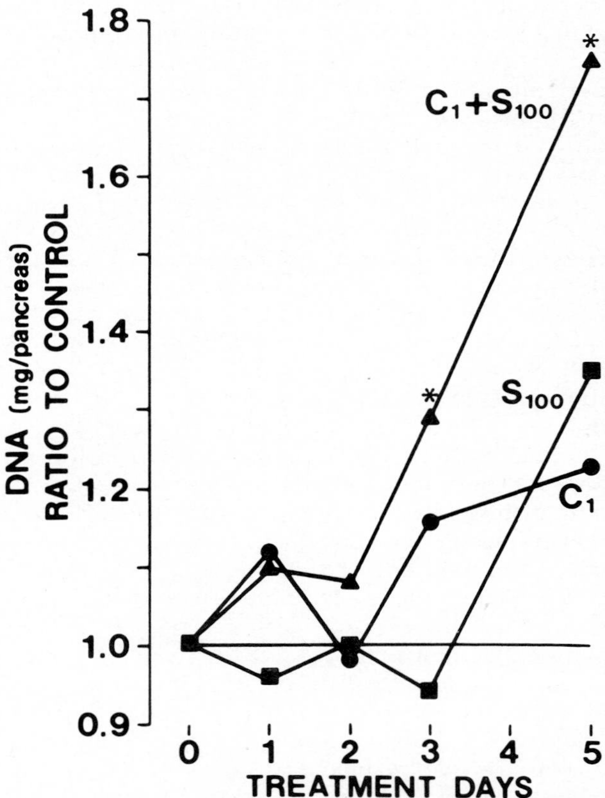

Figure 9-18. Total pancreatic DNA in rats treated with caerulein (C) and secretin (S), expressed as ratio of mean DNA of treated rats to mean DNA of control rats. N = 12 for each treatment group. Statistically significant (*) potentiation between caerulein and secretin was present after 3 and 5 days of treatment. (From Solomon et al [74], with permission of the American Physiological Society.)

for the pancreas [76]. There are conflicting results concerning the effect of cholecystectomy on pancreatic growth. Since we know that there is an increase in plasma CCK levels in dogs after cholecystectomy [77], we have studied the effect of cholecystectomy on pancreatic growth and duodenal CCK levels in the hamster and found no effect of the plasma or duodenal levels of CCK on pancreatic growth [unpublished studies]. In contrast, Rosenberg et al [78] showed an increase in plasma CCK that was correlated with hyperplasia of the pancreas after cholecystectomy in hamsters.

Caerulein and secretin also have effects on the endocrine pancreas [79]. They increase somatostatin content both in vitro and in vivo. Insulin content is unchanged, but glucagon content is increased. Islet DNA content is unchanged.

Pregnancy and lactation produce hypertrophy of the rat pancreas [80], which appears to be analogous to the effects of the hyperphagia of lactation on hypertrophy of the stomach due to hypergastrinemia [7].

Pentagastrin also exerts a trophic influence on the pancreas. Mayston and Barrowman [81] found that administration of pentagastrin to rats (in which hypophysectomy had caused pancreatic atrophy) returned pancreatic weight to normal.

Petersen et al [82] have demonstrated a trophic effect of pentagastrin and secretin on the rat pancreas and have confirmed the trophic effect of CCK. They concluded that the increase in pancreatic weight produced by CCK was accompanied by proportional increases in functional capacity (as demonstrated by maximal protein and bicarbonate output after CCK administration) and that chronic administration of secretin caused a decrease in the sensitivity of the pancreas to subsequent secretin challenge.

Dembinski and Johnson [83] produced hypogastrinemic rats by antrectomy and demonstrated a diminution in pancreatic weight as well as decreased RNA and DNA content. The pancreatic weight, as well as DNA and RNA content, was restored to that of controls by administration of exogenous pentagastrin.

Treatment with pentagastrin has also been shown to stimulate growth, as measured by weight, and RNA and DNA content in normal rats [73,84]. Production of endogenous hypergastrinemia by antral transposition has also been shown to increase pancreatic weight [85,86], and hypergastrinemia caused by fundusectomy causes an early increase in weight, RNA, and protein content that is transient and not apparent at 5–7 months after fundusectomy [54].

The administration of chronic cholinergic agonists causes an increase in the pancreatic content of protein and total DNA as well as in the output of pancreatic enzymes. Although the mechanism is not known, the changes may be due to increased gastrin [37,65].

Other hormones that have been studied in relation to a pancreatic trophic effect include EGF and neurotensin. Dembinski et al [87] have shown that EGF, given intraperitoneally but not intragastrically, increases pancreatic weight as well as the uptake of tritiated thymidine in rats. Are all hormones that stimulate pancreatic secretion trophic for the pancreas? Marx et al [88] found that neurotensin (alone or combined with caerulein), in doses equimolar to trophic doses of secretin and caerulein, had no trophic effect on the hamster pancreas. Feurle et al [89], however, found that neurotensin treatment increased DNA content and stimulated uptake of tritiated thymidine in the rat pancreas.

Fasting decreases the total pancreatic content of protein, amylase, RNA, and water [90]. Short-term feeding causes further diminution, but continued refeeding returns the values to basal levels or even higher.

Ninety percent resection of the small bowel produces pancreatic hyperplasia (with proportional increases in weight, DNA, RNA, and protein content) in rats [91], but intestinal bypass does not [92]. Pancreatic hyperplasia produced by intestinal resection is unaltered by pyloroplasty, vagotomy, or antrectomy, indicating a dissociation of the growth response from changes in serum gastrin levels [93].

Clinically, administration of CCK-8 has been suggested as a treatment for chronic pancreatitis. In a study of 30 patients with chronic pancreatitis, Pap et al [94] administered CCK-8 intranasally three times a day and reported increases in pancreatic volume, trypsin, lipase, and amylase. Patients were treated for 3 weeks, and functional capacity of enzyme secretion remained elevated for 3 months after treatment. Somatostatin administration to rats caused a decrease in DNA, RNA, and protein synthesis in short-term experiments, and after longer treatment a diminution in the pancreatic content of DNA and enzymes [95].

The mechanism of hormone-stimulated growth of gut mucosa and pancreas is not entirely understood. Induction of ornithine decarboxylase activity and synthesis of polyamines (putrescine, spermine, and spermidine) appear to be important early steps in the induction of hypertrophic [96] as well as hyperplastic [97,98] growth responses. Increased activity of ornithine decarboxylase and of polyamine biosynthesis is found in the intestinal mucosa of the newborn rat during rapid maturation and is also seen during recovery from chemotherapy-induced injury to intestinal mucosa. α-Difluoromethylornithine (an irreversible ornithine decarboxylase inhibitor) delays intestinal mucosal maturation as well as recovery from injury [99]. Increases in ornithine decarboxylase activity are closely correlated with intestinal hyperplasia after small bowel resection in the rat [100]. Caerulein-stimulated growth of the pancreas is accompanied by increases in the level of polyamines [101].

Small Intestine

Trophic effects of gastrointestinal hormones on the duodenum and small intestine generally parallel those on the stomach. Pentagastrin increases protein synthesis in the duodenum [10,11], as in the fundus. Antrectomy reduces duodenal RNA and DNA, which can be reversed by exogenous pentagastrin [19,83].

The hypertrophic mucosal response to gastrin seems to be limited in the small intestine to the duodenum, and antrectomy (with resultant decrease in serum gastrin levels) does not decrease DNA, RNA, or the weight of small intestinal mucosal in the jejunum [102]. Secretin itself has no trophic effect on any intestinal tissue; however, when administered with pentagastrin, it blocks trophic effects on the duodenum [13] and colon [103].

CCK and secretin have been implicated as trophic hormones for the small intestine, primarily because of their ability to prevent mucosal hypoplasia in dogs receiving total parenteral nutrition [104]. However, a recent study by Fine et al [105] suggests that the trophic effects of CCK and secretin seen in animals on total parenteral nutrition were attributable to trophic actions of pancreatic secretions themselves and are therefore indirect actions. After jejunoileal bypass in rats, no hypertrophy was seen in bypassed segments of intestine in animals treated with CCK and secretin, whereas in areas of intestine exposed to pancreatic secretions, increases in mucosal weights, protein, and DNA content were measured.

For many years, growth of gastrointestinal mucosa has been noted during lactation [7] and has been ascribed to hyperphagia [106,107]. Gastrin levels are known to be elevated at this time [108]. However, Lichtenberger and Trier [109] have examined the time course of duodenal hyperplasia, correlated with hyperphagia and elevated gastrin levels, and have concluded that the increase in cell proliferation during lactation is a direct response to food and is not mediated by hypergastrinemia.

Maturation of the small intestine is thought to be mediated by hormones. Mucosal hypertrophy is found at weaning, a period associated with an increase in gastrin [59] but not glucagon levels [110]. Saliva, which contains nerve growth factor and EGF, is known to produce a trophic response in the small intestine [111]. EGF/urogastrone, when given to suckling but not weanling mice, in doses sufficient to cause precocious eyelid opening, produces increases in intestinal weight [112]. EGF may be a strong factor for maturation of the immature intestine.

EGF also increases activity of hydrolytic enzymes and of DNA synthesis along the entire small bowel [113]. However, ornithine decarboxylase activity is stimulated by EGF only in the stomach and duodenum, not in the midgut or colon [36]. Ornithine decarboxylase is the rate-limiting enzyme in the polyamine biosynthetic pathway. Polyamine production is closely related to the burst of intracellular activity preceding cell synthesis.

Starvation produces a decrease in small intestinal content of DNA, RNA, and protein in rats, which is partially reversible by administration of pentagastrin [114].

Hypertrophy and hyperplasia are found in the small intestine after intestinal resection [51,115]. A number of gastrointestinal hormones are known to increase in concentration with small bowel resection [48]. Concentrations of gastrin, motilin, pancreatic polypeptide, and enteroglucagon are all elevated. Although gastrin is known to be trophic for portions of the small intestine, the major actions seem to be in the duodenum, and hypergastrinemia does not appear to play a central role in adaption to massive resection [116]. At present, enteroglucagon seems to be the most promising candidate for postresection modulation of trophic effects [117,118]. Gleeson et al [119] and Bloom [120] have demonstrated the presence of hypertrophic small bowel in a patient with an enteroglucagon secreting tumor. The hypertrophy resolved with resection of the tumor.

Grey and Morin [121] have reported the presence of a heat-stable acidic extract from the proximal small bowel of rats after a resection of 50 percent of the small bowel, which acts to specifically stimulate DNA synthesis in jejunal explants in organ culture. This substance appears to be a peptide, as it is destroyed by protease. It does not stimulate lymphocyte, skin fibroblast, or colon adenocarcinoma proliferation.

Colon

Trophic effects on the colon are similar to those on the gastric fundus. Exogenous pentagastrin is known to stimulate synthesis of colonic DNA [27]. Colonic weight in the rat is diminished by antrectomy [83]. Administration of pentagastrin to an antrectomized rat results in a return of the colon to normal weight. Both atropine and vagotomy produce increased uptake of tritiated thymidine in colonic mucosa, but neither has an effect on stimulation by pentagastrin [15]. VIP has no effect on colonic mucosal DNA synthesis alone but inhibits pentagastrin-stimulated trophic effects [27]. Glucagon stimulates colonic synthesis of DNA but has no effect on pentagastrin stimulation of mucosa [27]. Secretin alone has no effect on colonic synthesis or content of DNA, but like VIP, its sister hormone, it inhibits pentagastrin-stimulated hypertrophy of the colon in a dose-related fashion [103].

Diet has an important effect on colonic hypertrophy. Ryan et al [122] have given rats an elemental diet, either IV or orally, and standard rat chow. Animals given an elemental diet, either IV or orally, have diminished serum and antral concentrations of gastrin, a 25 percent loss in colonic weight, and a decreased rate of mucosal synthesis of DNA. Administration of exogenous pentagastrin elevates colonic synthesis of DNA but not as much as standard oral feedings. Addition of bulk (cellulose mixed with petroleum jelly) increases colonic mucosal DNA synthesis as well. The time course of reduction of DNA synthesis after administration of a synthetic diet suggests that colonic mucosa is maintained by multiple factors, at least two of which are endogenous release of gastrin and dietary bulk [39].

Gallbladder

Both CCK-8 and caerulein produce trophic effects on gallbladder mucosa [123,124]. Acute and chronic administration of CCK-8 and caerulein produce epithelial hyperplasia of the mouse gallbladder, as measured by tritiated thymidine uptake. Pentagastrin has no effect, either with acute or chronic administration.

REFERENCES

1. Polacek MA, Ellison EH: Parietal cell mass and gastric acid secretion in the Zollinger-Ellison syndrome. Surgery 60:606, 1966.
2. Dragstedt LR, Oberhelman HA, Smith CA: Experimental hyperfunction of the gastric antrum with ulcer formation. Ann Surg 134:332, 1951.
3. Rosenlund ML, Crean GP, Johnson DG, et al: The Zollinger-Ellison syndrome in a 10-year-old boy. J Pediatr 75:443, 1969.
4. Crean GP, Hogg DF, Rumsey RDE: Hyperplasia of the gastric mucosa produced by duodenal obstruction. Gastroenterology 56:193, 1969.
5. Crean GP, Rumsey RDE: Hyperplasia of the gastric mucosa during pregnancy and lactation in the rat. J Physiol 215:181, 1971.
6. MacDonald WC, Rubin CE: Gastric biopsy—a critical evaluation. Gastroenterology 53:143, 1967.
7. Lees F, Grandjean LC: The gastric and jejunal mucosae in healthy patients with parietal gastrectomy. Arch Int Med 101:943, 1958.
8. Crean GP, Rumsey RDE, Hogg DF, et al: Experimental hyperplasia of the gastric mucosa, in Semb L, Myren J (eds): *The Physiology of Gastric Secretion*. Baltimore, Williams & Wilkins, 1968, pp 82–85.
9. Crean GP, Marshall MW, Rumsey RDE: Parietal cell hyperplasia induced by the administration of pentagastrin (ICI 50,123) to rats. Gastroenterology 57:147, 1969.
10. Johnson LR, Aures D, Yuen L: Pentagastrin-induced stimulation of protein synthesis in the gastrointestinal tract. Am J Physiol 217:251, 1969.
11. Johnson LR, Aures D, Hakanson R: Effect of gastrin on the in vivo incorporation of ^{14}C-leucine into protein of the digestive tract. Proc Soc Exp Biol Med 132:996, 1969.
12. Stanley MD, Coalson RE, Grossman MI, et al: Influence of secretin and pentagastrin on acid secretion and parietal cell number in rats. Gastroenterology 63:264, 1972.
13. Johnson LR, Guthrie PD: Secretin inhibition of gastrin-stimulated deoxyribonucleic acid synthesis. Gastroenterology 67:601, 1974.
14. Johnson LR, Guthrie PD: Mucosal DNA synthesis: A short term index of the trophic action of gastrin. Gastroenterology 67:453, 1974.
15. Ryan GP, Johnson LR: Role of gastrin in mucosal DNA synthesis after vagotomy and atropine in the rat. Am J Physiol 235:E565, 1978.
16. Hollinshead JW, Debas HT, Yamada T, et al: Hypergastrinemia develops within 24 hours of truncal vagotomy in dogs. Gastroenterology 88:35, 1985.
17. Miller LR, Jacobson ED, Johnson LR: Effect of pentagastrin on gastric mucosal cells grown in tissue culture. Gastroenterology 64:254, 1973.
18. Willems G, Vansteenkiste Y, Smets P: Effects of food ingestion on the cell proliferation kinetics in the canine fundic mucosa. Gastroenterology 61:323, 1971.
19. Johnson LR, Chandler AM: RNA and DNA of gastric and duodenal mucosa in antrectomized and gastrin-treated rats. Am J Physiol 224:937, 1973.
20. Enochs MR, Johnson LR: Endocrine control of DNA synthesis in rat gastrointestinal mucosa. Gastroenterology 72:1055, 1977.
21. Crean GP: Effect of hypophysectomy on the gastric mucosa of the rat. Gut 9:332, 1968.

22. Crean GP, Rumsey RDE, Wheeler SM: Further observations concerning the effects of hypophysectomy on the gastric mucosa of the rat. Gut 12:721, 1971.
23. Steiner M, Bourges HR, Freedman LS, et al: Effect of starvation on the tissue composition of the small intestine in the rat. Am J Physiol 215:75, 1968.
24. Muller D, Sewing K-Fr, Ruoff H-J: Effect of pentagastrin on gastric mucosal nucleic acid synthesis of fed guinea pigs. Pharmacology 20:106, 1980.
25. Dembinski A, Konturek SJ: Effects of E, F, and I series prostaglandins and analogues on growth of gastroduodenal mucosa and pancreas. Am J Physiol 248:G170, 1985.
26. Johnson LR, Guthrie P: Effect of cholecystokinin and 16,16-dimethyl prostaglandin E_2 on RNA and DNA of gastric and duodenal mucosa. Gastroenterology 70:59, 1976.
27. Johnson LR: New aspects of the trophic action of gastrointestinal hormones. Gastroenterology 72:788, 1977.
28. Lehy T, Dubrasquet M, Bonfils S: Effect of somatostatin on normal and gastric-stimulated cell proliferation in the gastric and intestinal mucosae of the rat. Digestion 19:99, 1979.
29. Lehy T, Dubrasquet M, Brazeau P, et al: Inhibitory effect of prolonged administration of long-acting somatostatin on gastrin-stimulated fundic epithelial cell growth in the rat. Digestion 24:246, 1982.
30. Johnson LR, Guthrie PD: Proglumide inhibition of trophic action of pentagastrin. Am J Physiol 246:G62, 1984.
31. Upp JR Jr, Glass EJ, Townsend CM Jr, et al: Proglumide stimulates fundic and pancreatic growth in the rat. Gastroenterology, 90:1674, 1986.
32. Beauchamp RD, Townsend CM Jr, Singh P, et al: Proglumide, a gastrin receptor antagonist, inhibits growth of colon cancer and enhances survival in mice. Ann Surg 202:303, 1985.
33. Winsett OE, Townsend CM Jr, Glass EJ, et al: Gastrin stimulates growth of colon cancer. Surgery 99:302, 1986.
34. Seidel ER, Tabata K, Dembinski AB, et al: Attenuation of trophic response to gastrin after inhibition of ornithine decarboxylase. Am J Physiol 249:G16, 1985.
35. Johnson LR, Guthrie PD: Stimulation of rat oxyntic gland mucosal growth by epidermal growth factor. Am J Physiol 238:G45, 1980.
36. Feldman EJ, Aures D, Grossman MI: Epidermal growth factor stimulates ornithine decarboxylase activity in the digestive tract of mouse. Proc Soc Exp Biol Med 159:400, 1978.
37. Morisset J, Jolicoeur L, Caussignac Y, et al: Trophic effects of chronic bethanechol on pancreas, stomach, and duodenum in rats. Can J Physiol Pharmacol 60:871, 1982.
38. Sircar B, Johnson LR, Lichtenberger LM: Effect of chemically defined diets on antral and serum gastrin levels in rats. Am J Physiol 238:G376, 1980.
39. Sircar B, Johnson LR, Lichtenberger LM: Effect of synthetic diets on gastrointestinal mucosal DNA synthesis in rats. Am J Physiol 244:G372, 1983.
40. Lichtenberger LM, Lechago J, Johnson LR: Depression of antral and serum gastrin concentration by food deprivation in the rat. Gastroenterology 68:1473, 1975.
41. Johnson LR, Copeland EM, Dudrick S, et al: Structural and hormonal alterations in the gastrointestinal tract of parenterally fed rats. Gastroenterology 68:1177, 1975.
42. Nygaard K: Resection of the small intestine in rats. III. Morphological changes in the intestinal tract. Acta Chir Scand 133:233, 1967.
43. Weser E, Hernandez MH: Studies of small bowel adaptation after intestinal resection in the rat. Gastroenterology 60:69, 1971.
44. Seelig LL, Jr, Winborn WB, Weser E: Effect of small bowel resection on the gastric mucosa in the rat. Gastroenterology 72:421, 1977.
45. Winborn WB, Seelig LL Jr, Nakayama H, et al: Hyperplasia of the gastric glands after small bowel resection in the rat. Gastroenterology 66:384, 1974.
46. Rius X, Guix M, Garriga J, et al: Parietal cell volume, hypergastrinemia, and gastric acid hypersecretion after small bowel resection. Am J Surg 144:269, 1982.
47. Meyers WC, Jones RS: Hyperacidity and hypergastrinemia following extensive intestinal resection. World J Surg 3:539, 1979.
48. Besterman HS, Adrian TE, Mallinson CN, et al: Gut hormone release after intestinal resection. Gut 23:854, 1982.
49. Bowen JC, Paddack GL, Bush JC, et al: Comparison of gastric responses to small intestinal resection and bypass in rats. Surgery 83:402, 1978.
50. Dembinski AB, Johnson LR: Role of gastrin in gastrointestinal adaptation after small bowel resection. Am J Physiol 243:G16, 1982.
51. Weser E: Nutritional aspects of malabsorption: short gut adaptation. Clinics Gastroenterol 12:443, 1983.
52. Oscarson JEA, Veen HF, Williamson RCN, et al: Compensatory postresectional hyperplasia and starvation atrophy in small bowel: Dissociation from endogenous gastrin levels. Gastroenterology 72:890, 1977.
53. Deveney CW, Owen RL, Deveney K, et al: Effect of acid secretory capacity and chronic endogenous hypergastrinemia on pancreatic secretion and intestinal morphology in the rat. Dig Dis Sci 28:65, 1983.
54. Beauchamp RD, Marx M, Townsend CM Jr, et al: Effect of endogenous hypergastrinemia after fundusectomy on growth of the rat pancreas and colon. Gastroenterology 88:1319, 1985.
55. Korman MG, Laver MC, Hansky J: Hypergastrinaemia in chronic renal failure. Br Med J 1:209, 1972.
56. Gordon EM, Johnson AG, Williams G: Gastric assessment of prospective renal-transplant patients. Lancet 1:226, 1972.
57. Franzin G, Musola R, Mencarelli R: Morphological changes of the gastroduodenal mucosa in regular

dialysis uraemic patients. Histopathology 6:429, 1982.
58. Takeuchi K, Johnson LR: Pentagastrin protects against stress ulceration in rats. Gastroenterology 76:327, 1979.
59. Lichtenberger L, Johnson LR: Gastrin in the ontogenic development of the small intestine. Am J Physiol 227:390, 1974.
60. Dodge JA: Production of duodenal ulcers and hypertrophic pyloric stenosis by administration of pentagastrin to pregnant and newborn dogs. Nature 225:284, 1970.
61. Dodge JA, Karim AA: Induction of pyloric hypertrophy by pentagastrin. Gut 17:280, 1976.
62. Lucey MR, McCann S, Weir DG: Is maternal gastrin important in congenital hypertrophic pyloric stenosis? Postgrad Med J 58:584, 1982.
63. Moazam F, Kolts BE, Rodgers BM: In pursuit of the etiology of congenital hypertrophic pyloric stenosis. J Pediatr Gastroenterol Nutr 1:97, 1982.
64. Rothman SS, Wells H: Enhancement of pancreatic enzyme synthesis by pancreozymin. Am J Physiol 213:215, 1967.
65. Mainz DL, Black O, Webster PD: Hormonal control of pancreatic growth. J Clin Invest 52:2300, 1973.
66. Barrowman JA, Mayston PD: The trophic influence of cholecystokinin on the rat pancreas. J Physiol 238:73, 1973.
67. Yamaguchi T, Tabata K, Johnson LR: Effect of proglumide on rat pancreatic growth. Am J Physiol 249:G294, 1985.
68. Anastasi A, Erspamer V, Endean R: Isolation and amino acid sequence of caerulein, the active decapeptide of the skin of *Hyla caerulae.* Arch Biochem Biophys 125:57, 1968.
69. Erspamer V, Bertaccini G, de Caro G, et al: Pharmacological actions of caerulein. Experientia 23:702, 1967.
70. Solomon TE, Petersen H, Elashoff J, et al: Interaction of caerulein and secretin on pancreatic size and composition in rat. Am J Physiol 235:E714, 1978.
71. Townsend CM Jr, Franklin RB, Watson LC, et al: Stimulation of pancreatic cancer growth by caerulein and secretin. Surg Forum 32:228, 1981.
72. Pfeiffer CJ, Chernenko GA, Kohli Y, et al: Trophic effects of cholecystokinin octapeptide on the pancreas of the Syrian hamster. Can J Physiol Pharmacol 60:358, 1982.
73. Dembinski AB, Johnson LR: Stimulation of pancreatic growth by secretin, caerulein, and pentagastrin. Endocrinology 106:323, 1980.
74. Solomon TE, Vanier M, Morisset J: Cell site and time course of DNA synthesis in pancreas after caerulein and secretin. Am J Physiol 245:G99, 1983.
75. Otsuki M, Williams JA: Amylase secretion by isolated pancreatic acini after chronic cholecystokinin treatment in vivo. Am J Physiol 244:G683, 1983.
76. Johnson LR, Dudrick SJ, Guthrie PD: Stimulation of pancreatic growth by intraduodenal amino acids and HCl. Am J Physiol 239:G400, 1980.
77. Wiener I, Walker JP, Greeley GH Jr, et al: Increased release of cholecystokinin with intraduodenal fat after cholecystectomy in dogs. Surg Forum 35:196, 1984.
78. Rosenberg L, Duguid WP, Brown RA, et al: The effect of cholecystectomy on plasma CCK and pancreatic growth in the hamster. Gastroenterology 84:1289, 1983.
79. Yamada T, Brunstedt J, Solomon T: Chronic effects of caerulein and secretin on the endocrine pancreas of the rat. Am J Physiol 244:G541, 1983.
80. McLaughlin CL, Baile CA, Peikin SR: Hyperphagia during lactation: Satiety response to CCK and growth of the pancreas. Am J Physiol 244:E61, 1983.
81. Mayston PD, Barrowman JA: Influence of chronic administration of pentagastrin on the pancreas in hypophysectomized rats. Gastroenterology 64:391, 1973.
82. Petersen H, Solomon T, Grossman MI: Effect of chronic pentagastrin, cholecystokinin, and secretin on pancreas of rats. Am J Physiol 234:E286, 1978.
83. Dembinski AB, Johnson LR: Growth of pancreas and gastrointestinal mucosa in antrectomized and gastrin-treated rats. Endocrinology 105:769, 1979.
84. Majumdar APN, Goltermann N: Chronic administration of pentagastrin. Effects on pancreatic protein and nucleic acid contents and protein synthesis in rats. Digestion 19:144, 1979.
85. Oscarson J, Håkanson R, Liedberg G, et al: Variated serum gastrin concentration: Trophic effects on the gastrointestinal tract of the rat. Acta Physiol Scand Suppl 475:2, 1979.
86. Reber HA, Johnson F, Deveney K, et al: Trophic effects of gastrin on the exocrine pancreas in rats. J Surg Res 22:554, 1977.
87. Dembinski A, Gregory H, Konturek SJ, et al: Trophic action of epidermal growth factor on the pancreas and gastroduodenal mucosa in rats. J Physiol 325:35, 1982.
88. Marx M, Glass EJ, Townsend CM Jr, et al: Differential effect of caerulein and neurotensin on pancreatic growth. Dig Dis Sci 29:51S, 1984.
89. Feurle GE, Muller B, Ohnheiser G, et al: Action of neurotensin on size, composition, and growth of pancreas and stomach in the rat. Regul Pept 13:53, 1985.
90. Webster PD, Singh M, Tucerk PC, et al: Effects of fasting and feeding on the pancreas. Gastroenterology 62:600, 1972.
91. Haegel P, Stock C, Marescaux J, et al: Hyperplasia of the exocrine pancreas after small bowel resection in the rat. Gut 22:207, 1981.
92. Stock C, Haegel P, Marescaux J, et al: Effect of small bowel bypass on the rat exocrine pancreas. Lab Invest 46:231, 1982.
93. Stock-Damge C, Aprahamian M, Lhoste E, et al: Pancreatic hyperplasia after small bowel resection in the rat: Dissociation from endogenous gastrin levels. Digestion 29:223, 1984.
94. Pap A, Berger Z, Varro V: Trophic effect of cholecystokinin-octapeptide in man—a new way in the

treatment of chronic pancreatitis. Digestion 21:163, 1981.

95. Morisset J, Genik P, Lord A, et al: Effects of chronic administration of somatostatin on rat exocrine pancreas. Regul Pept 4:49, 1982.
96. Russell DH, Byus CV, Manen C-A: Proposed model of major sequential biochemical events of a trophic response. Life Sci 19:1297, 1976.
97. Janne J, Poso H, Raina A: Polyamines in rapid growth and cancer. Biochim Biophys Acta 473:241, 1978.
98. Raina A, Eloranta T, Pajula R-L, et al: Polyamines in rapidly growing animal tissues, in Gaugas JM (ed): *Polyamines in Biomedical Research.* New York, John Wiley & Sons, 1980, pp 38–49.
99. Luk GD, Marton LJ, Baylin SB: Ornithine decarboxylase is important in intestinal mucosal maturation and recovery from injury in rats. Science 210:195, 1980.
100. Luk GD, Baylin SB: Polyamines and intestinal growth—increased polyamine biosynthesis after jejunectomy. Am J Physiol 245:G656, 1983.
101. Morisset J, Benrezzak O: Polyamines and pancreatic growth induced by caerulein. Life Sci 35:2471, 1984.
102. Lorenz-Meyer H, Volker J-A, Friedel N, et al: Effect of antrectomy on small intestinal structure and function in the rat. Digestion 26:17, 1983.
103. Johnson LR, Guthrie PD: Effect of secretin on colonic DNA synthesis. Proc Soc Exp Biol Med 158:521, 1978.
104. Hughes CA, Bates T, Dowling RH: Cholecystokinin and secretin prevent the intestinal mucosal hypoplasia of total parenteral nutrition in the dog. Gastroenterology 75:34, 1978.
105. Fine H, Levine GM, Shiau Y-F: Effects of cholecystokinin and secretin on intestinal structure and function. Am J Physiol 245:G358, 1983.
106. Campbell RM, Fell BF: Gastro-intestinal hypertrophy in the lactating rat and its relation to food intake. J Physiol 171:90, 1964.
107. Cripps AW, Williams VJ: The effect of pregnancy and lactation on food intake, gastrointestinal anatomy and the absorptive capacity of the small intestine in the albino rat. Br J Nutr 33:17, 1975.
108. Lichtenberger LM, Nance DM, Gorski RA: Sex-related difference in antral and serum gastrin levels in the rat. Proc Soc Exp Biol Med 151:785, 1976.
109. Lichtenberger LM, Trier JS: Changes in gastrin levels, food intake, and duodenal mucosal growth during lactation. Am J Physiol 237:E98, 1979.
110. Buts J-P, DeMeyer R, VanCraynest M-P, et al: Pancreatic glucagon does not alter mucosal growth and maturation of sucrase and thymidine kinase activity in rat small intestine. Biol Neonate 43:253, 1983.
111. Li AKC, Schattenkerk ME, Huffman RG, et al: Hypersecretion of submandibular saliva in male mice: trophic response in small intestine. Gastroenterology 84:949, 1983.
112. Oka Y, Ghishan FK, Greene HL, et al: Effect of mouse epidermal growth factor/urogastrone on the functional maturation of rat intestine. Endocrinology 112:940, 1983.
113. Malo C, Menard D: Influence of epidermal growth factor on the development of suckling mouse intestinal mucosa. Gastroenterology 83:28, 1982.
114. Lichtenberger L, Welsh JD, Johnson LR: Relationship between the changes in gastrin levels and intestinal properties in the starved rat. Am J Dig Dis 21:33, 1976.
115. Williamson RCN, Chir M: Intestinal adaptation (second of two parts). Mechanisms of control. N Engl J Med 298:1444, 1978.
116. Morin CL, Ling V: Effect of pentagastrin on the rat small intestine after resection. Gastroenterology 75:224, 1978.
117. Uttenthal LO, Batt RM, Carter MW, et al: Stimulation of DNA synthesis in cultured small intestine by partially purified enteroglucagon. Regul Pept 3:84, 1982.
118. Jacobs LR, Polak J, Bloom SR, et al: Does enteroglucagon play a trophic role in intestinal adaptation? Clin Sci Mol Med 50:14, 1976.
119. Gleeson MH, Bloom SR, Polak JM, et al: Endocrine tumour in kidney affecting small bowel structure, motility, and absorptive function. Gut 12:773, 1971.
120. Bloom SR: An enteroglucagon tumour. Gut 13:520, 1972.
121. Grey VL, Morin CL: Evidence for a growth-stimulating fraction in the rat proximal intestine after small bowel resection. Gastroenterology 89:1305, 1985.
122. Ryan GP, Dudrick SJ, Copeland EM, et al: Effects of various diets on colonic growth in rats. Gastroenterology 77:658, 1979.
123. Lamote J, Putz P, Willems G: Effect of cholecystokinin-octapeptide, caerulein, and pentagastrin on epithelial cell proliferation in the murine gallbladder. Gastroenterology 83:371, 1982.
124. Putz Ph, Bazira L, Willems G: The effect of caerulein on epithelial growth in the mouse gall bladder. Experientia 36:429, 1980.

Chapter 10

Aging and Gut Peptides

Talaat Khalil, M.D., and James C. Thompson, M.D.

Lengthening of life expectancy has brought new problems to medicine. Geriatrics plays a major role in the practice of medicine today. Our society is getting older, and with luck the trend will continue. A few decades ago, only about one out of 11 of our population was over 65; soon the proportion will be as high as one in five [1]. Descriptive information regarding age-induced changes is abundant, though incomplete [1–3], but little information is available regarding the exact alterations in the physiologic mechanisms that attend aging, a deficit noted in recent symposia [4–8]. This review will cover some of the effects of aging on gut function and on the little we know about these effects on gastrointestinal hormones.

We might consider initially the question of what is "old." We use the terms life span, life expectancy, and median length of life to define aspects of survival of a living organism. Life span refers to the maximum age to which a population lives. Life expectancy refers to the average individual length of life. The median length of survival refers to the length of life at which 50 percent of the population are alive. To illustrate these concepts, we might consider a theoretical population in which half of the members died at the age of 50 years but the other half lived to the age of 100 years. The life span would be 100 years, the life expectancy would be 75 years, and the median life length would be 50 years. The life span means the number of years an individual may be expected to live, provided no vicissitudes intervene to cut life short. We could assume that the term life span denotes the maximum survival of an individual if death occurs as a result of senescence, while life expectancy denotes the survival of an individual if death occurs because of senescence or anticipated causes such as accidents or disease. Both indexes are important when considering a certain population in an aging study. Nonetheless, neither of these two parameters tells us what is an aged population or when aging starts.

In most studies on aging, "old" animals are defined as having achieved the age at which one half the population ordinarily dies [9]. We have used that definition, but it does create some problems. That age in humans in the United States, for example, is 77.4 years. Recruitment of 77-plus-year-old volunteers is difficult, and most studies in humans make an arbitrary assumption that an old person has reached some given age, usually 60.

We have listed the median survival time (or population half-life) for some common laboratory animals and for humans in Table 10-1. Much information is not available; for example, the median half-life for common dogs and cats and pigs and rabbits is not known. The age given for beagles is for highly inbred laboratory-raised animals. Information for pigs and rabbits is anecdotal, and the figures we give are based on personal communications from authorities.

We will summarize information available regarding changes in gut function with age.

Aging is associated with secretory and morphologic changes within the stomach. There is general agreement that both basal and stimulated secretions of gastric acid diminish with age in humans [10–19]. The most common explanation is a loss of parietal cells due to atrophic gastritis, the incidence of which increases steadily with age [16,20–25]. Acid secretion appears to remain normal in those elderly individuals with normal gastric mucosa [26]. We recently found that basal and stimulated acid secretions in rats decrease with aging (unpublished data) (Fig 10-1).

Studies on intestinal absorption in humans reveal general agreement that absorption of fat [27–34] and carbohydrates [35–40] diminishes

Table 10-1. How old is "old"? Age at which one-half of the population dies

Animal	*Median survival*	*Animal*	*Median survival*
BALB/c mice [156]		Rabbits [157]	Population half-life unknown. Normal life span of lab rabbit is 7 yr; retired breeders 18–20 mo. Any rabbit >3 yr is considered "old."
Male	23–25 mo		
Female	27 mo		
Fischer rats [158]			
Male	28 mo		
Female	26 mo		
Long-Evans rats [158]		Dogs (beagles [159])	
Male	28 mo	Male	14 yr
Female	28 mo	Female	14 yr
Sprague-Dawley rats [158]		Pigs [160]	Population half-life unknown. Domestic pigs usually killed at 3 yr. Maximal age of minipig colonies ranges from 10–15 yr, and this is ca 2/3 normal life span.
Male	25 mo		
Female	28 mo		
Syrian hamsters [161]			
Male	24 mo		
Female	19 mo		
Guinea pigs [162]		Humans [163] (1980, USA)	
Male	46 mo	Male, female, all races	77.4 yr
Female	30 mo		

(Adapted from [9].)

with age, but information regarding protein absorption is conflicting [6]. Older subjects have been reported to be in positive nitrogen balance [41], or to require an increased intake of protein in order to maintain a positive nitrogen balance [42,43], or to be no different in this respect from the young [44,45]. The uptake of specific amino acids in aged rats was found to be reduced [46]. Secretion of intestinal enzymes is assumed to be diminished in the elderly, but data are scarce [6]. The concentration and content of several enzymes in the proximal small bowel are reduced with aging in the rat [47], and study of enzyme kinetics in old mice revealed a diminished V_{max} but no difference in K_m values [48]. Several gut peptides—vasoactive intestinal peptide, gastric inhibitory polypeptide (GIP),

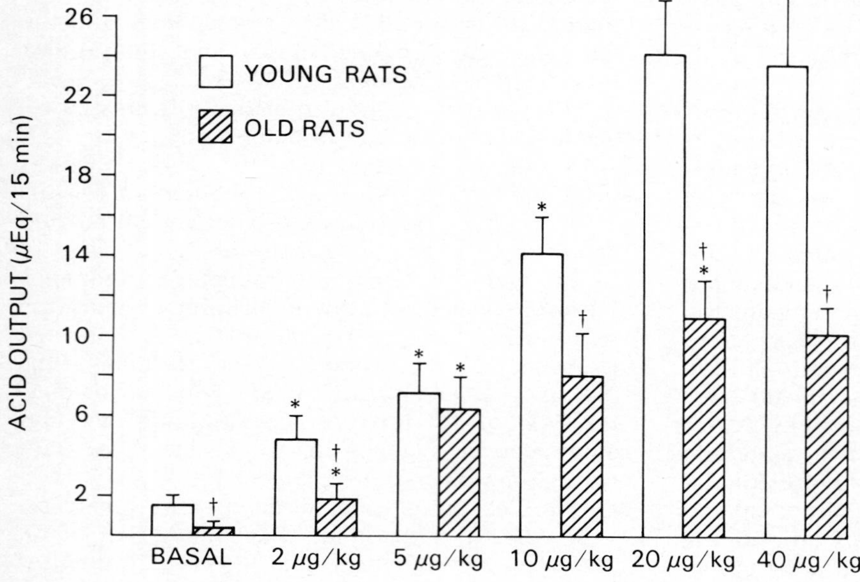

Figure 10-1. Effect of aging on fasting and gastrin-stimulated acid secretion in Fisher 344 rats. Young rats are 3 months old and old rats are 32 months old. (* = $p < 0.05$ vs basal; + = $p < 0.05$ vs young.)

glucagon, and pentagastrin (among others)— stimulate small bowel secretion [49–52], but the effect of aging on humoral stimulation of intestinal secretion is unknown.

Information regarding the effect of aging on intestinal motility is fragmentary and conflicting. Aged rats do not appear to have any major abnormality in gastrointestinal transit after a meal [53], and healthy elderly human subjects have a normal migrating motor complex during fasting, but the postprandial activity of the small intestine may be diminished compared to that of young adults [54].

Biliary disease is common in our society and increases with age [55–57]. Early studies on gallbladder emptying, using oral cholecystography images, showed that the gallbladder appears to empty more rapidly in older subjects [58–61]. Recent studies using more accurate techniques for measuring gallbladder volumes showed that the gallbladder emptying in response to intravenous cholecystokinin (CCK) [62] or to oral Lipomul [63] is similar in old and young individuals (Fig 10-2). Moreover, both fasting and maximally contracted gallbladder volumes and the percentage of reduction of gallbladder volume are the same in young and old humans [63]. However, the sensitivity of the gallbladder to endogenously released CCK in humans in vivo [63] or to CCK-8 in rabbits in vitro [64] decreases significantly with aging (Figs 10-3 and 10-4).

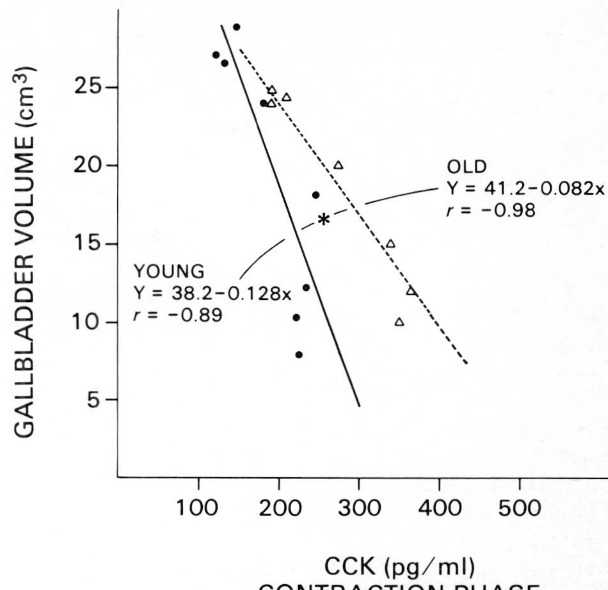

Figure 10-3. Linear regression analysis of gallbladder volume versus plasma. Concentrations of CCK 0–30 minutes after Lipomul ingestion in young and old humans. * = significant difference between slopes of regression. (From Khalil et al [63], by permission of The C. V. Mosby Co.)

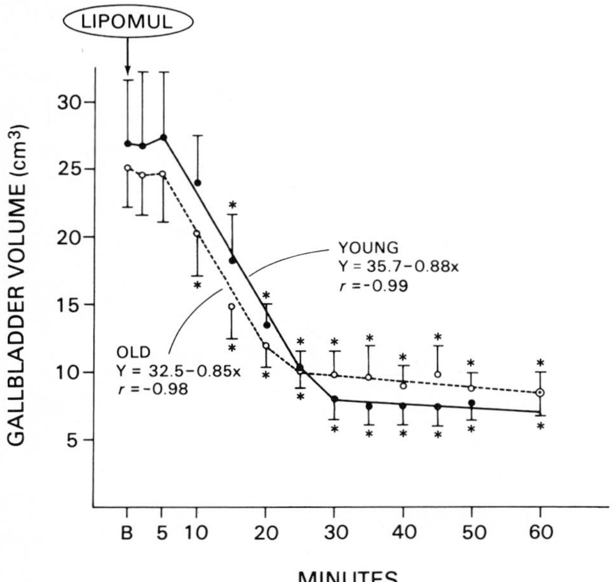

Figure 10-2. Gallbladder volume in response to oral Lipomul in young (mean age 32) and old (mean age 64) humans. Correlation between gallbladder size and time after Lipomul. * = significant decrease from basal volume. (From Khalil et al [63], by permission of The C. V. Mosby Co.)

Several investigators have described specific degenerative changes in the pancreas of dogs, rats, and humans that might be a normal accompaniment of senility [65–70]. These include metaplasia of the duct epithelium and degenerative changes in the alveoli that consist of general loss of basophilic staining quality in acinar cells, nuclear atrophy, increase in nucleolar substance, and dilatation of the acini and ducts that leads to flattening of the epithelium, resulting in minute cysts surrounded by a layer of extremely thin epithelium. The entire series of changes appears to be essentially destructive in regard to the functional capacity of the pancreas.

Exocrine pancreatic secretion is usually little changed by age in most individuals [71,72], except for a small subset with senile pancreatitis. In one study, trypsin and lipase concentrations from old patients were actually elevated [73]. Pancreatic flow and bicarbonate output after administration of secretin were unchanged in old subjects [71,74]. Recently, we have shown (Fig 10-5) that both basal and stimulated pancreatic volume and bicarbonate and protein output are all significantly diminished

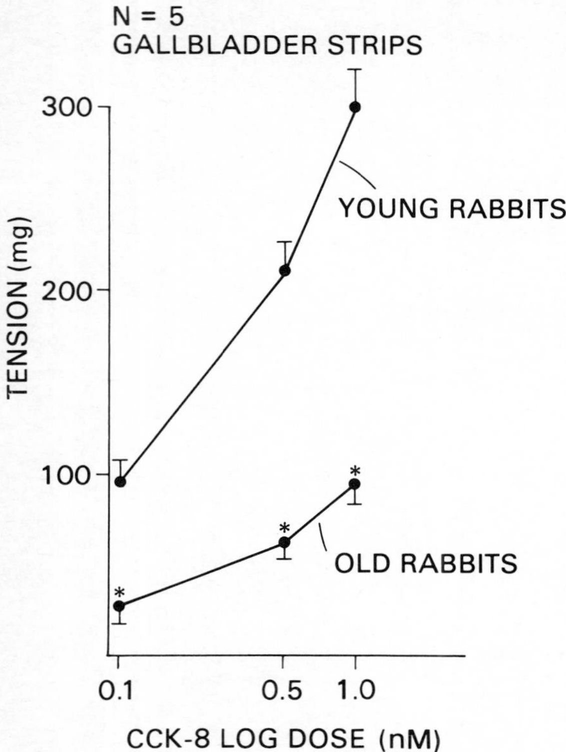

Figure 10-4. Gallbladder responses to CCK-8 in vitro in young and old rabbits. (* = $p < 0.05$ vs young.)

in old rats in vivo [75]. The secretion of amylase by isolated pancreatic acini from aged rats in response to secretagogues, carbamylcholines, CCK-8, and secretin is significantly decreased compared to that from young rats (Fig 10-6) [76].

There are no reports on the effect of age on release of hormones stimulating pancreatic secretion. We have preliminary evidence (Fig 10-7) that fasting and stimulated levels of CCK-33 are significantly higher in old individuals [63]. Serum concentrations of pancreatic polypeptide (PP) have been shown to increase with age in humans [77–80]. However, we found no increased release with aging in rats [81].

The effect of aging on the endocrine pancreas has been documented in a series of studies on glucose and the glucoregulatory hormones [5,82–90]. Serum insulin levels appear to increase with age, but the sensitivity to insulin is diminished [91,92]. Glucose tolerance declines with age [83–86]. After oral glucose, insulin levels are elevated in older nondiabetic humans [76–79], but the insulin response to intravenous glucose is diminished [93]. After glucose administration, older rats exhibit an immediate hyperinsulinemia, followed by a delay in the second phase output [94]. Large islets secrete more insulin in response to glucose in vitro than do small islets; aging slightly reduces insulin secretion from large islets but practically abolishes the response from small islets [94]. On the other hand, glucagon and adrenal responsiveness to moderate reduction in blood glucose by constant intravenous infusion of insulin does not change with aging in humans [95].

In preliminary studies [96], we found no significant difference in the release of insulin from islets obtained from young and old rats. Further, we found no difference in plasma levels and pancreatic content of insulin between young and old rats [81]. (The numbers of animals were small, and we did not differentiate between large and small islets.) The glucagon response to intragastric glucose in rats greatly increases with age [94]. Comparison of the insulin responses from islets from young and old animals revealed no differences [97]. A summary of related studies reveals that older rats have more large islets than the young

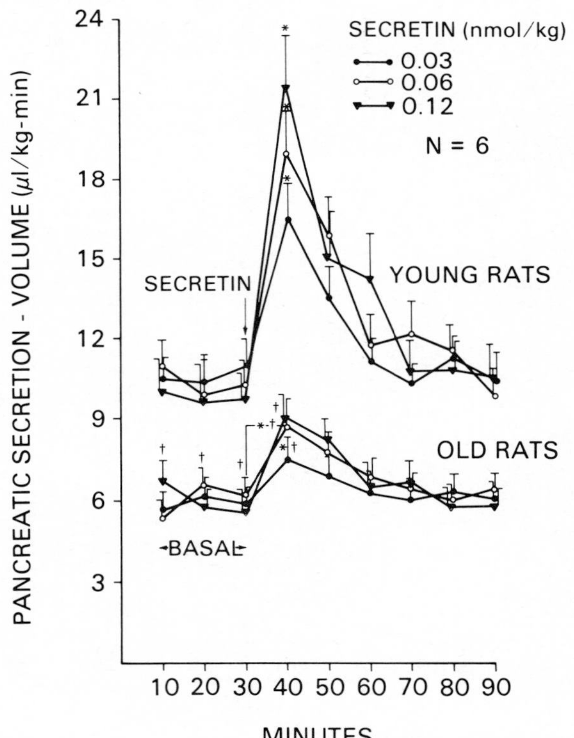

Figure 10-5. Effect of aging on basal and secretin-stimulated pancreatic secretion volume in Sprague-Dawley rats. (* = $p < 0.05$ vs basal; + = $p < 0.05$ vs young.) (From Khalil et al [75], by permission of Technical Publishing Co.)

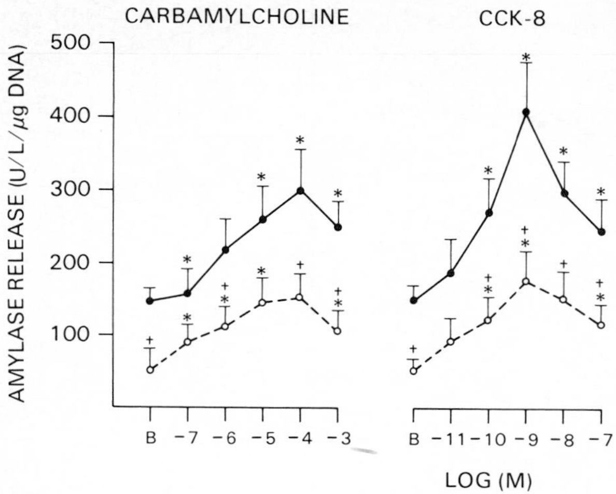
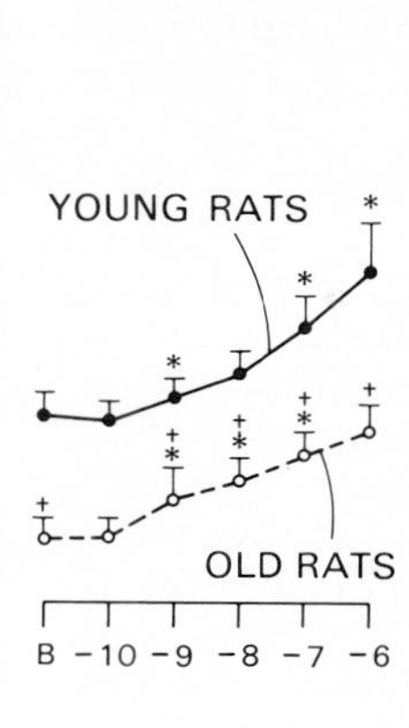

Figure 10-6. Effect of aging on response of rat isolated pancreatic acini to different secretagogues. (* = $p < 0.05$ vs control; + = $p < 0.05$ vs young.)

[98], more β cells in the islets [99], more insulin per β cell [100], and more insulin per islet [101] but a decrease in the glucose-stimulated release of insulin [102].

There is little information on the effects of aging on gastrointestinal hormones, and none whatsoever on its effect on the pharmacokinetics of gastrointestinal hormones. In addition to insulin

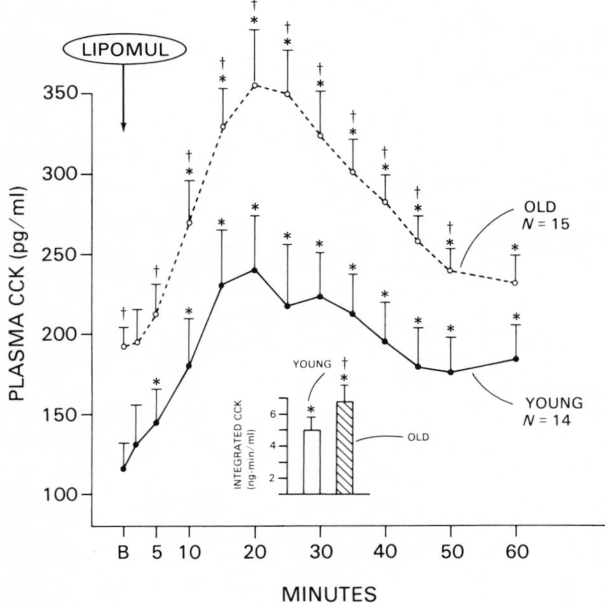

Figure 10-7. Effect of aging on fasting and Lipomul-stimulated CCK concentrations in humans. The inset shows the integrated CCK output during the 60 minutes after Lipomul ingestion. (* = $p < 0.05$ vs basal; + = $p < 0.05$ vs young.) (From Khalil et al [63], by permission of The C. V. Mosby Co.)

and glucagon (above), the only brain-gut peptide known to be associated with age is human pancreatic polypeptide (HPP), which is significantly increased in older individuals [103–105]. HPP response to both oral glucose [104] and oral Lipomul [105] is several times higher in the elderly. In contrast, in rats, the plasma levels of PP do not change with age, but the pancreatic tissue content decreases significantly [81]. Early studies reported that fasting serum gastrin concentrations in humans were increased with age [106,107], but in later studies fasting gastrin levels did not differ with age [108,109]. We found no difference in fasting gastrin between young and old rats, but the postprandial serum levels and antral gastrin were both lower in old rats [110].

Holt [6], in a discussion of altered pancreatic or intestinal secretion in the elderly, stated that there had been no studies on the release of CCK. We recently measured CCK release in young and old subjects and found that fasting and peak levels of CCK-33 were significantly higher in the old (see Fig 10-7) [63]. Both duodenal and jejunal tissue concentrations and content of CCK are higher in old rats compared to young rats. In contrast, duodenal tissue content of secretin is lower in old rats. Jejunal tissue content of secretin does not change with aging in rats [111]. After oral glucose, GIP levels showed little difference, but N-terminal glucagon was higher in the old than in the young [104]. However, β-cell sensitivity to endogenous GIP decreases with aging in humans [112].

In preliminary studies on the effect of aging on neurotensin levels in humans, we found that basal levels of neurotensin were significantly higher in the old and that fat was a strong stimulant of neurotensin release in the young but not in the old. Motilin, a hormone that has been shown to control gastric motility and the migration of intestinal myoelectric complex, particularly phase III, has been shown to increase in concentration with age in children [113]. However, it has no relation to age in elder groups [109].

There is no information on the effect of aging on hormone receptors in the gut. In a preliminary study [114], we found high affinity binding sites in the fundus of young but not old rats; conversely, the concentration of gastrin receptors in the duodenum and colon was 1.5 times higher in the old rats. In the mouse liver, there is no difference in the number of epidermal growth factor (EGF) receptors or the activity of associated tyrosine kinase between adults or senescent animals [115].

We found no reports on the effects of aging on the trophic actions of gastrointestinal hormones on normal and neoplastic tissues but a great deal of information on the effects of aging on carcinogenesis [91]. At age 25, one person out of 700 is at risk to develop cancer within the next 5 years, but at age 65, the risk is one out of 14 [116]. The risk for colorectal cancer doubles with each decade up to 75–80 years [117]. In a study of chemical carcinogenesis, the incidence of induction of tumor increased with duration of exposure but not with age [116], so that the increased incidence of cancer in older humans may be due simply to prolonged duration of exposure to carcinogens and not to aging itself.

In a study of gastric carcinogenesis, Kimura et al [118] found a higher rate of induction of cancer after application of *N*-methyl-*N*′-nitro-*N*-nitrosoguanidine in young than in old rats. Colon tumors induced by treatment with 1,2-dimethylhydrazine (DMH) had a similar incidence in young and old rats, but multiple tumors decreased with advancing age; larger, highly invasive malignant tumors were more common in old than in young animals [119]. Old and young mice treated with DMH showed the same frequency of tumor development, but the latent period was longer in the young [120].

Gastrin stimulates hyperplasia of normal colonic mucosa [121], and we have shown that chronic gastrin treatment stimulates the growth of a transplantable mouse colon carcinoma [122]. Other studies gave conflicting results, some reporting that gastrin does increase the incidence of carcinogen-induced gastric cancer [123] and others that it does not [124,125].

Physiologic events in many species are characterized by circadian rhythmicity, and changes in these rhythms have been reported with age [126–128]. These rhythms, carefully studied in the gut of the mouse and other species, are present in cell division [129–131], in release of enzymes [132–135], and in the concentrations of gastrointestinal hormones: CCK [135], gastrin [136], and GIP [137]. Rhythms exist in feeding and drinking [138] and may affect morphology, such as height and width of villi and thickness of mucosa [134]. Circadian stage-dependent effects on the synthesis of DNA in the gut have been reported to occur after administration of epidermal growth factor, insulin, glucagon, ACTH, and pentagastrin [139–143].

In confirmation of an observation made in 1917 [144], McCay et al made a series of observations beginning in 1935 [145–147] that restriction of food intake prolongs the life of laboratory rats. The phenomenon has been now reported in multiple species—crustaceans, fruit flies, fish, rats, mice, and hamsters [148]. Wistar rats fed ad lib had a 50 percent survivorship of 135 weeks; those fed only every other day had a 50 percent survivorship of 172 weeks [148]. Rats with restricted food intake were found to have an 80 percent survivorship at 800 days vs 48 percent of the ad lib fed animals [149]. In a group of rats given free dietary choice, the population half-life was found to be a strict inverse function of food intake [150]. Silverberg and Silverberg [151] concluded that in a variety of lower animals, life may be prolonged by restriction of food and that a high level of dietary fat has an adverse effect on the life span. Food restriction, even if initiated near weaning and maintained for only one year, caused a distinct prolongation of life [152]. Since life span can be affected by food restriction both early and late in life, it is likely that nutrition affects life span by way of a number of possible mechanisms [153]. One important question is whether dietary restriction extends the life span or whether free eating shortens it.

Masoro et al [154] developed a protocol in which one group of rats is fed ad libitum (median life span, 714 days [155]) and another group is fed 60 percent of the ad lib amount (median life span, 1,047 days [155]). Both groups are subdivided by thirds, one for longevity, one for longitudinal study of body mass, and the last for cross-sectional studies involving physiologic and biochemical measurements at 6-month intervals. The effects of the interaction of age and food deprivation on gastrointestinal hormones in this model for prolongation of life are not known.

As one begins to study possible mechanisms for age-related physiologic changes, one of the most striking findings is how little we know in terms of gross descriptive changes. That is, what is—exactly—the effect of aging on a specific physiologic process—say pancreatic secretion—in specific species—say the cat? No one knows.

This means that before we can determine exact mechanistic changes, we must accurately describe what happens with age. It is not possible to extrapolate and assume that everything slows down. For example, gallbladder emptying is more rapid in older humans [58–61]; age causes no change in intestinal motility in rats. Further, it is not always possible to generalize from species to species. Age causes an increase in basal and food-stimulated levels of PP in humans [77,80] but not in rats [81].

Many accurate observations on the effect of aging are now available [4–8,10], and we can look forward to studies that will clarify the mechanisms responsible for these changes.

REFERENCES

1. Adelman RC: Overview of the biology of aging, in Texter EC Jr (ed): *The Aging Gut. Pathophysiology, Diagnosis, and Management.* New York, Masson Publishing USA Inc, 1983, pp 1–3.
2. Sacher GA: Life table modification and life prolongation, in Finch CE, Hayflick L (eds): *Handbook of the Biology of Aging.* New York, Van Nostrand Reinhold, 1977, pp 582–638.
3. Harnes JR: Normal values with increasing age. J Chron Dis 33:593, 1980.
4. Adelman RC: Symposium—Overview of the biology of aging. Fed Proc 38:1955, 1979.
5. Adelman RC: Loss of adaptive mechanisms during aging. Fed Proc 38:1968, 1979.
6. Holt PR: Intestinal absorption and malabsorption, in Texter EC Jr (ed): *The Aging Gut. Pathophysiology, Diagnosis, and Management.* New York, Masson Publishing USA Inc, 1983, pp 33–56.
7. Masoro EJ: Symposium—Biology of aging. Introduction. Fed Proc 39:3162, 1980.
8. Texter EC Jr: Preface, in Texter EC Jr (ed): *The Aging Gut. Pathophysiology, Diagnosis, and Management.* New York, Masson Publishing USA Inc, 1983, p iii.
9. Walford RL: When is a mouse "old"? J Immunol 117:352, 1976.
10. Schuster MM: Disorders of the aging GI system. Hosp Prac Sept:95, 1976.
11. Keyrilainen O: Nature of gastric hypersecretion of acid in patients with duodenal ulcer. Ann Clin Res 29 (Suppl 1):1, 1980.
12. Baron JH: The clinical use of gastric function tests. Scand J Gastroenterol Suppl 6:9, 1970.
13. Grossman MI, Kirsner JB, Gillespie IE: Basal and histalog-stimulated gastric secretion in control subjects and in patients with peptic ulcer or gastric cancer. Gastroenterology 45:14, 1963.
14. Burhol PG, Myren J: Gastritis and gastric secretion, in Semb LS, Myren J (eds): *The Physiology of Gastric Secretion.* Baltimore, The Williams & Wilkins Co, 1968, pp 626–632.
15. Miyoshi A, Ohe K, Inagawa T, et al: A statistical study on the age distribution of gastric secretion in patients with peptic ulcer. Hiroshima J Med Sci 29:21, 1980.
16. Portis SA, King JC: The gastrointestinal tract in the aged. JAMA 148:1073, 1952.
17. Polland WS: Histamine test meals. An analysis of nine hundred and eighty-eight consecutive tests. Arch Intern Med 51:903, 1933.
18. Baron JH: Studies of basal and peak acid output with an augmented histamine test. Gut 4:136, 1963.
19. Berstad A, Petersen H, Myren J: Effect of secretin and pentagastrin on gastric secretion in man. Acta Hepatogastroenterol 19:277, 1972.
20. Siurala M, Isokoski M, Varis K, et al: Prevalence of gastritis in a rural population. Bioptic study of subjects selected at random. Scand J Gastroenterol 3:211, 1968.
21. Andrews GR, Haneman B, Arnold BJ, et al: Atrophic gastritis in the aged. Aust Ann Med 16:230, 1967.
22. Kimura K: Chronological transition of the fundic-pyloric border determined by stepwise biopsy of the lesser and greater curvatures of the stomach. Gastroenterology 63:584, 1972.
23. Strickland RG, Mackay IR: A reappraisal of the nature and significance of chronic atrophic gastritis. Am J Dig Dis 18:426, 1973.
24. Varis K, Ihamaki T, Harkonen M, et al: Gastric morphology, function, and immunology in first-degree relatives of probands with pernicious anemia and controls. Scand J Gastroenterol 14:129, 1979.
25. Villako K, Tamm A, Savisaar E, et al: Prevalence of antral and fundic gastritis in a randomly selected group of an Estonian rural population. Scand J Gastroenterol 11:817, 1976.
26. Kekki M, Samloff IM, Ihamaki T, et al: Age- and sex-related behaviour of gastric acid secretion at the population level. Scand J Gastroenterol 17:737, 1982.
27. Holt PR, Dominguez AA: Intestinal absorption of triglyceride and vitamin D_3 in aged and young rats. Dig Dis Sci 26:1109, 1981.
28. Kasper H: Faecal fat excretion, diarrhea, and subjective complaints with highly dosed oral fat intake. Digestion 3:321, 1970.
29. Pelz KS, Gottfried SP, Soos E: Intestinal absorption studies in the aged. Geriatrics 23:149, 1968.
30. Montgomery RD, Haeney MR, Ross IN, et al: The ageing gut: A study of intestinal absorption in relation to nutrition in the elderly. Quart J Med XLVII:197, 1978.
31. Becker GH, Meyer J, Necheles H: Fat absorption in young and old age. Gastroenterology 14:80, 1950.
32. Garcia P, Roderuck C, Swanson P: The relation of age to fat absorption in adult women together with observations on concentration of serum choles-

terol. Journal Paper J-2578, Ames, Iowa, Iowa Agricultural Experiment Station, Project 28, 1954, pp 601–609.
33. Webster SGP, Wilkinson EM, Gowland E: A comparison of fat absorption in young and old subjects. Age Ageing 6:113, 1977.
34. Citi S, Salvini L: The intestinal absorption of ^{131}I labelled olein and triolein, or ^{58}CO vit. B_{12} and ^{59}FE, in the aged subjects. Giorn Geront 12:123, 1964.
35. Phillips RA, Gilder H: Metabolism studies in the albino rat. The relation of age, nutrition and hypophysectomy on the absorption of dextrose from the gastrointestinal tract. Endocrinology 27:601, 1940.
36. Sapp OL, Sessions JT Jr, Rose JW Jr: Effect of aging on intestinal absorption of sugars. Clin Res 12:31, 1964.
37. Feibusch JM, Holt PR: Impaired absorptive capacity for carbohydrate in the aging human. Dig Dis Sci 27:1095, 1982.
38. Guth PH: Physiologic alterations in small bowel function with age. The absorption of D-xylose. Am J Dig Dis 13:565, 1968.
39. Kendall MJ: The influence of age on the xylose absorption test. Gut 11:498, 1970.
40. Webster SGP, Leeming JT: Assessment of small bowel function in the elderly using a modified xylose tolerance test. Gut 16:109, 1975.
41. Bogdonoff MD, Shock NW, Nichols MP: Calcium, phosphorus, nitrogen, and potassium balance studies in the aged male. J Gerontol 8:272, 1953.
42. Kountz WB, Hofstatter L, Ackermann P: Nitrogen balance studies in elderly people. Geriatrics 2:173, 1947.
43. Kountz WB, Hofstatter L, Ackermann PG: Nitrogen balance studies in four elderly men. J Gerontol 6:20, 1951.
44. Cheng AHR, Gomez A, Bergan JG, et al: Comparative nitrogen balance study between young and aged adults using three levels of protein intake from a combination wheat-soy-milk mixture. Am J Clin Nutr 31:12, 1978.
45. Zanni E, Calloway DH, Zezulka AY: Protein requirements of elderly men. J Nutr 109:513, 1979.
46. Navab F, Reis RJS, Konduri K, et al: Effect of aging on intestinal absorption of aromatic amino acids in the rat. Gastroenterology 86:1193, 1984.
47. Holt PR, Kotler DP: Aging does not impair upper intestinal adaptive responses to fasting and refeeding in the rat. Gastroenterology 86:1116, 1984.
48. Sayeed M: Age related changes in intestinal phosphomonoesterases. Fed Proc 26:259, 1967.
49. Barbezat GO, Grossman MI: Intestinal secretion: Stimulation by peptides. Science 174:422, 1971.
50. Schwartz CJ, Kimberg DV, Sheerin HE, et al: Vasoactive intestinal peptide stimulation of adenylate cyclase and active electrolyte secretion in intestinal mucosa. J Clin Invest 54:536, 1974.
51. Helman CA, Barbezat GO: The effect of gastric inhibitory polypeptide on human jejunal water and electrolyte transport. Gastroenterology 72:376, 1977.
52. Thompson JC, Marx M: Gastrointestinal hormones. Curr Prob Surg 21:1, 1984.
53. McDougal JN, Miller MS, Burks TF: Intestinal transit and gastric emptying in young and senescent rats. Dig Dis Sci 25:728, 1980.
54. Anuras S, Sutherland J: Jejunal manometry in healthy elderly subjects. Gastroenterology 86:1016, 1984.
55. Hermann RE: Biliary disease in the aging patient, in Texter EC Jr (ed): *The Aging Gut. Pathophysiology, Diagnosis, and Management.* New York, Masson Publishing USA Inc, 1983, pp 27–32.
56. Lund J: Surgical indications in cholelithiasis: Prophylactic cholecystectomy elucidated on the basis of long term follow-up on 526 nonoperated cases. Ann Surg 151:153, 1960.
57. Wenckert A, Robertson B: The natural course of gallstone disease. Gastroenterology 50:376, 1966.
58. Boyden EA: An analysis of the reaction of the human gall bladder to food. Anat Rec 40:147, 1928.
59. Boyden EA, Fuller AH: Anatomy and physiology of the gallbladder in children. A cholecystographic study. Am J Dis Child 48:565, 1934.
60. Boyden EA, Grantham SA Jr: Evacuation of the gall bladder in old age. Surg Gynecol Obstet 62:34, 1926.
61. Sacchetti G, Mandelli V, Roncoroni L, et al: Influence of age and sex on gallbladder emptying induced by a fatty meal in normal subjects. Am J Roentgenol Radium Ther Nucl Med 119:40, 1973.
62. Spellman SJ, Shaffer EA, Rosenthall L: Gallbladder emptying in response to cholecystokinin. A cholescintigraphic study. Gastroenterology 77:115, 1979.
63. Khalil T, Walker JP, Wiener I, et al: Effect of aging on gallbladder contraction and release of cholecystokinin-33 in humans. Surgery, 98:423, 1985.
64. Khalil T, Mate L, Greeley GH Jr, et al: Decreased gallbladder responsiveness to CCK-8 in aged rabbits. Gastroenterology 86:1134, 1984.
65. Morgan ZR, Feldman M: The liver, biliary tract and pancreas in the aged: An anatomic and laboratory evaluation. J Am Geriatr Soc 5:59, 1957.
66. Goodpasture EW: An anatomical study of senescence in dogs, with especial reference to the relation of cellular changes of age to tumors. J Med Res 38:127, 1918.
67. Andrew W: Senile changes in the pancreas of Wistar Institute rats and of man with special regard to the similarity of locule and cavity formation. Am J Anat 74:97, 1964.
68. Balo J, Ballon HC: Metaplasia of basal cells in the ducts of the pancreas: Its consequences. Arch Pathol 7:27, 1929.
69. Wallace SA, Ashworth CT: Early degenerative lesions of the pancreas. Tex State J Med 37:584, 1942.
70. Korpassy B: Die basalzellenmetaplasie der Ausfuhrungsgange des pankreas. Virchows Arch [A] 303:359, 1939.
71. Tiscornia OM: Human exocrine pancreatic re-

sponse with different types of secretin. Influence of sex, age, and previous intraduodenal sorbitol infusion. Am J Gastroenterol 69:166, 1978.
72. Gullo L, Priori P, Daniele C, et al: Exocrine pancreatic function in the elderly. Gerontology 29:407, 1983.
73. Mohiuddin J, Katrak A, Junglee D, et al: Serum pancreatic enzymes in the elderly. Ann Clin Biochem 21:102, 1984.
74. Rosenberg IR, Friedland N, Janowitz HD, et al: The effect of age and sex upon human pancreatic secretion of fluid and bicarbonate. Gastroenterology 50:191, 1966.
75. Khalil T, Fujimura M, Townsend CM Jr, et al: Effect of aging on pancreatic secretion in rats. Am J Surg 149:120, 1985.
76. Khalil T, Fujimura M, Townsend CM Jr, et al: Different secretagogue responses from pancreatic acini isolated from young and old rats. Dig Dis Sci 29:954, 1984.
77. Ryder JB: Steatorrhoea in the elderly. Gerontol Clin 5:30, 1963.
78. Floyd JC Jr, Fajans SS, Pek S, et al: A newly recognized pancreatic polypeptide; Plasma levels in health and disease. Recent Prog Horm Res 33:519, 1977.
79. Berger D, Crowther RC, Floyd JC Jr et al: Effect of age on fasting plasma levels of pancreatic hormones in man. J Clin Endocrinol Metab 47:1183, 1978.
80. Lonovics J, Divitt P, Watson LC, et al: Pancreatic polypeptide. A review. Arch Surg 116:1256, 1981.
81. Khalil T, Fujimura M, Alwmark A, et al: Effect of aging on plasma levels and pancreatic tissue content of insulin and pancreatic polypeptide in rats. Dig Dis Sci 29:954, 1984.
82. Davidson MB: The effect of aging on carbohydrate metabolism: A review of the English literature and a practical approach to the diagnosis of diabetes mellitus in the elderly. Metabolism 28:688, 1979.
83. Brandt RL: Decreased carbohydrate tolerance in elderly patients. Geriatrics 15:315, 1960.
84. Gottfried SP, Pelz KS, Clifford RC: Carbohydrate metabolism in healthy old men and women over 70 years of age. Am J Med Sci 242:475, 1961.
85. Bruch GE, O'Meallie LP: Senile diabetes. Am J Med Sci 254:602, 1967.
86. Streeten DHP, Gerstein MM, Marmor BM, et al: Reduced glucose tolerance in elderly human subjects. Diabetes 14:579, 1965.
87. Metz R, Surmaczynska B, Berger S, et al: Glucose tolerance, plasma insulin, and free fatty acids in elderly subjects. Ann Int Med 64:1042, 1966.
88. Jarrett RJ, Keen H: Glucose tolerance, age, and circulating insulin. Lancet 1:806, 1967.
89. Vinik A, Jackson WPU: Hyperglycemia in the elderly—Is it diabetes? Diabetes 17:348, 1968.
90. O'Sullivan JB, Mahan CM, Freedlender AE, et al: Effect of age on carbohydrate metabolism. J Clin Endocrinol 33:619, 1971.
91. Anisimov VN: Carcinogenesis and aging. Adv Cancer Res 40:365, 1983.
92. Silverstone FA, Brandfonbrener M, Shock NW, et al: Age differences in the intravenous glucose tolerance tests and the response to insulin. J Clin Invest 36:504, 1957.
93. Crockford PM, Harbeck RJ, Williams RH: Influence of age on intravenous glucose tolerance and serum immunoreactive insulin. Lancet 1:465, 1966.
94. Sartin J, Chaudhuri M, Obenrader M, et al: The role of hormones in changing adaptive mechanisms during aging. Fed Proc 39:3163, 1980.
95. Meneilly GS, Minaker KL, Young JB, et al: Counterregulatory responses to insulin-induced glucose reduction in the elderly. J Clin Endocrinol Metab 61:178, 1985.
96. Khalil T, Alwmark A, Fujimura M, et al: The effect of aging on the responsiveness of isolated rat pancreatic islets to glucose stimulation. Dig Dis Sci 29:954, 1984.
97. Reaven E, Solomon R, Azhar S, et al: Functional homogeneity of pancreatic islets of aging rats. Metabolism 31:859, 1982.
98. Kitahara A, Adelman RC: Altered regulation of insulin secretion in isolated islets of different sizes in aging rats. Biochem Biophys Res Commun 87:1207, 1979.
99. Reaven E, Gold G, Reaven G: Effect of age on leucine-induced insulin secretion by the β-cell. J Gerontol 35:324, 1980.
100. Coddling JA, Kalnins A, Haist RE: Effects of age and of fasting on the responsiveness of the insulin-secreting mechanism of the islets of Langerhans to glucose. Can J Physiol Pharmacol 53:716, 1975.
101. Reaven EP, Gold G, Reaven GM: Effect of age on glucose-stimulated insulin release by the β-cell of the rat. J Clin Invest 64:591, 1979.
102. Reaven E, Wright D, Mondon CE, et al: Effect of age and diet on insulin secretion and insulin action in the rat. Diabetes 32:175, 1983.
103. Rayford PL, Texter EC Jr: Brain-gut peptides, in Texter EC Jr (ed): *The Aging Gut. Pathophysiology, Diagnosis, and Management*. New York, Masson Publishing USA Inc, 1983, pp 173–194.
104. McConnell JG, Alam MJ, O'Hare MMT, et al: The effect of age and sex on the response of enteropancreatic polypeptides to oral glucose. Age Aging 12:54, 1983.
105. Khalil T, Walker JP, Greeley GH Jr, et al: Effect of aging on fasting and fat-stimulated plasma levels of pancreatic polypeptide in man. Gastroenterology 88:1445, 1985.
106. Trudeau WL, McGuigan JE: Serum gastrin levels in patients with peptic ulcer disease. Gastroenterology 59:6, 1970.
107. Blair EL, Greenwell JR, Grund ER, et al: Gastrin response to meals of different composition in normal subjects. Gut 16:766, 1975.
108. Archimandritis A, Alegakis G, Theodoropoulos G, et al: Serum gastrin concentrations in healthy

males and females of various ages. Acta Hepatogastroenterol 26:58, 1979.

109. Track NS, Watters LM, Gauldie J: Motilin, human pancreatic polypeptide (HPP) and gastrin plasma concentrations in fasting subjects. Clin Biochem 12:109, 1979.
110. Khalil T, Fujimura M, Greeley GH Jr, et al: Effect of aging on serum gastrin and antral gastrin content in Sprague-Dawley rats. Gastroenterology 88:1445, 1985.
111. Khalil T, Fujimura M, Greeley GH Jr, et al: Effect of aging on small intestinal tissue content of cholecystokinin and secretin in rats. Gastroenterology 88:1446, 1985.
112. Elahi D, Andersen DK, Muller DC, et al: The enteric enhancement of glucose-stimulated insulin release. The role of GIP in aging, obesity, and non-insulin-dependent diabetes mellitus. Diabetes 33:950, 1984.
113. Janik JS, Track NS, Filler RM: Motilin, human pancreatic polypeptide, gastrin, and insulin plasma concentrations in fasted children. J Pediatr 101:51, 1982.
114. Singh P, Khalil T, Thompson JC: Effect of aging on gastrin receptors in the rat gut. Dig Dis Sci 29:80S, 1984.
115. Finocchiaro L, Komano O, Loeb J: Epidermal growth factor stimulated protein kinase shows similar activity in liver of senescent and adult mice. FEBS Lett 187:96, 1985.
116. Peto R, Roe FJC, Lee PN, et al: Cancer and ageing in mice and men. Br J Cancer 32:411, 1975.
117. Tytgat GNJ, Mathus-Vliegen EMH, Offerhaus J: Value of endoscopy in the surveillance of high-risk groups for gastrointestinal cancer, in Sherlock P, Morson BC, Barbara L, Veronesi U (eds): *Precancerous Lesions of the Gastrointestinal Tract.* New York, Raven Press, 1983, pp 305–318.
118. Kimura M, Fukuda T, Sato K: Effect of aging on the development of gastric cancer in rats induced by N-methyl-N′-nitro-N-nitrosoguanidine. Gann 70:521, 1979.
119. Pozharisski KM: The significance of nonspecific injury for colon carcinogenesis in rats. Cancer Res 35:3824, 1975.
120. Turusov VS, Lanko NS, Parfenov YD: Effect of age on induction of intestinal tumors in mice by 1,2-dimethylhydrazine. Bull Exp Biol Med 92:1681, 1981.
121. Johnson LR: New aspects of the trophic actions of gastrointestinal hormones. Gastroenterology 72:788, 1977.
122. Winsett OE, Townsend CM Jr, Glass EJ, et al: Gastrin stimulates growth of colon cancer. Surg Forum 33:384, 1982.
123. Tahara E, Haizuka S: Effect of gastro-entero-pancreatic endocrine hormones on the histogenesis of gastric cancer in rats induced by N-methyl-N′-nitro-N-nitrosoguanidine; with special reference to development of scirrhous gastric cancer. Gann 66:421, 1975.
124. Tatsuta M, Itoh T, Okuda S, et al: Effect of prolonged administration of gastrin on experimental carcinogenesis in rat stomach induced by N-methyl-N′-nitro-N-nitrosoguanidine. Cancer Res 37:1808, 1977.
125. Deveney CW, Freeman H, Way LW: Experimental gastric carcinogenesis in the rat. Effects of hypergastrinemia and acid secretion. Am J Surg 139:49, 1980.
126. Touitou Y: Some aspects of the circadian time structure in the elderly. Gerontology 28 (Suppl 1):53, 1982.
127. Touitou Y, Fevre M, Lagoguey M, et al: Age- and mental health-related circadian rhythms of plasma levels of melatonin, prolactin, luteinizing hormone and follicle-stimulating hormone in man. J Endocrinol 91:467, 1981.
128. Yehuda S, Carasso RL: Changes in circadian rhythms of thermoregulation and motor activity in rats as a function of aging: Effects of d-amphetamine and α-MSH. Peptides 4:865, 1983.
129. Scheving LE, Burns ER, Pauly JE, et al: Circadian variation and cell division of the mouse alimentary tract, bone marrow and corneal epithelium. Anat Rec 191:479, 1978.
130. Neal JV, Potten CS: Circadian rhythms in the epithelial cells and the pericryptal fibroblast sheath in three different sites in the murine intestinal tract. Cell Tissue Kinet 14:581, 1981.
131. Rubin NH, Hokanson JA, Mayschak JB, et al: Several cytokinetic methods for showing circadian variation in normal murine tissue and in a tumor. Am J Anat 168:15, 1983.
132. Saito M, Murakami E, Suda M: Circadian rhythms in disaccharidases of rat small intestine and its relation to food intake. Biochim Biophys Acta 421:177, 1976.
133. Saito M, Murakami E, Nashida T, et al: Circadian rhythms of digestive enzymes in the small intestine of the rat. II. Effects of fasting and refeeding. J Biochem 80:563, 1976.
134. Stevenson NR, Sitren HS, Furuya S: Circadian rhythmicity in several small intestinal functions is independent of use of the intestine. Am J Physiol 238:G203, 1980.
135. Burhol PG, Rayford PL, Jorde R, et al: Radioimmunoassay of plasma cholecystokinin (CCK), duodenal release of CCK diurnal variation of plasma CCK and immunoreactive plasma CCK components in man. Hepatogastroenterology 27:300, 1980.
136. Nagata M, Osumi Y: Circadian rhythm of serum gastrin levels in rats. Jpn J Pharmacol 32:932, 1982.
137. Salera M, Giacomoni P, Pironi L, et al: Circadian rhythm of gastric inhibitory polypeptide (GIP) in man. Metabolism 32:21, 1983.
138. Zucker I: Light-dark rhythms in rat eating and drinking behavior. Physiol Behav 6:115, 1971.
139. Scheving LA, Yeh YC, Tsai TH, et al: Circadian-phase dependent stimulatory effects of epidermal growth factor on DNA synthesis in the tongue, esophagus and stomach of the adult male mouse. Endocrinology 105:1475, 1979.
140. Scheving LA, Yeh YC, Tsai TH, et al: Circadian-

phase dependent stimulatory effects of epidermal growth factor on DNA synthesis in the duodenum, jejunum, ileum, caecum, colon, and rectum of the adult male mouse. Endocrinology 106:1498, 1980.

141. Scheving LA, Scheving LE, Tsai TH, et al: Circadian stage-dependent effects of insulin and glucagon on incorporation of ^{3}H thymidine into deoxyribonucleic acid in the esophagus. Endocrinology 111:308, 1982.

142. Scheving LE, Tsai TH, Scheving LA: Chronobiology of the intestinal tract of the mouse. Am J Anat 168:433, 1983.

143. Vener K, Halberg F: Chronobiology and the digestive tract. Chronobiologia 9:335, 1982.

144. Osborne TB, Mendel LB, Ferry EL: The effect of retardation of growth upon breeding period and duration of life of rats. Science 45:294, 1917.

145. McCay CM, Crowell MF, Maynard LA: The effect of retarded growth upon the length of life span and upon the ultimate body size. J Nutr 10:63, 1935.

146. McCay CM, Maynard LA, Sperling G, et al: Retarded growth, life span, ultimate body size and age changes in the albino rat after feeding diets restricted in calories. J Nutr 18:1, 1939.

147. McCay CM, Maynard LA, Sperling G, et al: Nutritional requirements during the latter half of life. J Nutr 21:45, 1941.

148. Barrows CH, Kokkonen GC: Relationship between nutrition and aging. Adv Nutr Res 1:253, 1977.

149. Berg BN, Simms HS: Nutrition and longevity. II. Longevity and onset of disease with different levels of food intake. J Nutr 71:255, 1960.

150. Ross MH: Nutrition and longevity in experimental animals, in Winick M (ed): *Nutrition and Aging*, New York, Wiley, 1976, pp 43–57.

151. Silberberg M, Silberberg R: Diet and life span. Physiol Rev 35:347, 1955.

152. Stuchlikova E, Juricova-Horokova M, Deyl Z: New aspects of the dietary effects of life prolongation in rodents. What is the role of obesity in aging? Exp Gerontol 10:141, 1975.

153. Young VR: Diet as a modulator of aging and longevity. Fed Proc 38:1994, 1979.

154. Masoro EJ, Bertrand H, Liepa G, et al: Analysis and exploration of age-related changes in mammalian structure and function. Fed Proc 38:1956, 1979.

155. Masoro EJ, Yu BP, Bertrand HA, et al: Nutritional probe of the aging process. Fed Proc 39:3178, 1980.

156. From JM Holland, Oak Ridge Natl Lab, Oak Ridge, Tenn, in *Mammalian Models for Research in Aging*. NAS, Washington, D.C., 1981, pp 45–47.

157. Personal communication: Dr. Steven Weisbroth, AnMed Laboratory, 1804 Plaza Ave, New Hyde Park, NY 11040.

158. Hoffman HJ: Survival distributions for selected laboratory rat strains and stocks, in Gibson DC, Adelman RC, Finch C (eds): *Development of the Rodent As A Model System of Aging*. Book II. DHEW Pub No. (NIH) 79–161. US Department of Health, Education, and Welfare, Washington, DC, 1979, pp 19–34.

159. Redman HC: Survival distribution of beagle dogs maintained in laboratory colonies. Unpublished paper (1980) available from Dr. Hamilton Redman, Lovelace Inhalation Toxicology Research Institute, Albuquerque, NM.

160. Personal communication: Dr. Charles Middleton, Veterans Administration, 810 Vermont Ave NW, Washington, DC 20420.

161. Rampy LW, Nitschke KD, Bell TJ, et al: Interim results of two-year inhalation toxicologic studies of methylene chloride in rats and hamsters, page A185, Abstract #370. In Abstracts of Papers Presented at the 18th Annual Meeting of the Society of Toxicology, Held March 11–15, 1979, in New Orleans, La. New York, Academic Press, 1979.

162. Rust JH, Robertson RJ, Staffeldt EF, et al: Effects of lifetime periodic gamma-ray exposure on the survival and pathology of guinea pigs, in Lindop PJ, Sacher GA (eds): *Radiation and Aging*. Proceedings of a colloquium held June 23–24, 1966, in Semmerling, Austria. London, Taylor and Francis Ltd, 1967, pp 217–244.

163. National Center for Health Statistics: Vital Statistics, US, 1980, Vol II. See 6 Life Table DHHS Publ No (PHS) 84-1104, DHHS. Washington, DC, 1984, p. 3, Table 6C.

Chapter 11

Ontogeny of Gut Peptides

Keith T. Oldham, M.D., and James C. Thompson, M.D.

"Ontogeny recapitulates phylogeny."
Ernst Haeckel 1891

Descriptive embryology evolved slowly during the 19th century and more rapidly during the 20th. By the 1950s, most of the observations central to our understanding of human embryogenesis had been made. Only recently, however, has functional investigation in the area of gastrointestinal hormones been feasible. Development of electron microscopy, immunocytologic techniques, and specific radioimmunoassays has allowed a shift in emphasis from anatomy to function. This review covers observations, made chiefly in the last decade, that examine the ontogeny of peptide hormones, agents that perhaps govern gut embryogenesis and function. The gut is, of course, only one component in a complex system for processing nutrients that includes the liver, pancreas, and central and peripheral nervous systems. It is fair to say that these functional studies have begun.

EMBRYOLOGY REVIEW

Gut

The primitive human gut becomes recognizable 20 to 25 days after conception, at a stage when the embryo is only 2–3 mm in overall length [1]. Foregut and hindgut are identifiable as the cephalic and caudal segments of an undifferentiated endodermal tube [2,3]. The midgut opens ventrally into the yolk sac. During the fourth week, the primitive trachea and lung buds arise from a ventral foregut diverticulum. The liver can be recognized at this stage as a collection of endodermal cells at the level of the anterior intestinal portal where the transverse septum develops [4] (Fig 11-1). Shortly thereafter, during the fifth gestational week, the stomach becomes recognizable at a level corresponding to cervical vertebrae 3 through 5 as a dilatation of the foregut. The esophagus and stomach elongate and descend and achieve nearly adult position and appearance by the end of 7 weeks (Fig 11-2). Additional development, particularly of the gastric fundus, continues through the 12th week of gestation. At 7 weeks, gastric pits are seen initially in the midbody of the stomach on the lesser curvature. Parietal cells appear by 11 weeks, chief cells and mucous neck cells by 12 weeks. Surface epithelial cells appear simultaneously in the gastric cardia and pylorus at 11 weeks. They achieve complete coverage of the stomach by 13 weeks [1,5].

At 4 weeks, when the trachea and liver appear, the midgut is relatively quiescent. At 5 weeks the cecum develops in the distal midgut as a swelling caudal to the yolk sac stalk. Immediately following, there is remarkable growth and elongation of the midgut cephalad to the cecum, which causes herniation of the small intestine into the extra embryonic coelom by 6 weeks. Rotation and further elongation precede the small bowel's return to the abdomen, which is ordinarily completed between 10 and 12 weeks. The final step in midgut development is posterior fixation, achieved during the second and third trimesters.

The cecum is first seen at 5 to 6 weeks. The colon is somewhat slower than the small bowel to develop in length and diameter but is recognizable in adult form and location by 11 to 12 weeks. The anus and rectum have completed their separation from the urogenital sinus by 8 weeks.

Villi develop initially in the duodenum at 8 weeks and throughout the small bowel by 12 to 13 weeks [2,6]. These remain throughout adult life. Villi appear in the colon during the third gestational month and become more numerous for approximately 6 weeks but then disappear during

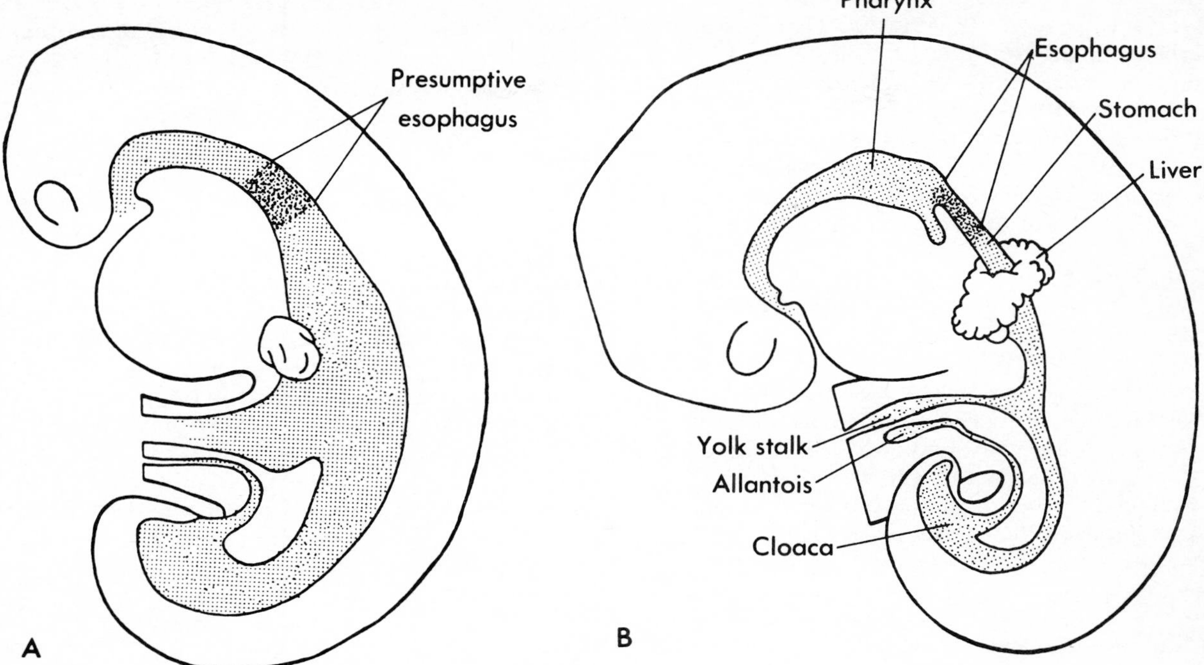

Figure 11-1. Elongation of the esophagus by cranial growth of the embryonic body. *A,* At 2.5 mm (fourth week); *B,* at 4.2 mm (fifth week). (From Gray and Skandalakis [8], by permission of W B Saunders Co.)

the final trimester. No colonic villi are found in human infants or adults [7]. Elements of the myenteric nerve plexus, which originates in the neural crest, reach the proximal gut by 6 weeks [2,8]. Innervation proceeds from the esophagus and reaches the small bowel by 7 weeks, the proximal colon by 8 weeks, and the distal colon by 12 weeks [9,10]. Species differences may be significant; neuronal tissues in the gut of guinea pigs appear to be much more mature at birth than those in the rat [11].

Pancreas

Gross Anatomy. Because of their complexity and importance, the endocrine pancreas and the exocrine pancreas deserve special note. The pancreas is first seen at 5 weeks' gestation as dorsal and ventral endodermal diverticula that emerge from the foregut at the level of the primitive duodenum. Both diverticula develop as ducts lined with cuboidal endodermal stem cells that multiply and segregate further into secondary and tertiary ducts. At 6 weeks these ducts are well developed and are surrounded by mesenchymal cells. By 7

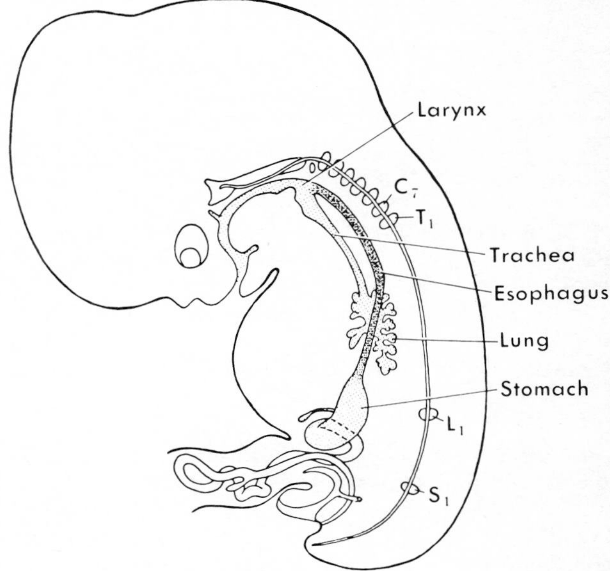

Figure 11-2. Elongation of the esophagus by cranial growth of the embryonic body at 17.5 mm (early eighth week). L_1, first lumbar segment; T_{12}, twelfth thoracic segment; T_1, first thoracic segment; C_7, seventh cervical segment; S_1, first sacral segment. (From Gray and Skandalakis [8], by permission of WB Saunders Co.)

weeks, after midgut rotation the dorsal and ventral anlagen fuse to form the adult pancreas. The dorsal anlage forms the body, tail, and the anterior portion of the head of the pancreas. The ventral anlage gives rise to the posterior portion of the head of the pancreas and the uncinate process. As the dorsal and ventral pancreatic segments fuse, they ordinarily form a single pancreatic duct of Wirsung draining into the duodenum with the common bile duct via the ampulla of Vater. The proximal dorsal duct may, however, remain patent as an accessory pancreatic duct [9,12–15].

Endocrine Pancreas

Light Microscopy. The process of islet formation during endocrine pancreatic differentiation occurs in five reasonably discrete stages seen with light microscopy [14–17]. Although evolution in electron microscopical and immunocytochemical techniques in the last two decades has allowed earlier recognition of secretory endocrine cells, this gross description remains useful. The first stage from 10 to 14 weeks' gestation is the "stage of budding islets." Early islets appear as clusters of cells budding from the primitive endodermal pancreatic ducts. Stage two (between 10 and 16 weeks) is the "stage of the central capillary cluster." Primitive endocrine clusters composed primarily of β cells engulf a central nutritive capillary. Discrete islets surrounded by recognizable exocrine acini become easily identifiable without connection to pancreatic ducts. In 1944 Hard [18] noted the appearance of β cell granules within hours of capillary engulfment. Ungranulated and α cells are arranged around the periphery of the islets. The stage between 16 and 20 weeks is the "stage of bipolar islets." Two cell populations, β and non-β, form opposite poles of the islet. Capillaries become numerous in each pole and most cells are granulated.

Next is the "mantle" stage, seen beyond 20 weeks' gestation [19]. The characteristic feature is β cells clustered centrally within the islet and the non-β cells draped around the core in a mantle configuration. The fifth and final "mature" stage is seen beyond 30 weeks' gestation in near term and newborn infants [14,16]. Here β and non-β cells are intermingled in an adult pattern with many capillaries. The islets are interspersed in connective tissue among acini and ducts. Interestingly, the mantle stage is the mature adult pattern seen in several nonprimate mammalian species, including the rat, mouse, rabbit, and hamster [14]. Although Robb's description of pancreatic islet development has wide acceptance [14], Liu and Potter [20] proposed the hypothesis that humans have a transient fetal population of primary islets early in development that involute by the second trimester and are replaced by mature adult islets prior to birth. This hypothesis might explain the observation that the α cell population diminishes in late fetal life [21].

Electron Microscopy, Immunocytology, Radioimmunoassay. At least four populations of endocrine cells of the human pancreatic islet can be identified by electron microscopic and immunohistochemical techniques [22–25]. α cells contain glucagon granules and are found primarily in the periphery and to a lesser extent intermingled within mature islets; β cells are insulin-producing granulated cells composing the largest proportion of pancreatic endocrine cells (about 70 percent) in the adult [26,27]. Mature D cells are found scattered among β cells and peripherally around the islets. They produce somatostatin. Pancreatic polypeptide (PP)-producing cells are found primarily in islets in the posterior portion of the head of the pancreas. In this PP-rich region, islets are largely composed of PP cells, although α, β, and D cells are present. There are relatively few PP cells found outside the head of the pancreas [28–30]. Within individual islets, the number of PP cells and α cells appears to be inversely related.

Both α and β cells are first identifiable by immunocytochemical staining at 9 weeks' gestation [27] (Table 11-1). They are initially located in the primitive "budding" islets or can be found as isolated cells next to the primitive ducts. Glucagon is detectable by radioimmunoassay as early as 6 weeks of gestation in fetal pancreatic extracts, though the α cells themselves are not yet identifiable [27,31]. Glucagon is measurable in serum by 8 weeks [16]. Insulin can be found in extracts of human fetal pancreas by 10 weeks, although release has not been shown prior to 12 weeks [27,32,33]. Differentiated β cells become recognizable with electron microscopy at 10 to 11 weeks, slightly later than the α cells, which appear at 9 weeks [22]. In early fetal development, the α cell population and the fetal pancreatic glucagon concentrations are significantly greater than the β cell population and the insulin concentrations. At birth, the α and β cell populations are approximately equal. In postnatal life there is a continued decrease in the α cell population, so that by adulthood there is a ratio of approximately 1:5 (α:β cells) [21,23,31] (Fig 11-3). Fetal release of glucagon is not stimulated by infusions of amino acids or induced hypoglycemia. Hill [34] has speculated that glucagon may therefore be more important in the metabolic adjustments to extrauterine life than in utero.

Table 11-1. Ontogeny of pancreatic peptide hormones in human fetal life (ages are in weeks of gestational age)

		Age of initial appearance		
Cell of origin	*Peptide*	*Pancreatic extracts*	*Plasma*	*Immunocytochemical staining*
α	Glucagon [16, 22, 26, 27, 31]	6	8	9
β	Insulin [16, 26, 27, 32]	10–11	12	9
D	Somatostatin [27, 36, 116]	8	—	9
PP	PP [26, 27, 35, 36]	8–9(?)	—	9

We do not know the intrauterine roles of glucagon and the α cell population. Fetal β cell development and the importance of insulin in utero are summarized in the section of this chapter on insulin.

Somatostatin-producing D cells appear in the human pancreas at approximately 8–9 weeks' gestation. PP cells are now reported in the gut and human fetal pancreas at 9–10 weeks' gestation, approximately the same as all other pancreatic endocrine cells [27,35,36]. The roles of PP and somatostatin in fetal growth and development are speculative; these roles are discussed in the respective sections.

The relative volume of endocrine tissue within the pancreas is greater in the fetus than in the mature infant. It reaches a peak at approximately 4–5 months' gestation but by birth had diminished by half. At 6 months of life the volume has decreased by another 50 percent and continues to diminish into adulthood. A full-term infant has an overall concentration of pancreatic endocrine cells that is approximately 6 times greater than that of an adult. This varies within specific regions of the gland. For example, the PP-rich region in the posterior pancreatic head in the fetus contains twice the islet concentration of a comparable region in the adult. The islet density in the glucagon-rich pancreatic body and tail in the fetus can be as high as 10 times that of the adult. In addition, the PP region is of greater relative size in the early fetus, in which it represents as much as 25 percent of the total endocrine gland volume; this diminishes to only 10 percent of the volume at birth. The significance of these shifting populations of fetal pancreatic endocrine cells remains unexplained [26,27,30,35].

Somatostatin-producing D cells are also more abundant in the fetus and infant than in the adult. Their highest relative volume is seen in infants, where they represent 40 percent of the total pancreatic endocrine cell mass. Somatostatin cell populations decrease through infancy to 8 percent of the total endocrine cell mass in the adult pancreas [27]. Further decreases of D cells are seen with aging. The importance of the high fetal concentration of D cells in the fetus is unexplained. Clark and Grant [27] speculated that somatostatin may have a role as a fetal paracrine inhibitor of pancreatic and gut hormone secretion, which is replaced by maturation of myenteric neural control mechanisms.

Exocrine Pancreas

Exocrine secretory acini are first seen at 8 to 10 weeks' gestation as solid clusters of cells around the primitive pancreatic ducts. At the end of the first trimester, they organize into discrete individual units, each associated with a small ductule. In the second trimester this irregular lobular arrangement with loose connective tissue gives way to a more compact, organized adult gland with individual lobes [15,17].

Central and Peripheral Nervous System

Eighteen days after conception, the developing human embryo has a recognizable neural plate under which lies the notochord. Differentiation of the neuroectoderm within the neural plate is rapid. By 22 days the neural tube is formed, although it is still open rostrally and caudally (Fig 11-4) [37,38]. An important additional collection of neural ectodermal cells, the neural crest, is easily seen at this stage. In simplest terms, the neural tube undergoes closure, elongation, and complex, rapid growth and maturation, ultimately forming

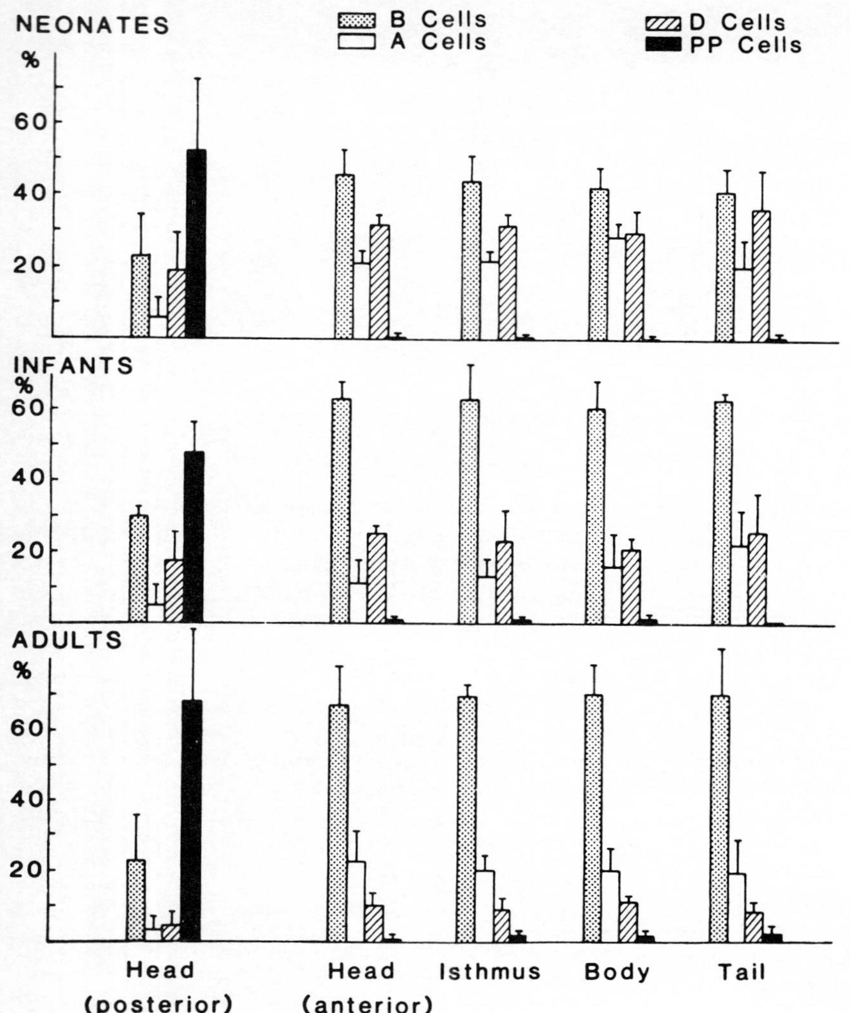

Figure 11-3. Percentage of each cell type in the endocrine tissue present in the various regions of the pancreas of six neonates, three infants, and three adults. Values are means ± SD. (From Rahier et al [23], by permission of Springer-Verlag.)

the brain and spinal cord. These are present and recognizable in adult form by 12 to 13 weeks, though the cerebral cortex in particular undergoes remarkable growth later in fetal life.

The neural crest gives rise to several elements of the peripheral nervous system, including the following: the afferent neurons of the dorsal root ganglia, Schwann cells, and portions of the autonomic ganglia and paraganglia, both sympathetic and parasympathetic [39,40]. Elements of neural crest origin contribute to the myenteric nervous system, which either produces or stores many brain-gut peptides, including gastrin, CCK, somatostatin, substance P, VIP, neurotensin, PP, and GRP. It is a striking phylogenetic observation that these identical peptides are produced in two organs by cell populations derived from different sources [39–41].

Neural crest cells further differentiate into specialized secretory cells with both paracrine and systemic endocrine roles. These include most notably the adrenal medullary cells, C calcitonin cells in the thyroid, and carotid body cells [39].

Two populations of endocrine epithelial cells coexist in the gut. The first, the argentaffin (chromaffin, 5-hydroxytryptamine, APUD) cell population, may have a neural crest origin; cells first appear in the duodenum at 8 to 9 weeks' gestation and by 12 weeks have spread to the entire gut, including the colon. The second is the nonargentaffin peptide-producing population of epithelial endocrine cells, with which we are primarily con-

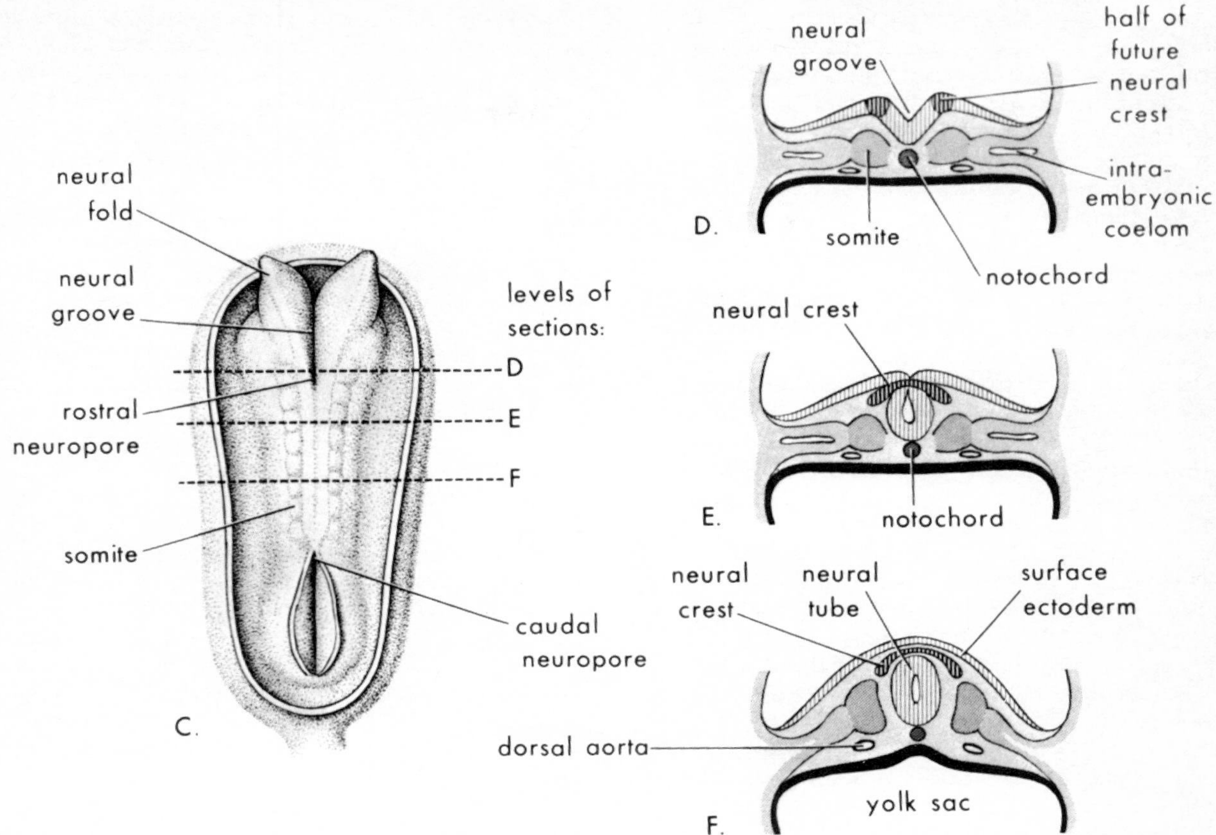

Figure 11-4. Diagrams illustrating formation of the neural crest and folding of the neural plate into the neural tube. **C.** Dorsal view of an embryo of about 22 days. The neural folds have fused opposite the somites but are widely spread out at both ends of the embryo. The rostral and caudal neuropores are indicated. **D–F.** Transverse sections of this embryo at the levels shown in C, illustrating formation of the neural tube and its detachment from the surface ectoderm. Note that some neuroectodermal cells are not included in the neural tube but remain between it and the surface ectoderm as the neural crest. These cells first appear as paired columns on the dorsolateral aspect of the neural tube but they soon become broken up into a series of segmental masses. (From Moore [38], by permission of WB Saunders Co.)

cerned. This includes cells in the gut, genitourinary tract, and respiratory tract. The weight of current evidence favors an intrinsic endodermal origin with differentiation into these endocrine cells [40,42,43].

Several invertebrate neuropeptides are phylogenetically similar to those of the mammalian enteroendocrine system. Solcia et al [39] have speculated that the early phylogenetic regulation of gut function through direct nervous system control via neurotransmitters has been in part supplanted and refined with the evolution of vertebrates, and more recently of mammals. The frequent reports of similarities in brain and gut neuropeptide structure and function tend to support this hypothesis [39–47].

PEPTIDE HORMONES

Gastrin (see also Chapter 14)

Gastrin-containing cells have been detected by means of immunohistochemical staining techniques in the human fetal duodenum at 10 to 11 weeks' gestation [48–50]. Both groups noted with surprise the appearance of duodenal gastrin at 14 (Dubois) to 20 (Larsson) weeks prior to its appearance in the antrum. Fetal pancreatic gastrin in humans is either absent or measurable only in small quantities [36,48,50]. A number of other mammalian species do have a significant amount of gastrin in the fetal pancreas [51,52].

The population of antral gastrin cells increases

in a roughly linear fashion from early stages of cell differentiation to near-adult levels at birth, and, despite early reports to the contrary, infant concentrations of duodenal gastrin are approximately 75 percent of those found in the adult [36,53]. The same general pattern appears to occur with the population of duodenal gastrin cells [53]. Low concentrations of gastrin are found in extracts of human fetal jejunum, and these remain low throughout fetal and adult life [53–55].

Investigations by Larsson et al [48] include gel chromatographic separation of fetal antral and duodenal extracts showing immunoreactive gastrin of two forms. The duodenal predominance of G-34 is in contrast to the antral predominance of G-17 [36,48,50,53]. Thus a striking early duodenal predominance of G cells producing G-34 is seen in early development of the gut. The large adult population of antral cells producing G-17 is well known [48,56,57]. The functional significance of these observations is not known, but they raise the question of a significant fetal role for G-34 at a time of critical growth and maturation of the fetal gastrointestinal tract. The question of the differential appearance and affinity of gastrin receptors in the fetal and the adult gut has not yet received attention.

Fasting concentrations of serum gastrin in newborns are substantially higher than in either mothers or normal adults [58–66]. Euler et al [63] reported mean serum gastrin levels of 137 pg/mL in newborn cord blood (n = 217) versus 40 pg/mL in normal adults (n = 802). Although significant variability is noted in infants, it is interesting that several infants had serum gastrin concentrations higher than 500 pg/mL, a level ordinarily associated with the Zollinger-Ellison syndrome in adults. Furthermore, 13 percent of all infants in the study had gastrin levels higher than 200 pg/mL. The possibilities that the high gastrin levels were associated with drugs, infant or maternal age, or obstetric complications were apparently eliminated in the study.

Gastric contents at birth have a neutral pH, but acid can be demonstrated simply by emptying the newborn stomach of the swallowed neutral amniotic fluid. This maneuver will immediately lower the pH to approximately 4.0 and often to levels of 2.0 or 3.0 within 24 hours [60–62]. With the first feeding, serum gastrin concentrations rise to levels that are actually higher than those at birth. Recent evidence from fetal rats in late gestation indicates that release of acid (both in vivo and in vitro) is possible with pentagastrin stimulation [67,68]. The observation that acid and gastrin are both present at birth is evidence that the gastric acid-gastrin regulatory mechanism is functional at birth or within the first hours of life [64,69].

There is, however, substantial evidence to the contrary. Miller [70] in 1941 reported gastric acid hypersecretion in the first 48 hours of life, which declined to near achlorhydria at one month of age. Soon afterwards, acid secretory capability rose to adult levels. The mechanism responsible for the transient achlorhydria is not clear. Euler et al [65] demonstrated that term infants have a basal acid output greater than that of adults and furthermore that it is unresponsive to pentagastrin stimulation.

Sann et al [64] have shown that mean fasting serum gastrin levels decline from newborn levels (130 pg/mL) during the first months of life but remain elevated above adult levels for at least several months. They confirmed postprandial gastrin elevations in infants and children, in whom they concluded that the adult pattern of release was present. However, Rodgers et al [71] and Rogers et al [72] have shown no significant difference in the gastrin release in newborn infants fed a protein meal or 5 percent glucose and water. This suggests that protein may not be as powerful a releaser of gastrin in the antrum of the newborn as it is in the adult.

Takeuchi, Johnson, and colleagues [73–75] showed that prior to weaning rats lack the expected acid secretory and DNA synthetic response of fundic mucosal gastrin. These deficiencies appear to be due to an absence of mucosal gastrin receptors in suckling rats. Typical adult patterns of response appear at the time of weaning, as do specific gastrin receptors [73–76]. Of interest also is the observation that development of gastrin receptors in rats is sex-related. Pubertal male and female rats have equal gastrin-binding capacities. After puberty, males develop significantly more receptor-binding capability than females and retain it through adult life [75].

Euler et al [65], in analyzing current information, offer explanations of the apparent unresponsiveness of the parietal cell population of newborns to gastrin stimulation: 1) the stomach is already maximally stimulated at birth for reasons we do not know, 2) an inactive molecular form of gastrin may be circulating at birth, and 3) the parietal cell mass is unresponsive because it lacks functional gastrin receptors at this age. In humans, the role of gastrin receptors in newborns has not yet been investigated; we do not know the composition or significance of the several gastrin forms at birth. The interrelationships between acid, gastrin, and gastrin receptors and the maturation process are not fully known.

Cholecystokinin (CCK) (see also Chapter 15)

CCK appears in the duodenal and small intestinal mucosa in the human fetus at 10 weeks' gestation, the same time gastrin appears in the duodenum. No CCK has been reported in the human fetal antrum [49]. The concentrations of CCK progressively increase in the fetal duodenum and jejunum, achieving adult levels at a time as yet undefined. CCK is present in the gut in both mucosal endocrine cells and in neurons of the myenteric plexus.

Rats, like humans, have maximal CCK concentrations in the duodenum and jejunum. High concentrations in newborns are achieved during suckling, between 3 and 14 days of life, after which there is a remarkable decrease with weaning to low adult levels at 28 days. The 14-day peak may reflect a summation of increasing amounts of myenteric neural CCK and the decreasing content of mucosa [77,78].

The neuronal tissue levels of CCK in the myenteric plexus are relatively low initially, increasing progressively with age to adult levels. The mucosal endocrine levels of CCK are highest in the fetus and newborn, after which they fall to adult levels. Extracts of rat brain show that CCK appears between birth and 3 days of age and increases to an adult plateau at 28 days [79]. The rate of increase is maximal at weaning, between 7 and 21 days. The ontogeny of CCK in the human nervous system and the role of CCK in fetal development of the brain and the gut are unknown.

Secretin (see also Chapter 16)

Secretin is detectable by radioimmunoassay in human fetal duodenal extracts by 8 weeks' gestation [53]. Thereafter it increases in a linear fashion to term, when levels are 20 times greater than those detected initially. Secretin appears in the jejunum by 12 weeks' gestation, increasing 3-fold at term. Secretin concentrations at birth are approximately 10 percent lower in the duodenum and jejunum than in the mature adult. Secretin-producing cells are found in the ileum in some adult mammals, but the ontogeny and function of this distal gut secretin are still unknown [80,81].

Serum secretin levels are higher at birth (and for at least the first four days of life) than are maternal or control adult levels. For the first days or weeks of life, secretin is apparently not released in response to feeding. However, by 24 days of life, postprandial release of secretin does occur [82]. Rogers et al [83] suggested that neonates could have 1) elevated secretin production, 2) diminished (renal) clearance, or 3) alternative, inactive, molecular forms of secretin. This last possibility is unlikely because of repeated failure to demonstrate other molecular forms of secretin. Moazam et al [84] demonstrated that concentrations of secretin in neonatal and adult gut extracts are equal, which suggests that increased production is not the likely mechanism for the hypersecretinemia. They also demonstrated that the secretin half-life is prolonged in newborn piglets by approximately 50 percent over adult values (3.6 min vs. 2.6 min). This is reasonably suggestive that one mechanism of secretin elevation in newborns is diminished renal clearance.

What is the significance of simultaneously elevated serum gastrin and secretin levels in newborn humans [82,83]? One possibility is that the normal regulatory mechanisms are not yet functional. The situation is clouded by the observation that serum secretin in newborn swine does in fact respond to some stimuli. Intraduodenal acid infusion produces dramatic secretin release [84]. The mechanisms of control of secretin release and its function once released are not completely understood. Regulation of secretin may be mediated by somatostatin, which in turn is not yet functional in this newborn pig model. There may be intrinsic differences between the mechanisms for release of secretin in humans and those in pigs.

The distribution, release, and maturation of secretin appear to be species-specific. Rats have a gastrointestinal tract that undergoes significant postnatal maturation with weaning at approximately 18 days of life. High levels of serum secretin at birth fall to near zero at 10 days, then rise with weaning to adult levels [85]. Guinea pigs are somewhat different, having a gastrointestinal tract that is nearly mature at birth. They have an adult distribution of secretin at birth. The regulatory mechanisms, including acid stimulation, appear to be intact in the newborn guinea pig as well as in the newborn pig. The relationship in fetal and newborn humans is largely unknown.

Glucagon (see also Chapter 17)

Pancreatic Glucagon. Human pancreatic glucagon-producing α cells are recognizable at 8 weeks' gestation [27,31,86,87]. They are located initially in the early "budding" islets or can be found as isolated cells next to the primitive pancreatic ducts. Glucagon is detectable by radioimmunoassay as early as 7 weeks' gestation in pancreatic extracts. Serum glucagon is measurable by 8 weeks. Insulin appears slightly later and is measurable in pancreatic extracts by 8 to 10 weeks. Differentiated β cells become recognizable with electron microscopy at 10 to 11 weeks [27,32,33,86,88]. Characteristic adult islet-cell morphology is not achieved until the third trimester; the β cells have been functional for 20 weeks when this occurs.

Recent reports suggest that glucagon, identical in character to that derived from the pancreatic α cells, is also found in the human fetal stomach [89–91]. The earliest detection was at 16 weeks' gestation. The role of this fundal (pancreatic) glucagon is unclear.

In early fetal development, the α cell population and fetal concentrations of pancreatic glucagon are significantly greater than the β cell population and the concentrations of insulin. At birth, the populations are about equal. In postnatal life there is a continued decrease in the α cell population, so that by adulthood there is a ratio of approximately 1 to 5 (α:β) cells [21,31]. The significance of this fetal glucagon predominance during growth and development is unclear. Exogenous pancreatic glucagon, when administered to suckling rats, does not induce maturation of the gastrointestinal tract, either in terms of growth or of enzyme maturation, as do insulin and hydrocortisone. Furthermore, exogenous pancreatic glucagon has no effect on the growth of adult rat intestine [89,92]. The fact that pancreatic glucagon concentrations are high in utero and that serum glucagon increases at birth and remains high throughout neonatal life in rats may be related to the delayed appearance of glucagon receptors. These receptors are known to be low in fetal and newborn rats but increase to approximately 25 percent of adult levels by 2 days of age.

Enteroglucagon. In the pancreas, glicentin-producing cells are apparent at 8 weeks' gestation in the walls of primitive pancreatic ducts. By 12 weeks, these are interspersed within the islet cell "clusters," and by 16 weeks they are contained within the recognizable islets of Langerhans. This pattern closely follows development of the α cell [16,93,94].

The extrapancreatic glicentin-producing cells appear initially in the ileum at 8 weeks' gestation. By 10 weeks, they appear in the oxyntic mucosa and in the proximal small bowel, and they are apparent in the colon by 11 to 12 weeks [53,93,94].

The importance of enteroglucagon in embryogenesis and gut maturation is uncertain. The early appearance of enteroglucagon and particularly its possible role as a mediator of gut growth are suggestive of an important role.

Gastric Inhibitory Polypeptide (GIP) (see Chapter 18)

Human GIP is found initially at 8 to 11 weeks' gestation in approximately equal concentrations in the fetal duodenum and jejunum [53]. A 10-fold increase to adult concentrations occurs prior to birth. Duodenal concentrations are slightly but consistently higher than those found in the jejunum throughout fetal and adult life [95]. Ultrastructural analysis confirms these findings; the K cell is recognizable by 9 to 10 weeks [86,96].

Rat GIP is found in small intestinal extracts late in gestation (20 days). In the duodenum and small intestine, GIP increases significantly throughout the first month of life [97]. This increase is similar to that of many of the gut peptides, which are seen (in phylogenetically more primitive animals) to rise in the immediate postnatal period. In humans, this increase occurs during late gestation, and adult levels are present at birth.

The developmental function of GIP in humans is unknown, but its early appearance, its known physiologic importance, and particularly its relationship to insulin (a critical known determinant of intrauterine growth) suggest a significant role in the embryo.

Vasoactive Intestinal Peptide (VIP) (see also Chapter 19)

Chayvialle et al [98] found VIP in extracts of human fundus and duodenum between 8 and 9.5 weeks' gestation, at a time when it is absent from the pancreas and small bowel. VIP-immunoreactive neurons appear proximally in the gut and migrate distally, cephalad to caudad. In chickens, this proximal appearance is at 13 days' incubation, with migration to the distal colon by 19 days just prior to hatching [99].

By 10 weeks of age, VIP-immunoreactive nerve fibers are present in the entire human gastrointestinal tract [53,98,100]. Early in fetal development, few VIP nerves are seen in the pancreas. Between 15 and 21 weeks, an adult pattern of distribution of

VIP within the gut is present, with the highest concentration in the duodenum and small bowel and smaller concentrations in the stomach and pancreas. Thereafter, VIP concentrations increase 2- to 3-fold and achieve adult levels by birth.

Beyond 25 weeks' gestation, the significant event in humans is not an increase in the number of VIP-containing nerve fibers but rather an ingrowth from the intermuscular myenteric plexus to the submucosal nerve plexus [98]. This ingrowth is particularly remarkable in the proximal gut, where the association between the VIP-positive fibers from nerve cells and the base of the secretory glands becomes an intimate one. The non-VIP immunoreactive cell bodies of the secretory glandular cells become surrounded by VIP-positive fibers. In the distal gut, particularly the colon, the VIP fibers appear to be more limited to the circular and longitudinal smooth muscle.

Sundler et al [99], in 1979, elegantly showed a similar process in chickens that was achieved in the postnatal period. At hatching, VIP neurons are present only in the myenteric plexus, after which neural fibers approach the base of the secretory epithelial gland, and by 1 to 2 days of life the fibers invade the core of each villus to achieve intimate contact with VIP-positive and negative enteric endocrine cells by 2–4 weeks.

Rats have a similar postpartum maturation of the VIP nervous system [101]. VIP concentrations in the small bowel increase significantly between birth and 9 weeks of age, most significantly after weaning with gut maturation. This is different from humans, in whom VIP immunoreactive nerves are present and thought to be functionally important in the regulation of the growth and development of fetal digestive structures from the third month of pregnancy onward. The relationship in the proximal gut may be more important for regulation of mucosal blood flow and regulation of epithelial function, with the distal anatomic arrangement perhaps more important for the development of gut motility.

Preterm infants (mean gestational age 33 weeks) have serum VIP levels five times those seen in adults [102]. Interestingly, these levels are approximately twice those found in normal term infants (mean gestational age 39 weeks). VIP appears to remain elevated in humans throughout the neonatal period. Serum VIP levels do not change with feeding in human infants, though bottle-fed term infants have higher serum VIP levels than full-term infants who are breast-fed.

One concern about perinatal observations of serum VIP levels is that the placenta itself has significant extractable VIP [103], and placental production or regulation of fetal VIP is possible. Although the adult VIP half-life is short (about 1 minute), the fetal and newborn VIP half-lives are unknown, so that the placental contribution to high levels of VIP in newborns cannot be excluded. Whether the high VIP level in term and preterm neonates is important developmentally is not known.

Pancreatic Polypeptide (PP) (see also Chapter 20)

Early studies describing pancreatic polypeptide are difficult to interpret because of molecular heterogeneity, which is especially true of cross-reactivity with the more recently recognized peptide YY (PYY) from the pancreas. Information regarding this peptide is summarized separately.

Larsson et al [104], in 1975, reported PP cells in human fetal pancreas at 18–20 weeks' gestation, the earliest stage evaluated. Malaisse-Lagae et al [29] found PP cells in the human pancreas at 33 weeks' gestation and noted a fetal pancreatic cell population approximately 50 percent of the eventual adult levels. PP cells are recognizable earlier than this by means of ultrastructural techniques (other islet cells appear functional as early as 7 to 8 weeks) [86]. Recent reports show PP immunoreactivity in the pancreas at 10 weeks [27,35,36].

In the human gut, PP immunoreactivity is seen in ileal and colonic mucosal cells at 10 weeks [105,106]. PP cells are present in the fundus by 12 weeks. Paulin and Dubois [30], in 1978, reported scattered PP cells in the human fetal antrum and duodenum but a significant cell population in the distal ileum. PP-positive cells have been reported in the stomach, duodenum, and proximal small intestine [105], but most authors agree that the primary population of PP-producing cells in fetal humans is in the pancreas.

In rats, no PP cells are found before birth. They begin to appear at birth, which is significantly later than seen with insulin, glucagon, or somatostatin. PP cells are initially scattered among the exocrine acini and endocrine islets. Seven days postnatally, the number of PP cells increases within the islets, with decreasing numbers in the acini. By 8 to 10 days postnatally, adult cell populations are seen. PP cells appear in the rat colon two days following birth [107,108]; they increase in numbers between days 7 and 14 and thereafter decrease to reasonably low adult levels. PP cells are seen transiently in the rat pylorus and rectum at 14 days, but none are present before or after this. In both rats and humans, PP appears somewhat later than the other pancreatic endocrine peptides; the developmental significance of this is unclear.

Peptide YY. PYY is a relatively new candidate hormone isolated in 1980 by Tatemoto and Mutt [109] from extracts of swine duodenum; it was characterized in 1982 [110]. Similar to PP, PYY is a 36 amino acid peptide that is found in epithelial endocrine cell populations in the gut of birds, mammals, amphibians, reptiles, and fish. In adult primates, PYY immunoreactive cells are present in the ileum, colon, and rectum in significant concentrations. PYY is thought to have a paracrine function [56].

PYY appears at 19 days in the duodenum, colon, and rectum in rat embryos [107,111]. The concentration increases, and the population spreads to the pylorus and the ileum. The duodenal concentration falls sharply after birth, though colon and rectal concentrations of PYY cells remain high from 19 days' gestation through weaning at 3 weeks. The colon concentration in adults is significant, but the rectal concentration is quite low. El-Salhy et al [107] note significant concentrations of PYY cells in the pylorus, ileum, and rectum of adult rats.

The physiologic roles of PYY are not yet clear in adults and the fetus; we (and others) have shown in unpublished studies that PYY inhibits pancreatic (and probably gastric) secretion. Ontogeny in humans is unreported.

Somatostatin (see also Chapter 21)

Somatostatin immunoreactive D cells are numerous in the fetal human pancreas and gut. In the gut, these cells appear quite early. They are seen in low concentrations in the small and large intestine by 8 to 11 weeks. At this time, the concentration is highest in the proximal small bowel, duodenum, and jejunum [53,112]. Somatostatin appears in the antrum at 12 weeks and the fundus at 14 weeks. Thereafter, it increases in the gut 10- to 20-fold by birth, at which time it is 80–90 percent of mature adult levels [113,114].

Pancreatic somatostatin is initially found in humans at 8 weeks' gestation [36,115–117]. It increases with gestational age and achieves concentrations at birth that are five times higher than those in adults.

In the rat, somatostatin-producing cells first appear in the pancreas at 14 days [118] and in the duodenum by 16 to 17 days. A roughly linear increase then occurs in the gut with age. Somatostatin-producing cells appear after birth in the fundus. An adult distribution is reached 3 weeks postnatally (after weaning). The concentration of somatostatin in the pancreas of rats is low at birth but increases 7-fold by 3 days of life, after which a plateau is reached [119–122]. Significant increases in concentrations of somatostatin in the gastric fundus are seen at weaning (21 days of age). Both McIntosh et al [118] and Koshimuizu [121] concluded that somatostatin is a likely modulator of maturation of the gut in rats.

In rats, the population of somatostatin cells in both the thyroid and cerebellum increases in the first postnatal week and then diminishes [123,124]. A transient, possibly developmental role for somatostatin in these two organs is possible.

Human infants have an arteriovenous concentration gradient for plasma somatostatin in cord blood at birth [125,126]. Concentrations of somatostatin in amniotic fluid vary during pregnancy; they are 4 to 5 times higher in midgestation than at near term [127]. These observations suggest a fetal production of somatostatin. Early human fetal production in the brain, gut, and pancreas suggests that somatostatin plays a developmental role for the gut in utero.

Neurotensin (see also Chapter 22)

Human fetal neurotensin first appears at 12 weeks' gestation in the jejunum, ileum, and colon, with a progressive increase in the population of N cells, such that by 20 weeks of age, neurotensin appears as far proximal as the distal duodenum. During development, jejunal, ileal, and colonic neurotensin content increases 4-fold, and peak levels reached in the ileum are two to three times greater than those found in colon and jejunum, respectively. Adult levels are achieved during the third trimester. Between 20 weeks of gestation and term, there is a diminution of the cell population of the distal duodenum [53,128–130] (Fig 11-5).

Eluted fetal neurotensin in humans appears to have two molecular forms (Fig 11-5) [130]. During early embryonic development, peak A, a fetal form, is predominant at 12–15 weeks of life [131] (Fig 11-6). By 31–40 weeks, this predominance has shifted to the adult, late gestational form. The importance of the transient duodenal cell population and of a fetal molecular form is unknown but a role in gut embryogenesis is suggested.

Motilin (see also Chapter 23)

In humans, low concentrations of motilin are found in the duodenum and jejunum, initially between 8 and 11 weeks' gestation. Thereafter, there

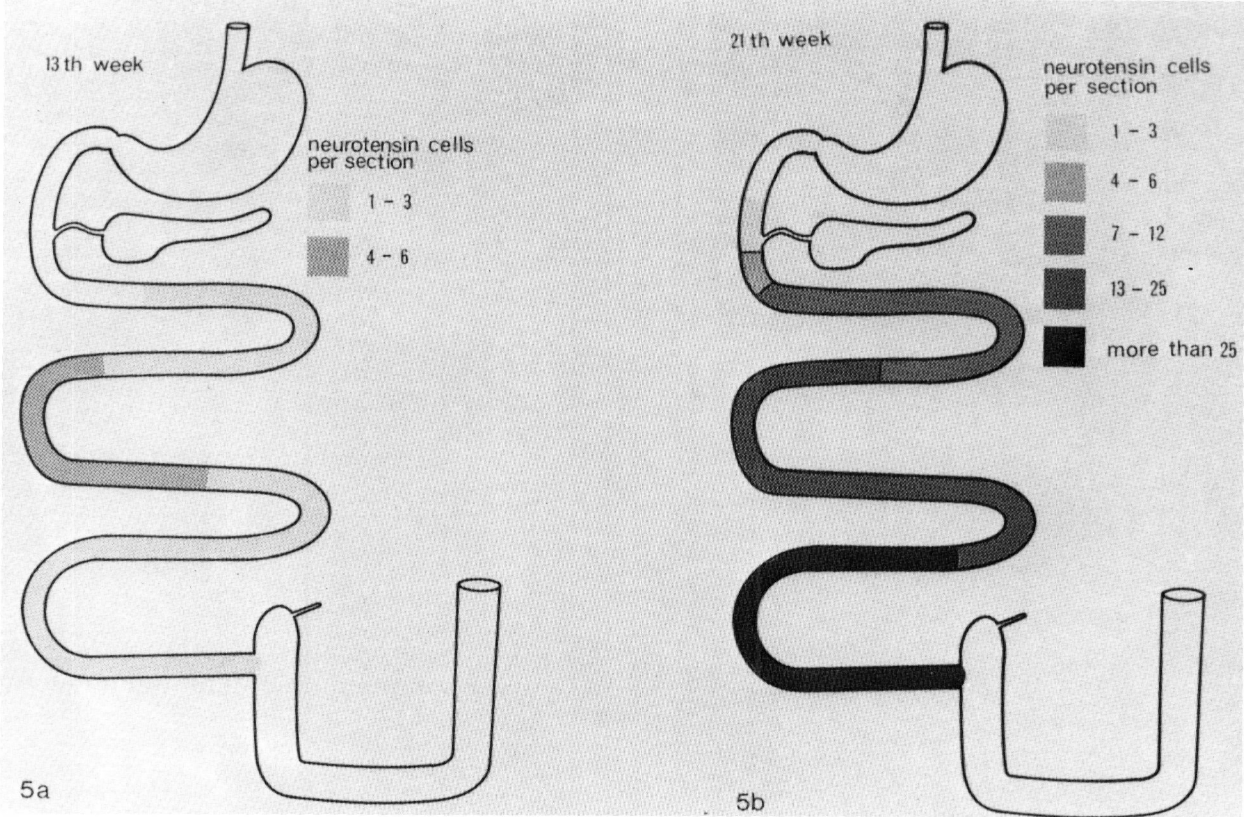

Figure 11-5. Schematic drawing of the distribution of neurotensin cells in embryos of 13 and 21 weeks. Note the shift of a higher frequency of neurotensin cells toward the terminal ileum. (From Helmstaeder et al [130], by permission of Springer-Verlag.)

is a roughly linear 25-fold increase in tissue concentrations during fetal life, to nearly adult levels at term. Duodenal concentrations are consistently twice those of the jejunum. The role of motilin in fetal development and maturation of the gut is unknown [53,132].

Substance P (see also Chapter 24)

Substance P is found in the human brain stem at 18 to 25 weeks' gestation [133]. Its development, time of appearance, and function in the gut are unknown in humans.

In the mouse, scattered endocrine epithelial cells containing immunoreactive substance P are found in the small intestine and colon at 17 days' gestation. These cells increase progressively until 10 days of life, when the adult pattern is achieved. Nerve fibers but no nerve cell bodies appear in the colon myenteric plexus the fourth postnatal day and reach adult levels by day 10 [134]. This sequence of postnatal maturation of the rat gut is frequently completed before birth in the human fetus.

Bombesin (and Gastrin-Releasing Peptide [GRP]) (see also Chapter 25)

Bombesin-like immunoreactive cells are found in human fetal bronchial mucosa [135]. They are not present in the adult lung. Similarly, immunoreactive GRP cells are found in extracts of human fetal lung in significant concentrations, but most adult lung extracts do not possess this GRP-like activity [136]. The assay used in this investigation discriminated between bombesin and GRP. Normal fetal human lung contains GRP reactive cells in the fetal bronchi by 12 weeks' gestation [137]. During development, these coalesce in small clusters around the bronchi. By term, they appear as "neuroepithelial bodies" either in bronchi or in bronchioles [137–139]. In human infants at the

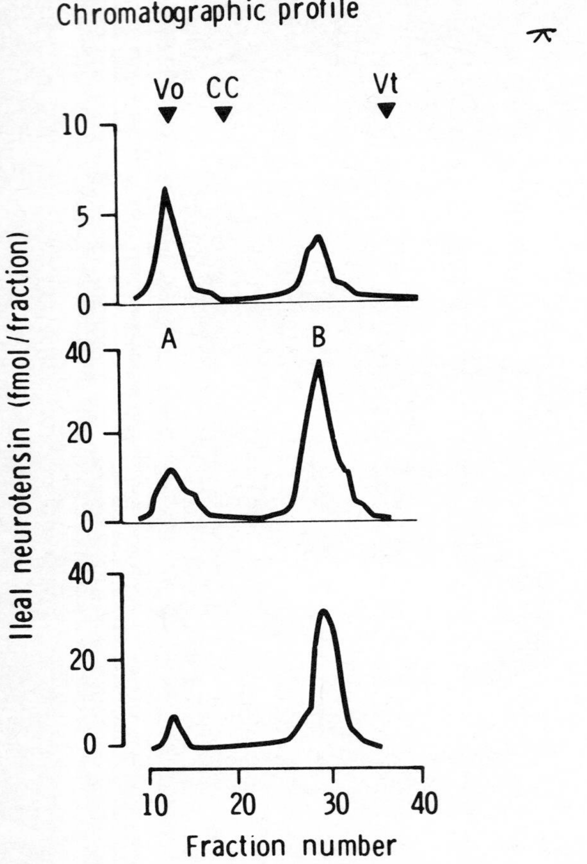

Figure 11-6. Representative gel permeation chromatography profiles of neurotensin immunoreactivity from different regions of fetal and adult gut (water extracts). The top panel is the profile obtained from fetuses aged 12–15 weeks. The central panel is obtained from fetuses aged 31 weeks to term, and the bottom panel is obtained from adult extracts. (From Polak and Bloom [131], by permission of The New York Academy of Sciences.)

ages of 2, 6, and 7 months, there are fewer GRP immunoreactive cells, and in adult humans, GRP-containing cells are present only in a few isolated bronchial mucosal cells. Neuroepithelial bodies may function as hypoxia-sensitive chemoreceptors in the lung [135,140]. A role in local regulation of the pulmonary vascular bed has been suggested.

The ontogeny and significance of bombesin-like and GRP peptides in the human embryonic gut are unknown.

Epidermal Growth Factor (EGF) (Urogastrone) (see also Chapter 26)

The ontogeny of urogastrone in humans is currently unknown. A single recent report documents the presence, by radioimmunoassay, of EGF in human amniotic fluid at 16 to 24 weeks' gestation [141]. The time of appearance, distribution, and effects in the embryo have not been investigated.

Exogenous EGF given to suckling rats and mice will induce precocious maturation of brush border hydrolytic enzymes. These effects appear limited to those enzymes associated with cell membrane receptors, including the disaccharidases, sucrase, trehalase, and lactase, and amylase, alkaline phosphatase, and peptidase [142,143]. However, when given to the fetus at 15 to 17 days' gestation, EGF does not produce changes in DNA concentration or in fetal weight or gut length [144].

Postnatally EGF given to suckling rats does increase growth of intestinal mucosa, including increased weight:length ratios [143].

EGF stimulates growth, DNA synthesis, and mitosis of neonatal rat hepatocytes in vitro. This effect is potentiated by low concentrations of insulin and glucagon [145].

In summary, in experimental animals, EGF is known to induce precocious maturational changes in intestinal brush border enzymes, normally seen with weaning. EGF will induce DNA synthesis in some portions of the gastrointestinal tract, including rat gastric and duodenal mucosa and pancreas [146,147]. A period of nonresponse to exogenous EGF is apparent in mice in late gestation. The physiologic significance of these observations is unknown. EGF does appear to have a potential regulatory function in growth and development, particularly in regard to maturation of intestinal mucosa.

Insulin

Insulin is a 51 amino acid peptide first isolated by Banting and Best in 1922; it is produced by pancreatic islet β cells and is known to have a critically important role as the chief regulator of carbohydrate metabolism. One role of potential developmental importance is its effect on the maturation of gut epithelium in newborn animals. Exogenous insulin will induce precocious sucrase and hydrolytic brush border enzymatic capability in the immature rat intestine [148–150]. Probably the most important embryologic action, however, is insulin's striking but nonspecific effect as an anabolic agent in utero [16,151].

Ontogeny. Extracts of human fetal pancreas have been shown to possess insulin by 8 to 10 weeks' gestation. Thereafter, the content increases progressively. Serum insulin is detectable by 12 weeks [23,26,27,33] and is thought to be entirely fetal in origin, since placental transport of insulin has not been shown. Although insulin appears at 10 to 12 weeks in the fetus, typical release with glucose does not appear to develop in vivo until approximately 28 to 32 weeks' gestation [147]. In vitro organ cultures of 12 week fetal pancreatic β cells show a similar lack of response to glucose [152,153]. Concentrations of insulin in the human fetal pancreas are variable but are usually greater than those found in adults [33].

By 11.5 days' gestation, β cells appear in the rat pancreas. Insulin release is detectable in serum between 12.5 days and 14 days [24], but it does not appear sensitive to glucose-stimulated release or increase in biosynthetic rate until later. As in humans, the appearance of insulin precedes that of somatostatin, which is seen in rats at 15.5 days. Adult morphology of rat islets and acini is apparent by 18.5 days.

Interesting clinical correlation for the fetal insensitivity to insulin is seen in infants of diabetic mothers (IDM) [151]. Hypersomatism and overgrowth involving every organ system, particularly related to lipogenesis, are characteristic in term infants of diabetic mothers. Pederson [154] first observed that chronic elevations in maternal serum glucose levels are reflected transplacentally by the fetus, with β cell hyperplasia and fetal hyperinsulinemia. Though hyperinsulinemia may be present by the first trimester, infants appear unresponsive until approximately 28 to 30 weeks' gestation. Preterm infants of diabetic mothers are seldom large, while term infants are usually so [151].

The hypersomatism of IDM can be controlled or eliminated by compulsive control of maternal concentrations of serum glucose [151]. Positive correlation has been shown between endocrine cell mass, β cell volume, and body weight with IDM [16]. Positive correlation exists between the degree of β cell hyperplasia and fetal and maternal glucose levels [16]. Increased insulin content of the pancreas, as well as of microdissected islets, is also seen in IDM.

Clinical conditions associated with hyperinsulinemia (or possibly increased end-organ sensitivity to insulin)—insulinoma, nesidioblastosis, and the Beckwith-Wiedemann syndrome [155]—all show characteristic hypersomatism. Conversely, intrauterine growth failure accompanies clinical situations in which there is absent or diminished serum insulin in the fetus. These conditions include 1) "transient diabetes mellitus," thought to be associated with intrauterine viral infections [156], 2) pancreatic agenesis [157], a rare disorder, and 3) leprechaunism with deficiencies in tissue response to insulin [158,159]. The last group of patients have significant elevations of serum insulin but apparent end-organ unresponsiveness. Infants who are small for gestational age have decreased endocrine mass, decreased β cell numbers, and decreased cord blood insulin levels [16]. In summary, it appears that insulin is a critical but nonspecific regulator of human fetal growth after 28 to 30 weeks' gestation [160–164].

Receptors. Insulin receptors in membrane preparations of rabbit hepatic cells appear late in gestation, peak at birth, and decline thereafter. Insulin receptor activity in rat tissue is high in late fetal and early neonatal life, apparently reflecting a combination of high affinity and increased numbers. This activity declines to adult levels within a relatively short time after birth [165]. Insulin receptors on human erythrocytes are high at birth and persist at high levels throughout the neonatal period. Their concentration diminishes during the first year of life to levels seen with older children and adults [166]. Whether this reflects changes in receptor affinity or number is unclear. The concentration of glucagon and insulin receptors appears to be inversely related [166–168].

The fetal β cells in all animals investigated show a different pattern of response to glucose in prenatal and postnatal life. The lack of sensitivity to glucose in utero may be an example of receptor immaturity.

Somatomedin

The somatomedins are a family of peptides widely distributed in mammals and other vertebrates that appear to have physiologic growth-stimulating properties at multiple sites. Though initially isolated from mammalian brain extracts, the somatomedins are present throughout the body, especially in the liver. Somatomedins are structurally similar to insulin. The named somatomedin peptides confirmed in humans include somatomedin A, somatomedin C, insulin-like growth factor 1, and insulin-like growth factor 2. The primary proposed role for all somatomedins is regulation of growth in conjunction with growth hormone, presumably including the fetus and newborn. To date, there appears no evidence that somatomedins have a specific direct effect on the gastrointestinal tract [169–171].

Ontogeny. The ontogeny of the somatomedins in humans has been difficult to dissect because of the multiple molecular forms present and the variability in the different bioassays [169,170]. Mouse liver embryonic cells produce somatomedin C in vivo and in vitro. Somatomedin C in cell culture stimulates fibroblast proliferation and has been shown to induce growth in vivo in amphibians [172].

Concentrations of somatomedin in human maternal serum show a positive correlation with birth weight and length [170,173]. Maternal serum somatomedin C, insulin-like growth factor 2, and insulin-like growth factor 1 all increase progressively during gestation and fall significantly after birth [172–174]. Levels of somatomedin A are low in the serum of human fetuses and newborns but increase to adult concentrations by 6 to 10 years of age. This, of course, makes a role as a growth modulator in utero and early life unlikely for somatomedin A.

Sara et al [173], in 1981, reported a specific radioimmunoassay for yet another "human embryonic" form of somatomedin. This somatomedin is present in human fetal and early postnatal life. It is first reported at 16 to 22 weeks' gestation. After rising through the third trimester, it diminishes near birth and is virtually gone at the age of 2 months. The presence of an embryonic molecular form during development that "involutes" with aging is similar to some of the gastrointestinal hormones and suggests a developmental role during embryogenesis [173,175,176].

Several clinical conditions manifested by failure of intrauterine growth or CNS development are known to be characterized by lower than expected levels of human embryonic somatomedin. These conditions include thalassemia, hemophilia, anencephaly, and Down's syndrome [173].

REFERENCES

1. Gray SW, Skandalakis JE: The stomach, in Gray SW, Skandalakis JE (eds): *Embryology for Surgeons. The Embryologic Basis for the Treatment of Congenital Defects.* Philadelphia, W B Saunders Co, 1972, pp 101–127.
2. Johnson FP: The development of the mucous membrane of the oesophagus, stomach and small intestine in the human embryo. Am J Anat 10:521, 1910.
3. Lewis FT: The development of the stomach, in Keibel F, Mall FP (eds): *Manual of Human Embryology.* Philadelphia, J B Lippincott Co, 1912, pp 368–381.
4. Moore KL: The embryonic period. The fourth to seventh weeks, in Moore KL: *The Developing Human. Clinically Oriented Embryology.* 3rd Ed. Philadelphia, W B Saunders Co, 1982.
5. Salenius P: On the ontogenesis of the human gastric epithelial cells. A histologic and histochemical study. Acta Anat (Suppl 46) 50:1, 1962.
6. Gray SW, Skandalakis JE: The small intestines, in Gray SW, Skandalakis JE (eds): *Embryology for Surgeons. The Embryologic Basis for the Treatment of Congenital Defects.* Philadelphia, W B Saunders Co, 1972, pp 129–186.
7. Gray SW, Skandalakis JE: The colon and rectum, in Gray SW, Skandalakis JE (eds): *Embryology for Surgeons. The Embryologic Basis for the Treatment of Congenital Defects.* Philadelphia, W B Saunders Co, 1972, pp 187–216.
8. Gray SW, Skandalakis JE: The esophagus, in Gray SW, Skandalakis JE (eds): *Embryology for Surgeons. The Embryologic Basis for the Treatment of Congenital Defects.* Philadelphia, W B Saunders Co, 1972, pp 63–100.
9. Moore KL: The digestive system. Esophagus, stomach, intestines and major digestive glands, in Moore KL: *The Developing Human. Clinically Oriented Embryology.* 3rd Ed. Philadelphia, W B Saunders Co, 1982.
10. Okamoto E, Ueda T: Embryogenesis of intramural ganglia of the gut and its relation to Hirschsprung's disease. J Pediatr Surg 2:437, 1967.
11. Huang CG, Eng J, Yalow RS: Ontogeny of immunoreactivity cholecystokinin, vasoactive intestinal peptide, and secretin in guinea pig brain and gut. Endocrinology 118:1096, 1986.
12. Dawson W, Langman J: An anatomical-radiological study on the pancreatic duct pattern in man. Anat Rec 139:59, 1961.
13. Gray SW, Skandalakis JE: The pancreas, in Gray SW, Skandalakis JE (eds): *Embryology for Surgeons. The Embryologic Basis for the Treatment of Congenital Defects.* Philadelphia, W B Saunders Co, 1972, pp 263–281.
14. Robb P: The development of the islets of Langerhans in the human foetus. Quart J Exp Physiol 46:335, 1961.
15. Conklin JL: Cytogenesis of the human fetal pancreas. Am J Anat 111:181, 1962.
16. Van Assche FA, Aerts L: The fetal endocrine pancreas. Contrib Gynecol Obstet 5:44, 1979.
17. Falkmer S, Patent GJ: Comparative and embryological aspects of the pancreatic islets, in Geiger SR (ed): *Handbook of Physiology. Section 7: Endocrinology.* Washington, D.C., American Physiological Society, 1972, pp 1–23.
18. Hard WL: The origin and differentiation of the alpha and beta cells in the pancreatic islets of the rat. Am J Anat 15:369, 1944.
19. Ferner H, Kern H: The islet organ of selachians, in Brolin SE, Hellman B, Knutson H (eds): *The Structure and Metabolism of the Pancreatic Islets.* Oxford, Pergamon Press, 1964, pp 3–10.
20. Liu HM, Potter EL: Development of the human pancreas. Arch Pathol 74:439, 1962.
21. Wirdnam PK, Milner RDG: Quantitation of the B and A cell fractions in human pancreas from early fetal life to puberty. Early Hum Dev 5:299, 1981.
22. Deconinck JF, Van Assche FA, Potvliege PR, et al: The ultrastructure of the human pancreatic islets. II. The islets of neonates. Diabetologia 8:326, 1972.
23. Rahier J, Wallon J, Henquin J-C: Cell populations in the endocrine pancreas of human neonates and infants. Diabetologia 20:540, 1981.
24. Yoshinari M, Daikoku S: Ontogenetic appearance of

immunoreactive endocrine cells in rat pancreatic islets. Anat Embryol 165:63, 1982.

25. Bjorkman N, Hellerstrom C, Hellman B, et al: The cell types in the endocrine pancreas of the human fetus. Zellforschung 72:425, 1966.
26. Stefan Y, Grasso S, Perrelet A, et al: A quantitative immunofluorescent study of the endocrine cell populations in the developing human pancreas. Diabetes 32:293, 1983.
27. Clark A, Grant AM: Quantitative morphology of endocrine cells in human fetal pancreas. Diabetologia 25:31, 1983.
28. Orci L, Malaisse-Lagae F, Baetens D, et al: Pancreatic-polypeptide-rich regions in human pancreas. Lancet 2:1200, 1978.
29. Malaisse-Lagae F, Stefan Y, Cox J, et al: Identification of a lobe in the adult human pancreas rich in pancreatic polypeptide. Diabetologia 17:361, 1979.
30. Paulin C, Dubois PM: Immunohistochemical identification and localization of pancreatic polypeptide cells in the pancreas and gastrointestinal tract of the human fetus and adult man. Cell Tissue Res 188:251, 1978.
31. Assan R, Boillot J: Pancreatic glucagon and glucagon-like material in tissues and plasma from human fetuses 6–26 weeks old. Pathol Biol 21:149, 1973.
32. Rastogi GK, Letarte J, Fraser TR: Immunoreactive insulin content of 203 pancreases from foetuses of healthy mothers. Diabetologia 6:445, 1970.
33. Wellmann KF, Volk BW, Brancato P: Ultrastructure and insulin content of the endocrine pancreas in the human fetus. Lab Invest 25:97, 1971.
34. Hill DE: Effect of insulin on fetal growth. Semin Perinatol 2:319, 1978.
35. Orci L, Stefan Y, Malaisse-Lagae F, et al: Instability of pancreatic endocrine cell populations throughout life. Lancet 1:615, 1979.
36. Track NS, Creutzfeldt C, Litzenberger J, et al: Appearance of gastrin and somatostatin in the human fetal stomach, duodenum and pancreas. Digestion 19:292, 1979.
37. Dawson W, Langman J: An anatomical-radiological study on the pancreatic duct pattern in man. Anat Rec 139:59, 1961.
38. Moore KL: The nervous system, in Moore KL (ed): *The Developing Human. Clinically Oriented Embryology*. 3rd Ed. Philadelphia, W B Saunders Co, 1982.
39. Solcia E, Capella C, Buffa R, et al: Endocrine cells of the digestive system, in Johnson LR (ed): *Physiology of the Gastrointestinal Tract*. New York, Raven Press, 1981, pp 39–58.
40. Le Douarin NM, Teillet M-AM: Experimental analysis of the migration and differentiation of neuroblasts of the autonomic nervous system and of neurectodermal mesenchymal derivatives, using a biological cell marking technique. Develop Biol 41:162, 1974.
41. Solcia E, Buffa R, Capella C, et al: Immunohistochemical characterization of gastroenteropancreatic endocrine cells and related multihormonal cells. Problems, pitfalls and facts, in Miyoshi A (ed): *Gut Peptides. Secretion, Function and Clinical Aspects*. Tokyo, Kodansha Ltd, and New York, Elsevier/North-Holland Biomedical Press, 1979, pp 303–309.
42. Solcia E, Vasallo G, Sampietro R: Endocrine cells in the antro-pyloric mucosa of the stomach. Z Zellforsch 81:474, 1967.
43. Pearse AGE: Cell migration and the alimentary system: Endocrine contributions of the neural crest to the gut and its derivatives. Digestion 8:372, 1973.
44. Singh I: The prenatal development of enterochromaffin cells in the human gastro-intestinal tract. J Anat (Lond) 97:377, 1963.
45. Singh I: The distribution of cells of the enterochromaffin system in the gastrointestinal tract of human foetuses. Acta Anat 64:544, 1966.
46. Josephson RL, Altmann GG: Distribution of diazopositive (argentaffin) cells in the small intestine of rats of various ages. Am J Anat 136:15, 1973.
47. Cole JW, McKalen A: Argentaffin cells in the intestinal epithelium of human embryos. Nature 193:198, 1962.
48. Larsson L-I, Rehfeld JF, Goltermann N: Gastrin in the human fetus. Distribution and molecular forms of gastrin in the antro-pyloric gland area, duodenum and pancreas. Scand J Gastroenterol 12:869, 1977.
49. Dubois PM, Paulin C, Chayvialle JA: Identification of gastrin-secreting cells and cholecystokinin-secreting cells in the gastrointestinal tract of the human fetus and adult man. Cell Tissue Res 175:351, 1976.
50. Larsson L-I: Ontogeny of peptide-producing nerves and endocrine cells of the gastro-duodeno-pancreatic region. Histochemistry 54:133, 1977.
51. Larsson L-I, Rehfeld FJ, Sundler F, et al: Pancreatic gastrin in foetal and neonatal rats. Nature 262:609, 1976.
52. Braaten JT, Greider MH, McGuigan JE, et al: Gastrin in the perinatal rat pancreas and gastric antrum: Immunofluorescence localization of pancreatic gastrin cells and gastrin secretion in monolayer cell cultures. Endocrinology 99:684, 1976.
53. Bryant MG, Buchan AMJ, Gregor M, et al: Development of intestinal regulatory peptides in the human fetus. Gastroenterology 83:47, 1982.
54. Stein BA, Buchan AMJ, Morris J, et al: The ontogeny of regulatory peptide-containing cells in the human fetal stomach: An immunocytochemical study. J Histochem Cytochem 31:1117, 1983.
55. Lehy T, Gres L, Ferreira de Castro E: Quantitation of gastrin and somatostatin cell populations in the antral mucosa of the rat. Cell Tissue Res 198:325, 1979.
56. Walsh JH: Gastrointestinal hormones and peptides, in Johnson LR (ed): *Physiology of the Gastrointestinal Tract*. New York, Raven Press, 1981, pp 59–144.
57. Larsson L-I, Håkanson R, Rehfeld JF, et al: Occurrence and neonatal development of gastrin im-

munoreactivity in the digestive tract of the rat. Cell Tissue Res 149:275, 1974.
58. Attia RR, Ebeid AM, Fischer JE, et al: Maternal fetal and placental gastrin concentrations. Anaesthesia 37:18, 1982.
59. von Berger L, Henrichs I, Raptis S, et al: Gastrin concentration in plasma of the neonate at birth and after the first feeding. Pediatrics 58:264, 1976.
60. Avery GB, Randolph JG, Weaver T: Gastric acidity in the first day of life. Pediatrics 37:1005, 1966.
61. Griswold C, Shohl AT: Gastric digestion in newborn infants. Am J Dis Child 30:541, 1925.
62. Hess AF: The gastric secretion of infants at birth. Am J Dis Child 6:264, 1913.
63. Euler AR, Ament ME, Walsh JH: Human newborn hypergastrinemia: An investigation of prenatal and perinatal factors and their effects on gastrin. Pediatr Res 12:652, 1978.
64. Sann L, Chayvialle JAP, Bremond A, et al: Serum gastrin level in early childhood. Arch Dis Child 50:782, 1975.
65. Euler AR, Byrne WJ, Meis PJ, et al: Basal and pentagastrin-stimulated acid secretion in newborn human infants. Pediatr Res 13:36, 1979.
66. Euler AR, Byrne WJ, Cousins LM, et al: Increased serum gastrin concentrations and gastric acid hyposecretion in the immediate newborn period. Gastroenterology 72:1271, 1977.
67. Garzon B, Ducroc R, Onolfo J-P, et al: Biphasic development of pentagastrin sensitivity in rat stomach. Am J Physiol 242:G111, 1982.
68. Garzon B, Ducroc R, Geloso JP: Ontogenesis of gastric response to agonists and antagonists of acid secretion in fetal rat. J Dev Physiól 4:195, 1982.
69. Lari J, Lister J, Duthie HL: Response to gastrin pentapeptide in children. J Pediatr Surg 3:682, 1968.
70. Miller RA: Desoxycorticosterone acetate and oestradiol dipropionate therapy in the newborn infant. Arch Dis Child 16:113, 1941.
71. Rodgers BM, Dix PM, Talbert JL, et al: Fasting and postprandial serum gastrin in normal human neonates. J Pediatr Surg 13:13, 1978.
72. Rogers IM, Davidson DC, Lawrence J, et al: Neonatal secretion of gastrin and glucagon. Arch Dis Child 49:796, 1974.
73. Speir GR, Takeuchi K, Peitsch W, et al: Mucosal gastrin receptor. VII. Up- and downregulation. Am J Physiol 242:G243, 1982.
74. Peitsch W, Takeuchi K, Johnson LR: Mucosal gastrin receptor. VI. Induction by corticosterone in newborn rats. Am J Physiol 240:G442, 1981.
75. Johnson LR, Peitsch W, Takeuchi K: Mucosal gastrin receptor. VIII. Sex-related differences in binding. Am J Physiol 243:G469, 1982.
76. Ackerman SH: Ontogeny of gastric acid secretion in the rat: Evidence for multiple response systems. Science 217:75, 1982.
77. Larsson L-I, Rehfeld JF, Sundler F, et al: Pancreatic gastrin in foetal and neonatal rats. Nature 262:609, 1976.
78. Noyer M, Bui ND, Deschodt-Lanckman M, et al: Postnatal development of the cholecystokinin-gastrin family of peptides in the brain and gut of rat. Life Sci 27:2197, 1980.
79. Brand SJ: The post-natal development of cholecystokinin-like activity in the brain and small intestine of the rat. J Physiol 326:425, 1982.
80. Chey WY, Escoffery R: Secretin cells in the gastrointestinal tract. Endocrinology 98:1390, 1976.
81. Straus E, Yalow RS: Immunoreactive secretin in gastrointestinal mucosa of several mammalian species. Gastroenterology 75:401, 1978.
82. Lucas A, Adrian TE, Bloom SR, et al: Plasma secretin in neonates. Acta Paediatr Scand 69:205, 1980.
83. Rogers IM, Davidson DC, Lawrence J, et al: Neonatal secretion of secretin. Arch Dis Child 50:120, 1975.
84. Moazam F, Rodgers BM, Wheeldon S, et al: Secretin levels in plasma and tissue of the neonatal swine. Biol Neonate 42:1, 1982.
85. Paquette TL, Shulman DF, Alpers DH, et al: Postnatal development of intestinal secretin in rats and guinea pigs. Am J Physiol 243:G511, 1982.
86. Moxey PC, Trier JS: Endocrine cells in the human fetal small intestine. Cell Tissue Res 183:33, 1977.
87. Larsson L-I, Holst J, Håkanson R, et al: Distribution and properties of glucagon immunoreactivity in the digestive tract of various mammals: An immunohistochemical and immunochemical study. Histochemistry 44:281, 1975.
88. Larsson L-I: Ontogeny of peptide-producing nerves and endocrine cells of the gastro-duodeno-pancreatic region. Histochemistry 54:133, 1977.
89. Buts J-P, DeMeyer R, VanCraynest M-P, et al: Pancreatic glucagon does not alter mucosal growth and maturation of sucrase and thymidine kinase activity in rat small intestine. Biol Neonate 43:253, 1983.
90. Buchan AMJ, Bryant MG, Stein BA, et al: Pancreatic glucagon in human foetal stomach. Histochemistry 74:515, 1982.
91. Ravazzola M, Unger RH, Orci L: Demonstration of glucagon in the stomach of human fetuses. Diabetes 30:879, 1981.
92. Weser E: Nutritional aspects of malabsorption: Short gut adaptation. Clinics Gastroenterol 12:443, 1983.
93. Leduque P, Moody AJ, Dubois PM: Ontogeny of immunoreactive glicentin in the human gastrointestinal tract and endocrine pancreas. Regul Pept 4:261, 1982.
94. Stefan Y, Ravazzola M, Grasso S, et al: Glicentin precedes glucagon in the developing human pancreas. Endocrinology 110:2189, 1982.
95. Leduque P, Gespach C, Brown JC, et al: Ontogeny of gastric inhibitory peptide in the human gastrointestinal tract and endocrine pancreas. Acta Endocrinol 99:112, 1982.
96. El-Salhy M, Wilander E, Grimelius L: Immunocytochemical localization of gastric inhibitory peptide (GIP) in the human foetal pancreas. Ups J Med Sci 87:81, 1982.

97. Gespach C, Bataille D, Jarrousse C, et al: Ontogeny and distribution of immunoreactive gastric inhibitory polypeptide (IR-GIP) in rat small intestine. Acta Endocrinol 90:307, 1979.
98. Chayvialle J-A, Paulin C, Descos F, et al: Ontogeny of vasoactive intestinal peptide in the human fetal digestive tract. Regul Pept 5:245, 1983.
99. Sundler F, Alumets J, Fahrenkrug J, et al: Cellular localization and ontogeny of immunoreactive vasoactive intestinal polypeptide (VIP) in the chicken gut. Cell Tissue Res 196:193, 1979.
100. Buffa R, Capella C, Solcia E, et al: Vasoactive intestinal peptide (VIP) cells in the pancreas and gastrointestinal mucosa. An immunohistochemical and ultrastructural study. Histochemistry 50:217, 1977.
101. Laburthe M, Bataille D, Rosselin G: Vasoactive intestinal peptide (VIP): Variation of the jejuno-ileal content in the developing rat as measured by radioreceptorassay. Acta Endocrinol 84:588, 1977.
102. Lucas A, Bloom SR, Aynsley-Green A: Vasoactive intestinal peptide (VIP) in preterm and term neonates. Acta Paediatr Scand 71:71, 1982.
103. Ebeid AM, Attia R, Murray P, et al: The placenta as a possible source of gut peptide hormones. Gastroenterology 70:A99/957, 1976.
104. Larsson L-I, Sundler F, Håkanson R: Immunohistochemical localization of human pancreatic polypeptide (HPP) to a population of islet cells. Cell Tissue Res 156:167, 1975.
105. Leduque P, Paulin C, Dubois PM: Immunocytochemical evidence for a substance related to the bovine pancreatic polypeptide-peptide YY group of peptides in the human fetal gastrointestinal tract. Regul Pept 6:219, 1983.
106. Lehy T, Cristina ML: Ontogeny and distribution of certain endocrine cells in the human fetal large intestine. Histochemical and immunocytochemical studies. Cell Tissue Res 203:415, 1979.
107. El-Salhy M, Wilander E, Juntti-Berggren L, et al: The distribution and ontogeny of polypeptide YY (PYY)- and pancreatic polypeptide (PP)-immunoreactive cells in the gastrointestinal tract of rat. Histochemistry 78:53, 1983.
108. Sundler F, Håkanson R, Larsson L-I: Ontogeny of rat pancreatic polypeptide (PP) cells. Cell Tissue Res 178:303, 1977.
109. Tatemoto K, Mutt V: Isolation of two novel candidate hormones using a chemical method for finding naturally occurring polypeptides. Nature 285:417, 1980.
110. Tatemoto K: Isolation and characterization of peptide YY (PYY), a candidate gut hormone that inhibits pancreatic exocrine secretion. Proc Natl Acad Sci USA 79:2514, 1982.
111. El-Salhy M, Wilander E, Abu-Sinna G, et al: On the ontogeny of polypeptide YY (PYY) in the gut of chickens. Biomed Res 3:680, 1982.
112. Alumets J, Sundler F, Håkanson R: Distribution, ontogeny and ultrastructure of somatostatin immunoreactive cells in the pancreas and gut. Cell Tissue Res 185:465, 1977.
113. Dubois PM, Paulin C: Gastrointestinal somatostatin cells in the human fetus. Cell Tissue Res 166:179, 1976.
114. Dubois MP: Immunoreactive somatostatin is present in discrete cells of the endocrine pancreas. Proc Natl Acad Sci USA 72:1340, 1975.
115. Rahier J, Wallon J, Henquin JC: Abundance of somatostatin cells in the human neonatal pancreas. Diabetologia 18:251, 1980.
116. Chayvialle JA, Paulin C, Dubois PM, et al: Ontogeny of somatostatin in the human gastro-intestinal tract, endocrine pancreas and hypothalamus. Acta Endocrinol 94:1, 1980.
117. Dubois PM, Paulin C, Assan R, et al: Evidence for immunoreactive somatostatin in the endocrine cells of human foetal pancreas. Nature 256:731, 1975.
118. McIntosh C, Arnold R, Bothe E, et al: Gastrointestinal somatostatin: Extraction and radioimmunoassay in different species. Gut 19:655, 1978.
119. Dupouy JP, Chatelain A, Dubois MP: Normal development of cells with somatostatin immunoreactivity in the pancreas and duodenum of the rat fetus and newborn. Cell Tissue Res 231:463, 1983.
120. Ghirlanda G, Bataille D, Dubois MP, et al: Variations of the somatostatin content of gut, pancreas, and brain in the developing rat. Metabolism 27 (Suppl 1):1167, 1978.
121. Koshimizu T: The development of pancreatic and gastrointestinal somatostatin-like immunoreactivity and its relationship to feeding in neonatal rats. Endocrinology 112:911, 1983.
122. Lehy T, Dubrasquet M, Brazeau P, et al: Inhibitory effect of prolonged administration of long-acting somatostatin on gastrin-stimulated fundic epithelial cell growth in the rat. Digestion 24:246, 1982.
123. Inagaki S, Shiosaka S, Takatsuki K, et al: Ontogeny of somatostatin-containing neuron system of the rat cerebellum including its fiber connections: An experimental and immunohistochemical analysis. Devel Brain Res 3:509, 1982.
124. Alumets J, Håkanson R, Lundqvist G, et al: Ontogeny and ultrastructure of somatostatin and calcitonin cells in the thyroid gland of the rat. Cell Tissue Res 206:193, 1980.
125. Saito H, Saito S, Sano T, et al: Fetal and maternal plasma levels of immunoreactive somatostatin at delivery: Evidence for its increase in the umbilical artery and its arteriovenous gradient in the fetoplacental circulation. J Clin Endocrinol Metab 56:567, 1983.
126. Furuhashi N, Takahashi T, Fukaya T, et al: Plasma somatostatin and growth hormone in the human fetus and its mother at delivery. Gynecol Obstet Invest 16:59, 1983.
127. Fitz-Patrick D, Patel YC: Measurement, characterization, and source of somatostatin-like immunoreactivity in human amniotic fluid. J Clin Invest 64:737, 1979.
128. Sundler F, Håkanson R, Hammer RA, et al: Immunohistochemical localization of neurotensin in en-

docrine cells of the gut. Cell Tissue Res 178:313, 1977.

129. Sundler F, Håkanson R, Leander S, et al: Light and electron microscopic localization of neurotensin in the gastrointestinal tract. Ann NY Acad Sci 400:94, 1982.
130. Helmstaedter V, Muhlmann G, Feurle GE, et al: Immunohistochemical identification of gastrointestinal neurotensin cells in human embryos. Cell Tissue Res 184:315, 1977.
131. Polak JM, Bloom SR: The central and peripheral distribution of neurotensin. Ann NY Acad Sci 400:75, 1982.
132. Leduque P, Paulin C, Chayvialle JA, et al: Immunocytological evidence of motilin- and secretin-containing cells in the human fetal gastro-entero-pancreatic system. Cell Tissue Res 218:519, 1981.
133. Nomura H, Shiosaka S, Inagaki S, et al: Distribution of substance P-like immunoreactivity in the lower brainstem of the human fetus: An immunohistochemical study. Brain Res 252:315, 1982.
134. Sundler F, Håkanson R, Larsson L-I, et al: Substance P in the gut: An immunochemical and immunohistochemical study of its distribution and development, in von Euler US, Pernow B (eds): *Substance P.* New York, Raven Press, 1977, pp 59–65.
135. Wharton J, Polak JM, Bloom SR, et al: Bombesin-like immunoreactivity in the lung. Nature 273:769, 1978.
136. Yamagushi K, Abe K, Kameya T, et al: Production and molecular size heterogeneity of immunoreactive gastrin-releasing peptide in fetal and adult lungs and primary lung tumors. Cancer Res 43:3932, 1983.
137. Tsutsumi Y, Osamura RY, Watanabe K, et al: Immunohistochemical studies on gastrin-releasing peptide- and adrenocorticotropic hormone-containing cells in the human lung. Lab Invest 48:623, 1983.
138. Lauweryns JM, Cokelaere M, Deleersnyder M, et al: Intrapulmonary neuro-epithelial bodies in newborn rabbits. Influence of hypoxia, hyperoxia, hypercapnia, nicotine, reserpine, L-DOPA and 5-HTP. Cell Tissue Res 182:425, 1977.
139. Track NS, Cutz E: Bombesin-like immunoreactivity in developing human lung. Life Sci 30:1553, 1982.
140. Lauweryns JM, Goddeeris P: Neuroepithelial bodies in the human child and adult lung. Am Rev Resp Dis 111:469, 1975.
141. Barka T, van der Noen H, Gresik EW, et al: Immunoreactive epidermal growth factor in human amniotic fluid. Mt Sinai J Med 45:679, 1978.
142. Malo C, Menard D: Influence of epidermal growth factor on the development of suckling mouse intestinal mucosa. Gastroenterology 83:28, 1982.
143. Oka Y, Ghishan FK, Greene HL, et al: Effect of mouse epidermal growth factor/urogastrone on the functional maturation of rat intestine. Endocrinology 112:940, 1983.
144. Calvert R, Beaulieu J-F, Menard D: Epidermal growth factor (EGF) accelerates the maturation of fetal mouse intestinal mucosa in utero. Experientia 38:7, 1982.
145. Draghi E, Armato U, Andreis PG, et al: The stimulation by epidermal growth factor (urogastrone) of the growth of neonatal rat hepatocytes in primary tissue culture and its modulation by serum and associated pancreatic hormones. J Cell Physiol 103:129, 1980.
146. Johnson LR, Guthrie PD: Stimulation of rat oxyntic gland mucosal growth by epidermal growth factor. Am J Physiol 238:G45, 1980.
147. Dembinski A, Gregory H, Konturek SJ, et al: Trophic action of epidermal growth factor on the pancreas and gastroduodenal mucosa in rats. J Physiol 325:35, 1982.
148. Menard D, Malo C: Insulin-evoked precocious appearance of intestinal sucrase activity in suckling mice. Dev Biol 69:661, 1979.
149. Menard D, Malo C, Calvert R: Insulin accelerates the development of intestinal brush border hydrolytic activities of suckling mice. Dev Biol 85:150, 1981.
150. Kumegawa M, Takuma T, Ikeda E, et al: Precocious differentiation of chick embryo pancreas in vitro. Biochim Biophys Acta 585:554, 1979.
151. Hill DE: Fetal effects of insulin. Obstet Gynecol Annu 11:133, 1982.
152. Mandel TE, Hoffman L, Collier S, et al: Organ culture of fetal mouse and fetal human pancreatic islets for allografting. Diabetes 31 (Suppl 4):39, 1982.
153. Hoffman L, Mandel TE, Carter WM, et al: Insulin secretion by fetal human pancreas in organ culture. Diabetologia 23:426, 1982.
154. Pedersen J: Weight and length at birth of infants of diabetic mothers. Acta Endocrinol 16:330, 1954.
155. Herzberg V, Boughter M, Seyed S, et al: Possible etiologic mechanism for the overgrowth and hypoglycemia in patients with Beckwith-Wiedemann syndrome. Clin Res 27:812A, 1979.
156. Schiff D, Colle E, Stern L: Metabolic and growth patterns in transient neonatal diabetes. N Engl J Med 287:119, 1972.
157. Lemons JA, Ridenour R, Orsini EN: Congenital absence of the pancreas and intrauterine growth retardation. Pediatrics 64:255, 1979.
158. Donohue WL, Uchida I: Leprechaunism. A euphemism for a rare familial disorder. J Pediatr 45:505, 1954.
159. Schilling EE, Rechler MM, Grunfeld C, et al: Primary defect of insulin receptors in skin fibroblasts cultured from an infant with leprechaunism and insulin resistance. Proc Natl Acad Sci USA 76:5877, 1979.
160. Vorherr H: Factors influencing fetal growth. Am J Obstet Gynecol 142:577, 1982.
161. Campbell IL, Hellquist LNB, Taylor KW: Insulin biosynthesis and its regulation. Clin Sci 62:449, 1982.
162. Milner RDG, Leach FN, Ashworth MA: The ontogeny of insulin secretion mechanisms. Biochim Biophys Acta 304:225, 1973.
163. Grillo TAI: The occurrence of insulin in the pan-

creas of foetuses of some rodents. J Endocrinol 31:67, 1964.

164. Asplund K: Effects of glucose on insulin biosynthesis in foetal and newborn rats. Horm Metab Res 5:410, 1973.

165. Puukka R, Puukka M, Knip M, et al: Erythrocyte insulin binding in normal infants, children and adults. Horm Res 17:185, 1983.

166. Polychronakos C, Ruggere MD, Benjamin A, et al: The role of cell age in the difference in insulin binding between adult and cord erythrocytes. J Clin Endocrinol Metab 55:290, 1982.

167. Ganguli S, Sinha MK, Sterman B, et al: Ontogeny of hepatic insulin and glucagon receptors and adenylate cyclase in rabbit. Am J Physiol 244:E624, 1983.

168. Sara VR, Hall K, Misaki M, et al: Ontogenesis of somatomedin and insulin receptors in the human fetus. J Clin Invest 71:1084, 1983.

169. Heinrich UE, Schalch DS, Jawadi MH, et al: Nsila and foetal growth. Acta Endocrinol 90:534, 1979.

170. Kastrup KW, Andersen HJ, Lebech P: Somatomedin in newborns and the relationship to human chorionic somatotropin and fetal growth. Acta Paediatr Scand 67:757, 1978.

171. Sara VR, Gennser G, Persson P-H: Radioreceptor-assayable somatomedins during pregnancy and their relationship to fetal growth. J Dev Physiol 4:187, 1982.

172. D'Ercole AJ, Underwood LE, Clemmons DR, et al: Somatomedin-C: Molecular structure, biological actions and role in post-natal and fetal growth, in Cumming IA, Funder JW, Mendelsohn FAO (eds): *Endocrinology*. Canberra, AAS, 1980, pp 215–218.

173. Sara VR, Hall K, Rodeck CH, et al: Human embryonic somatomedin. Proc Natl Acad Sci USA 78:3175, 1981.

174. Bennett A, Wilson DM, Liu F, et al: Levels of insulin-like growth factors I and II in human cord blood. J Clin Endocrinol Metab 57:609, 1983.

175. Kurtz A, Jelkmann W, Bauer C: A new candidate for the regulation of erythropoiesis. Insulin-like growth factor I. FEBS Lett 149:105, 1982.

176. Underwood LE, D'Ercole AJ, Furlanetto RW, et al: Somatomedin and growth: A possible role for somatomedin C in fetal growth, in Giordano G, Van Wyk JJ, Minuto F (eds): *Somatomedins and Growth*. New York, Academic Press, 1979, pp 215–223.

Chapter 12

Possible Role of Gut Hormones in Cancer

Courtney M. Townsend, Jr., M.D., Pomila Singh, Ph.D., and James C. Thompson, M.D.

In the United States alone, carcinomas of the large bowel, stomach, and pancreas account for over 150,000 new cases and cause the death of 75,000 patients yearly [1]. Treatment of these cancers relies heavily upon adequate tumor resection. This is effective only when localized tumor is present. There is no widely effective systemic treatment for metastatic colon, stomach, or pancreatic cancer. Breast cancers are often successfully palliated by endocrine manipulation when specific receptors for hormone(s) (estrogen and progesterone) that are known to stimulate growth of the normal breast are present in the cancer.

The Scottish surgeon Beatson first demonstrated endocrine control of cancer growth [2]. On June 15, 1895, he performed bilateral salpingo-oophorectomy on a 33 year old woman with massive recurrence of breast carcinoma involving the left chest wall. Complete and dramatic regression of the tumor occurred over 4 months and the patient lived for 44 months after this operation. She eventually succumbed to her disease. In 1951, Huggins and Bergenstal reported that bilateral adrenalectomy caused regression of breast and prostatic cancer in humans [3]. Since that time, many studies have confirmed these original observations.

The evolution of the concept that cancers which arise from classic hormone target tissues are either hormone-dependent or -independent (terminology first used in 1945 by Huggins and Scott [4]) has allowed the development of successful, although temporary, strategies to arrest growth of hormone-responsive cancers. Hormone-responsive cancers may be inhibited either by hormone deprivation or by the administration of excessive amounts of trophic hormones. Although the ground-breaking studies involved cancers under control of female or male sex hormones, cancers of other endocrine target tissue, namely thyroid [5], may also be successfully treated by hormone manipulation, and leukemias and lymphomas may be arrested by administration of glucocorticoids [6].

In 1902, Bayliss and Starling [7] identified the first hormone, secretin. These investigators found that irrigation of a denervated loop of proximal small intestine with hydrochloric acid caused a prompt increase in output of pancreatic juice. The major hormones responsible for pancreatic exocrine secretion in humans and animals are secretin, which primarily stimulates volume and bicarbonate output, and cholecystokinin (CCK), which stimulates the output of pancreatic digestive enzymes [8].

Gastrin is produced by G cells of the antrum of the stomach. The primary physiologic action of gastrin is to stimulate acid secretion from parietal cells of the stomach. In addition, gastrin stimulates growth of mucosal cells of the gastrointestinal tract [9]. Similar to other peptide hormones, gastrin acts via a specific membrane receptor (GR). Gastrin receptors are present in fundic and colonic mucosa of frogs, rats, and dogs [10–15].

GROWTH EFFECTS OF GUT PEPTIDES ON NORMAL GUT AND PANCREAS

Patients with Zollinger-Ellison syndrome (ZES) who have hypergastrinemia due to a gastrin-producing islet cell (non-β cell) tumor of the pancreas [16] have significantly increased (4–6 times greater than normal) parietal cell mass [17–19]. Pentagastrin (a pentapeptide that is a biologically active fragment of gastrin) stimulates growth of gastric and colonic mucosa of chronically treated rats; this trophic effect can be blocked by secretin [9,20]. Somatostatin, a cyclic tetradecapeptide, inhibits gastrin-stimulated gastric, intestinal, and pancreatic DNA synthesis [21–23]. Proglumide, a glutamic acid derivative that is both a gastrin and a CCK receptor antagonist, inhibits the trophic effect of pentagastrin on rat stomach by blocking the binding of gastrin to its GR [24].

Secretin and CCK are the most potent known humoral stimulants of pancreatic secretion; given simultaneously, each potentiates the action of the other [25]. Bombesin is a peptide from amphibian skin that has direct effects upon isolated pancreatic acini [26] and that releases gastrin and CCK in dogs [27,28] and rats [29]. Receptors for secretin [30], CCK [31,32], and bombesin [33] have been identified in dispersed cells from the pancreatic acini of guinea pigs.

Barrowman and Mayston [34] demonstrated that daily administration of CCK for 9 days produced hypertrophy (increased weight and RNA content) and hyperplasia (increased content of DNA) of the rat pancreas. The data concerning the effects of secretin (given alone) on pancreatic growth are conflicting. Solomon et al [35], studying adult rats, have shown that administration of secretin alone produced hypertrophy but not hyperplasia of the pancreas. On the other hand, we have shown that when given alone, secretin stimulates hyperplasia of the hamster pancreas [36]. Other investigators [37] have reported that chronic treatment with secretin produced both hypertrophy and hyperplasia in rat pancreas. Epidermal growth factor (EGF) produces hyperplasia of the oxyntic gland mucosa of the stomach [38], and of the pancreas in the rat [39]. Removal of the major source of EGF in mice (the submandibular salivary glands) protects them against chemical induction of carcinoma of the colon [40].

GROWTH EFFECT OF GUT PEPTIDES ON GUT AND PANCREATIC CANCER

Endogenous hypergastrinemia produced by either antral exclusion or by small bowel resection in rats causes increased DNA synthesis in colon tumors or an increased incidence of tumors of the bowel, respectively, in carcinogen-treated rats [41–46]. Tahara and Haizuka [47] have reported that gastrin increased the incidence of carcinogen-induced gastric cancer in rats. Others have found that elevated gastrin levels inhibit the incidence of carcinogen-induced stomach cancers in rats [48,49].

We have reported that chronic treatment with the combination of caerulein (an analogue of CCK) and secretin stimulates the growth of hamster H2T pancreatic cancer in vivo [36]. Takahashi et al [50] found that gastrin enhanced stomach and colon cancer growth in nude mice; this growth was inhibited by secretin. We have found that chronic administration of pentagastrin stimulated the growth of MC-26 cancer in vivo and significantly decreased survival due to accelerated tumor growth that occurred in gastrin-treated animals (Table 12-1) [51]. Sumiyoshi et al [52] found that pentagastrin stimulated the growth of a human gastric adenocarcinoma xenograft in athymic mice. In addition, they found that pentagastrin stimulated protein kinase activity in this tumor cell line, both in vivo and in vitro. Hudd et al [53] reported that CCK-8 stimulated production of CEA by a human cholangiocarcinoma (SLU-132) implanted in nude mice and also appeared to inhibit growth of this tumor.

Pentagastrin increases DNA synthesis in cultured rat gastric and duodenal mucosal cells [54]. Growth of the human colon carcinoma cell line, HC84S, is mildly stimulated by gastrin and EGF in vitro [55]. We have shown increased DNA synthesis in a cell line from a human stomach carcinoma (AGS) treated with pentagastrin [56]. Tetragastrin and caerulein cause hyperplasia of BV-9 rat gastric cancer in vitro [57].

The significance of these observations is that normal gastric and colon mucosal cell proliferation and pancreatic growth may be controlled by gas-

Table 12-1. Response of fundic mucosa and tumor from mice inoculated with 5×10^4 cells (MC-26 mouse colon cancer)

Treatment	*N*	*Fundus wt (mg)*	*Fundus DNA (mg)*	*Tumor wt (mg)*	*Tumor DNA (mg)*
Control	12	10.3 ± 1.2	0.16 ± 0.02	480 ± 64	2.73 ± 0.31
PG (125 μg/kg)	11	19.4 ± 2.2*	0.22 ± 0.02*	785 ± 85*	4.33 ± 0.43*
PG (250 μg/kg)	10	45.9 ± 6.3*	0.35 ± 0.04*	815 ± 113*	4.18 ± 0.33*
PG (500 μg/kg)	11	63.1 ± 6.4*	0.48 ± 0.04*	783 ± 100*	4.14 ± 0.31*

* = $p < 0.05$; mean ± SEM; significance determined by Student's *t* test; control mice received saline; PG = pentagastrin.

trointestinal hormones, and that growth of colon, stomach, and pancreatic cancers may also be affected by gastrointestinal hormones.

ROLE OF PEPTIDE HORMONE RECEPTORS IN GUT CANCER

Receptors for steroid and peptide hormones have been detected in a wide variety of human tumors. However, not all cancers of endocrine-responsive tissue possess specific receptors for hormones. The reasons for this are unknown. There are specific receptors for vasoactive intestinal polypeptide (VIP) in human colon [58], human pancreatic [59], and human gastric [60] carcinoma cell lines. Secretin and caerulein receptors have been described in a human pancreatic cancer cell line [61]. Korc et al [62] have recently described EGF receptors in two human pancreatic cell lines.

We have assayed cultured cells from mouse colon as well as human colon and cell lines from stomach cancer for GR [56]. We have found gastrin receptors in MC-26 mouse colon cancer cells in vitro and in vivo [63,64]. Of two colon carcinoma cell lines, one, LoVo, has specific GR, while the other, HT-29, does not. The parent line of a human stomach carcinoma (AGS), as well as three of 12 separate clones derived from the parent line, have specific gastrin receptors. We have detected GR in the plasma membrane fraction of biopsy specimens from freshly resected human colon, rectal, and stomach cancers and from normal gastrointestinal mucosa [65]. The concentration of GR was similar in both the cancers and normal mucosa.

Pentagastrin is not only trophic for normal gut cells but also is trophic for some gut cancer cells. We found that pentagastrin in young (10-day-old) rats was ineffective in stimulating gastric mucosal DNA synthesis but stimulated synthesis of DNA in 28-day-old rat stomachs. This differential response is probably due to the absence of gastrin receptors in the young rats, since they are detected only in rats over 28-days old [66].

We have developed a highly sensitive assay for the measurement of gastrin receptors in normal and neoplastic gastrointestinal tissues [66]. We have found high affinity gastrin receptors on gut cancer cell lines in vitro [66] and in freshly resected human stomach and colon cancers [65]. Of the 12 different gastrointestinal cancer cell lines we have screened for the presence of gastrin receptors, so far we have identified one human stomach cancer cell line (AGS, as well as four of the seven different clones derived from this cell line), one human colon cancer cell line (LoVo), and one mouse colon cancer cell line (MC-26) that possess gastrin receptors. Additionally, a hamster pancreatic (H2T) and a human duodenal (HUTU) cancer cell line have low amounts of gastrin receptors. The affinity of these gastrin-binding sites on the cancer cell lines, interestingly, appears to be similar to that observed for normal cells from the fundic mucosa of rats.

We have found that the trophic effects of gastrin on MC-26 mouse colon cancers are mediated by the interaction of gastrin with its receptors [63,64,66]. Using our gastrin receptor assay, we have demonstrated the presence of specific, high affinity (K_d 0.5 nM) gastrin receptors on MC-26 cell lines [64]. We have previously demonstrated that the in vivo growth rate of MC-26 cells is significantly increased in the presence of pentagastrin [51]. There is a strong possibility that the trophic effect is mediated by gastrin receptors. We have found that gastrin receptors are sensitive to circulating levels of gastrin [63,67].

Human breast cancers with abundant estrogen and progesterone receptors respond to endocrine manipulation while some with low concentrations of receptors (and almost all of those without receptors) do not respond to hormone treatment [68]. We expect to find a spectrum of concentrations of GR in colon and stomach cancers. Some cancers will possess specific gastrin receptors and some will not; in tumors with GR, growth may be manipulated (stimulated or inhibited) by gastrin or antigastrin compounds. By assaying tumors for GR and studying the effects of gastrin both on tumors that do and that do not possess GR, we should be able to more clearly define the role of gastrin in growth control of gastrointestinal cancers.

Beauchamp et al [69] from our laboratory have recently shown that proglumide, a gastrin receptor antagonist, inhibits growth of the MC-26 mouse colon cancer (Fig 12-1). This suggests that antihormone treatment for colon cancer may become useful in a manner similar to that in which the antihormone (tamoxifen) is currently employed in the treatment of breast cancer. Analysis of gastrointestinal tumors for gastrointestinal hormone receptors may allow us to select those patients with gastrointestinal cancers who would respond to treatment with antihormones or hormone ablation. It may be possible in the future to develop therapeutic strategies for patients with gastrointestinal cancers that are based upon manipulation of the serum concentrations or effects of gastrointes-

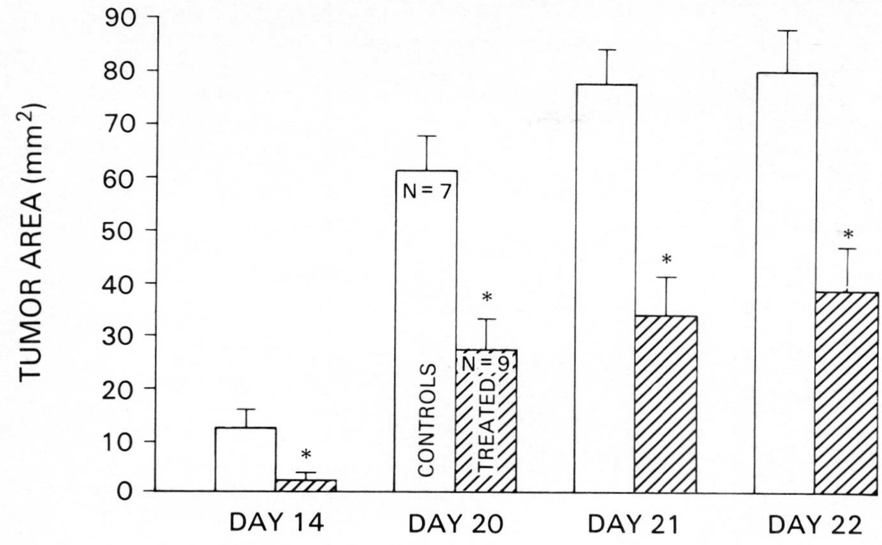

Figure 12-1. Tumor size in saline-treated controls compared to proglumide-treated (250 mg/kg tid) mice beginning on the day of inoculation of 5×10^4 tumor cells. (* = $p < 0.05$.) Mice received 5×10^4 MC-26 cells subcutaneously on day 1. (From Beauchamp et al [69], by permission of the JB Lippincott Co.)

tinal hormones in a manner similar to current strategies that are successfully employed in the treatment of patients with breast cancer.

The mitogenic effect of gastrointestinal hormones for colon, stomach, and pancreatic cancers could have important clinical applications. We speculate that it may one day be possible to affect growth of human tumors by manipulation of the serum concentrations of gastrointestinal hormones or by specific inhibition of their trophic action.

REFERENCES

1. CA—A Cancer Journal for Clinicians. 34:14, 1984.
2. Beatson GT: On the treatment of inoperable cases of carcinoma of the mamma: Suggestions for a new method of treatment, with illustrative cases. Lancet 2:104, 1896.
3. Huggins C, Bergenstal DM: Inhibition of human mammary and prostatic cancers by adrenalectomy. Cancer Res 12:134, 1952.
4. Huggins C, Scott WW: Bilateral adrenalectomy in prostatic cancer. Clinical features and urinary excretion of 17-ketosteroids and estrogen. Ann Surg 122:1031, 1945.
5. Balme HW: Metastatic carcinoma of the thyroid successfully treated with thyroxine. Lancet 1:812, 1954.
6. Lippman ME, Halterman RH, Leventhal BG, et al: Glucocorticoid-binding proteins in human acute lymphoblastic leukemic blast cells. J Clin Invest 52:1715, 1973.
7. Bayliss WM, Starling EH: The mechanisms of pancreatic secretion. J Physiol (Lond) 28:325, 1902.
8. Thompson JC, Marx M: Gastrointestinal hormones. Curr Probl Surg 21:1, 1984.
9. Johnson LR: New aspects of the trophic action of gastrointestinal hormones. Gastroenterology 72:788, 1977.
10. Brown J, Gallager ND: A specific gastrin receptor site in the rat stomach. Biochem Biophys Acta 538:42, 1978.
11. Soumarmon A, Cheret AM, Lewin MJM: Localization of gastrin receptors in intact isolated and separated rat fundic cells. Gastroenterology 73:900, 1977.
12. Takeuchi K, Speir GR, Johnson LR: Mucosal gastrin receptor. II. Physical characteristics of binding. Am J Physiol 237:E295, 1979.
13. Takeuchi K, Speir GR, Johnson LR: Mucosal gastrin receptor. III. Regulation by gastrin. Am J Physiol 238:G135, 1980.
14. Peitsch W, Takeuchi K, Johnson LR: Mucosal gastrin receptor. VI. Induction by corticosterone in newborn rats. Am J Physiol 240:G442, 1981.
15. Soll AH, Amirian DA, Thomas LP, et al: Gastrin receptors on isolated canine parietal cells. J Clin Invest 73:1434, 1984.
16. Townsend CM Jr, Thompson JC: Gastrinoma. Curr Probl Cancer 7:1, 1982.
17. Polacek MA, Ellison EH: Parietal cell mass and gastric acid secretion in the Zollinger-Ellison syndrome. Surgery 60:606, 1966.
18. Rosenlund ML, Crean GP, Johnson DG, et al: The Zollinger-Ellison syndrome in a 10-year-old boy. J Pediatr 75:443, 1969.
19. Sum P, Perey BJ: Parietal-cell mass (PCM) in a man with Zollinger-Ellison syndrome. Can J Surg 12:285, 1969.
20. Johnson LR, Guthrie PD: Effect of secretin on colonic DNA synthesis. Proc Soc Exp Biol Med 158:521, 1978.
21. Lehy T, Dubrasquet M, Bonfils S: Effect of somatostatin on normal and gastric-stimulated cell prolifer-

ation in the gastric and intestinal mucosae of the rat. Digestion 19:99, 1979.
22. Lehy T, Dubrasquet M, Brazeau P, et al: Inhibitory effect of prolonged administration of long-acting somatostatin on gastrin-stimulated fundic epithelial cell growth in the rat. Digestion 24:246, 1982.
23. Morisset J, Genik P, Lord A, et al: Effects of chronic administration of somatostatin on rat exocrine pancreas. Regul Pept 4:49, 1982.
24. Johnson LR, Guthrie PD: Proglumide inhibition of trophic action of pentagastrin. Am J Physiol 246:G62, 1984.
25. Petersen H, Grossman MI: Pancreatic exocrine secretion in anesthetized and conscious rats. Am J Physiol 233:E530, 1977.
26. Lee PC, Jensen RT, Gardner JD: Bombesin-induced desensitization of enzyme secretion in dispersed acini from guinea pig pancreas. Am J Physiol 238:G213, 1980.
27. Fender HR, Curtis PJ, Rayford PL, et al: Effect of bombesin on serum gastrin and cholecystokinin in dogs. Surg Forum 27:414, 1976.
28. Miyata M, Rayford PL, Thompson JC: Hormonal (gastrin, secretin, cholecystokinin) and secretory effects of bombesin and duodenal acidification in dogs. Surgery 89:209, 1980.
29. Obie JF, Cooper CW: Bombesin stimulates gastrin secretion in the rat without increasing serum calcitonin. Proc Soc Exp Biol Med 162:437, 1979.
30. Jensen RT, Charlton CG, Adachi H, et al: Use of ^{125}I-secretin to identify and characterize high-affinity secretin receptors on pancreatic acini. Am J Physiol 245:G186, 1983.
31. Sankaran H, Deveney CW, Goldfine ID, et al: Preparation of biologically active radioiodinated cholecystokinin for radioreceptor assay and radioimmunoassay. J Biol Chem 254:9349, 1979.
32. Jensen RT, Lemp GF, Gardner JD: Interaction of cholecystokinin with specific membrane receptors on pancreatic acinar cells. Proc Natl Acad Sci USA 77:2079, 1980.
33. Jensen RT, Moody T, Pert C, et al: Interaction of bombesin and litorin with specific membrane receptors on pancreatic acinar cells. Proc Natl Acad Sci USA 75:6139, 1978.
34. Barrowman JA, Mayston PD: The trophic influence of cholecystokinin on the rat pancreas. J Physiol 238:73P, 1973.
35. Solomon TE, Petersen H, Elashoff J, et al: Interaction of caerulein and secretin on pancreatic size and composition in rat. Am J Physiol 235:E714, 1978.
36. Townsend CM Jr, Franklin RB, Watson LC, et al: Stimulation of pancreatic cancer growth by caerulein and secretin. Surg Forum 32:228, 1981.
37. Dembinski AB, Johnson LR: Stimulation of pancreatic growth by secretin, caerulein, and pentagastrin. Endocrinology 106:323, 1980.
38. Johnson LR, Guthrie PD: Stimulation of rat oxyntic gland mucosal growth by epidermal growth factor. Am J Physiol 238:G45, 1980.
39. Dembinski A, Gregory H, Konturek SJ, et al: Trophic action of epidermal growth factor on the pancreas and gastroduodenal mucosa in rats. J Physiol 325:35, 1982.
40. Li AKC, Schattenkerk ME, deVries JE, et al: Submandibular sialadenectomy retards dimethylhydrazine-induced colonic carcinogenesis. Gastroenterology 78:1207, 1980.
41. Tilson MD: Colonic carcinogenesis after partial resection of small bowel and a single dose of dimethylhydrazine in rats. Surg Forum 31:413, 1980.
42. Oscarson JEA, Veen HF, Ross JS, et al: Ileal resection potentiates 1,2-dimethylhydrazine-induced colonic carcinogenesis. Ann Surg 189:503, 1979.
43. Williamson RCN, Bauer FLR, Oscarson JEA, et al: Promotion of azoxymethane-induced colonic neoplasia by resection of the proximal small bowel. Cancer Res 38:3212, 1978.
44. Harte PJ, Rayner AA, Munroe A, et al: Potentiation of dimethylhydrazine-induced adenocarcinoma at the suture line by major bowel resection. Surg Forum 31:411, 1980.
45. Celik C, Mittelman A, Lewis D, et al: Effect of colectomy on carcinogenicity of symmetrical dimethylhydrazine in rats. Surg Forum 31:415, 1980.
46. McGregor DB, Jones RD, Karlin DA, et al: Trophic effects of gastrin on colorectal neoplasms in the rat. Ann Surg 195:219, 1982.
47. Tahara E, Haizuka S: Effects of gastro-entero-pancreatic endocrine hormones on the histogenesis of gastric cancer in rats induced by N-methyl-N′-nitro-N-nitrosoguanidine; with special reference to development of scirrhous gastric cancer. Gann 66:421, 1975.
48. Tatsuta M, Itoh T, Okuda S, et al: Effect of prolonged administration of gastrin on experimental carcinogenesis in rat stomach induced by N-methyl-N′-nitro-N-nitrosoguanidine. Cancer Res 37:1808, 1977.
49. Deveney CW, Freeman H, Way LW: Experimental gastric carcinogenesis in the rat. Effects of hypergastrinemia and acid secretion. Am J Surg 139:49, 1980.
50. Takahashi T, Yamaguchi T, Bando K, et al: International Cancer Congress, Seattle, Washington, 1982, p 97 (abstract).
51. Winsett OE, Townsend CM Jr, Glass EJ, et al: Gastrin stimulates growth of colon cancer. Surgery, 99:302, 1986.
52. Sumiyoshi H, Yasui W, Ochiai A, et al: Effects of gastrin on tumor growth and cyclic nucleotide metabolism in xenotransplantable human gastric and colonic carcinomas in nude mice. Cancer Res 44:4276, 1984.
53. Hudd C, Euhus DM, LaRegina MC, et al: Effect of cholecystokinin on metabolism and growth of human cholangiocarcinoma. Gastroenterology 86:1118, 1984.
54. Lichtenberger L, Miller LR, Erwin DN, et al: Effect of pentagastrin on adult rat duodenal cells in culture. Gastroenterology 65:242, 1973.
55. Murakami H, Masui H: Hormonal control of human

colon carcinoma cell growth in serum-free medium. Proc Natl Acad Sci USA 77:3464, 1980.

56. Rae-Venter B, Simon PM, Townsend CM Jr, et al: Gastrin receptors in cultured human cells derived from carcinoma of the colon. Endocrinology 108:A153, 1981.
57. Kobori O, Vuillot M-T, Martin F: Growth responses of rat stomach cancer cells to gastro-entero-pancreatic hormones. Intl J Cancer 30:65, 1982.
58. Laburthe M, Rousset M, Chevalier G, et al: Vasoactive intestinal peptide control of cyclic adenosine 3′:5′-monophosphate levels in seven human colorectal adenocarcinoma cell lines in culture. Cancer Res 40:2529, 1980.
59. Estival A, Mounielou P, Trocheris V, et al: Presence of VIP receptors in human pancreatic adenocarcinoma cell line. Modulation of the cAMP response during cell proliferation. Biochem Biophys Res Commun 111:958, 1983.
60. Emami S, Gespach C, Forgue-LaFitte M-E, et al: Histamine and VIP interactions with receptor-cyclic AMP systems in the human gastric cancer cell line HGT-1. Life Sci 33:415, 1983.
61. Estival A, Clemente F, Ribet A: Adenocarcinoma of the human exocrine pancreas: Presence of secretin and caerulein receptors. Biochem Biophys Res Commun 102:1336, 1981.
62. Korc M, Meltzer PS, Trent J: Enhanced expression of the receptor for epidermal growth factor correlates with alterations of the short arm of chromosome 7 in human pancreatic cancer. Dig Dis Sci 30:978, 1985.
63. Singh P, Walker JP, Townsend CM Jr, et al: Mouse colon cancer and trophic effects of pentagastrin in relation to gastrin receptor levels in vivo. Dig Dis Sci 29:80S, 1984.
64. Singh P, Townsend CM Jr, Walker JP, et al: Gastrin receptors in a mouse colon cancer cell line responsive to trophic effects of gastrin. Surg Forum 35:205, 1984.
65. Rae-Venter B, Simon PM, Townsend CM Jr, et al: Receptors in human colon carcinoma. Gastroenterology 80:1256, 1981.
66. Singh P, Rae-Venter B, Townsend CM Jr, et al: Gastrin receptors in normal and malignant gastrointestinal mucosa: Age-associated changes. Am J Physiol 249:G761, 1985.
67. Singh P, Walker JP, Townsend CM Jr, et al: Role of gastrin and gastrin receptors on the growth of a transplantable mouse colon carcinoma (MC-26), in Balb/c mice. Cancer Res, 46:1612, 1986.
68. Horwitz KG, McGuire WL, Pearson OH, et al: Predicting response to endocrine therapy in human breast cancer: A hypothesis. Science 189:726, 1975.
69. Beauchamp RD, Townsend CM Jr, Singh P, et al: Proglumide, a gastrin receptor antagonist, inhibits growth of colon cancer and enhances survival in mice. Ann Surg 202:303, 1985.

Chapter 13

Circadian Rhythms of Gut Peptides

James N. Pasley, Ph.D., Norma H. Rubin, Ph.D., and Phillip L. Rayford, Ph.D.

Circadian rhythms are a major feature of an organism's adaptation to its environment. These rhythms represent important processes through which events in the internal environment are organized in time to permit maximal adaptation to the external environment [1]. The concepts of chronobiology have great potential application in research and in the practice of medicine [2]. Chronobiologic studies and recognition of the temporal organization of body function in humans may provide a baseline for what constitutes "normal" function as distinct from disease states.

The existence of regular rhythms of motor activity, secretion, and possibly absorption in the digestive tract is a concept that is receiving increasing acceptance. Although there is not much information concerning the rhythmic nature of gastrointestinal peptides in humans and experimental animals, available results suggest that changing plasma levels of gastrointestinal peptides signal changing levels of activity within target tissues and their control systems. In this chapter, we will summarize current knowledge concerned with the chronobiology of gastrointestinal peptides.

TERMINOLOGY

The range of frequencies of rhythms that has been found in living systems extends from cycles of less than a second to cycles of a year or more. Rhythms that occur with a frequency of about 24 $\pm$ 4 hours are called circadian (circa, about; diem, day). Ultradian rhythms have a frequency that is shorter than circadian; examples are electroencephalogram (EEG), rapid eye movement (REM), and peristalsis. Infradian rhythms have frequencies longer than circadian. The infradian domain has been subdivided into several regions such as circaseptan, a rhythm of about 7 days, and circannual, a rhythm of about one year. Regions in the ultradian and circadian domain have not as yet been delineated, except for the "specific ranges" of the electroencephalogram (cycles per second; delta, theta, alpha, and beta). This chapter will concentrate on rhythms with a frequency roughly corresponding to the 24-hour rotation of the earth, the circadian. The word diurnal is sometimes used synonymously with circadian, but diurnal is better used to describe animals that are active by day, as opposed to nocturnal animals, which are active by night.

STATISTICAL ANALYSIS

The statistical analysis of chronobiologic data is accomplished by conventional methods as well as by the cosinor procedure, an inferential statistical technique for assessing rhythms in time series [3]. In this technique, data are fitted to a 24-hour cosine curve by the method of least squares, and the rhythmic components are objectively determined [3]. The cosinor procedure objectively determines the following information. First, a probability value (P), which indicates the significance of the fit of the cosine curve to the data; if the P value is 0.05 or less, the fluctuation of the variable studied is presumed to be cyclic, not random. Second, the method determines point and interval estimates of the rhythm components: mesor, amplitude, and acrophase. The mesor is the rhythm-adjusted mean that is equivalent to the 24-hour arithmetic mean, provided that the data points are equidistant and cover an integral number of cycles. The amplitude is defined as one half the total extent of predictable change; it represents the distance between the mesor and the crest of the cosine function used to approximate the rhythm. We should recognize that the amplitude represents only one half of the total predictable extent of change and that it is not equivalent to the difference between the actual peak and trough of the time plot. The acrophase corresponds to the time when mean measured values are highest; however, it is not necessarily identical to the time when the "peak" value was recorded.

The acrophase is frequently expressed in negative degrees; if 360° = 24 hours, then −15° = 1 hour. Thus, if the reference point is local midnight, −15° would represent 0100 hour. The reason why negative degrees are used is in keeping with trigonometric convention. The cosinor permits one to compare the rhythm components objectively. For example, the acrophase of a variable under study may be shifted to an earlier or a later occurrence by some experimental manipulation. A substance or physical agent capable of causing such a "phase advance" or "phase delay" is called a phase-resetter.

The time plot of individual or averaged display of data as a function of time is called a chronogram. Often data will not be expressed in "clock hours" but will instead be expressed as HALO (hour after lights on), with the beginning of light being 0 hour. All other times are referred to this. Thus, 2 hours after lights on = 2 HALO, 14 hours after lights on = 14 HALO.

RHYTHMIC NATURE OF GASTROINTESTINAL PEPTIDES

Gastrin

Although periodic activity of the digestive tract is now well recognized, there is little information concerning circadian variation of gastrointestinal peptides in serum and tissue [4–8]. Gastrin has been the most extensively studied, but reports on circadian rhythms of gastrin in serum vary [5–7]. These differences in fluctuations of gastrin may result from differences in radioimmunoassay (RIA) or from the molecular form of gastrin measured by different antibodies [5]. Generally, circadian rhythm of serum gastrin in mice and rats with continuous access to food is characterized by high levels in the dark period and low levels during the light period [6,7].

In humans, gastrin concentrations reach their maximum from 8 PM to midnight and their nadir toward the end of the dark period [5,8]. Feeding may play a significant role, since it has been shown that the circadian rhythm of gastrin is dependent upon the feeding schedule [8,9]. Fasting humans have, in fact, been reported to have no rhythmic variation of serum gastrin [8].

In rats and mice deprived of food for at least 14 hours before sampling, serum gastrin levels were generally highest at the end of the dark period or very early in the light period and reached their lowest values at the end of the light period or very early in the dark period [4,6]. A 12-hour fast in rats resulted in lowering the mesor (rhythm-adjusted mean) and delayed the acrophase (time of occurrence of highest value) in serum gastrin [10]. Thus, the acrophase was shifted and the mesor was reduced by fasting, but the rhythm remained, in the sense that the highest levels occurred during the time of greatest feeding activity and the lowest levels during times of rest. In addition, a circadian rhythm of immunoreactive gastrin in brain tissue from fasting mice has also been identified (unpublished data) (Fig 13-1), with similar characteristics to that observed in serum from fasted mice. Thus, in both humans and mice, peak gastrin levels are related to feeding; the largest caloric intake is associated with the largest quantity of gastrin. Similarly, the lowest gastrin levels during the light period are associated with the smallest food and protein intake of the 24-hour period. The circadian rhythm of epinephrine appears to be nearly identical to the rhythm of gastrin, and epinephrine has been shown to induce the release of gastrin [9].

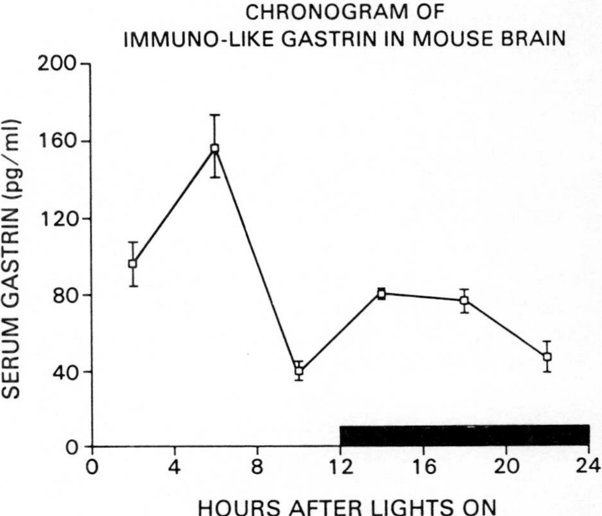

Figure 13-1. Circadian rhythm of immunolike gastrin extracted from mouse brain tissue. Data presented as hours after lights on (HALO). Bar from 12 to 24 hours = darkness.

The circadian variations of serum gastrin and pepsinogen in healthy individuals, duodenal ulcer patients, and pregnant women have been reported [11]. Patients with duodenal ulcers showed decreased gastrin mesors and increased serum pepsinogen compared to controls [11]. Pregnant women, on the other hand, showed increased mesors of serum gastrin and decreased mesors of serum pepsinogen. Thus, the pepsinogen/gastrin ratio may be a discriminatory marker of gastrin secretory capacity and may improve the physiologic significance of single gastrin or pepsinogen serum levels.

Periodic motor activity occurs in the fasting gut in humans and animals [12]. Trout et al [13] have provided evidence for a circadian rhythm in gastric emptying rates in rats. Temporal oscillations of activity in the proximal portion of the gastrointestinal tract, which includes gastric, pancreatic, and biliary secretory mechanisms, appear intimately related to the release of peptides [12]. The periodic activity of the gut ceases with feeding in animals and humans [12]. The rise in plasma levels of gastrin after feeding appears to be a part of this inhibition of activity in the proximal bowel but may not play a role in the inhibition of the distal bowel [14,15].

Gastrin is an important trophic hormone stimulating DNA synthesis in the small intestinal mucosa in vivo and in vitro, and this trophic action of gastrin is apparently necessary for maintaining a homeostatic environment along the gastrointestinal tract [16]. Feeding stimulates the release of gastrin, which has a stimulatory effect on intestinal cell proliferation [17]. All cells of the alimentary tract from tongue to anus divide with a circadian frequency, and this phenomenon has been demonstrated repeatedly by many investigators who have used several different techniques.

The common finding in all regions of the gut is that both DNA synthesis and mitosis are least active around the time of transition from light to darkness, but both increase in activity during the dark to reach a peak around the transition of darkness to light [18,19]. The phasing of rhythms is similar from one region of the gut to another, but the amplitude may vary considerably.

Cholecystokinin (CCK)

A diurnal variation in plasma CCK has been reported in six human subjects fed a standard diet [20]. The study did not, however, involve sampling over a 24-hour span. As might be expected, mean plasma CCK levels rose after each meal and remained elevated 2–3 hours after each meal. We have found a circadian rhythm in plasma CCK in rats fasted for 24 hours, with the acrophase occurring around midnight during the dark phase and the low point occurring in the early afternoon during the light phase. This would again indicate that CCK levels would be highest when the animals are normally feeding and are active [21].

Periodic motor activity in the foregut is inhibited by feeding in animals, and this inhibition of oscillatory activity has been correlated with increasing plasma levels of CCK [22]. Exogenous administration of CCK, however, does not suppress the periodic activity in the distal bowel [15]. Fasting for 24 hours or more has been reported to decrease tissue levels of CCK in the jejunum and ileum in the rat [23].

Pancreatic Polypeptide (PP)

A circadian variation in plasma levels of human PP (hPP) has been reported for humans fed a strictly controlled diet [24]. As with CCK, the plasma levels of hPP showed sharp peaks after each meal and were relatively stable during the night [24]. Periodic oscillations in the foregut of the dog are marked by cyclic rises in plasma levels of PP [25].

Secretin

In humans, plasma levels of secretin rose transiently after a meal and were highest during the dark period. Peak levels were measured some 7 hours after the evening meal before returning to basal levels by morning (Fig 13-2) [26]. The reason for the increase in plasma secretin some 7 hours after the last meal is unknown. Secretin has been reported to inhibit the circadian rhythm of intestinal cell renewal in rats [27] but has little effect on the incidence of cyclic migrating myoelectric complex in the small intestine [15].

Gastric Inhibitory Polypeptide (GIP)

In fed humans, serum GIP levels peak after each meal; they appear to remain elevated after meals until late evening, then fall to basal levels (Fig 13-3) [28,29]. A heavy late meal or a prolonged fast may alter the phasing of this rhythm the next day [29]. GIP is known to be released by the oral ingestion of glucose, fat, and amino acids [30,31]. In one study in which the male subjects were fed

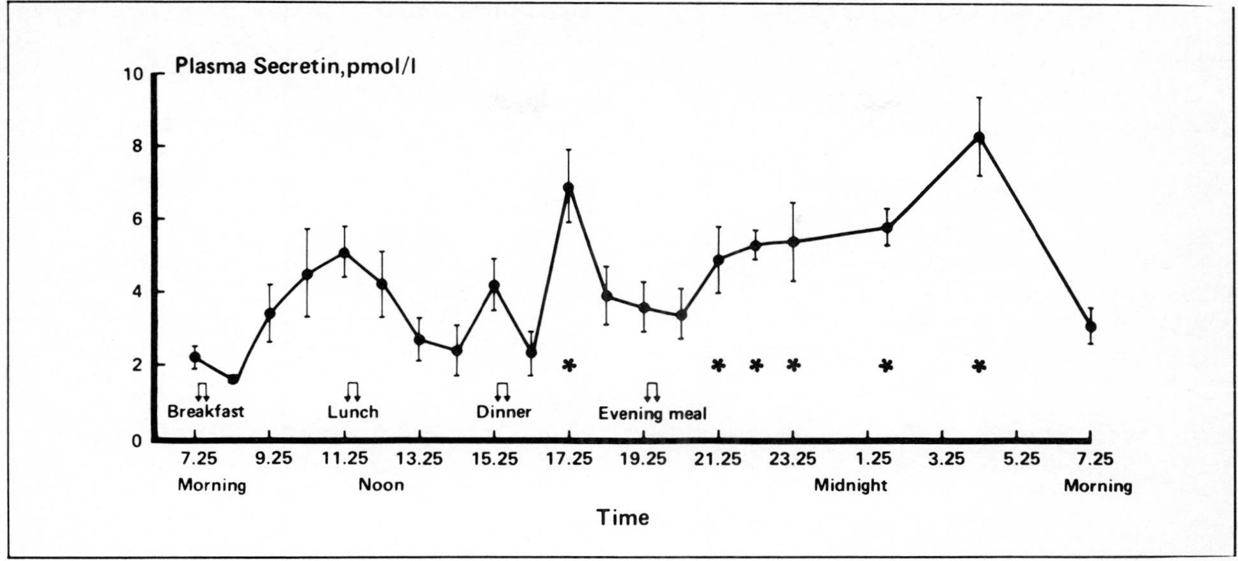

Figure 13-2. Diurnal profile of plasma secretin. Each point represents the mean of one examination in each of six healthy young males. The vertical bars are the standard errors of the means, and the asterisks indicate that the corresponding mean values differ significantly from the initial mean basal value ($p < 0.05$). (From Burhol et al [26], by permission of S. Karger AG, Basel.)

carbohydrate- and fat-rich meals, the GIP variations appeared to parallel the diurnal triglyceride changes [28].

In young adult rats on various feeding schedules, serum GIP levels (measured over a 24-hour period) varied significantly with time [32]. The re-

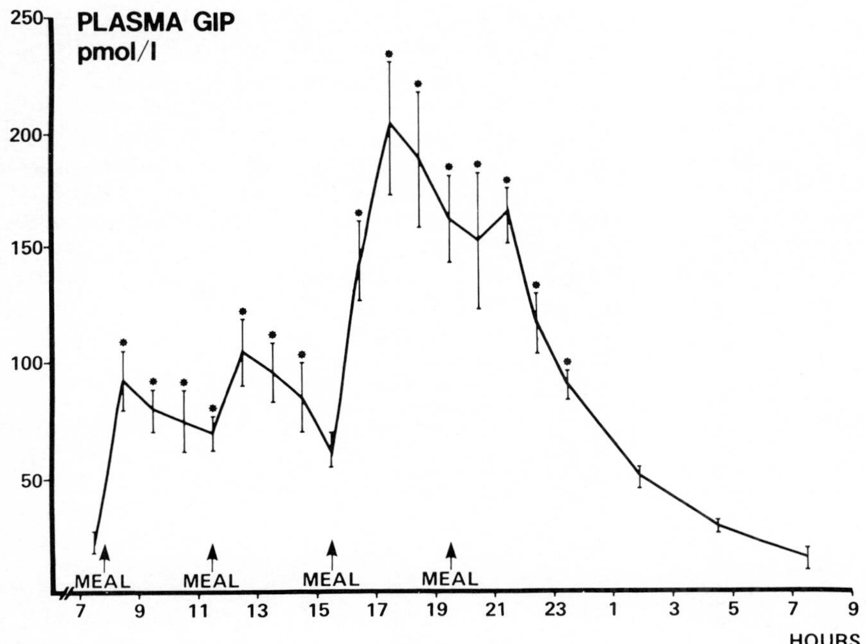

Figure 13-3. Plasma GIP during the 24-hour test period. Each point represents the mean of one examination in each of the six subjects. The vertical bars indicate the standard errors of the mean, and the asterisks indicate that the corresponding mean value differs significantly from the mean basal value ($p = 0.031$). (From Jorde et al [29], by permission of Universitetsforlaget.)

lease of GIP, however, was stimulated by food ingestion when food was presented in the 24-hour cycle. No circadian rhythm was detected in fasted rats, which suggested that this circadian rhythm is not endogenous but food-related.

Vasoactive Intestinal Peptide (VIP)

No significant alterations in plasma VIP levels were observed in fed women over a 24-hour period, even after meals [33]. Fasting levels of VIP are low and are relatively unchanged after food [34]. Since VIP is widely distributed in many tissues throughout the body, and since evidence suggests that it may act as a peptidergic neurotransmitter, plasma concentrations of VIP may reflect a wide variety of different activities from various parts of the body, not just the gastrointestinal tract [34]. Circadian variations of this peptide may, therefore, be difficult to detect.

VIP has widespread distribution throughout the gastrointestinal tract, with receptors in crypt and villus cells of the small intestine [35,36]. VIP can elicit accumulation of cyclic AMP in intestinal cells and thus may act as a potential mediator of crypt cell proliferation [37]. Consistent with the role of cyclic AMP as an inhibitor of intestinal cell proliferation, VIP has been found to inhibit incorporation of [^{3}H]thymidine in isolated intestinal segments in the rat [38].

Motilin

The motor activity of the gastrointestinal tract consists of two different patterns over a 24-hour period—one digestive, and the other interdigestive [39]. The interdigestive period is characterized by a migrating myoelectric complex (MMC), which is a cyclic caudal-moving band of contractions, interrupted by long-lasting motor quiescence. The interdigestive MMCs in the proximal portion of the gut are accompanied by rises in plasma motilin and can be induced by administration of motilin [12,39]. The ingestion of food causes the MMCs to cease. Thus, the circadian interdigestive gastrointestinal motor activity over a 24-hour period may be regulated by circulating concentrations of plasma motilin [12,39].

Epidermal Growth Factor (EGF)

EGF is found in human saliva [40], amniotic fluid [41], milk [42], and in Brunner's glands in duodenal mucosa [43]. A circadian rhythm of EGF concentrations has been demonstrated in the submandibular gland of the rat [43]. The absence of circadian periodicity of immunoreactive EGF, however, has been reported in plasma and urine of humans [43]. EGF may play an important role in the control of rhythms in cell proliferation in the digestive tract [19]. EGF stimulates oxyntic mucosal growth, as measured by in vitro incorporation of [^{3}H]thymidine, and it produces a circadian phase-dependent stimulation of DNA synthesis in duodenal, jejunal, ileal, cecal, colonic, and rectal tissues of male mice [44].

An increase in DNA synthesis in tongue and esophagus was noted at 4, 8, and 12 hours after injection of EGF in mice, while the stomach and colon responded only at 8 and 12 hours after injection [44]. The response to EGF in regard to cell proliferation of the gastrointestinal tract thus appears to be tissue-specific and related to the circadian stage at which it is administered [19].

Glucagon and Insulin

Circadian rhythms in the plasma concentrations of insulin and glucagon have been demonstrated in humans and in laboratory mammals kept under standardized conditions [24,45]. With insulin, these patterns are characterized in rodents by low levels during the light period and peaks during the dark [45]. A somewhat opposite variation occurs in humans, with high levels associated with daytime peaks and decreasing levels after midnight [24]. The circadian rhythm of glucagon is one of low amplitude, with peak levels occurring toward the end of the dark period in rodents [24]; in humans, peaks occur after food ingestion, followed by a trough in the early morning hours [45]. The circadian rhythms of insulin and glucagon are altered by constituents of the diet [45]. A high-protein diet results in a 3-fold increase in glucagon levels and a more pronounced circadian rhythm characterized by highest levels that occur during the dark period in rats [45]. A high-carbohydrate diet resulted in elevated insulin levels during the dark, whereas a high-protein diet did not induce a marked change [45].

SYNCHRONIZATION OF GASTROINTESTINAL RHYTHMS

Light-Dark Cycle Effects

The circadian rhythms of any system can be synchronized to periodic environmental events such as the light-dark cycle of nature. Thus, an investigator can synchronize the circadian system of a rodent to the light-dark cycle of the laboratory, which can follow a reasonably precise 24-hour frequency. Although the circadian system of humans is more likely to be synchronized to their social cycle, human circadian rhythms can be entrained by light-dark cycles [46]. Several rhythmic variables show internal synchronization in humans and rodents [2] (for example, the body temperatures of both are normally high when they are active and low when they are resting). In general, the approximate time when any phase of a rhythm will occur is quite predictable in relation to local time. If the exogenous synchronizing force such as constant light or constant darkness is removed, the circadian rhythm will follow its innate frequency, and the phasing will continuously change from day to day in relation to local clock time. Oscillations under these conditions are said to free-run.

Effects of Feeding and Meal Timing

Behavioral responses or components of ingested food may influence the phasing control of a particular circadian variable [46]. In singly housed mice exposed to cold stress and restricted to feeding one time per day, the timing of the meal affects their short-term survival [47]. When feeding occurs only in the first part of the light stage, most animals die, whereas if feeding is permitted during the first part of the dark cycle, most animals survive. The circadian stage at which the food is presented is important in determining whether or not an animal can adjust to such restriction [48].

Human subjects who consumed all of their daily calories at either breakfast or dinner lost weight when on the breakfast-only regime and gained weight when consuming only dinner, even though the caloric intakes were the same [48]. The circadian rhythms of insulin and glucagon differed on these two feeding regimens. Peak levels of insulin and glucagon appeared less than an hour apart on the breakfast-only regimen, but on the dinner-only regimen, there was a 5-hour difference in the peaks, with the insulin peak occurring earlier [48]. The consumption of food appears to play a vital role in the circadian rhythms of gastrointestinal hormones. The highest levels of many gastrointestinal peptides, however, occur in late evening, not just after dinner, so that meal-taking may not be the most important factor in the regulation of circadian variation of these peptides [49].

Diet content is also important in the rhythmicity of enzyme activities of the gastrointestinal tract. When one diet containing all carbohydrate and then another containing all protein were fed in alternate 12-hour periods, rhythms with 24-hour cycles were observed. Monosaccharide transport increased with the all carbohydrate meal and decreased when the protein meal started. Disaccharidase activities and mucosal protein and DNA levels all increased at the beginning of the protein meal, decreasing again at the onset of the carbohydrate meal [50]. Thus, protein feeding appears to cue a rise in enzyme activity that is independent of the clock time at which feeding occurs.

A circadian rhythm for exocrine pancreatic secretion has been reported in the rat and the chicken [51,52]. Circadian morphologic alterations identified in the rat pancreatic acinar cell appear to coincide with secretory variations [53]. A circadian rhythm of pancreatic lipase and amylase secretion that does not seem to be linked with circadian intestinal enzyme release has also been identified [54].

Meal timing also appears to affect circadian variations in cell proliferation in the gastrointestinal tract. In animals synchronized to a 12:12 light-dark cycle, feeding behavior, motor activity, and DNA synthesis begin to rise around the time of the light-dark transition [19]. When feeding is limited to a 4-hour period, the peak rhythms of DNA synthesis in organs such as the duodenum, esophagus, and tongue shift to coincide with the time food is presented [19].

Neural Control Factors

Central nervous system rhythms may play a role in the control of rhythmic fluctuations of gastrointestinal peptides. The vagus has been suggested as a possible controlling factor for the circadian variations in serum gastrin levels [6]. A loss of circadian rhythmicity of serum gastrin levels was reported in male Wistar rats after vagotomy, which suggested that the central nervous system controls the rhythm of serum gastrin via the vagus [6]. Christensen et al [5] showed that serum gastrin concentrations are increased by anticholinergic therapy and are decreased by beta-adrenergic blockade, even though the circadian rhythm of gastrin was maintained.

In mammals, a pacemaking system has been proposed whose function is to maintain daily order in physiologic processes, such as enzyme activities, body temperature, feeding, drinking behavior, the sleep-wake cycle, and hormone secretion [55,56]. The two suprachiasmatic nuclei (SCN) of the anterior hypothalamus are thought to be the most important pacemaker system involved in the generation of circadian rhythms. The circadian rhythms integrated by the SCN can be entrained (synchronized in phase and period) by time cues (Zeitgebers), such as the daily cycle of light of day and the dark of night. The Zeitgeber, or entraining stimulus, regulates the period of the endogenous oscillating system to 24 hours. In mammals, a visual pathway from the retina (retinohypothalamic tract) to the brain is necessary for mediating entrainment. The retinohypothalamic pathway terminates in the SCN area, which appears to mediate entrainment [55].

Lesions of the SCN have been found to disrupt circadian rhythmicity in a wide variety of physiologic variables, including locomotor activity, sleep-wakefulness cycle, adrenal corticosteroid release, pineal enzyme activity, body core temperature, and corneal mitotic index [57–60].

There has been some doubt as to whether humans possess an SCN. Recent evidence has shown a pair of neuronal clusters apparently homologous to the SCN in the human brain [56]. The human SCN may play the same functional role in the circadian system. Destruction of the area containing the human SCN by tumors disrupts the sleep-wake cycle [56] in a manner similar to that observed from lesion studies in animals.

We have studied the role of the suprachiasmatic nuclei in the coordination of rhythms in cell proliferation in various regions of the mouse intestinal tract, as measured by the incorporation of [^{3}H]thymidine into deoxyribonucleic acid [57,61]. The most consistent effect of SCN lesions was a phase advance in the rhythms in cell proliferation in the tongue (Fig 13-4), esophagus, gastric stomach, and colon. A reduction in rhythm amplitude occurred in the tongue and esophagus, while an amplitude increase was observed in the stomach and colon. The mesor rhythm (adjusted mean) was

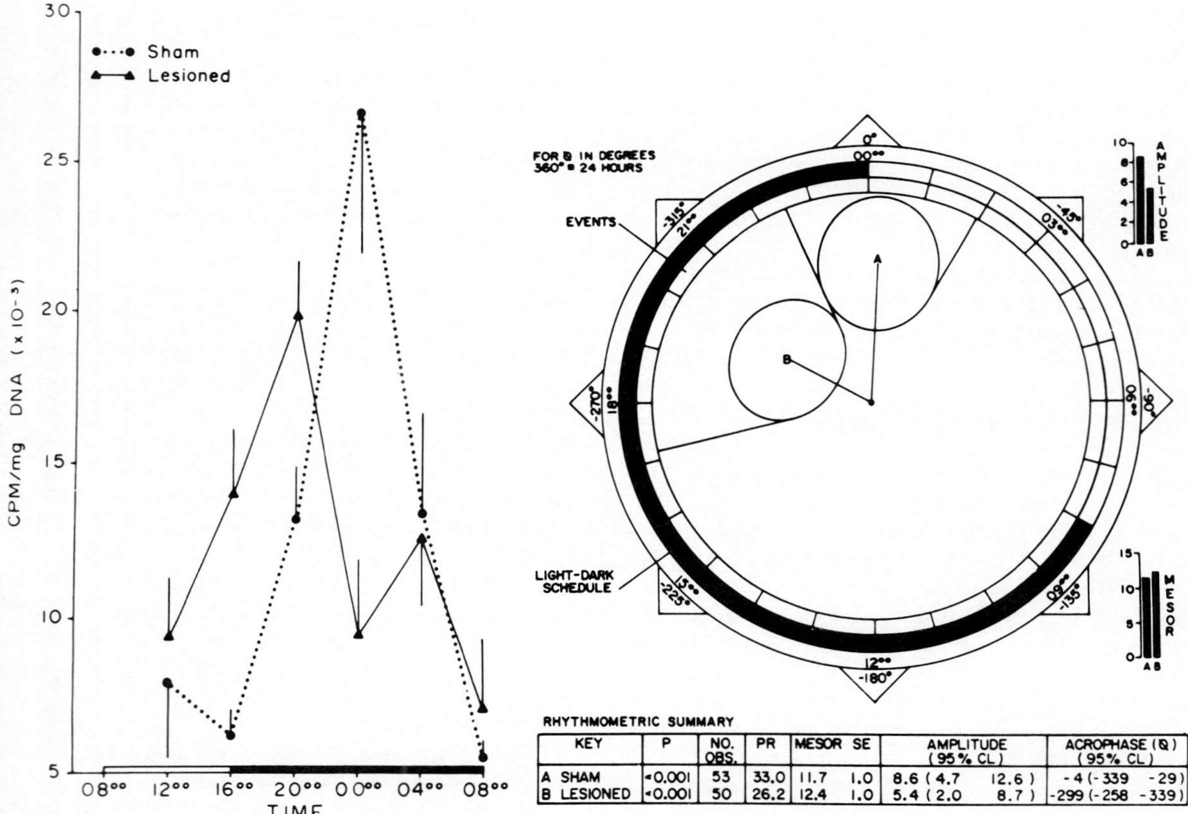

RHYTHMOMETRIC SUMMARY

KEY	P	NO. OBS.	PR	MESOR	SE	AMPLITUDE (95% CL)	ACROPHASE (ϴ) (95% CL)
A SHAM	<0.001	53	33.0	11.7	1.0	8.6 (4.7 12.6)	-4 (-339 -29)
B LESIONED	<0.001	50	26.2	12.4	1.0	5.4 (2.0 8.7)	-299 (-258 -339)

Figure 13-4. Circadian rhythm of [^{3}H]TdR incorporation into DNA of tongue; rhythm was phase-advanced by about 4 hours in experimental animals. Dots and vertical bars = mean and standard error (SE). Results of cosinor analysis are presented in polar plot, in which the rhythm's acrophase is indicated by the direction of the vector (in relation to circadian time scale). (From Scheving et al [58], by permission of Alan R. Liss, Inc.)

increased by SCN lesions in all tissues. Thus, we concluded that the SCN acts as a phase-resetter and amplitude modulator for cell proliferation in the gastrointestinal tract.

ENDOCRINE CONTROL FACTORS

The endocrine system has also been implicated as a possible controlling factor of circadian rhythms of the gastrointestinal tract.

Adrenocortical Hormones

Adrenalectomy has been shown to increase levels of serum gastrin in rats [62]. In addition, injections of pentagastrin produced a significant decrease in plasma corticosterone levels but had no effect on the normal evening increase in plasma corticosterone levels that is associated with circadian periodicity in rats [63]. Furthermore, a gastrin-like peptide may be involved in the modulation of ACTH secretion [63]. The rhythms of certain blood cell counts, enzyme levels, cell mitosis, and electrolytes are obliterated by adrenalectomy and are reinstated by periodic administration of adrenocortical hormones [47].

A short-chain synthetic analogue of ACTH, ACTH-17, has circadian stage (time of day)-dependent effects on cell proliferation in the rodent intestinal tract [19]. When given at different times, ACTH-17 may induce either an increase, a decrease, or no response in DNA synthesis in the tongue, esophagus, and stomach of mice [19].

REPRODUCTIVE HORMONES

Gonadal steroids have been shown to affect the normal circadian rhythm of locomotor activity [64]. Sex differences in circadian rhythms have been reported in mice in the weights of lymphoreticular organs, liver, kidney, and in the mitotic index of corneal epithelium [65]. The differences, if any, in gastrointestinal hormone production between sexes are unclear. The incidence of human gastric carcinoma is higher in men than in women [66–68], and the dominant histologic type in male patients is well-differentiated adenocarcinoma. In addition, female, castrated male, and estrogen-treated male rats showed a lower incidence of gastric cancer induced by *N*-methyl-*N*′-nitro-*N*-nitrosoguanidine (MNNG) than did nontreated male rats [69]. Others have reported that estrogens may protect against metaplastic change [70]. Moreover, female sex steroids have been reported to reduce gastrin levels in cats [71]. In contrast, serum gastrin levels in humans have been reported to be elevated during pregnancy compared to nonpregnant controls [72]. We have recently reported sex differences in the circadian rhythm of serum gastrin in rats, with male rats exhibiting higher levels and increased amplitude of serum gastrin compared to females [73]. Neurohypophyseal CCK has been reported to be higher in the male than in the female rat [74]. Neurohypophyseal CCK apparently varies according to the estrus cycle in the rat, with the highest content being during proestrus and estrus [75]. Although the roles of estradiol and testosterone in facilitating integrated circadian rhythmicity of gastrointestinal peptides may be subtle, the effects of their circadian rhythms on gastrointestinal peptides may be important.

REFERENCES

1. Rusak B, Zucker I: Neural regulation of circadian rhythms. Physiol Rev 59:449, 1979.
2. Scheving LE: Temporal variation in man, in Lassman G, Seitelberger F (eds): *Rhythmische Funktionen in Biologischen Systemen*. Vienna, Facultas-Verlag, 1977, pp 49–74.
3. Halberg F, Johnson EA, Nelson W, et al: Autorhythmometry procedures for physiologic self-measurements and their analysis. Physiol Teacher 1:1, 1972.
4. Ganguli PC, Forrester JM: Circadian rhythm in plasma level of gastrin. Nature 236:127, 1972.
5. Christensen KC, Stadil F, Malmstrom J, et al: The effect of beta-adrenergic and cholinergic blockade on the circadian rhythm of gastrins in serum. Scand J Gastroenterol 13:263, 1978.
6. Nagata M, Osumi Y: Circadian rhythm of serum gastrin level in rats. Jpn J Pharmacol 32:932, 1982.
7. Barnes CL, Pasley JN, Rayford PL: Circadian rhythm of serum gastrin in fed and fasted female Balb/C mice. Proc Soc Exp Biol Med 178:186, 1985.
8. Moore JG, Wolfe M: Circadian plasma gastrin patterns in feeding and fasting man. Digestion 11:226, 1974.
9. Feurle G, Ketterer H, Becker HD, et al: Circadian serum gastrin concentrations in control persons and in patients with ulcer disease. Scand J Gastroenterol 7:177, 1972.
10. Bosshard A, Pansu D, Chayvialle JA, et al: Effect of fasting and somatostatin administration on circadian rhythms of jejunal cell renewal and plasma gastrin level in rats. Digestion 23:245, 1982.
11. Tarquini B, Benvenuti M, Cavallini V, et al: Pepsinogen gastrin mesor ratio: A potential simple marker for gastric secretory function. Chronobiologia 11:11, 1984.
12. Wingate DL: Complex clocks. Dig Dis Sci 28:1133, 1983.
13. Trout DL, Aparicio P: Evidence of circadian variation

in gastric emptying rates in rats. Fed Proc 43:726, 1984.
14. Thomas PA, Schang J-C, Kelly KA, et al: Can endogenous gastrin inhibit canine interdigestive gastric motility? Gastroenterology 78:716, 1980.
15. Wingate DL, Pearce EA, Hutton M, et al: Quantitative comparison of the effects of cholecystokinin, secretin, and pentagastrin on gastrointestinal myoelectric activity in the conscious fasted dog. Gut 19:593, 1978.
16. Johnson LR: The trophic action of gastrointestinal hormones. Gastroenterology 70:278, 1976.
17. Korman MG, Soveny C, Hansky J: Effect of food on serum gastrin evaluated by radioimmunoassay. Gut 12:619, 1971.
18. Rubin NH, Hokanson JA, Mayschak JW, et al: Several cytokinetic methods for showing circadian variation in normal murine tissue and in a tumor. Am J Anat 168:15, 1983.
19. Scheving LE, Tsai TH, Scheving LA: Chronobiology of the intestinal tract of the mouse. Am J Anat 168:433, 1983.
20. Burhol PG, Rayford PL, Jorde R, et al: Radioimmunoassay of plasma cholecystokinin (CCK), duodenal release of CCK, diurnal variation of plasma CCK and immunoreactive plasma CCK components in man. Hepatogastroenterology 27:300, 1980.
21. Pasley JN, Barnes CL, Rayford PL: Circadian rhythms of serum gastrin and plasma CCK in rodents. Chronobiologia 12:263, 1985.
22. Schang J-C, Kelly KA: Inhibition of canine interdigestive proximal gastric motility by cholecystokinin-octapeptide (CCK-OP). Gastroenterology 78:1253, 1980.
23. Fujimura M, Sakamoto T, Greeley GH Jr, et al: Effect of fasting on secretin and cholecystokinin levels in the rat small intestine. Fed Proc 43:1072, 1984.
24. Tasaka Y, Inoue S, Maruno K, et al: Twenty-four hour variations of plasma pancreatic polypeptide, insulin and glucagon in normal human subjects. Endocrinol Jpn 27:495, 1980.
25. Keane FB, DiMagno EP, Dozois RR, et al: Relationships among canine interdigestive exocrine pancreatic and biliary flow, duodenal motor activity, plasma pancreatic polypeptide, and motilin. Gastroenterology 78:310, 1980.
26. Burhol PG, Jorde R, Lygren I, et al: Diurnal profile of plasma secretin in man. Digestion 22:192, 1981.
27. Pansu D, Berard A, Dechelette MA, et al: Influence of secretin and pentagastrin on the circadian rhythm of cell proliferation in the intestinal mucosa in rats. Digestion 11:266, 1974.
28. Salera M, Giacomoni P, Pironi L, et al: Circadian rhythm of gastric inhibitory polypeptide (GIP) in man. Metabolism 32:21, 1983.
29. Jorde R, Burhol PG, Waldum HL, et al: Diurnal variation of plasma gastric inhibitory polypeptide in man. Scand J Gastroenterol 15:617, 1980.
30. Brown JC, Dryburgh JR, Ross SA, et al: Identification and actions of gastric inhibitory polypeptide. Rec Prog Horm Res 31:487, 1975.
31. Thomas FB, Mazzaferri EL, Crockett SE, et al: Stimulation of secretion of gastric inhibitory polypeptide and insulin by intraduodenal amino acid perfusion. Gastroenterology 70:523, 1976.
32. Alinder G, Rubin NH, Greeley GH Jr, et al: Circadian variation in gastric inhibitory polypeptide in serum and tissue in the rat. Surg Forum 36:168, 1985.
33. Ottesen B, Ulrichsen H, Fahrenkrug J, et al: Vasoactive intestinal polypeptide and the female genital tract: Relationship to reproductive phase and delivery. Am J Obstet Gynecol 143:414, 1982.
34. Mitchell SJ, Bloom SR: Measurement of fasting and postprandial plasma VIP in man. Gut 19:1043, 1978.
35. Laburthe M, Bataille D, Rosselin G: Vasoactive intestinal peptide (VIP): Variation of the jejuno-ileal content in the developing rat as measured by radioreceptorassay. Acta Endocrinol 84:588, 1977.
36. Laburthe M, Prieto J, Amiranoff B, et al: VIP receptors in intestinal epithelial cells: Distribution throughout the intestinal tract, in Rosselin G, Fromageot P, Bonfils S (eds): *Hormone Receptors in Digestion and Nutrition*. New York, Elsevier/North-Holland Biomedical Press, 1979, pp 241–254.
37. Klein RM, McKenzie JC: The role of cell renewal in the ontogeny of the intestine. II. Regulation of cell proliferation in adult, fetal, and neonatal intestine. J Pediatr Gastroenterol Nutr 2:204, 1983.
38. Craven PA, DeRubertis FR: Cyclic nucleotide metabolism in rat colonic epithelial cells with different proliferative activities. Biochim Biophys Acta 676:155, 1981.
39. Itoh Z, Honda R, Hiwatashi K, et al: Motilin-induced mechanical activity in the canine alimentary tract. Scand J Gastroenterol 11 (Suppl 39):93, 1976.
40. Starkey RH, Orth DN: Radioimmunoassay of human epidermal growth factor (urogastrone). J Clin Endocrinol Metab 45:1144, 1977.
41. Carpenter G: Epidermal growth factor is a major growth-promoting agent in human milk. Science 210:198, 1980.
42. Barka T, van der Noen H, Gresik EW, et al: Immunoreactive epidermal growth factor in human amniotic fluid. Mt Sinai J Med 45:679, 1978.
43. Krieger DT, Hauser H, Liotta A, et al: Circadian periodicity of epidermal growth factor and its abolition by superior cervical ganglionectomy. Endocrinology 99:1576, 1976.
44. Scheving LA, Yeh YC, Tsai TH, et al: Circadian phase-dependent stimulatory effects of epidermal growth factor on deoxyribonucleic acid synthesis in the duodenum, jejunum, ileum, caecum, colon, and rectum of the adult male mouse. Endocrinology 106:1498, 1980.
45. Tiedgen M, Seitz HJ: Dietary control of circadian variations in serum insulin, glucagon and hepatic cyclic AMP. J Nutr 110:876, 1980.
46. Aschoff J: Circadian timing. Ann NY Acad Sci 423:442, 1984.
47. Halberg F: Implications of biologic rhythms for clinical practice. Hosp Prac 12:139, 1977.

48. Halberg F, Halberg E, Carandente F: Chronobiology and metabolism in the broader context of timely intervention and timed treatment, in Schattaner FK (ed): *Diabetes Research Today*. Symp. Med. Hoechst 12. Stuttgart, Thieme Verlag, 1976, pp 1–51.
49. Jorde R, Burhol PG: Diurnal profiles of gastrointestinal regulatory peptides. Scand J Gastroenterol 20:1, 1985.
50. Stevenson NR: Feeding and intestine digestive-absorptive rhythmicity, in Vener K (ed): *Chronobiology and the Digestive System*. NIH Publ. #84-857, 1984, pp 5–17.
51. Barrowman J, Brogan D, Fordham J, et al: A possible diurnal rhythm in rat pancreatic secretion. J Physiol 208:14P, 1970.
52. Salido GM, Madrid JA, Martin EA, et al: Circadian rhythmicity in the 'basal' pancreatic secretion of the domestic fowl. Chronobiologica Int 1:173, 1984.
53. Muller OM, Gerber HB: Circadian changes of the rat pancreas acinar cell. A quantitative morphological investigation. Scand J Gastroenterol 20 (Suppl 112):12, 1985.
54. George DE, Lebenthal E, Landis M, et al: Circadian rhythm of the pancreatic enzymes in rats: Its relation to small intestinal disaccharidase. Nutr Res 5:651, 1985.
55. Moore RY: Organization and function of a central nervous system circadian oscillator: The suprachiasmatic hypothalamic nucleus. Fed Proc 42:2783, 1983.
56. Moore-Ede MC: The circadian timing system in mammals: Two pacemakers preside over many secondary oscillators. Fed Proc 42:2802, 1983.
57. Halberg F, Lubanovic WA, Sothern RB, et al: Nomifensine chronopharmacology schedule shifts and circadian temperature rhythms in di-suprachiasmatically lesioned rats—modelling emotional chronopathology and chronotherapy. Chronobiologia 6:405, 1979.
58. Scheving LE, Tsai TH, Powell EW, et al: Bilateral lesions of suprachiasmatic nuclei affect circadian rhythms in [^{3}H]-thymidine incorporation into deoxyribonucleic acid in mouse intestinal tract, mitotic index of corneal epithelium, and serum corticosterone. Anat Rec 205:239, 1983.
59. Powell EW, Halberg F, Pasley JN, et al: Suprachiasmatic nucleus and circadian core temperature rhythm in the rat. J Therm Biol 5:189, 1980.
60. Powell EW, Pasley JN, Scheving LW, et al: Amplitude-reduction and acrophase-advance of circadian mitotic rhythm in corneal epithelium of mice with bilaterally lesioned suprachiasmatic nuclei. Anat Rec 197:277, 1980.
61. Pasley JN, Powell EW, Tsai TH: Alterations of circadian rhythms in cell division of the mouse gastrointestinal tract after bilateral suprachiasmatic nuclear lesions. Physiologist 26:A-78, 1983.
62. Majumdar APN: Bilateral adrenalectomy: Effects of hydrocortisone and pentagastrin on some structural and functional properties of the stomach of weanling rats. Scand J Gastroenterol 16:151, 1981.
63. Itoh S, Hirota R, Katsuura G, et al: Suppressive effect of pentagastrin on pituitary-adrenocortical secretion. Endocrinol Jpn 26:741, 1979.
64. Morin LP: Effect of ovarian hormone on synchrony of hamster circadian rhythms. Physiol Behav 24:741, 1980.
65. Tsai TH, Scheving LE, Scheving LA, et al: Sex differences in circadian rhythms of several variables in lymphoreticular organs, liver, kidney and corneal epithelium in adult CD2F1 mice. Anat Rec 211:263, 1985.
66. Sigdestad CP, Lesher S: Photo-reversal of the circadian rhythm in the proliferative activity of the mouse small intestine. J Cell Physiol 78:121, 1972.
67. Griffith GW: The sex ratio in gastric cancer and hypothetical considerations relative to aetiology. Br J Cancer 22:163, 1968.
68. Fujimoto I: Role of population-based cancer registry. Jpn J Cancer Clin 23:557, 1977.
69. Furukawa H, Iwanaza T, Koyama H, et al: Effect of sex hormones on the experimental induction of cancer in rat stomach—a preliminary study. Digestion 23:151, 1982.
70. Kirschbaum A: The role of hormones in cancer: Laboratory animals. Cancer Res 17:432, 1957.
71. Albinus M, Blair EL, Hirst F, et al: Effects of female sex hormones and adrenocorticotropin on feline gastrin and gastric secretions. J Endocrinol 69:449, 1976.
72. Steen J, Westergaard L: Gastrin and gastrointestinal dyspepsia in pregnancy. Acta Obstet Gynecol Scand 62:155, 1983.
73. Pasley JN, Barnes CL, Rayford PL: Sex differences in circadian rhythms of serum gastrin in rats. Dig Dis Sci 30:394, 1985.
74. Deschepper C, Lotstra F, Vandesande F, et al: Cholecystokinin varies in the posterior pituitary and external eminence of the rat according to factors affecting vasopressin and oxytocin. Life Sci 32:2571, 1983.
75. Goldman S, Van Reeth O, Schiffmann S, et al: Changes in neurohypophysial cholecystokinin content during oestrus cycle in the rat. Neurochem Int 6:779, 1984.

Section Four

Gastrin-CCK Family

Chapter 14

Gastrin

Isidoro Wiener, M.D., Talaat Khalil, M.D., James C. Thompson, M.D., and Phillip L. Rayford, Ph.D.

The science of endocrinology may well have begun on an afternoon in 1902 when Bayliss and Starling [1] demonstrated that acid introduced into the denervated loop of the small intestine caused the pancreas to secrete. The blood-borne chemical messenger released by the acidified intestine was named secretin, and later, according to Babkin [2], the word "hormone" was introduced by Starling at the suggestion of Hardy [3].

Edkins [4,5] reported in 1905 that extracts of antral mucosa stimulated acid secretion from the gastric fundus. He named the active principal in this extract gastrin. A long controversy followed over whether gastrin was contaminated with or was identical to histamine. The first method [6] for chemical extraction of gastrin that was free of histamine was not published until almost 60 years after Edkin's report, when Gregory and Tracy [7] isolated pure gastrin from the antral mucosa of hogs. The chemical structure and physiologic actions of gastrin were determined, and the compound has been synthesized [8,9]. Gastrin has been the subject of many reviews [10–17].

FORMS AND DISTRIBUTION

Studies on the molecular forms and tissue distribution of gastrin have served as prototypes for other regulatory peptides.

Chemistry of Gastrin

Several molecular forms of gastrin have been isolated and characterized. The gastrin molecule originally isolated by Gregory et al [9] consists of 17 linearly arranged L-amino acids, with a molecular weight of around 2100 daltons. The peptide exists in two near-identical variants, gastrin I without and gastrin II with an esterified sulfate attached to the tyrosyl residue at position 12. The N-terminal of the molecule is blocked by pyroglutamyl, and the C-terminal is blocked by an amide. The molecule has no basic amino acids, is strongly acidic, and is only slightly soluble in dilute acid [9]. Gastrin heptadecapeptides G-17-I and G-17-II have been isolated and purified from the antral mucosa of humans [18], hogs, dogs, cats, sheep, and cows (Table 14-1) [19].

Another larger form of gastrin has been isolated from serum and tumor tissue of patients with the Zollinger-Ellison (ZE) syndrome [7,20–23]. This form of big gastrin was found to exist in nonsulfated and sulfated forms, each form consisting of 34 amino acid residues, G-34-I and G-34-II, with molecular weights of 3800 to 3900 daltons [23,24]. The C-terminal 17 amino acid sequence of big gastrin, G-34, is identical to the structure of little gastrin (G-17) and possesses all the biologic actions of the heptadecapeptide. The amino acid sequence of G-34 from human gastrinoma and from hog antral mucosa has been determined (Table 14-1) [25].

A small form of gastrin has been detected in the serum of normal persons, in patients with pernicious anemia [26], and in mucosal extracts of patients with gastrinoma [25,27]. This form of gastrin, named minigastrin, was initially reported to contain 13 amino acid residues but now is known to have 14. It exists in unsulfated and sulfated forms, G-14-I and G-14-II. The amino acid composition of this pair of polypeptides is identical to the C-terminal tetradecapeptide of G-34 and G-17 (Table 14-1), and G-14 possesses all the physiologic actions of G-34 and G-17 [27].

Other forms of gastrin have been identified in serum and tissue of humans and animals. Big-big gastrin of Yalow et al [28,29] and component I of Rehfeld et al [26] are both, by chromatography and

Table 14-1. Amino acid sequences of gastrin*

Gastrin	Approximate molecular weight I	Approximate molecular weight II	
Little gastrin (G-17)			
Man	2098	2178	pGlu-Gly-Pro-Trp-Leu-Glu-Glu-Glu-Glu-Glu-Ala-Tyr[a]-Gly-Trp-Met-Asp-Phe-NH_2
Hog	2116	2196	pGlu-Gly-Pro-Trp-Met-Glu-Glu-Glu-Glu-Glu-Ala-Tyr[a]-Gly-Trp-Met-Asp-Phe-NH_2
Dog	2058	2138	pGlu-Gly-Pro-Trp-Met-Glu-Glu-Glu-Ala-Glu-Ala-Tyr[a]-Gly-Trp-Met-Asp-Phe-NH_2
Cow and sheep	2026	2106	pGlu-Gly-Pro-Trp-Val-Glu-Glu-Glu-Glu-Ala-Ala-Tyr[a]-Gly-Trp-Met-Asp-Phe-NH_2
Cat	2040	2120	pGlu-Gly-Pro-Trp-Val-Glu-Glu-Glu-Ala-Glu-Ala-Tyr[a]-Gly-Trp-Met-Asp-Phe-NH_2
Minigastrin (G-14-I, 5-17)			
Man	1833		pGlu-Gly-Pro-Trp-Leu-Glu-Glu-Glu-Glu-Glu-Ala-Tyr-Gly-Trp-Met-Asp-Phe-NH_2
Big gastrin (G-34-I)			
Man	3839		pGlu-Leu-Gly-Pro-Gln-Gly-His-Pro-Ser-Leu-Val-Ala-Asp-Pro-Ser-Lys-Lys-[b]Gln-Gly-Pro-Trp-Leu-Glu-Glu-Glu-Glu-Glu-Ala-Tyr-Gly-Trp-Met-Asp-Phe-NH_2
Hog	3883		pGlu-Leu-Gly-Leu-Gln-Gly-Pro-Pro-His-Leu-Val-Ala-Asp-Leu-Ala-Lys-Lys-[b]Gln-Gly-Pro-Trp-Met-Glu-Glu-Glu-Glu-Glu-Ala-Tyr-Gly-Trp-Met-Asp-Phe-NH_2
Pentagastrin	768		N-t-butyloxycarbonyl-β-Ala-Trp-Met-Asp-Phe-NH_2

* Except where noted, the amino acid sequences for gastrins of different species are identical.
[a] Gastrin of each species exists in forms I and II; in form I, there is no SO_3H attached to Tyr in position 12.
[b] Point of cleavage by trypsin.

RIA analyses, larger molecules than big gastrin. Big-big gastrin and component I have not been characterized chemically or assigned biologic actions. A crude form of big-big gastrin has been isolated from tumor tissue [23]. A pair of inactive gastric fragments is present in hog antral mucosa that was demonstrated to have the *N*-tridecapeptide sequence of G-17 [9]. Repeated filtrations of serum on large Sephadex columns suggest the existence of no less than 20 different gastrins (6 component I, 6 G-34, 4 G-17, 4 G-14) [30].

Some fragments of G-34 found in plasma in humans do not occur in antral extracts and are not produced when G-34 or its N-terminal fragments are incubated in plasma in vitro. These fragments are presumed to be generated from the 1-17 sequences by the action of peptidases found on capillary walls. This 1-17 fragment of G-34 did not influence acid secretion when administered to humans alone or in combination with hG-17 [31].

Two gastrins, comprising the N-terminal 1 to 13 portion of the heptadecapeptide (G-1-13, I and II), have been isolated from the antral mucosa of hogs [25], and material that corresponds immunologically and chromatographically to this was isolated from the serum and tumor of patients with gastrinoma [32,33]. These gastrins lack the active C-terminal tetradecapeptide and are not known to be biologically active. After intravenous infusion of secretin, the concentration of G-1-13 in the serum of patients with Zollinger-Ellison tumors was found to increase rapidly, which led Dockray [32] to suggest that this form of gastrin may be stored by the tumor together with G-17 and G-34.

A variety of abnormally processed gastrins are synthesized and released to the circulation during the active period of duodenal ulcer disease, including component I, G-34, G-17, G-14, and the tridecapeptide, and all of them appear in sulfated and nonsulfated forms. In addition, a C-terminal glycine-extended peptide corresponding to each (nonsulfated and sulfated) molecular form of gastrin has been reported in high concentrations during active but not inactive periods of duodenal ulcer disease. These glycine-extended forms are inhibitors of gastric acid secretion and may participate in the regulation of acid secretion during the active periods of duodenal ulcer disease [34]. In duodenal ulcer patients, fasting serum concentrations of G-34 are twice those of G-17; however, both components increase similarly after a meal. In duodenal ulcer patients with previous subtotal gastrectomy and gastroduodenostomy, concentrations of all gastrin components, except G-34, are significantly lower compared to those of unoperated ulcer patients [35].

The antral concentration of the N-terminal gastrin fragment is higher in patients with active duodenal ulcer compared to that of normal controls or patients with gastric ulcers or pernicious anemia. On the other hand, there is no difference in duodenal gastrin forms among these groups [36]. After a meal, the serum concentrations of the N-terminal tridecapeptide-like fragment of G-1-13 increase markedly in patients with active duodenal ulcer compared to those of healthy subjects. The infusion of G-1-13 into healthy subjects, in doses that result in concentrations similar to those measured in duodenal ulcer patients, inhibits the acid response to a meal and to exogenous G-34, G-17, and pentagastrin but not to G-4 [37].

Sulfation of gastrin forms in serum, antrum, and duodenum is reduced in patients with hypergastrinemia associated with gastric ulcer or pernicious anemia when compared to healthy humans or patients with duodenal ulcer [38].

The larger forms of gastrin appear to be less active and are less sensitive to catabolism. Whether the larger forms are precursors of the smaller forms is controversial. Gregory and Tracy [25] did suggest that G-34 is a precursor of G-17, but Rehfeld et al [30] reported the conversion of G-17 to G-34 in circulation. Walsh et al [39], in studies in which G-34 and G-17 were infused into humans, found no evidence of conversion of G-34 to G-17 in plasma, nor were there increases in G-34 after the infusion of G-17. Since the three smaller forms of gastrin plus component I and big-big gastrin may react equally on a molar basis with gastrin antiserum, measurements of total gastrin may not correlate with biologic activity. We should further bear in mind that endogenous G-17 may be cleaved during passage from the gastrin cells to the antral vein; the products of this conversion, rather than G-17 itself, are considered by Dockray et al [40] to most likely be the physiologically important form of gastrin in dogs.

Distribution

In all species investigated, antral mucosa is the richest source of gastrin. Gastrin is apparently synthesized by the G cells located in the pyloric glands of antral mucosa [41] and in the proximal part of the small intestine [42,43]. The G cell population of the pyloric antrum of cats has been reported to range from 10.3 to 15.4 million cells [44]. Antral gastrin content correlates well with mucosal pH [45], but not enough is known of the histologic structure of gastric mucosa to answer the crucial question of whether G cells begin at the point that parietal cells end. The total mass of gastrin in the human duodenum is estimated to be as much as that in the human antrum [42], but a study by Rehfeld et al [30] suggests that the antrum contains five to ten times more gastrin than the duodenum. The concentration of gastrin in the antrum in normal humans has been reported to be slightly greater than that found in patients with duodenal ulcer [46]. The ratio of gastrin (G) and somatostatin (D) cells appears to be controlled by the antral pH; the G:D ratio increases in states of reduced acid secretion and decreases in massive hyperchlorhydria [47].

The duodenum reportedly accounts for all basal gastrin in antrectomized patients, 40–50 percent of basal gastrin in unoperated patients, and up to 33 percent of gastrin released by a meal in unoperated subjects. These results suggest that the duodenum is a major source of extra-antral gastrin.

Gastrin extracted from human antral mucosa and jejunum contains a greater amount of G-17, whereas duodenal extracts have been reported to consist of amounts of G-34 greater than [46,48] or equal to amounts of G-17 [30]. Considerable amounts of gastrin-like immunoreactivity are found in human gastric juice, and on characterization these are similar to gastrin 1-17 [49]. Biologically active luminal pentagastrin has no effect on gastric mucosa, even at nonphysiologic concentrations [50]. In other species, such as dogs [40,51] and rats [52], an even greater portion of gastrin is situated in antral tissue, with diminishing concentrations in the mucosa of the small intestine from duodenum to ileum [40,51]. Little gastrin, G-17, is a predominant immunoreactive form found in antral mucosa extracts of dogs, whereas a smaller gastrin, probably G-14, is the principal form found in duodenal extracts [53]. Fragments of little gastrin have been found to react with the extracts of homogenates of brain, especially the cortical gray matter of humans, dogs, pigeons, trout, and frogs [54].

Molecular Genetic Studies

Both porcine and human gastrin cDNA have been cloned [55,56]. The human gastrin gene is about 4100 base pairs long and contains two intervening sequences. A 3500 base pair intervening sequence is located five base pairs proximal to the ATG initiator codon, while a 129 base pair sequence separates the region coding for the principal hormonal form of gastrin, the heptadecapeptide, from the region coding for the major N-terminal portion of gastrin precursor [57,58]. The primary translation product of gastrin mRNA consists of 101 and 104 amino acids in humans [55] and pigs [56], respectively. The post-translational modifications of this product involve cleavages of peptide bonds and derivations of amino acids [59]. A trypsin-like enzyme cleaves the precursor peptide at the C-terminal site of the pairs' basic residues (e.g., Lys-Lys or Arg-Arg). An important modification in the C-terminal of gastrin is the amidation of phenylalanine, which renders the peptide biologically active. Sulfation of the tyrosyl residue occurs in less than half of the gastrins [60]. Recently, Sugano et al [61] suggested that active G-17 is formed by the amidation of its glycine-extended form rather than by the cleavage of G-34. Furthermore, they proposed that the initial step in the post-translational processing may involve amino-terminal processing of progastrin into each of the C-terminal extended components. There is no direct evidence available for the existence of progastrin in tissues, but Sugano and Yamada [62] recently identified and characterized progastrin-like immunoreactivity in porcine stomach using antisera that recognized a synthetic progastrin peptide as deduced from the nucleotide sequence of gastrin mRNA. Two peptides purified from a human gastrinoma, peptides A and B, were found to correspond to the amino acid sequence deduced for the amino-terminal portion of human and porcine progastrin [63,64]. Immunochemical studies with antibodies to these two peptides have shown that they are localized predominantly in the antral mucosa in pigs, ferrets, dogs, and cats but not in humans, guinea pigs, rats, or mice [65].

ASSAY

Concentrations of gastrin in test samples have been measured by bioassay, using stimulation of gastric acid secretion as an indicator [66]. The sensitivity of bioassays is insufficient to detect the small quantities of gastrin in serum of normal individuals or in most patients. In addition, the gastrin bioassays may lack specificity.

After the initial success of McGuigan [67], several sensitive, specific, and precise radioimmunoassays were developed that are capable of detecting concentrations of gastrin in serum

[21,26,68–71]. Gastrin radioimmunoassays have been used to study changes in serum gastrin levels that occur under physiologic conditions. Fasting serum gastrin levels have been reported to range from 20 to 400 pg/mL [72,73]. Results of a cooperative study between several laboratories indicated that there was a wide interlaboratory variation in gastrin measurements [74]. These variations may be due to the use of different assay methods, iodination techniques, gastrin standard or gastrin antisera, or any combination of these [21,26,74,75].

PHARMACOKINETICS AND CATABOLISM

Heptadecapeptide gastrins from different species are similar except for the substitution of one or two amino acids (see Table 14-1) [76]. The C-terminal tetradecapeptide portion of the gastrin molecule has all the known biologic actions of the whole molecule [77,78], and the C-terminal tripeptide amide has distinct biologic activity [79,80]. The N-terminal G-17 fragment plays a significant role in the regulation of gastric acid secretion in patients with active duodenal ulcers [37].

Expressed as the exogenous dose required to obtain a given response, the molar potency of gastrin increases with chain length, that is, from G-14 to G-34 [11,81]. In contrast to this, Valenzuela et al [82] found that exogenous doses of G-17 and G-34 were approximately equipotent in stimulating gastric and pancreatic protein secretion in dogs. The ratio of potency of gastrin on gallbladder and pancreatic secretion to potency for acid secretory effect does not vary with chain length; these are essentially constant for G-4 through G-34. In terms of the blood level needed to give definitive response, however, G-17 has been reported to be more potent than either G-14 or G-34 [83]. On a molar basis, the relative potencies of exogenous G-34, G-17, and G-14 are 3:2:1, and the relative potencies based upon increments of serum concentrations are 1:4:2, respectively [81,83]. In the fasting state, the ratio of G-34 and G-17 is about 2:1. Postprandially, the ratio is 1:1. G-14 is about 5 percent of the total gastrin concentration [84]. The number of gastrin receptors decreases during fasting without altering the affinity of the receptor for the hormone [85]. In a cytochemical bioassay with induced carbonic anhydrase response as the indicator of acid secretion in guinea pig parietal cells, G-34 had a higher overall carbonic anhydrase activity than G-13 and G-17 [86].

Gastrin has been shown, by direct measurement, to disappear rapidly from the circulation after it has been injected intravenously [87] or after its release has been blocked by acidification of the antrum [21]. The disappearance half-time (T½) of the various molecular forms of exogenously infused gastrin has been reported [88]. The half-life of heptadecapeptide gastrin in dogs is 2.1 minutes [89], that of big gastrin is 15 minutes [81], and that of minigastrin is 1.8 minutes [90]. Yalow and Berson [21] demonstrated a disappearance half-time of 7 minutes for endogenous plasma gastrin after antral acidification in patients with pernicious anemia. We found that endogenously released, mixed-molecular gastrin in dogs has a half-life of 8.6 minutes (Fig 14-1); however, two different half-times, 2.8 and 15.4 minutes, could be calculated, probably corresponding to the times of G-17 and G-34 [91].

The effects of vascular transit of the liver, kidney, small intestine, lung, and hind limb on exogenously administered and endogenously released gastrin have been studied in dogs [88,92–94]. Mackie et al [95] showed, in monkeys, that the rate of catabolism of exogenous gastrin is not decreased after distal small bowel resection. A single passage through the liver resulted in reduction of the concentrations of G-17 and pentagastrin by 46 and 95 percent, respectively [96]. Later studies on the hepatic uptake of gastrin showed that diminution of heptadecapeptide gastrin during portal transit was not significant when the mass of gastrin entering and leaving the liver and the concentration of gastrin in bile were measured and calculated. Gastrin fragments comprising less than 8 amino acid residues are more than 90 percent inactivated by portal transit [89]. The degree of hepatic inactivation decreases with increasing chain length (G-9, G-10, and G-14), and no significant inactivation of G-17 and G-34 is found in humans [97] and dogs [98] in vivo and in rats in vitro [99]. In contrast, Gimmon et al [100] found that an apparent clearance of gastrin by the liver or lung or both is enhanced by the administration of intravenous hypercaloric nutrients.

The kidney was thought to be the most important known site of the catabolism of gastrin. Significantly elevated plasma gastrin concentrations were found in anephric patients and patients with acute and chronic renal failure, which decreased to normal after kidney transplantation or when kidney function returned to normal [101]. Radioimmunoassay measurements of arterial and venous concentrations after gastrin was injected into dogs showed that passage through the kidney resulted in approximately 40 percent diminution

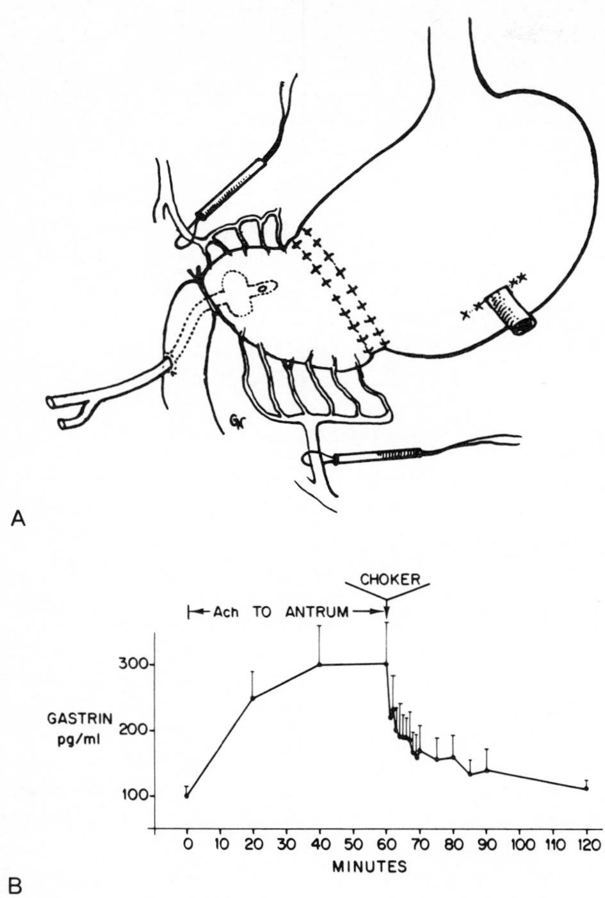

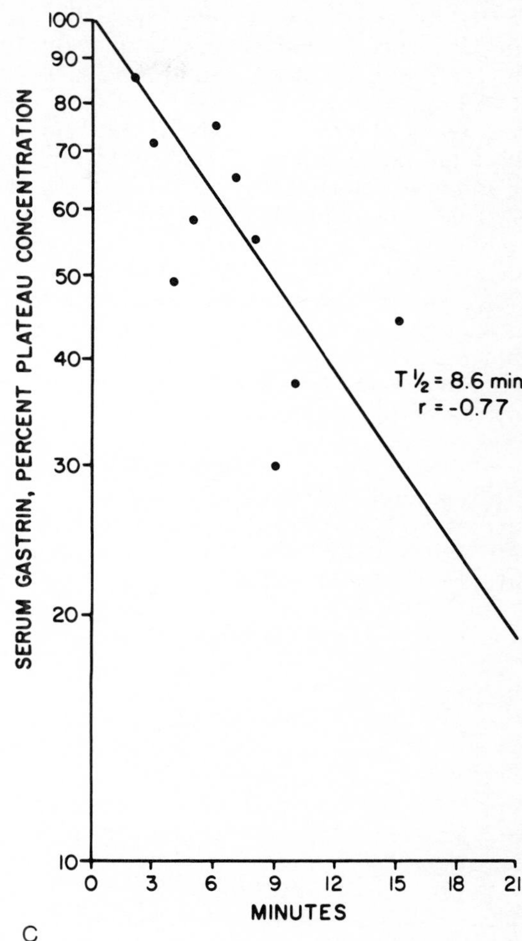

Figure 14-1. Calculations of metabolic half-life (T½) of circulating endogenous gastrin in dogs. ***A.*** Diagram of preparation of isolated antral pouch and gastric fistula. Total blood supply of antrum was isolated on the greater and lesser curvatures; each pedicle was encircled with a choker. (From Villar et al [91], with permission of the CV Mosby Co.) ***B.*** Absolute gastrin values before, during stimulation, and after the chokers were tightened. (From Villar et al [91], with permission of the CV Mosby Co.) ***C.*** Semilogarithmic plot of the half-time (T½) of endogenous gastrin. The points represent actual percent values of each time period. The solid line is the best-fitted curve calculated by linear regression analysis (r = correlation coefficient). (From Villar et al [91], with permission of the CV Mosby Co.)

of gastrin concentration [88]. In studies on the uptake of endogenous gastrin by the kidney, there was no significant difference in the mass of gastrin in the renal artery and the renal vein during basal and suppressed states, but the mass of gastrin leaving the kidney during periods of endogenous release was significant, about 35 percent less than the mass of gastrin presented to the kidney. Urinary gastrin excretion was less than 0.4 percent of that entering the kidney [102].

Bilateral nephrectomy in rats results in increased serum gastrin levels without any changes in basal acid secretion [103]. Increases in gastrin levels were found after nephrectomy in rats with and without antrums, which suggests that the kidney catabolizes both antral and duodenal gastrin. Taylor et al [104] found the human kidney to be unimportant in the metabolism of G-17, since circulating G-17 is six times more potent than G-34 in stimulating acid secretion. They suggest that raised gastrin concentrations observed in patients with chronic renal failure are of little significance in terms of the increased incidence of duodenal ulcer disease in these patients.

Temperly et al [105] showed that the gastric secretory response to synthetic human gastrin was diminished when gastrin was given by infusion into the mesenteric artery as compared with administration through a peripheral vein. Becker et al [106] found that during the basal state, endogenous levels of gastrin in the mesenteric vein of dogs were not significantly different from those in the abdominal aorta, but when gastrin release was stimulated by nutrient irrigation of the antrum, concentrations of gastrin in the mesenteric vein were significantly less than those in the aorta. Some evidence exists that the gastric fundus eliminates gastrin and that the extraction rate increases when acid is secreted by the stomach [107], and it has been suggested that the lung may be [108] and may not be [92] an important site for the removal of gastrin [108].

The NH_2-terminal tridecapeptide fragment of G-17 is known to circulate in higher concentrations than other forms of gastrin in gastrinoma patients and in patients with acute duodenal ulcers and gastritis. Peterson [109] suggested that the increasing NH_2-terminal (1-13) of G-17 was not caused by a decreased metabolism of this fragment. He also showed that it reduced gastric acid secretion. Lilja et al [110] found that 6 weeks after 75 percent intestinal resection, meal-stimulated concentrations of serum gastrin were significantly increased. They returned to preoperative levels within 10 weeks. Transient postresectional hypergastrinemia may result from a loss of a distal inhibitor.

Thompson et al [94] found that the integrated uptake of endogenous and exogenous gastrin by the kidney, hind leg, and the head was similar in dogs and concluded that extraction of gastrin occurs during transit of all capillary beds and appears to be a nonspecific process. Peterson et al [111] could not demonstrate extraction of gastrin in any vascular beds of the head, lung, liver, kidney, and legs in patients with mild hepatic parenchymatous disease. They suggested that gastrin degradation is not confined to certain specific organs but takes place in many organs or perhaps in the total volume of distribution of gastrin. Recently, Movsas et al [112] reported the presence of an enzyme (gastrinase) in tissue extracts of rat kidney, liver, and brain that is specific for degradation of G-34. The liver and brain enzymes appear less specific than the kidney enzyme [112].

Grossman [10] maintained that removal of gastrin from the circulation was too rapid to be caused by extraction by any specific organ but rather must be due to some nonspecific widespread catabolic process, probably existing in circulating serum. When we restudied the problem, we did find similar uptake across a peripheral muscle bed to that we found across the kidney [94]. As usual, Grossman was right, but there are some lingering bits of evidence to suggest that although all capillary beds may extract gastrin equally, the renal bed may be first among equals.

RELEASE

Gastrin is released by mechanical, neural, or chemical stimuli that act on the G cell (Table 14-2) [76]. Chemicals that release gastrin are either carried by blood, released from nerve endings, or contained in ingested food substances that bathe the luminal projections of the G cell. Some of the chemicals that have been reported to release gas-

Table 14-2. **Release of gastrin**

Chemical
- Bile salts
- Bombesin
- Calcium
- Epinephrine
- Ethanol
- Gastrin-releasing factor
- Glycine alanine
- L-Arginine
- Magnesium
- Phenylalanine
- Topical application of acetylcholine
- Topical application of partially digested proteins
- Tryptophan

Mechanical
- Distention of antrum
- Distention of fundus

Neural
- Cephalic stimulation
- Sham feeding
- Vagotomy

Suppression
- Atropine (except food)
- Acidification of antrum
- Bethanechol
- Calcitonin
- GIP
- Glucagon
- Hyperglycemia
- Secretin
- Somatostatin
- Some synthetic prostaglandin analogues, e.g., enprostil
- VIP

trin in humans are calcium [113,114], magnesium [115],epinephrine [116], and L-arginine hydrochloride [117]. In patients with gastrinoma and hyperparathyroidism, release of gastrin is attributable to elevated blood levels of calcium [118]. We showed that calcium given either intravenously [113,114] or orally [119] (Fig 14-2) may play a role in gastrin-stimulated acid secretion in humans. Patients with duodenal ulcers are more sensitive to this calcium-dependent mechanism than nonduodenal ulcer subjects [120]. The interrelations among gastrin, calcium, and calcitonin are covered in Chapter 32.

In dogs, insulin-induced hypoglycemia [121], sham feeding [122], topical application of acetylcholine to the antral mucosa [71,123], duodenum, and jejunum [124], distention of the antrum [125], distention of the fundus [126], and topical application of partially digested proteins [127], ethanol [128], bile salts [129], some amino acids [127], and food [122] have been shown to stimulate the release of gastrin. In contrast, Service et al [130] found that insulin-induced hypoglycemia resulted in no change in gastrin levels, and using the euglycemic clamp, insulin was found to have a direct suppressive effect on gastrin. Johnson and Guthrie [131] found in rats that food in the gastrointestinal tract is not required for either gastrin release or synthesis.

The release of gastrin in humans may be more complex. Proteins, peptones, and amino acids have all been demonstrated to release significant amounts of gastrin [132–135]. Hirschowitz [136] found that effectiveness in stimulating gastrin release was coffee = mannitol < Sustacal = Vivonex < solid food. The specific amino acids that are most potent gastrin releasers in humans are tryptophan and phenylalanine. Both are also the most potent amino acid stimulants of acid secretion [137]. The position and availability of the amino groups seem to be critical for the ability of the amino acids to act in a stimulatory way. Glycine, for example, is a potent stimulant but is considerably less active when the amino group is methylated, yielding sarcosine. Also, the stimulatory action of alanine is reduced when the amino group is present in the alpha instead of the beta position [138]. Iso-osmolar ethanol releases gastrin, probably by a specific effect on gastrin cells. However, the release of gastrin by hyperosmolar solutions of ethanol, sucrose, and urea is probably a nonspecific effect and is caused by damage of gastric mucosa [139]. The effect of a hypo-osmolar solution of sodium taurocholate—a well-known gastric mu-

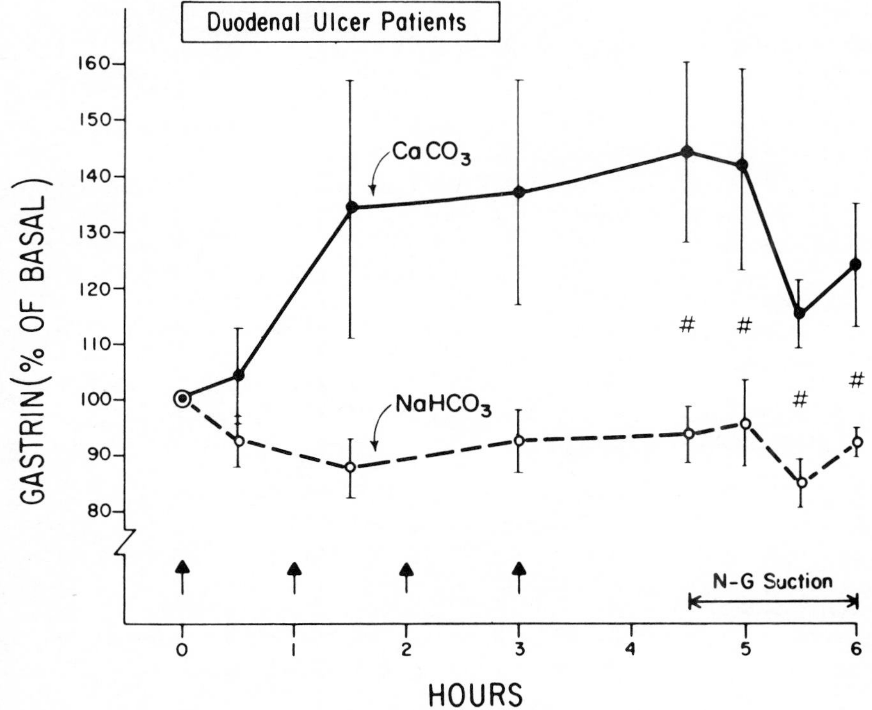

Figure 14-2. Changes in serum concentration of gastrin (expressed as percent of basal gastrin concentration) following ingestion of either $CaCo_3$ or $NaHCO_3$. Values represent the mean ± SE for 12 duodenal ulcer patients. Arrows denote times of administration of the antacid. Significant differences ($p = 0.05$) between the two curves are indicated by #. (From Reeder et al [119], with permission of the American College of Surgeons.)

cosal barrier breaker—on gastrin release supports this hypothesis.

Vagal release of gastrin is more important in some species, such as dogs [121] and rats [140], than in others, such as humans [141] and chickens [140]. Atropine administered to cats has been reported to decrease gastrin levels and the gastric acid response to food, but the effect appears to be a transient one, lasting for only one hour [142]. Basal and food-stimulated serum gastrin levels increase after vagotomy in humans and dogs [143] and in the isolated perfused rat stomach [144]. The post-vagotomy basal hypergastrinemia may result from increased stimulation of a normal G cell population at the ganglionic level [144]. After vagotomy in dogs, atropine suppresses but does not abolish the gastrin response to food [145]. Atropine abolishes gastrin release in dogs after all stimuli except food [122,146]. Atropine increases rather than inhibits stimulated gastrin release in humans [114,147]. The mechanism responsible for this increase is unclear but does not appear to be related to changes in intragastric pH, since atropine continues to invoke a significant gastrin response, even when the pH is held constant [147]. The major effect of atropine is probably cholinergic, whereas the mechanism for food-induced release of gastrin is either noncholinergic or highly resistant to atropine [122]. There seems to be support for the existence of intracerebral cholinergic mechanisms involved in the release of gastrin and peripheral cholinergic mechanisms mediating inhibitory effects on gastrin release [148]. Gastrin response to cephalic stimulation in humans is enhanced by low doses of atropine [149].

In humans, distention of the intact stomach stimulates acid secretion, not accompanied by a rising serum gastrin level [150]. Schubert et al [151] suggested a model in which gastric secretion is regulated by two interdependent intramural neurons: cholinergic neurons that stimulate gastric secretion indirectly by inhibition of somatostatin secretion, and a noncholinergic neuron that stimulates gastric secretion directly by release of a peptide stimulant, probably bombesin. Noncholinergic, vagal release of gastrin may be mediated by bombesin-containing peptidergic nerves, since bombesin-like activity has been found in postganglionic vagal fibers in the rat stomach [152]. Cholinergic mechanisms normally facilitate meal-stimulated gastrin release in humans, since unlike gastrin release stimulated by sham feeding or distention, gastrin release stimulated by an amino-acid meal is reduced by low doses of atropine [153]. Hirschowitz et al [154] found a muscarinic cholinergic pathway leading to gastrin release by food. Debas et al [155] showed that vagal stimulation of gastrin release is mediated along direct antral vagal pathways, while vagal inhibition requires intact vagal fibers from the proximal stomach. We found an increase in stimulated levels of gastrin release in humans after proximal selective vagotomy in studies in which the pH of the stomach was kept constant by intragastric titration [156]. This is evidence for an inhibitor of gastrin release that is activated by vagal stimulation of the proximal stomach.

Further evidence of cholinergically mediated mechanisms of inhibition of gastrin release were found by Taylor et al [157], who observed that bethanechol inhibits the release of gastrin by bombesin in dogs. Walsh and Lam [14] suggested that cholinergic inhibitory fibers were present in the gastric fundus and that the origin of the increased basal gastrin after vagotomy was from the antrum. Although cholinergic mechanisms appear to mediate most forms of gastrin release in dogs, the role in human physiology requires clarification. Vagal inhibition of gastrin release in humans may be more potent than stimulation of release.

Epinephrine stimulates serum gastrin secretion in the basal state and in response to a meal [158]. Furthermore, since vagotomy in humans [141] does not abolish gastrin release in response to insulin-induced hypoglycemia, other noncholinergic mechanisms, perhaps adrenergic [159], appear to mediate this response. Plasma gastrin and norepinephrine concentrations were reported to be higher in duodenal ulcer patients than in normal controls, both during and after a meal [160]. A peptide meal in the intestine of humans increased acid output without increasing circulating serum levels of gastrin.

Ayalon et al [161] found that gastrin was released from the antrum in dogs during the intestinal phase of gastric acid secretion; significantly increased levels of gastrin were detected in both antral and peripheral venous blood. This finding had previously been rejected [162].

Konturek et al [163,164] reported that a liver extract meal kept selectively in the stomach or the duodenum of dogs caused an increase in serum gastrin levels and in acid output. The gastric meal was about twice as potent in releasing gastrin when compared with an intestinal meal. The amount of gastrin decreased stepwise upon acidification of the meal, and it was suggested that secretin might inhibit release of endogenous gastrin, since duodenal acidification releases secretin [165].

The peptide bombesin (see Chapter 25) stimulates gastrin release in humans, dogs, and cats when injected intravenously [166,167]. Gastrin-releasing peptide (GRP) also stimulates gastrin release in dogs [168] and rats [169]. Chronic bombesin administration in rats causes antral gastrin cell hyperplasia and increases both gastrin release and antral gastrin content [131,170], independent of the presence of food in the gastrointestinal tract. This suggests that either bombesin itself or the actual release of gastrin is a sufficient stimulus for increasing gastrin biosynthesis [131].

In patients with duodenal ulcers, bombesin produces an increase in plasma gastrin output similar to that obtained in normal subjects; this is in contrast to gastrin stimulated by a meal, which causes significantly higher release in duodenal ulcer patients [171]. Bombesin antiserum inhibits neurally mediated gastrin release from the isolated perfused rat stomach, and its effect is additive to that of atropine, indicating that bombesin and acetylcholine are the main intramural neural regulators of gastrin [172]. Acetylcholine acts predominantly to decrease the paracrine secretion of somatostatin, thereby perhaps eliminating the continuous restraint of somatostatin on gastrin secretion and enabling bombesin to exert its potent stimulatory effect on gastrin release [172].

Antrectomy has been reported to abolish the rise in serum gastrin levels that follows introduction of liver extract into the intestine [173]. We found that introduction of liver extract into an isolated duodenal pouch caused an increase in gastrin concentration in the venous effluent of an isolated antrum; duodenal acidification abolished this response [174]. Patients with moderate pancreatic exocrine dysfunction tend to show high acid outputs and low serum gastrin levels, while those with severe dysfunction have slightly lower acid outputs and higher serum gastrin levels [175].

Release of gastrin is suppressed by acidification of the antral mucosa [176]. A typical endocrine closed-loop relation exists between gastrin and hydrogen ions. Gastrin causes secretion of hydrogen ions from parietal cells and, once the antral pH reaches about 1.5, hydrogen ions suppress release of gastrin from antral G cells (see Fig 9-3). Acid suppression of gastrin release is dose-related [123] and, even with strong stimuli, may not be complete [136]. Continuous gastric alkalinization for 5 hours increases serum gastrin levels in humans [177].

Infusion of somatostatin inhibits both gastrin release and gastric acid secretion [178]. The inhibition of gastrin release by somatostatin may be a direct effect on the G cells, since it abolishes the in vitro responses of the gastric antrum to arginine [179]. Somatostatin suppresses both gastrin-stimulated [180] and food-stimulated [181] gastric acid secretion, which suggests that the inhibitory effects might also be caused by a different influence on the secretory cells of the stomach [180]. Thomas [182] found that somatostatin is a strong inhibitor of pentagastrin-stimulated acid secretion and of gastrin release, but it is a weak inhibitor of acid secretion stimulated by histamine.

The mechanism by which somatostatin exerts its negative control over gastrin release and gastric acid secretion is not completely understood. The inhibitory action of somatostatin on stimulated gastrin release in rat antral organ cultures may be at least in part by interrupting a cyclic AMP-dependent component of the secretory process [183]. Whether somatostatin inhibits acid secretion by mechanisms independent of gastrin is not certain. Intravenous infusion of pharmacologic doses of somatostatin into humans [178], dogs [182], and rats [184] inhibits pentagastrin-stimulated gastric acid secretion, suggesting a direct action on the parietal cells. When antibodies to somatostatin are perfused into isolated rat stomachs in the presence of pentagastrin, acid output increases significantly over controls without concomitant significant changes in gastrin concentration [185]. In rats, the inhibitory effect of somatostatin on acid secretion is prevented by indomethacin pretreatment, suggesting that somatostatin may act indirectly via endogenous prostaglandins [184].

Suppression of gastrin release is brought about by all members of the secretin family of hormones —secretin [186], glucagon [187,188], GIP [189], and VIP [189]. The inhibitory action of these agents in the isolated perfused rat stomach is mediated, at least partially, through the release of antral somatostatin [190–192]. These same peptides inhibit the action of gastrin on oxyntic cells. In humans, both gastrin release and gastric secretion in response to a test meal are diminished by hyperglycemia [193], which may be attributed to the release of GIP by glucose. On the other hand, the hypergastrinemia observed in type II diabetes is probably due to autonomic dysfunction with slow gastric emptying [194]. Although natural prostaglandins may not affect gastrin release, some synthetic prostanoids (for example, enprostil [195,196]) do inhibit gastrin release. Calcitonin has also been shown to inhibit the release of gastrin and its action on hydrogen ion secretion in normal humans [197], cats [198], and patients with peptic ulcer disease [199] and parathyroid adenoma

[200]. Secretin and calcitonin significantly inhibit the serum gastrin and gastric acid responses to bombesin [201]. Although calcitonin gene-related peptide does inhibit gastric secretion, it does not alter gastrin release after bombesin or a meal (unpublished data from our laboratory [202]. Moreover, gastrin and pentagastrin stimulate calcitonin secretion, which appears to be a pharmacologic rather than a physiologic phenomenon [203].

Secretin stimulates gastrin release in patients with ZE tumors [186,204]. In these patients, secretin infusion causes a brisk increase in circulating levels of gastrin, compared with a depression of postprandial gastrin levels in normal patients and in patients with a usual form of ulcer disease. Secretin releases gastrin in vitro from tissue cultures of gastrinoma tissue [205]. Imamura et al [206] suggested that gastrinoma cells have receptors that bind with secretin, resulting in the release of gastrin.

Evidence of pituitary control of gastrin synthesis and release has been obtained from studies in which hypophysectomy caused significant atrophy of gastric and intestinal mucosa and a reduction in parietal cell population [207,208]. Crean [209] suggested that this effect is caused by a specific pituitary deprivation, since it could not be accounted for by inhibition of somatic growth. It is probably not related to deprivation of adenocorticotropic hormone, in rats at least, since adrenalectomy did not cause reduction in mucosal growth [209]. Surgical removal of a pheochromocytoma resulted in a significant decrease in both serum epinephrine and gastrin concentrations in the basal state and after food stimulation [158]. Acid secretion increases in rats when small amounts of pentagastrin are administered to the hypothalamus [210]. Pawlikowski et al [211] found coexistence of acromegaly and gastrinoma in two patients who were free of peptic symptoms.

Since elevated serum calcium levels are known to release gastrin, the role of parathormone (PTH) in the mild hypergastrinemia seen in some patients with hyperparathyroidism has been unclear. PTH was recently found to induce gastrin release from the gastric antrum without concomitant systemic hypercalcemia [212] or any change in the somatostatin level in antral venous blood [213].

Gastrin levels have been found to vary directly with thyroid function in patients with hyper- and hypothyroidism [214–216], and treatment with T_4 has been shown to be trophic for gastrin cells and to release gastrin in the rat [217]. We have found that acute and chronic hyperthyroidism in the rat causes hypergastrinemia, along with elevations in antral mucosal concentrations of gastrin-releasing peptide and diminished antral concentrations of somatostatin (unpublished studies by G. Greeley).

Inoue et al [218] found increases in integrated gastrin release in response to a meal 2 and 3 weeks after total colectomy in dogs. Following removal of the antrum, gastrin content in the proximal duodenum was increased several fold as compared with controls [219]. Prior to pancreaticoduodenectomy, gastrin secretory function was within the normal range; it was significantly reduced postoperatively [220]. Cimetidine blocked the stimulation of oxygen uptake and aminopyrine accumulation in isolated canine parietal cells caused by histamine. Cimetidine prevents the enhancement caused by histamine but had no effect on the direct stimulation of gastrin [221].

Basal levels of gastrin are higher in neonates and in elderly subjects [222]. During pregnancy, there is a progressive increase in gastrin levels, reaching peak levels during labor [223]. The mean serum gastrin concentrations in maternal and cord blood are significantly higher than serum gastrin levels found in normal, healthy, nonpregnant women [224], with umbilical gastrin concentrations higher than maternal levels [223]. The higher fetal gastrin concentrations are attributable to the advanced state of development of the gastrointestinal system of the newborn [223]. Gastrin and several other gut hormones rise steeply after early enteral feeding in newborns, reaching concentrations higher than those seen in fasting adults [225]. (For further information regarding gastrin metabolism in the fetal and newborn periods, see Chapter 11.) Feldman et al [226] found that, compared with men, women release greater amounts of gastrin but at the same time are less sensitive to stimulation of acid secretion by gastrin.

ACTIONS

The major physiologic action of gastrin is to stimulate acid secretion from the stomach. Gastrin stimulates acid secretion by at least three separate actions: direct stimulation of parietal cell activity; potentiating interaction with histamine, a paracrine stimulus; and, quantitatively, by the release of histamine. None of the actions of gastrin appears to involve a change in cyclic AMP metabolism [227]. Proglumide inhibits gastrin-stimulated gastric acid secretion; it appears to be a specific competitive gastrin receptor blocker [228].

Johnson [229] has provided clear evidence that

gastrin is a trophic hormone for gastric, fundic, and intestinal mucosa and for the pancreas. Gastrin directly stimulates those biochemical processes, deoxyribonucleic acid and ribonucleic acid synthesis, that are involved in tissue growth. Pentagastrin has been shown to prevent pancreatic atrophy that is normally seen in rats after hypophysectomy [230]. Rats subjected to hypophysectomy were found to have low levels of serum and antral gastrin [231,232]. Administration of growth hormone resulted in significantly higher levels of gastrin in serum and mucosa and reversal of gastrointestinal atrophy, suggesting that growth hormone acts through gastrin to produce its gastrointestinal effects.

The trophic effects of gastrin on the stomach and pancreas may be physiologic. Gastrin administered parenterally to adult rats promotes growth of the gastrointestinal tract, as evidenced by increases in DNA and RNA content and DNA synthesis [233]. In patients with gastrin-secreting tumors, hypertrophy and hyperplasia of gastric mucosa have been observed [234]. Chronic endogenous hypergastrinemia in rats produced by implantation of gastric antrum into the colon causes pancreatic and colonic hypertrophy independent of acid secretion and small bowel enlargement only when gastric hyperacidity is present [235]. Gastrin administered directly into the lumen of the small intestine of rats produces trophic effects without changes in circulating gastrin [236]. No effect was observed when gastrin was infused into the stomach, indicating no physiologic role for luminal gastrin in the normal acid-secreting stomach. In contrast to adults, gastrin is present in significantly higher concentrations in fetal sheep gastric juice than in plasma [237]. Gastrin in the lumen of the fetal gastrointestinal tract may have a unique maturational role [238]. Proglumide blocks the trophic action of exogenous gastrin in rats, which suggests that the trophic effect of gastrin is mediated by the gastrin receptor [239].

Gastrin also stimulates pepsin secretion and increases gastric mucosal blood flow. It causes electrolyte and water secretion by the stomach [7], pancreas [240,241], liver [242], and Brunner's glands [243]. Gastrin stimulates the function of parietal cells isolated from canine fundic mucosa [244,245]. These effects of gastrin are potentiated by interaction with histamine [246,247]. Whether gastrin effects on parietal cells are direct or through a second mediator is controversial. Gastrin stimulates histamine release from isolated gastric glands in rabbits [248] and increases histamine formation in the rat fundic mucosa but not in the dog [247]. It causes minimal, if any, direct stimulation of parietal cell function in isolated gastric glands of rabbits [227]. Soll et al [249] recently showed the presence of specific receptors for gastrin in the canine parietal cells.

A controversy over the role of gastrin in lower esophageal sphincter (LES) contraction smoldered for years. Most students agree that gastrin causes LES contraction but only when given in supraphysiologic amounts. In achalasia, no change was found in serum gastrin concentrations after somatostatin infusion; however, LES pressure was decreased significantly [250]. Dennis et al [251] found that the LES response to a protein stimulus was not altered by endogenous hypergastrinemia, which suggested that endogenous gastrin does not play a major role in the regulation of LES pressure. Jensen et al [252] found that total change in serum G-17 and G-34 after a peptone meal approached the threshold stimulation of LES pressure for these forms of gastrin but was not accompanied by a significant increase in LES pressure. Supraphysiologic doses of G-17 and G-34, however, have similar potencies for stimulation of human LES pressure.

REFERENCES

1. Bayliss WM, Starling EH: The mechanisms of pancreatic secretion. J Physiol (Lond) 28:325, 1902.
2. Babkin BP: *Secretory Mechanism of the Digestive Glands.* 2nd Ed. New York, Paul B. Hoeber Inc, 1950, p 560.
3. Bayliss WM: *Principles of General Physiology.* 4th Ed. London, Longmans, Green and Co, 1924, p 112.
4. Edkins JS: On the chemical mechanism of gastric secretion. Proc Roy Soc Lond 76:376, 1905.
5. Edkins JS: The chemical mechanism of gastric secretion. J Physiol 34:133, 1906.
6. Komarov SA: Gastrin. Proc Soc Exp Biol Med 38:514, 1938.
7. Gregory RA, Tracy HJ: The constitution and properties of two gastrins extracted from hog antral mucosa. Part 1. The isolation of two gastrins from hog antral mucosa. Gut 5:103, 1964. Part II. The properties of two gastrins isolated from hog antral mucosa. Gut 5:107, 1964.
8. Anderson JC, Barton MA, Gregory RA, et al: Synthesis of gastrin. Nature 204:933, 1964.
9. Gregory H, Hardy PM, Jones DS, et al: The antral hormone gastrin. Structure of gastrin. Nature 204:931, 1964.
10. Grossman MI (ed): *Gastrin: Proceedings of a Conference Held in September 1964.* Berkeley, University of California Press, 1966.
11. Walsh JH, Grossman MI: Gastrin. N Engl J Med 292:1324; 1377, 1975.
12. Rayford PL, Thompson JC: Gastrin. Surg Gynecol Obstet 145:257, 1977.

13. Rehfeld JF, Amdrup E (eds): *Gastrins and the Vagus.* New York, Academic Press, 1979.
14. Walsh JH, Lam SK: Physiology and pathology of gastrin. Clinics Gastroenterol 9:567, 1980.
15. Walsh JH: Gastrin, in Bloom SR, Polak JM (eds): *Gut Hormones.* New York, Churchill Livingstone, 1981, pp 163–170.
16. Walsh JH: Gastrointestinal hormones and peptides. Gastrin, in Johnson LR (ed): *Physiology of the Gastrointestinal Tract.* New York, Raven Press, 1981, pp 60–72.
17. Bribian Amengual J, Alastrue Tierra MA, Criado I Gabarro M: Actualizacion de la gastrina. Rev Esp Enferm Apar Dig 61:519, 1982.
18. Bentley PH, Kenner GW, Sheppard RC: Human gastrin: Isolation, structure and synthesis; structures of human gastrins I and II. Nature 209:583, 1966.
19. Kenner GW, Sheppard RC: Gastrins of various species, in Andersson S (ed): *Frontiers in Gastrointestinal Hormone Research.* Stockholm, Almqvist & Wiksell, 1973, pp 137–142.
20. Yalow RS, Berson SA: Size and charge distinctions between endogenous human plasma gastrin in peripheral blood and heptadecapeptide gastrins. Gastroenterology 58:609, 1970.
21. Yalow RS, Berson SA: Radioimmunoassay of gastrin. Gastroenterology 58:1, 1970.
22. Yalow RS, Berson SA: Further studies on the nature of immunoreactive gastrin in human plasma. Gastroenterology 60:203, 1971.
23. Gregory A, Tracy HJ: Isolation of two "big gastrins" from Zollinger-Ellison tumour tissue. Lancet 2:797, 1972.
24. Gregory RA, Tracy HJ: Big gastrin. Mt. Sinai J Med NY 40:359, 1973.
25. Gregory RA, Tracy HJ: The chemistry of the gastrins: Some recent advances, in Thompson JC (ed): *Gastrointestinal Hormones.* Austin, University of Texas Press, 1975, pp 13–24.
26. Rehfeld JF, Stadil F, Vikelsoe J: Immunoreactive gastrin components in human serum. Gut 15:102, 1974.
27. Gregory RA, Tracy HJ: Isolation of two minigastrins from Zollinger-Ellison tumour tissue. Gut 15:683, 1974.
28. Yalow RA, Berson SA: And now, "big, big" gastrin. Biochem Biophys Res Commun 48:391, 1972.
29. Yalow RS, Wu N: Additional studies on the nature of big big gastrin. Gastroenterology 65:19, 1973.
30. Rehfeld JF, Stadil F, Malmstrom J, et al: Gastrin heterogeneity in serum and tissue. A progress report, in Thompson JC (ed): *Gastrointestinal Hormones.* Austin, University of Texas Press, 1975, pp 43–58.
31. Pauwels S, Dockray GJ, Walker R, et al: N-terminal tryptic fragment of big gastrin. Metabolism and failure to influence gastrin 17-evoked acid secretion in humans. Gastroenterology 86:86, 1984.
32. Dockray GJ: Patterns of serum gastrin at rest and after stimulation in man and dogs, in Thompson JC (ed): *Gastrointestinal Hormones.* Austin, University of Texas Press, 1975, pp 59–73.
33. Dockray GJ, Walsh JH: Amino terminal gastrin fragment in serum of Zollinger-Ellison syndrome patients. Gastroenterology 68:222, 1975.
34. Petersen B: Abnormally processed gastrins in active duodenal ulcer disease. Scand J Clin Lab Invest 44(Suppl 168):25, 1984.
35. Lamers CB, Walsh JH, Jansen JB, et al: Evidence that gastrin 34 is preferentially released from the human duodenum. Gastroenterology 83:233, 1982.
36. Petersen B, Andersen BN: Abnormal processing of antral gastrin in active duodenal ulcer disease. Eur J Clin Invest 14:214, 1984.
37. Petersen B, Christiansen J, Rehfeld JF: The N-terminal tridecapeptide fragment of gastrin-17 inhibits gastric acid secretion. Regul Pept 7:323, 1983.
38. Andersen BN, Petersen B, Borch K: Decreased sulfation of serum and tissue gastrin in hypergastrinemia of antral origin. Digestion 31:17, 1985.
39. Walsh JH, Isenberg JI, Ansfield J, et al: Clearance and acid-stimulation action of human big and little gastrins in duodenal ulcer subjects. J Clin Invest 57:1125, 1976.
40. Dockray GJ, Gregory RA, Tracy HJ, et al: Postsecretory processing of heptadecapeptide gastrin: Conversion to C-terminal immunoreactive fragments in the circulation of the dog. Gastroenterology 83:224, 1982.
41. Creutzfeldt W, Tract NS, Creutzfeldt C, et al: The secretory cycle of the G-cell. Ultrastructural and biochemical investigations of the effect of feeding in rats, in Thompson JC (ed): *Gastrointestinal Hormones.* Austin, University of Texas Press, 1975, pp 197–211.
42. Nilsson G, Yalow RS, Berson SA: Distribution of gastrin in the gastrointestinal tract of human, dog, cat and hog, in Andersson S (ed): *Frontiers in Gastrointestinal Hormone Research.* Stockholm, Almqvist & Wiksell, 1973, pp 95–101.
43. Walsh JH, Richardson CT, Fordtran JS: pH dependence of acid secretion and gastrin release in normal and ulcer patients. J Clin Invest 55:462, 1975.
44. Cowley DJ, Ganguli PC, Polak JM, et al: The G cell population of the pyloric antrum of the cat. Digestion 12:25, 1975.
45. Jackson BM, Reeder DD, Searcy JR, et al: Correlation of the surface pH, histology, and gastrin concentration of gastric mucosa. Ann Surg 176:727, 1972.
46. Malmstrøm J, Stadil F, Rehfeld JF: Concentration and component pattern in gastric, duodenal, and jejunal mucosa of normal human subjects and patients with duodenal ulcer. Gastroenterology 70:697, 1976.
47. Arnold R, Hulst MV, Neuhof CH, et al: Antral gastrin-producing G-cells and somatostatin-producing D-cells in different states of gastric acid secretion. Gut 23:285, 1982.
48. Berson SA, Yalow RS: Nature of immunoreactive

gastrin extracted from tissues of gastrointestinal tract. Gastroenterology 60:215, 1971.
49. Hengels KJ, Muller JE, Scholten T, et al: Evidence for the secretion of gastrin into human gastric juice. Gut 21:760, 1980.
50. Ayalon A, Yazigi R, Devitt P, et al: Does luminal gastrin stimulate gastric acid secretion? Am J Surg 141:94, 1981.
51. Watson LC, Reeder DD, Becker HD, et al: Gastrin concentrations in upper gastrointestinal mucosa in dogs. Surgery 76:419, 1974.
52. Reeder DD, Watayou T, Booth RAD, et al: Depletion of antral gastrin after food in rats. Am J Surg 129:67, 1975.
53. Rayford PL, Curtis PJ, Hill FL, et al: Molecular heterogeneity of gastrin in dog antral and duodenal mucosa. Abstract #42, Endocrinology Program Booklet, 58th Annual Meeting of the Endocrine Society, June, 1976.
54. Vanderhaeghen JJ, Signeau JC, Gept SW: New peptide in the vertebrate CNS reacting with antigastrin antibodies. Nature 257:604, 1975.
55. Boel E, Vuust J, Norris F, et al: Molecular cloning of human gastrin cDNA: Evidence for evolution of gastrin by gene duplication. Proc Natl Acad Sci USA 80:2866, 1983.
56. Yoo OJ, Powell CT, Agarwal KL: Molecular cloning and nucleotide sequence of full-length cDNA coding for porcine gastrin. Proc Natl Acad Sci USA 79:1049, 1982.
57. Wiborg O, Berglund L, Boel E, et al: Structure of a human gastrin gene. Proc Natl Acad Sci USA 81:1067, 1984.
58. Ito R, Sato K, Helmer T, et al: Structural analysis of the gene encoding human gastrin: The large intron contains an *Alu* sequence. Proc Natl Acad Sci USA 81:4662, 1984.
59. Habener JF, Potts JT Jr: Biosynthesis of parathyroid hormone. N Engl J Med 299:580, 1978.
60. Andersen BN, Petersen B, Borch K, et al: Variations in the sulfation of circulating gastrins in gastrointestinal diseases. Scand J Gastroenterol 18:565, 1983.
61. Sugano K, Aponte GW, Yamada T: Identification and characterization of glycine-extended posttranslational processing intermediates of progastrin in porcine stomach. J Biol Chem 260:1724, 1985.
62. Sugano K, Yamada T: Progastrin-like immunoreactivity in porcine antrum: Identification and characterization with region-specific antisera. Biochem Biophys Res Commun 126:72, 1985.
63. Reeve JR Jr, Walsh JH, Tompkins RK, et al: Amino terminal fragments of human progastrin from gastrinoma. Biochem Biophys Res Commun 123:404, 1984.
64. Desmond H, Dockray GJ, Spurdens M: Identification by specific radioimmunoassay of two novel peptides derived from the C-terminus of porcine preprogastrin. Regul Pept 11:133, 1985.
65. Jonsson A-C, Dockray GJ: Immunohistochemical localization to pyloric antral G cells of peptides derived from porcine preprogastrin. Regul Pept 8:283, 1984.
66. Lai KS: Studies on gastrin. Gut 5:327, 1964.
67. McGuigan JE: Immunochemical studies with synthetic human gastrin. Gastroenterology 54:1005, 1968.
68. Charters AC, Odell WD, Davidson WD, et al: Development of a radioimmunoassay for gastrin. Arch Surg 99:361, 1969.
69. Charters AC, Odell WD, Davidson WD, et al: Gastrin. Immunochemical properties and measurement by radioimmunoassay. Surgery 66:104, 1969.
70. Hansky J, Cain MD: Radioimmunoassay of gastrin in human serum. Lancet 2:1388, 1969.
71. McGuigan JE, Jaffe BM, Newton WT: Immunochemical measurements of endogenous gastrin release. Gastroenterology 59:499, 1970.
72. Berson SA, Yalow RS: Radioimmunoassay in gastroenterology. Gastroenterology 62:1061, 1972.
73. Pointner H: Normal serum gastrin levels in patients with liver cirrhosis. Digestion 13:372, 1975.
74. Rayford PL, Reeder DD, Thompson JC: Interlaboratory reproducibility of gastrin measurements by radioimmunoassay. J Lab Clin Med 86:521, 1975.
75. Walsh JH: Validation of radioimmunoassay, in Thompson JC (ed): *Gastrointestinal Hormones.* Austin, University of Texas Press, 1975, pp 251–255.
76. Thompson JC: Chemical structure and biological actions of gastrin, cholecystokinin, and related compounds, in Holton P (ed): *International Encyclopedia of Pharmacology and Therapeutics.* New York, Pergamon Press, 1973, pp 261–286.
77. Morley JS, Tracy HJ, Gregory RA: Structure-function relationships in the active C-terminal tetrapeptide sequence of gastrin. Nature 207:1356, 1965.
78. Tracy HJ, Gregory RA: Physiological properties of a series of synthetic peptides structurally related to gastrin I. Nature 204:935, 1964.
79. Lin TM: Gastrointestinal actions of the C-terminal tripeptide of gastrin. Gastroenterology 63:922, 1972.
80. Lin TM, Southard GL, Spray GF: Stimulation of gastric acid secretion in the dog by C-terminal penta-, tetra-, and tripeptides of gastrin and their O-methyl esters. Gastroenterology 70:733, 1976.
81. Walsh JH, Debas HT, Grossman MI: Pure human big gastrin. Immunochemical properties, disappearance half time, and acid-stimulating action in dogs. J Clin Invest 54:477, 1974.
82. Valenzuela JE, Bugat R, Grossman MI: Effect of big and little gastrins on pancreatic and gastric secretion. Proc Soc Exp Biol Med 159:237, 1978.
83. Walsh JH, Trout HH, Debas HT, et al: Immunochemical and biological properties of gastrins obtained from different species and of different molecular species of gastrin, in Chey WY, Brooks FP (eds): *Endocrinology of the Gut.* Thorofare, NJ, Charles B. Slack Inc, 1974, pp 277–289.

84. Lamers C, Harrison A, Ippoliti A, et al: Molecular forms of circulating gastrin in normal subjects and duodenal ulcer patients. Gastroenterology 76:1179, 1979.
85. Speir GR, Takeuchi K, Johnson LR: Characterization of the interaction between gastrin and its receptor in rat oxyntic gland mucosa. Biochim Biophys Acta 716:308, 1982.
86. Askew AR, Napier BJ: The biological activity of different gastrin peptides assessed using a cytochemical section bioessay. Aust NZ J Surg 51:341, 1981.
87. Reeder DD, Jackson BM, Brandt EN Jr, et al: Rate and pattern of disappearance of exogenous gastrin in dogs. Am J Physiol 222:1571, 1972.
88. Thompson JC, Rayford PL, Ramus NI, et al: Patterns of release and uptake of heterogeneous forms of gastrin, in Thompson JC (ed): *Gastrointestinal Hormones.* Austin, University of Texas Press, 1975, pp 125–151.
89. Reeder DD, Brandt EN Jr, Watson LC, et al: Pre- and post-hepatic measurements of mass of endogenous gastrin. Surgery 72:34, 1972.
90. Debas HT, Walsh JH, Grossman MI: Pure human minigastrin. Secretory potency and disappearance rate. Gut 15:686, 1974.
91. Villar HV, Reeder DD, Rayford PL, et al: Rate of disappearance of circulating endogenous gastrin in dogs. Surgery 81:404, 1977.
92. Thompson JC, Becker HD, Evans JCW, et al: Studies on the catabolism of gastrin, in Chey WY, Brooks FP (eds): *Endocrinology of the Gut.* Thorofare, NJ, Charles B Slack Inc, 1974, pp 295–303.
93. Thompson JC, Reeder DD, Davidson WD, et al: Studies on the metabolism of gastrin, in Andersson S (ed): *Frontiers in Gastrointestinal Hormone Research.* Stockholm, Almqvist & Wiksell, 1973, pp 111–135.
94. Thompson JC, Llanos OL, Teichmann RK, et al: Catabolism of gastrin and secretin. World J Surg 3:469, 1979.
95. Mackie CR, Lewis MH, Go VLW, et al: Exogenous gastrin in Rhesus monkeys. The effect of 50% distal small-bowel resection on its rate of disappearance. Arch Surg 116:297, 1981.
96. Thompson JC, Reeder DD, Davidson WD, et al: Effect of hepatic transit of gastrin, pentagastrin and histamine measured by gastric secretion and by assay of hepatic vein blood. Ann Surg 170:493, 1969.
97. Tranberg K-G, Hagander P, Schenck HV: Hepatic uptake of synthetic human gastrin I (1-17) in humans. Surgery 93:747, 1983.
98. Strunz UT, Thompson MR, Grossman MI: Hepatic inactivation of gastrin fragments of various chain lengths. Gastroenterology 70:941, 1976.
99. Doyle JW, Wolfe MM, McGuigan JE: Hepatic clearance of gastrin and cholecystokinin peptides. Gastroenterology 87:60, 1984.
100. Gimmon Z, Murphy RF, Chen M-H, et al: The effect of parenteral and enteral nutrition on portal and systemic immunoreactivities of gastrin, glucagon and vasoactive intestinal polypeptide (VIP). Ann Surg 196:571, 1982.
101. Wesdorp RIC, Falcao HA, Banks PB, et al: Gastrin and gastric acid secretion in renal failure. Am J Surg 141:334, 1981.
102. Booth RAD, Reeder DD, Hjelmquist UB, et al: Renal inactivation of endogenous gastrin in dogs. Arch Surg 106:851, 1973.
103. El Munshid HA, Liedberg G, Rehfeld JF, et al: Effect of bilateral nephrectomy on serum gastrin concentration, gastric histamine content, histidine decarboxylase activity, and acid secretion in the rat. Scand J Gastroenterol 11:87, 1976.
104. Taylor IL, Sells RA, McConnell RB, et al: Serum gastrin in patients with chronic renal failure. Gut 21:1062, 1980.
105. Temperly JM, Stagg BH, Wyllie JH: Disappearance of gastrin and pentagastrin in the portal circulation. Gut 12:372, 1971.
106. Becker HD, Reeder DD, Thompson JC: Extraction of circulating endogenous gastrin by the small bowel. Gastroenterology 65:903, 1973.
107. Evans JCW, Reeder DD, Becker HD, et al: Extraction of circulating endogenous gastrin by the gastric fundus. Gut 15:112, 1974.
108. Korman MG, Hansky J, Ritchie BC, et al: Disappearance of gastrin across the lung. Aust J Exp Biol Med Sci 51:679, 1973.
109. Petersen B: Metabolism of the NH_2-terminal tridecapeptide of gastrin-17 in normal subjects and duodenal ulcer patients. Scand J Gastroenterol 18:613, 1983.
110. Lilja P, Wiener I, Inoue K, et al: Changes in circulating levels of cholecystokinin, gastrin, and pancreatic polypeptide after small bowel resection in dogs. Am J Surg 145:157, 1983.
111. Petersen B, Henriksen JH, Rehfeld JF, et al: Removal of endogenous gastrin in man. Scand J Gastroenterol 16:727, 1981.
112. Movsas B, Mannor GE, Yalow RS: Degradation of the 34 amino acid gastrin by rat tissue homogenates. Life Sci 36:89, 1985.
113. Reeder DD, Jackson BM, Ban JL, et al: Influence of hypercalcemia on gastric secretion and serum gastrin concentrations in man. Ann Surg 172:540, 1970.
114. Reeder DD, Becker HD, Thompson JC: Effect of intravenously administered calcium on serum gastrin and gastric secretion in man. Surg Gynecol Obstet 138:847, 1974.
115. Fender HR, Thompson JC: The effect of magnesium on gastrin levels in duodenal ulcer and Zollinger-Ellison patients. Fed Proc 34:442, 1975.
116. Stadil F, Rehfeld JF: Release of gastrin by epinephrine in man. Gastroenterology 65:210, 1973.
117. Kalk WJ, Vinik AI, Bank S, et al: Plasma gastrin responses to arginine in chronic pancreatitis. Diabetes 23:264, 1974.
118. Christiansen J: Primary hyperparathyroidism and peptic ulcer disease. Scand J Gastroenterol 9:111, 1974.

119. Reeder DD, Conlee JL, Thompson JC: Calcium carbonate antacid and serum gastrin concentration in duodenal ulcer. Surg Forum 22:308, 1971.
120. Christiansen J, Kirkegaard P, Olsen PS, et al: Interaction of calcium and gastrin on gastric acid secretion in duodenal ulcer patients. Gut 25:174, 1984.
121. Jaffe BM, McGuigan JE, Newton WT: Immunochemical measurement of the vagal release of gastrin. Surgery 68:196, 1970.
122. Csendes A, Walsh JH, Grossman MI: Effects of atropine and of antral acidification on gastrin release and acid secretion in response to insulin and feeding in dogs. Gastroenterology 63:257, 1972.
123. Jackson BM, Reeder DD, Thompson JC: Dynamic characteristics of gastrin release. Am J Surg 123:137, 1972.
124. Becker HD, Reeder DD, Thompson JC: Direct measurement of gastrin release from duodenum and jejunum in dogs. Am J Physiol 227:897, 1974.
125. Grossman MI, Robertson CR, Ivy AC: Proof of a hormonal mechanism for gastric secretion: The humoral transmission of the distention stimulus. Am J Physiol 153:1, 1948.
126. Debas HT, Walsh JH, Grossman MI: Evidence for oxyntopyloric reflex for release of antral gastrin. Gastroenterology 68:687, 1975.
127. Debas HT, Csendes A, Walsh JH, et al: Release of antral gastrin, in Chey WY, Brooks FP (ed): *Endocrinology of the Gut.* Thorofare, NJ, Charles B. Slack Inc, 1974, pp 222–232.
128. Becker HD, Reeder DD, Thompson JC: Gastrin release by ethanol in man and in dogs. Ann Surg 179:906, 1974.
129. Nahrwold DL: Bile as a gastric secretory stimulant. Surgery 71:157, 1972.
130. Service FJ, Nelson RL, Rubenstein AH, et al: Direct effect of insulin on secretion of insulin, glucagon, gastric inhibitory polypeptide, and gastrin during maintenance of normoglycemia. J Clin Endocrinol Metab 47:488, 1978.
131. Johnson LR, Guthrie PD: Regulation of antral gastrin content. Am J Physiol 245:G725, 1983.
132. Ganguli PC: The effect of protein, carbohydrate, or fat on plasma gastrin concentration in human subjects. Gut 11:1061, 1970.
133. Jaffe BM, Clendinnen BG, Clarke RJ, et al: Effect of selective and proximal gastric vagotomy on serum gastrin. Gastroenterology 66:944, 1974.
134. Korman MG, Soveny C, Hansky J: Serum gastrin in duodenal ulcer. Gut 12:899, 1971.
135. Walsh JH, Yalow RS, Berson SA: The effect of atropine on plasma gastrin response to feeding. Gastroenterology 60:16, 1971.
136. Hirschowitz BI: Gastrin release in fistula dogs with solid compared to nutrient and nonnutrient liquid meals. Dig Dis Sci 28:705, 1983.
137. Byrne WJ, Christie DL, Ament ME, et al: Acid secretory response in man to 18 individual amino acids. Clin Res 25:108, 1977.
138. Elwin C-E: Gastric acid responses to antral application of some amino acids, peptides, and isolated fractions of a protein hydrolysate. Scand J Gastroenterol 9:239, 1974.
139. Eysselein VE, Singer MV, Wentz H, et al: Action of ethanol on gastrin release in the dog. Dig Dis Sci 29:12, 1984.
140. Kokue E, Hayama T: Doubtful role of endogenous gastrin in chicken gastric secretion by vagal stimulation. Experientia 31:197, 1975.
141. Stadil F, Rehfeld JF: Gastrin response to insulin after selective, highly selective, and truncal vagotomy. Gastroenterology 66:7, 1974.
142. Svensson S-O, Emås S, Dorner M, et al: Cholinergic release of gastrin by feeding in cats. Gastroenterology 70:742, 1976.
143. McGuigan JE, Trudeau WL: Serum gastrin levels before and after vagotomy and pyloroplasty or vagotomy and antrectomy. N Engl J Med 286:184, 1972.
144. Pederson RA, Kwok YN, Buchan AMJ, et al: Gastrin release from isolated perfused rat stomach after vagotomy. Am J Physiol 247:G248, 1984.
145. Debas HT, Walsh JH, Grossman MI: After vagotomy atropine suppresses gastrin release by food. Gastroenterology 70:1082, 1976.
146. Debas HT, Walsh JH, Grossman MI: Mechanisms of release of antral gastrin, in Thompson JC (ed): *Gastrointestinal Hormones.* Austin, University of Texas Press, 1975, pp 425–435.
147. Farooq O, Walsh JH: Atropine enhances serum gastrin response to insulin in man. Gastroenterology 68:662, 1975.
148. Nilsson G: Gastrin: Isolation, characterization, and functions, in Jerzy Glass GB (ed): *Gastrointestinal Hormones.* New York, Raven Press, 1980, pp 127–167.
149. Feldman M, Richardson CT, Taylor IL, et al: Effect of atropine on vagal release of gastrin and pancreatic polypeptide. J Clin Invest 63:294, 1979.
150. Soares EC, Zaterka S, Walsh J: Acid secretion and serum gastrin at graded intragastric pressures in man. Gastroenterology 72:676, 1977.
151. Schubert ML, Bitar KN, Makhlouf GM: Regulation of gastrin and somatostatin secretion by cholinergic and noncholinergic intramural neurons. Am J Physiol 243:G442, 1982.
152. Dockray GJ, Vaillant C, Walsh JH: The neuronal origin of bombesin-like immunoreactivity in the rat gastrointestinal tract. Neuroscience 4:1561, 1979.
153. Schiller LR, Walsh JH, Feldman M: Effect of atropine on gastrin release stimulated by an amino acid meal in humans. Gastroenterology 83:267, 1982.
154. Hirschowitz BI, Gibson R, Molina E: Atropine suppresses gastrin release by food in intact and vagotomized dogs. Gastroenterology 81:838, 1981.
155. Debas HT, Hollinshead J, Seal A, et al: Vagal control of gastrin release in the dog: Pathways for stimulation and inhibition. Surgery 95:34, 1984.
156. Thompson JC, Lowder WS, Peurifoy JT, et al: Effect of selective proximal vagotomy and truncal vagotomy on gastric acid and serum gastrin responses to

a meal in duodenal ulcer patients. Ann Surg 188:431, 1978.
157. Taylor IL, Dockray GJ, Calam J, et al: Big and little gastrin responses to food in normal and ulcer subjects. Gut 20:957, 1979.
158. Tatsuta M, Baba M, Itoh T: Increased gastrin secretion in patients with pheochromocytoma. Gastroenterology 84:920, 1983.
159. Olbe L: Gastrin release in man as determined by bioassay and immunoassay, in Thompson JC (ed): *Gastrointestinal Hormones.* Austin, University of Texas Press, 1975, pp 461–466.
160. Angeras U, Farnebo L-O, Graffner H, et al: Effects of food on plasma catecholamine and gastrin levels in patients with duodenal ulcer and normal volunteers. Digestion 25:205, 1982.
161. Ayalon A, Devitt P, Guzman S, et al: Release of antral gastrin in response to an intestinal meal in dogs. Surgery 91:399, 1982.
162. Kauffman GL Jr, Grossman MI: Serum gastrin during intestinal phase of acid secretion in dogs. Gastroenterology 77:26, 1979.
163. Konturek SJ, Adair TH, Rayford PL, et al: pH profile of gastric acid, serum gastrin and secretin responses to gastric and intestinal meals in the dog. Gastroenterology 70:903, 1976.
164. Konturek SJ, Rayford PL, Thompson JC: Effect of pH of gastric and intestinal meals on gastric acid, plasma gastrin and secretin responses in the dog. Am J Physiol 233:E537, 1977.
165. Lee KY, Tai HH, Chey WY: Plasma secretin and gastrin responses to a meat meal and duodenal acidification in dogs. Am J Physiol 230:784, 1976.
166. Bertaccini G, Erspamer V, Melchiorri P, et al: Gastrin release by bombesin in the dog. Br J Pharmacol 52:219, 1974.
167. Erspamer V, Melchiorri P: Actions of bombesin on secretions and motility of the gastrointestinal tract, in Thompson JC (ed): *Gastrointestinal Hormones.* Austin, University of Texas Press, 1975, pp 575–589.
168. Inoue K, McKay D, Yajima H, et al: Effect of synthetic porcine gastrin-releasing peptide on plasma levels of immunoreactive cholecystokinin, pancreatic polypeptide and gastrin in dogs. Peptides 4:153, 1983.
169. Greeley GH Jr, Thompson JC: Insulinotropic and gastrin-releasing action of gastrin-releasing peptide (GRP). Regul Pept 8:97, 1984.
170. Lehy T, Accary JP, Labeille D, et al: Chronic administration of bombesin stimulates antral gastrin cell proliferation in the rat. Gastroenterology 84:914, 1983.
171. Delle Fave G, Kohn A, de Magistris L, et al: Effects of bombesin on gastrin and gastric acid secretion in patients with duodenal ulcer. Gut 24:231, 1983.
172. Schubert ML, Saffouri B, Walsh JH, et al: Inhibition of neurally mediated gastrin secretion by bombesin antiserum. Am J Physiol 248:G456, 1985.
173. Thompson MR, Debas HT, Walsh JH, et al: Release of gastrin from an antral pouch by liver extract bathing oxyntic and intestinal mucosa. Physiologist 19:390, 1976.
174. Llanos OL, Villar HV, Konturek SJ, et al: Release of antral and duodenal gastrin in response to an intestinal meal. Ann Surg 186:614, 1977.
175. Sato T, Kameyama J, Sasaki I, et al: Gastric acid secretion and serum gastrin levels in chronic pancreatitis. Gastroenterol Jpn 16:93, 1981.
176. Woodward ER, Dragstedt LR: Role of the pyloric antrum in regulation of gastric secretion. Physiol Rev 40:490, 1960.
177. Peters MN, Feldman M, Walsh JH, et al: Effect of gastric alkalinization on serum gastrin concentrations in humans. Gastroenterology 85:35, 1983.
178. Bloom SR, Mortimer CH, Thorner MO, et al: Inhibition of gastrin and gastric-acid secretion by growth-hormone release-inhibiting hormone. Lancet 2:1106, 1974.
179. Isenberg JI, Walsh JH, Grossman MI: Zollinger-Ellison syndrome. Gastroenterology 65:140, 1973.
180. Raptis S, Dollinger HC, von Berger L, et al: Effects of somatostatin on gastric secretion and gastrin release in man. Digestion 13:15, 1975.
181. Konturek SJ, Tasler J, Cieszkowski M, et al: Effect of growth hormone release-inhibiting hormone on gastric secretion, mucosal blood flow, and serum gastrin. Gastroenterology 70:737, 1976.
182. Thomas WEG: Inhibitory effect of somatostatin on gastric acid secretion and serum gastrin in dogs with and without duodenogastric reflux. Gut 21:996, 1980.
183. Harty RF, Maico DG, McGuigan JE: Postreceptor inhibition of antral gastrin release by somatostatin. Gastroenterology 88:675, 1985.
184. Morz R, Prager-Petz J, Pointner H: Effect of luminal somatostatin on pentagastrin-stimulated gastric acid secretion in the rat. Am J Physiol 245:G297, 1983.
185. Short GM, Doyle JW, Wolfe MM: Effect of antibodies to somatostatin on acid secretion and gastrin release by the isolated perfused rat stomach. Gastroenterology 88:984, 1985.
186. Thompson JC, Reeder DD, Bunchman HH, et al: Effect of secretin on circulating gastrin. Ann Surg 176:384, 1972.
187. Becker HD, Reeder DD, Thompson JC: Effect of glucagon on circulating gastrin. Gastroenterology 65:28, 1973.
188. Konturek SJ, Biernat J, Kwiecien N, et al: Effect of glucagon on meal-induced gastric secretion in man. Gastroenterology 68:448, 1975.
189. Villar HV, Fender HR, Rayford PL, et al: Suppression of gastrin release and gastric secretion by gastric inhibitory polypeptide (GIP) and vasoactive intestinal polypeptide (VIP). Ann Surg 184:97, 1976.
190. Chiba T, Taminato T, Kadowaki S, et al: Effects of glucagon, secretin, and vasoactive intestinal polypeptide on gastric somatostatin and gastrin release from isolated perfused rat stomach. Gastroenterology 79:67, 1980.

191. Wolfe MM, Reel GM, McGuigan JE: Inhibition of gastrin release by secretin is mediated by somatostatin in cultured rat antral mucosa. J Clin Invest 72:1586, 1983.
192. McIntosh CHS, Pederson RA, Koop H, et al: Gastric inhibitory polypeptide stimulated secretion of somatostatinlike immunoreactivity from the stomach: Inhibition by acetylcholine or vagal stimulation. Can J Physiol Pharmacol 59:468, 1981.
193. MacGregor IL, Deveney C, Way LW, et al: The effect of acute hyperglycemia on meal-stimulated gastric, biliary, and pancreatic secretion, and serum gastrin. Gastroenterology 70:197, 1976.
194. Sasaki H, Nagulesparan M, Dubois A, et al: Hypergastrinemia in obese noninsulin-dependent diabetes: A possible reflection of high prevalence of vagal dysfunction. J Clin Endocrinol Metab 56:744, 1983.
195. Mahachai V, Walker K, Sevelius H, et al: Enprostil, a dehydro-prostaglandin E_2, has potent antisecretory and antigastrin properties in patients with duodenal ulcer disease. Gastroenterology 86:1171, 1984.
196. Davis GR, Walsh JH, Santa Ana CA, et al: Effect of cimetidine and enprostil (a syntex investigational prostaglandin E_2) on gastric acidity and serum gastrin concentration in normal subjects. Gastroenterology 86:1058, 1984.
197. Fahrenkrug J, Schaffalitzky de Muckadell OB, Hornum I, et al: The mechanism of hypergastrinemia in achlorhydria; effect of food, acid, and calcitonin on serum gastrin concentrations and component pattern in pernicious anemia, with correlation to endogenous secretin concentrations in plasma. Gastroenterology 71:33, 1976.
198. Becker HD, Konturek SJ, Reeder DD, et al: Effect of calcium and calcitonin on gastrin and gastric secretion in cats. Am J Physiol 225:277, 1973.
199. Becker HD, Reeder DD, Scurry MT, et al: Inhibition of gastrin release and gastric secretion by calcitonin in patients with peptic ulcer. Am J Surg 127:71, 1974.
200. Mollerup C, Cartensen HE, Bruun E, et al: Possible antagonists to gastrin in parathyroid adenomas. Br J Surg 67:890, 1980.
201. Jansen JBMJ, Lamers CBHW: Calcitonin and secretin inhibit bombesin-stimulated serum gastrin and gastric acid secretion in man. Regul Pept 1:415, 1981.
202. Pappas TN, Debas HT, Walsh JH, et al: Calcitonin gene related peptide (CGRP) selectivity inhibits acid secretion in the dog. Gastroenterology 88:1530, 1985.
203. Heynen G, Brassine A, Daubresse JC, et al: Lack of clinical and physiological relationship between gastrin and calcitonin in man. Eur J Clin Invest 11:331, 1981.
204. Isenberg JI, Walsh JH, Passaro E Jr, et al: Unusual effect of secretin on serum gastrin, serum calcium and gastric acid secretion in a patient with suspected Zollinger-Ellison syndrome. Gastroenterology 62:626, 1972.
205. Track NS, Creutzfeldt C, Junge U, et al: Gastrin turnover in gastrinoma tissue; in vitro incubation, subcellular fraction and monolayer culture studies, in Thompson JC (ed): *Gastrointestinal Hormones.* Austin, University of Texas Press, 1975, pp 403–424.
206. Imamura M, Adachi H, Takahashi K, et al: Gastrin release from gastrinoma cells stimulated with secretin. Dig Dis Sci 27:1130, 1982.
207. Crean GP: Effect of hypophysectomy on the gastric mucosa of the rat. Gut 9:332, 1968.
208. Haeger K, Jacobsohn D, Kahlson G: Atrophy of the gastrointestinal mucosa following hypophysectomy or adrenalectomy. Acta Physiol Scand 30 (Suppl 3):161, 1953.
209. Crean GP: A comparison between the effects of hypophysectomy and adrenalectomy on the gastric mucosa of rats. Gut 9:343, 1968.
210. Tepperman BL, Evered MD: Gastrin injected into the lateral hypothalamus stimulates secretion of gastric acid in rats. Science 209:1142, 1980.
211. Pawlikowski M, Owczarczyk I, Stepien H: Serum gastrin levels in patients with acromegaly. Horm Metab Res 13:714, 1981.
212. Bolman RM III, Cooper CW, Garner SC, et al: Stimulation of gastrin secretion in the pig by parathyroid hormone and its inhibition by thyrocalcitonin. Endocrinology 100:1014, 1977.
213. Selking O, Gustavsson S, Johansson H, et al: Effect of parathyroid hormone on gastrin and somatostatin release from the gastric antrum. Ups J Med Sci 86:259, 1981.
214. Seino Y, Matsukura S, Miyamoto Y, et al: Hypergastrinemia in hyperthyroidism. J Clin Endocrinol Metab 43:852, 1976.
215. Seino Y, Matsukura S, Inoue Y, et al: Hypogastrinemia in hypothyroidism. Am J Dig Dis 23:189, 1978.
216. Dahlberg PA, Karlsson FA, Lundqvist G: High serum gastrin levels in thyrotoxic patients. Clin Endocrinol 14:125, 1981.
217. Mulholland MW, Quigley T, Bonsack M, et al: Relationship of antral gastrin cells and serum gastrin to thyroid function in the rat. Endocrinology 114:840, 1984.
218. Inoue K, Wiener I, Fried GM, et al: Effect of colectomy on cholecystokinin and gastrin release. Ann Surg 196:691, 1982.
219. Nilsson G, Brodin K: Increase of gastrin concentration in duodenal mucosa of dogs following resection of the gastric antrum. Acta Physiol Scand 99:510, 1977.
220. Sudo T, Ishiyama K, Kawamura M, et al: Changes in plasma gastrin and secretin levels after pancreaticoduodenectomy. Surg Gynecol Obstet 158:133, 1984.
221. Soll AH, Walsh JH: Regulation of gastric acid secretion. Ann Rev Physiol 41:35, 1979.
222. Archimandritis A, Alegakis G, Theodoropoulos G, et al: Serum gastrin concentrations in healthy

males and females of various ages. Acta Hepatogastroenterol 26:58, 1979.
223. Attia RR, Ebeid AM, Fischer JE, et al: Maternal fetal and placental gastrin concentrations. Anaesthesia 37:18, 1982.
224. Dokumov S, Tarkolev N, Shterev A, et al: Serum gastrin I concentrations of mother and newborn immediately after birth. Br J Obstet Gynaecol 88:126, 1981.
225. Lucas A, Adrian TE, Christofides N, et al: Plasma motilin, gastrin, and enteroglucagon and feeding in the human newborn. Arch Dis Child 55:673, 1980.
226. Feldman M, Richardson CT, Walsh JH: Sex-related differences in gastrin release and parietal cell sensitivity to gastrin in healthy human beings. J Clin Invest 71:715, 1983.
227. Chew CS, Hersey SJ: Gastrin stimulation of isolated gastric glands. Am J Physiol 242:G504, 1982.
228. Rovati AL: The relationship between chemical structure of a new dicarboxylic amino-acid derivative and antigastrin activity in the rat. Br J Pharmacol 34:677P, 1968.
229. Johnson LR: Trophic action of gastrointestinal hormones, in Thompson JC (ed): *Gastrointestinal Hormones.* Austin, University of Texas Press, 1975, pp 215–230.
230. Barrowman JA, Mayston PD: The trophic effect of pentagastrin on the pancreas, in Thompson JC (ed): *Gastrointestinal Hormones.* Austin, University of Texas Press, 1975, pp 231–247.
231. Enochs MR, Johnson LR: Growth hormone; a possible regulation of gastrin. Gastroenterology 68:889, 1975.
232. Enochs MR, Johnson LR: Effect of hypophysectomy and growth hormone on serum and antral gastrin levels in the rat. Gastroenterology 70:727, 1976.
233. Johnson LR: New aspects of the trophic action of gastrointestinal hormones. Gastroenterology 72:788, 1977.
234. Neuburger P, Lewin M, de Recherche C, et al: Parietal and chief cell populations in four cases of Zollinger-Ellison syndrome. Gastroenterology 63:937, 1972.
235. Deveney CW, Owen RL, Deveney K, et al: Effect of acid secretory capacity and chronic endogenous hypergastrinemia on pancreatic secretion and intestinal morphology in the rat. Dig Dis Sci 28:65, 1983.
236. Johnson LR, Guthrie PD, Dudrick SJ: Effects of luminal gastrin on the growth of rat intestinal mucosa. Gastroenterology 81:71, 1981.
237. Shulkes A, Chick P, Hardy KJ: Presence and stability of gastrin in the gastric juice of the fetal sheep. Clin Exp Pharmacol Physiol 11:45, 1984.
238. Grand RJ, Watkins JB, Torti FM: Development of the human gastrointestinal tract. A review. Gastroenterology 70:790, 1976.
239. Johnson LR, Guthrie PD: Proglumide inhibition of trophic action of pentagastrin. Am J Physiol 246:G62, 1984.
240. Preshaw RM, Cooke AR, Grossman MI: Stimulation of pancreatic secretion by a humoral agent from the pyloric gland area of the stomach. Gastroenterology 49:617, 1965.
241. Preshaw RM, Cooke AR, Grossman MI: Pancreatic secretion induced by stimulation of the pyloric gland area of the stomach. Science 148:1347, 1965.
242. Nahrwold DL, Cooke AR, Grossman MI: Choleresis induced by stimulation of the gastric antrum. Gastroenterology 52:18, 1967.
243. Stening GF, Grossman MI: Hormonal control of Brunner's glands. Gastroenterology 56:1047, 1969.
244. Soll AH: The actions of secretagogues on oxygen uptake by isolated mammalian parietal cells. J Clin Invest 61:370, 1978.
245. Soll AH: Secretagogue stimulation of [^{14}C]aminopyrine accumulation by isolated canine parietal cells. Am J Physiol 238:G366, 1980.
246. Soll AH: Potentiating interactions of gastric stimulants on [^{14}C]aminopyrine accumulation by isolated canine parietal cells. Gastroenterology 83:216, 1982.
247. Soll AH: The interaction of histamine with gastrin and carbamylcholine on oxygen uptake by isolated mammalian parietal cells. J Clin Invest 61:381, 1978.
248. Bergqvist E, Obrink KJ: Gastrin-histamine as a normal sequence in gastric acid stimulation in the rabbit. Ups J Med Sci 84:145, 1979.
249. Soll AH, Amirian DA, Thomas LP, et al: Gastrin receptors on isolated canine parietal cells. J Clin Invest 73:1434, 1984.
250. Greco AV, Bianco A, Altomonte L, et al: Effect of somatostatin on lower esophageal sphincter (LES) pressure and serum gastrin in normal and achalasic subjects. Horm Metab Res 14:26, 1982.
251. Dennis MA, Maher JW, Crandall-Moore V, et al: Response of the canine lower esophageal sphincter to endogenous hypergastrinemia. J Surg Res 31:400, 1981.
252. Jensen DM, McCallum RW, Corazziari E, et al: Human lower esophageal sphincter responses to synthetic human gastrins 34 (G-34) and 17 (G-17). Gastroenterology 79:431, 1980.

Chapter 15

Cholecystokinin

Marilyn Marx, M.D., Guillermo Gomez, M.D., Janos Lonovics, M.D., and James C. Thompson, M.D.

HISTORY

In 1928, Ivy and Oldberg [1] found that instillation of fat into the proximal small intestine caused brisk contraction of the gallbladder. They reasoned that a blood-borne agent from the gut was responsible for the contraction, and they named the substance cholecystokinin (CCK). Fifteen years later, Harper and Raper [2] discovered an agent that, when released from the duodenal mucosa, stimulated pancreatic enzyme secretion. They named this substance pancreozymin. Purification of the two agents by Jorpes and Mutt (summarized by Jorpes [3]) demonstrated that both were actually a single substance that proved to be a peptide having 33 residues. Since its first described action was gallbladder contraction, the hormone was called cholecystokinin.

CCK is a linear 33 amino acid peptide hormone with a molecular weight of 3918 daltons [4] (see Appendix). CCK exhibits both macro- and microheterogeneity. It occurs in several molecular forms (CCK-58 [5,6], CCK-39, CCK-33, CCK-8, CCK-5 [7], CCK-4, and probably CCK-21 and CCK-12 as well) and may be sulfated or desulfated. The sulfated tyrosine residue of position 7, counting from the C-terminal (in CCK-33), governs the potency of gallbladder contraction [8]. It has been reported that the C-terminal octapeptide portion of CCK is 2½ times more potent on a molar basis than the entire CCK-33 molecule, and the C-terminal pentapeptide is identical to that of gastrin [4,9]. CCK-4 is, therefore, identical to gastrin 4. In a recent study that re-evaluated the bioactivity of CCK analogues, Solomon et al [10] concluded that CCK-8 was not more potent than CCK-33.

CCK appears to be a heterogeneous system of peptides (among which there is a biosynthetic relationship) produced from a single precursor [7]. By means of recombinant DNA techniques, PRE-PRO-CCK, a 115 amino acid precursor of CCK with a molecular weight of about 13,000 daltons, has been identified in the rat brain [11] as well as in porcine brain and gut [12]. The sequences of porcine and rat PRE-PRO-CCK show an overall homology of 75 percent. This CCK precursor possesses several features common to secreted proteins and by peptidase cleavage would generate a PRO-CCK of 95 amino acids. Distribution and characterization of immunoreactive PRO-CCK in the rat brain have been reported recently [13].

DISTRIBUTION

CCK is present throughout the small intestine; a study by Ogden et al from our laboratory has reported relative mucosal concentrations of CCK throughout the digestive tract of the dog [14]. Concentrations are highest in the duodenum, but the largest mass of CCK is in the jejunum [14]. The regional differences reflect the localization of CCK to endocrine cells in the proximal gut, while CCK in the ileum and colon is localized in nerves. The myenteric plexus of Auerbach and the submucosal plexus of Meissner in the colon are particularly rich in CCK-containing nerves; these nerves appear to innervate ganglionic cell bodies that do not contain CCK immunoreactivity [15]. CCK-8 and CCK-4 predominate in the intestine.

CCK is widely distributed throughout both the central and peripheral nervous systems [7]. In the brain, CCK exists in at least five forms, and it is the most abundant peptide system [16]. Although there is controversy concerning the major forms of CCK in the brain (due to differences in extraction techniques), Morley [17] concluded that the predominant form is CCK-8 (60–70 percent), with approximately 15 percent being CCK-33. Studies from our laboratory, however, suggest that in the rat and cow, at least, CCK-33 may in fact predominate, and that there is a progressive decrease, going from rostral to caudal portions of the brain, in both bio- and radioimmunoassayable quantities of CCK-8 and CCK-33 [18].

Using immunocytochemistry, CCK-like immunoreactivity has been localized in the nerve cells of the coelenterate hydra, which has the most primitive nervous system in the animal kingdom [19]. This information provides evidence in support of the early evolutionary emergence of the gastrin/CCK family, with CCK most probably being phylogenetically older than gastrin [20].

In the mammalian central nervous system, all regions except the pineal body, the pituitary, and the cerebellum contain significant amounts of CCK [21]. The CCK-containing nerves are particularly numerous in the neocortex, the hippocampus, the amygdaloid nuclei, the hypothalamus, and the dorsal horns of the spinal cord [15].

In the peripheral nervous system, in addition to the major CCK innervation of the colon and ileum, occasional CCK-containing nerves also innervate the muscle wall of the urinary bladder and the distal part of the uterus [15,21].

RADIOIMMUNOASSAY

The development of sensitive and specific radioimmunoassay techniques has made it possible to measure physiologic levels of CCK in tissues and body fluids of humans and other mammals. Early assays were reported a decade ago [22,23]; at least ten assays are now available that recognize CCK-8 or CCK-33 [24–33]. Our current assay recognizes CCK-33 with great sensitivity but cross-reacts hardly at all with CCK-8 and with gastrin [32].

PHARMACOKINETICS AND CATABOLISM

The disappearance half-life of endogenous CCK has been found to be 5–7 minutes in humans [23], but the half-life of exogenous CCK is between 2 and 3 minutes in both humans and dogs [34]. Both the kidney and the liver play important roles in the metabolism of CCK. The CCK-destroying enzyme of kidney cortex acts on the C-terminal part of the molecule, while the mechanism of CCK inactivation by the liver is not yet fully understood [35]. Pancreas, lung, and small intestine also possess CCK-8 destroying activities, although these were significantly lower than the activity found in the kidney cortex [35]. In humans, both hepatic cirrhosis and chronic renal failure are clinical conditions that result in significant prolongation of the disappearance half-time of CCK-8 [36].

Sakamoto et al [37] from our laboratory have prepared dogs with portacaval transposition and found that about 50 percent of CCK-8 is destroyed, as measured by both bioassay and radioimmunoassay, on a single passage through the liver, whereas RIA concentrations and bioactivity of CCK-33 are unaffected on hepatic transit.

Deficiencies in proteolysis of CCK have been postulated to have a role in fetal abnormalities observed in cystic fibrosis disease [38].

RELEASE

The release of CCK is initiated by products of fat and protein digestion within the intestinal lumen. The classic agents for release are L-isomers of amino acids, especially tryptophan and phenylalanine, and straight-chain fatty acids with chain lengths of C_{10-18}. Food releases CCK [39]. Duodenal acidification appears to release CCK [39,40], although we have repeatedly been unable to demonstrate it [41]. Divalent cations, such as magnesium, zinc, and calcium, are also potent stimulants for CCK release [42,43]. We believe that both the cholecystokinetic and cathartic effects of magnesium are related to its release of CCK. Verapamil, a calcium antagonist, does not affect CCK-33 release [44]. CCK also has a diurnal profile. In healthy humans, CCK increases stepwise during the day, peaking 2 hours after the evening meal [45,46].

Wiener et al [47] from our laboratory were the first to show correlation between bioactivity (gallbladder contraction measured by ultrasonography) and release of CCK (measured by RIA) in humans (Fig 15-1). Lilja et al [48] compared the concentrations of plasma CCK in pigs, dogs, and humans after food or intraduodenal fat intake. They found that postprandial release of CCK occurred after 5 minutes in humans, after 20 minutes in pigs, and after 120 minutes in dogs. CCK release was probably related to gastric emptying, as CCK was released within 20 minutes after introduction of intraduodenal fat in all three species.

Many studies have provided controversial evidence on the question of whether CCK-8 or CCK-33 is the predominant molecular form of cholecystokinin released after a meal. The present consensus

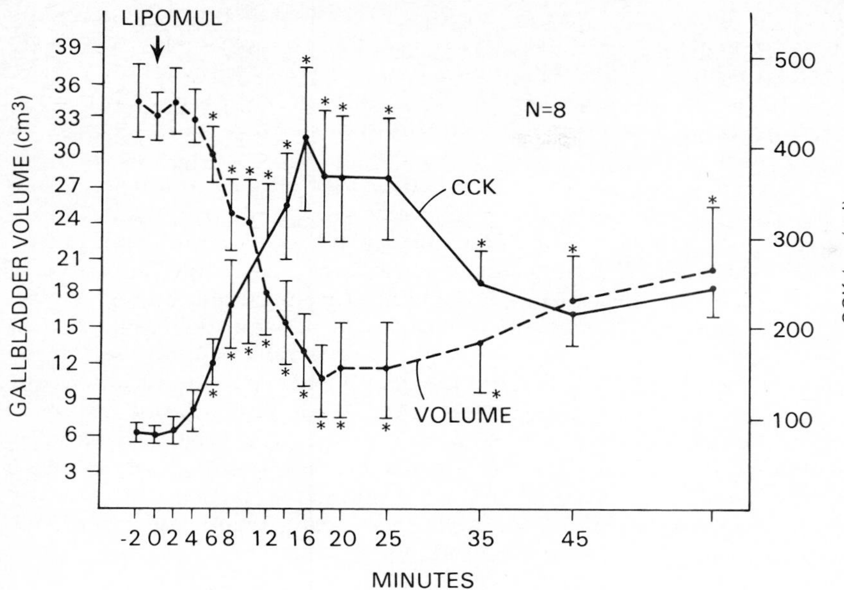

Figure 15-1. Concentrations of plasma CCK (solid line) (mean ± SE) and gallbladder volume (broken line) in eight normal men before and after intraduodenal instillation of Lipomul (* = $p < 0.05$). (From Wiener et al [47], by permission of the J B Lippincott Co.)

appears to be that the two forms are released in about equal amounts, as measured in peripheral blood. Somatostatin inhibits the release of CCK stimulated by fat [49].

Release of CCK does not depend upon the presence or absence of vagal stimulation [50,51]. Vagotomy does not interfere with release of CCK in dogs [52], but in humans it increases the secretion of CCK in response to nutrients [53]. We found that atropine can depress the stimulated release of CCK in dogs. In human studies, Hopman et al [54] concluded that atropine delays but does not inhibit the CCK-stimulated secretion. Partial gastrectomy in humans also leads to greater plasma CCK response after oral intake of fat [55]. CCK levels are increased by bombesin [56–59].

Thompson et al [34] described studies in normal humans, in preoperative and postoperative patients with duodenal ulcers, in diabetic patients, and in postoperative patients with the Zollinger-Ellison syndrome in which CCK levels were found to increase significantly in response to the ingestion of food. The CCK response to food was more rapid in patients with duodenal ulcers and in diabetic patients than in normal subjects. There was a greater prolongation of elevated CCK levels in normal subjects than in patients with duodenal ulcers or diabetes.

In celiac disease there is a reversible defect of secretion of CCK that correlates with the altered gallbladder emptying observed in this illness [60].

Inoue et al [61] found an increase in CCK release and in mucosal CCK stores after pancreatic duct ligation in dogs. This suggests that postprandial release of CCK is normally suppressed by the presence of pancreatic enzymes in the duodenum, which in turn supports the possibility that CCK may be involved in a feedback loop. Despite several attempts, so far we have been unsuccessful in providing direct evidence that introduction of pancreatic enzymes into the duodenum suppresses release of CCK in dogs. Folsch et al [62] found that the negative feedback control of pancreatic enzyme secretion in rats may be mediated by release of CCK.

Increased release of CCK after small bowel resection has been shown in dogs [63] and is probably secondary to accelerated gastric emptying and intestinal transit. In rats, plasma levels and intestinal content of CCK are elevated after small bowel resection [64]. Resection of the colon also leads to an increase in release of CCK after food stimulation in dogs [65], providing evidence that the colon contains a factor that inhibits release of CCK.

Increased release of CCK has been found after cholecystectomy in hamsters [66] and dogs [67], which suggests that the gallbladder may be involved in feedback inhibitory mechanisms. In humans, we reported [68,69] that in patients with gallstones whose gallbladders contract, the release of CCK is diminished and gallbladder sensitivity to CCK is increased.

Gomez et al [70] from our group investigated the effect of endogenous bile on the release of CCK in dogs and found that fat-stimulated release of CCK is considerably enhanced when bile is totally diverted from the intestinal lumen. In contrast, both basal and fat-stimulated levels of plasma CCK are depressed in the presence of excessive bile. These findings support the hypothesis that bile exerts a physiologic negative feedback effect on the release of CCK. Bile is not necessary in order for fat to stimulate CCK endocrine cells in the intestinal mucosa [70].

General anesthesia inhibits gastrointestinal and pancreatic secretion. Lilja et al [71] investigated the effects of anesthetic agents on the release of CCK in dogs and found a pronounced inhibition of fat-induced CCK release by pentobarbital and abolition of CCK release by halothane. In contrast, chloralose anesthesia had little effect on fat-stimulated release of CCK. These findings re-emphasized the need to consider the effects of anesthetic agents in all physiologic studies. Fried et al [72] reported that alcohol decreased the CCK plasma levels in dogs but not in healthy humans.

ACTIONS

The principal physiologic actions of CCK are stimulation of contraction of the gallbladder [8] and of pancreatic enzyme secretion [73]. The classic bioassay for CCK is contraction of an isolated strip of rabbit gallbladder (see Fig 4-3). In addition, CCK stimulates pancreatic bicarbonate secretion [74] and insulin release [75] from the pancreas; it also stimulates intestinal motility [76,77], contraction of the resting stomach and pyloric sphincter [78–80], flow of hepatic bile [81–83], secretion of Brunner's glands [84], blood flow in the superior mesenteric artery [85], bicarbonate secretion from the stomach and duodenum [86], secretion of pepsinogen from gastric glands [87], and growth of the pancreas [88]. On the other hand, CCK decreases systemic arterial pressure [89], and it inhibits contraction of the lower esophageal sphincter [79] and of the sphincter of Oddi [90] as well as motility in the active stomach [78].

CCK is a weak stimulant of gastric acid secretion and inhibits pentagastrin-stimulated acid secretion in dogs and humans [73,91]. Soll et al [92] recently reported that activation of somatostatin-mediated acid inhibitory mechanisms by CCK may account for the poor stimulatory effect of CCK on gastric acid secretion. The mechanism underlying the action of CCK on pancreatic exocrine function at the cellular level seems to be via binding to a receptor on the acinar cell membrane. The receptor binding releases membrane-bound calcium [93], which coincides with an increase in cellular cyclic GMP [94]. CCK does not stimulate adenylate cyclase activity [21] but, in fact, noncompetitively inhibits the increase in adenylate cyclase activity caused by secretin and VIP [95]. Pancreatic protein secretion, stimulated by CCK, is increased by neurotensin [96–98].

The CCK-stimulatory effects on intestinal motility may differ according to the route of administration of the peptide; intraluminal infusion caused an increase in migrating action potentiation, but IV infusion did not [99]. Measured quantities of physiologically released CCK have been correlated with gallbladder contraction in normal humans [47] and in gallstone patients [68]. Nearly identical correlation was seen after exogenous administration of pure CCK-33 in humans [100]. We have also recently correlated levels of physiologically released CCK in dogs with simultaneous bioassay measurements of gallbladder contraction and pancreatic protein secretion [32].

Women are more likely to develop cholesterol gallstones than men, and it has been suggested that elevated levels of estrogen and progesterone may increase the risk of gallbladder disease in women. Several studies [101–103] have examined the male-female differences in CCK-stimulated gallbladder contraction. Fried et al [102] found that the gallbladder showed diminished sensitivity to endogenously released CCK during the estrogen peak of the menstrual cycle. They concluded that this hormonal motility disorder may predispose premenopausal women to the formation of gallstones. Zhu et al [103], studying the effect of estrogen and progesterone on CCK-stimulated gallbladder contraction in vitro, showed no significant difference between the contractility of gallbladder strips from normal males and females. They found that castration in males inhibited gallbladder contraction in response to CCK. Estrogen, but not progesterone, inhibited gallbladder contraction. In addition, they found that the gallbladder of the pregnant rabbit showed diminished sensitivity to CCK. Ryan [104] reported that the contractile response of the gallbladder to CCK is diminished in pregnant guinea pigs and concluded that pregnancy might reduce the contribution of the intracellular calcium pool to the contractile process. Mate et al (unpublished data from our laboratory) have found that luteinizing hormone releasing hormone, in concentrations of 10^{-6} to 10^{-8} g/mL alone or in combination with CCK-8, has no effect on rabbit gallbladder contraction in vitro.

CCK has been shown to act in the control of the intestinal phase of pancreatic polypeptide release [105] and is an effective humoral releaser of pancreatic polypeptide in humans [106]. PP is also released after intracerebroventricular administration of CCK-8 [107].

The satiety effect of CCK was first observed in rats [108] and has now been extended to include similar observations in a number of laboratory animals as well as in humans [109,110]. The mechanism of the effect is unclear, but gastric vagal fibers appear to be required, and there is evidence that opiate receptors in the CNS are involved [111]. CCK administration to specific abdominal organs during meals suggests that the bed of the cranial mesenteric or celiac arteries is the major site of CCK satiety action [112]. CCK receptors have been localized to the circular smooth muscle layer of the pylorus, and gastric distention may be one of the possible mechanisms for CCK-induced satiety [113].

Possible Mechanisms of CCK-Induced Gallbladder Contraction

CCK is the most potent cholecystokinetic agent. The mechanisms by which CCK stimulates gallbladder contraction are not completely understood. It has been postulated that CCK acts directly on receptors in the gallbladder smooth muscle cells, since contraction is not inhibited by sympatholytic or parasympatholytic agents or by tetrodoxin [114–116]. The existence of a specific CCK receptor has been recently demonstrated on bovine gallbladder muscularis membranes [117].

Calcium channels and nucleotide systems of the gallbladder muscle cells are connected to CCK receptors in some way or may even be part of these receptors. In the development of gallbladder contraction, extracellular calcium seems to be more important, since removal of extracellular calcium from the Kreb's solution causes 80 percent inhibition in the CCK-induced contraction. The effect of CCK is also inhibited both by CCK-receptor antagonists and by the calcium channel blocker verapamil (Lonovics, unpublished data), which suggests that CCK stimulates gallbladder contraction (at least in rabbits) through receptor-operated calcium channels. Since the effect of CCK is also inhibited by aminophylline, a phosphodiesterase inhibitor, and isoproterenol, which activates adenyl cyclase [118], the cyclic nucleotide system is almost certainly involved in the mechanical response of CCK, as has been previously proposed by Andersson et al [119]. Phenothiazine, a calmodulin inhibitor, has also been shown to inhibit CCK response in this laboratory. Therefore, calmodulin may serve as an important link among CCK receptors, the cyclic nucleotide system, and the contractile proteins of gallbladder muscle. To focus our own ideas and, possibly, to facilitate further research activity, we have constructed a hypothetical model in which we try to explain the possible mechanism of the stimulation-contraction coupling process taking place in the rabbit gallbladder muscle during CCK stimulation (Fig 15-2).

CCK RECEPTOR ANTAGONISTS

The existence of several classes of CCK receptor antagonists has been recently documented [120–125]. In order to be a fully competitive CCK receptor antagonist, a substance must be devoid of agonist activity, must inhibit the interaction of CCK with its cell surface receptors, and must cause a parallel rightward shift in the dose-response curve for the stimulation of enzyme secretion caused by CCK.

One class of CCK antagonists is composed of derivatives of cyclic nucleotides [120,121]. Of the various nucleotides tested, dibutyryl cGMP is the most potent CCK receptor antagonist [121]. A second class of CCK receptor antagonist is composed of derivatives of amino acids such as proglumide (a derivative of glutaramic acid) and benzotript (a derivative of tryptophan) [122]. These two are equipotent but three times less potent than dibutyryl cGMP in antagonizing the action of CCK [125].

Recently, a third class of CCK receptor antagonists has been discovered. Spanarkel et al [123] first noted that a peptide can function as a fully competitive CCK receptor antagonist. They synthesized CCK-27-32-NH_2, a peptide that represents the COOH-terminal heptapeptide of CCK minus the COOH-terminal phenylalanine residue, and found that its CCK antagonist action is 30 times more potent than that of dibutyryl cGMP and approximately 100 times more potent than that of proglumide or benzotript [123]. They also showed that the COOH-terminal phenylalanine residue of CCK was not an essential requirement for the binding of CCK or structurally related peptides to the CCK receptor but was essential for intrinsic CCK-like biologic activity [123]. Although the COOH-terminal phenylalanine residue was not essential for binding, it apparently influences the affinity with which the peptide is bound to its receptors [123]. When the COOH-terminal phenylalanine residue is removed from CCK-27-33, there is a 3,000-fold decrease in the apparent affinity of the peptide for its receptor [124].

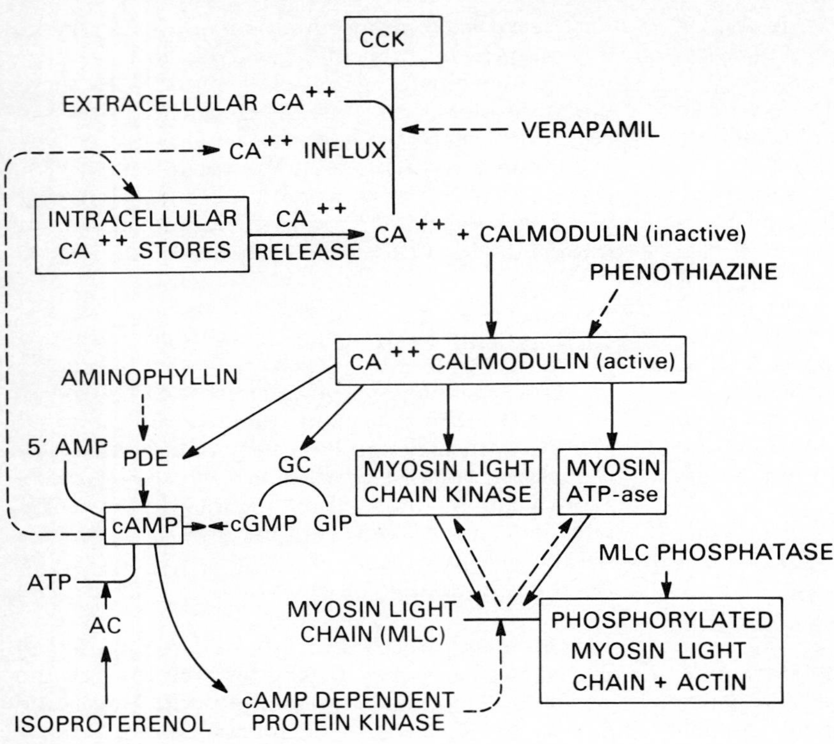

Figure 15-2. Hypothetical model proposed by Lonovics for mechanism of action of CCK on gallbladder muscle cells. CCK appears to stimulate gallbladder contraction through receptor-activated calcium channels rather than by activating cAMP. Calmodulin appears to play a central role in the stimulation-contraction coupling mechanism. Calmodulin activates a series of intracellular enzymes, leading to the phosphorylation of the myosin light chain, which in turn interacts with actin to produce gallbladder contraction.

In addition to CCK-27-32-NH_2, fragments of CCK varying in length from 1 to 3 amino acids and their NH_2-terminal butyloxycarbonyl (Boc) derivatives can be added to the class of new peptide CCK receptor antagonists [125]. Jensen et al [125] found that Boc-Met-Asp-Phe-NH_2 antagonized the action of CCK and was as potent as proglumide (and approximately three times less potent than dibutyryl cGMP) in antagonizing the interaction of CCK with its receptors. They also showed that shorter COOH-terminal derivatives of CCK could antagonize the action of CCK. Boc-Asp-Phe-NH_2, Boc-Phe-NH_2, and Met-Asp-Phe-NH_2 also acted as CCK antagonists. Boc-Asp-Phe-NH_2 was approximately seven times less potent than Boc-Met-Asp-Phe-NH_2, and Boc-Phe-NH_2 was approximately 27 times less potent than Boc-Met-Asp-Phe-NH_2. Removal of the butyloxycarbonyl moiety substantially reduced the potency with which the peptide inhibited the action of CCK. In antagonizing the action of CCK, Met-Asp-Phe-NH_2 was approximately 40 times less potent than Boc-Met-Asp-Phe-NH_2 and, in contrast to their corresponding butyloxycarbonyl derivatives, Asp-Phe-NH_2 and Phe-NH_2 do not antagonize the action of CCK [125].

An alternative to the concept of competitive antagonism of dibutyryl cGMP at the level of the CCK receptor has been suggested by Miller et al [126]. Rather than binding to the CCK receptor, cGMP may interact directly with CCK, thereby blocking the region of the peptide that binds to the receptor. Their findings support the possibility of a soluble interaction between dibutyryl cGMP and the peptides of the CCK-gastrin family that is specific for the COOH-terminal (receptor binding) region of these peptides. This interaction is dependent on the concentration of dibutyryl cGMP and correlates with concentrations that inhibit biologic activity. The proposed complex is dispersed by gel filtration chromatography and is prevented from being formed by certain detergents.

REFERENCES

1. Ivy AC, Oldberg E: A hormone mechanism for gallbladder contraction and evacuation. Am J Physiol 86:599, 1928.

2. Harper AA, Raper HS: Pancreozymin, a stimulant of the secretion of pancreatic enzymes in extracts of the small intestine. J Physiol 102:115, 1943.
3. Jorpes JE: Memorial lecture: The isolation and chemistry of secretin and cholecystokinin. Gastroenterology 55:157, 1968.
4. Rayford PL, Thompson JC. Gastrin. Surg Gynecol Obstet 145:257, 1977.
5. Eysselein VE, Deveney CW, Sankaran H, et al: Biological activity of canine intestinal cholecystokinin-58. Am J Physiol 245:G313, 1983.
6. Eysselein VE, Reeve JR Jr, Shively JE, et al: Partial structure of a large canine cholecystokinin (CCK_{58}): Amino acid sequence. Peptides 3:687, 1982.
7. Brownstein MJ, Rehfeld JF: Molecular forms of cholecystokinin in the nervous system. Ann NY Acad Sci 448:9, 1985.
8. Amer MS: Studies with cholecystokinin. II. Cholecystokinetic potency of porcine gastrins I and II and related peptides in three systems. Endocrinology 84:1277, 1969.
9. Thompson JC: Chemical structure and biological actions of gastrin, cholecystokinin, and related compounds, in Holton P (ed): *International Encyclopedia of Pharmacology and Therapeutics.* New York, Pergamon Press, 1973, pp 261–286.
10. Solomon TE, Yamada T, Elashoff J, et al: Bioactivity of cholecystokinin analogues: CCK-8 is not more potent than CCK-33. Am J Physiol 247:G105, 1984.
11. Deschenes RJ, Haun RS, Sunkel D, et al: Modulation of cholecystokinin gene expression. Ann NY Acad Sci 448:53, 1985.
12. Gubler U, Chua AO, Hoffman BJ, et al: Cloned cDNA to cholecystokinin mRNA predicts an identical preprocholecystokinin in pig brain and gut. Proc Natl Acad Sci USA 81:4307, 1984.
13. Beinfeld MC: Cholecystokinin (CCK) gene-related peptides: Distribution and characterization of immunoreactive pro-CCK and an amino-terminal pro-CCK fragment in rat brain. Brain Res 344:351, 1985.
14. Ogden WD, Fried GM, Sakamoto T, et al: Distribution of cholecystokinin in the alimentary tract of dogs. Surg Forum 33:132, 1982.
15. Larsson L-I, Rehfeld JF: Localization and molecular heterogeneity of cholecystokinin in the central and peripheral nervous system. Brain Res 165:201, 1979.
16. Rehfeld JF, Hansen HF, Marley PD, et al: Molecular forms of cholecystokinin in the brain and the relationship to neuronal gastrins. Ann NY Acad Sci 448:11, 1985.
17. Morley JE: The ascent of cholecystokinin (CCK)—From gut to brain. Life Sci 30:479, 1982.
18. Simon-Assmann PM, Yazigi R, Greeley GH Jr, et al: Biologic and radioimmunologic activity of cholecystokinin in regions of mammalian brains. J Neurosci Res 10:165, 1983.
19. Grimmelikhuijzen CJP, Sundler F, Rehfeld JF: Gastrin/CCK-like immunoreactivity in the nervous system of coelenterates. Histochemistry 69:61, 1980.
20. Larsson L-I, Rehfeld JF: Evidence for a common evolutionary origin of gastrin and cholecystokinin. Nature 269:335, 1977.
21. Rehfeld JF: Cholecystokinin. Clinics Gastroenterol 9:593, 1980.
22. Reeder DD, Becker HD, Smith NJ, et al: Measurement of endogenous release of cholecystokinin by radioimmunoassay. Ann Surg 178:304, 1973.
23. Harvey RF, Hartog M, Dowsett L, et al: A radioimmunoassay for cholecystokinin-pancreozymin. Lancet 2:826, 1973.
24. Burhol PG, Jenssen TG, Lygren I, et al: Iodination with iodogen and radioimmunoassay of cholecystokinin (CCK) in acidified plasma, CCK release, and molecular CCK components in man. Digestion 23:156, 1982.
25. Byrnes DJ, Henderson L, Borody T, et al: Radioimmunoassay of cholecystokinin in human plasma. Clin Chim Acta 111:81, 1981.
26. Calam J, Ellis A, Dockray GH: Identification and measurement of molecular variants of cholecystokinin in duodenal mucosa and plasma. Diminished concentrations in patients with celiac disease. J Clin Invest 69:218, 1982.
27. Chang T-M, Chey WY: Radioimmunoassay of cholecystokinin. Dig Dis Sci 28:456, 1983.
28. Kothary PC, Vinik AI, Owyang C, et al: Immunochemical studies of molecular heterogeneity of cholecystokinin in duodenal perfusates and plasma in humans. J Biol Chem 258:2856, 1983.
29. Maton PN, Selden AC, Chadwick VS: Large and small forms of cholecystokinin in human plasma: Measurement using high pressure liquid chromatography and radioimmunoassay. Regul Pept 4:251, 1982.
30. Rehfeld JF, Holst JJ, Lindkaer Jensen S: The molecular nature of vascularly released cholecystokinin from the isolated perfused porcine duodenum. Regul Pept 3:15, 1982.
31. Schafmayer A, Werner M, Becker H-D: Radioimmunological determination of cholecystokinin in tissue extracts. Digestion 24:146, 1982.
32. Fried GM, Ogden WD, Swierczek J, et al: Release of cholecystokinin in conscious dogs: Correlation with simultaneous measurements of gallbladder pressure and pancreatic protein secretion. Gastroenterology 85:1113, 1983.
33. Walsh JH, Lamers GB, Valenzuela JE: Cholecystokinin-octapeptidelike immunoreactivity in human plasma. Gastroenterology 82:438, 1982.
34. Thompson JC, Fender HR, Ramus NI, et al: Cholecystokinin metabolism in man and dogs. Ann Surg 182:496, 1975.
35. Lonovics J, Hajnal F, Suddith RL, et al: Metabolism of different molecular forms of cholecystokinin. Adv Physiol Sci 12:383, 1981.
36. Kanayama S, Himeno S, Kurokawa M, et al: Marked prolongation in disappearance half-time of plasma cholecystokinin-octapeptide in patients with hepatic cirrhosis. Am J Gastroenterol 80:557, 1985.
37. Sakamoto T, Fujimura M, Newman J, et al: Comparison of hepatic elimination of different forms of

cholecystokinin in dogs. Bioassay and radioimmunoassay comparisons of cholecystokinin-8-sulfate and -33-sulfate. J Clin Invest 75:280, 1985.

38. Gosden CM, Gosden JR: Fetal abnormalities in cystic fibrosis suggest a deficiency in proteolysis of cholecystokinin. Lancet 2:541, 1984.
39. Meyer JH: Release of secretin and cholecystokinin, in Thompson JC (ed): *Gastrointestinal Hormones*. Austin, University of Texas Press, 1975, pp 475–489.
40. Chen YF, Chey WF, Chang T-M, et al: Duodenal acidification releases cholecystokinin. Am J Physiol 249:G29, 1985.
41. Miyata M, Rayford PL, Thompson JC: Hormonal (gastrin, secretin, cholecystokinin) and secretory effects of bombesin and duodenal acidification in dogs. Surgery 87:209, 1980.
42. Inoue K, Wiener I, Fagan CJ, et al: Effect of oral magnesium sulfate on gallbladder contraction and cholecystokinin release in man. Gastroenterology 80:1181, 1981.
43. Fried GM, Inoue K, Wiener I, et al: Effect of divalent cations on the release of cholecystokinin and gastrin. Surg Forum 32:209, 1981.
44. Mate L, Greeley GH Jr, Thompson JC: Effect of verapamil on bombesin-stimulated pancreatic and gastric secretion and release of gastrin and cholecystokinin. Dig Dis Sci 29:960, 1984.
45. Burhol PG, Rayford PL, Jorde R, et al: Radioimmunoassay of plasma cholecystokinin (CCK), duodenal release of CCK, diurnal variation of plasma CCK, and immunoreactive plasma CCK components in man. Hepatogastroenterology 27:300, 1980.
46. Jorde R, Burhol PG: Diurnal profiles of gastrointestinal regulatory peptides. Scand J Gastroenterol 20:1, 1985.
47. Wiener I, Inoue K, Fagan CJ, et al: Release of cholecystokinin in man. Correlation of blood levels with gallbladder contraction. Ann Surg 194:321, 1981.
48. Lilja P, Fried GM, Wiener I, et al: Comparison of concentrations of plasma cholecystokinin in pig, dog, and man after food or intraduodenal fat. Gastroenterology 82:1118, 1982.
49. Sakamoto T, Greeley GH Jr, Fujimura M, et al: Effect of fat and somatostatin on release of secretin and cholecystokinin in dogs. Dig Dis Sci 29:72S, 1984.
50. Rayford PL, Guzman S, Hill FLC, et al: The effects of vagotomy on bombesin-stimulated release of gastrin and cholecystokinin in dogs. Physiologist 21:97, 1978.
51. Guzman S, Chayvialle J-A, Banks WA, et al: Effect of vagal stimulation on pancreatic secretion and on blood levels of gastrin, cholecystokinin, secretin, vasoactive intestinal peptide, and somatostatin. Surgery 86:329, 1979.
52. Fried GM, Ogden WD, Greeley G, et al: Correlation of release and actions of cholecystokinin in dogs before and after vagotomy. Surgery 93:786, 1983.
53. Hopman WPM, Jansen JBMJ, Lamers CBHW: Plasma cholecystokinin response to a liquid fat meal in vagotomized patients. Ann Surg 200:693, 1984.
54. Hopman WPM, Jansen JBMJ, Lamers CBHW: Effect of atropine on the plasma cholecystokinin response to intraduodenal fat in man. Digestion 29:19, 1984.
55. Hopman WPM, Jansen JBMJ, Lamers CBHW: Plasma cholecystokinin response to oral fat in patients with Billroth I and Billroth II gastrectomy. Ann Surg 199:276, 1984.
56. Fender HR, Curtis PJ, Rayford PL, et al: Effect of bombesin on serum gastrin and cholecystokinin in dogs. Surg Forum 27:414, 1976.
57. Miyata M, Guzman SB, Rayfod PL, et al: Response of cholecystokinin, secretin, and pancreatic secretion to graded doses of bombesin. Surg Forum 29:390, 1978.
58. Lilja P, Greeley GH Jr, Thompson JC: Pancreatic exocrine secretion. Release of gastrin and cholecystokinin in response to bombesin in pigs. Arch Surg 138:825, 1984.
59. Rayford PL, Miller TA, Thompson JC: Secretin, cholecystokinin and newer gastrointestinal hormones. N Engl J Med 295:1093; 1157, 1976.
60. Maton PN, Selden AC, Fitzpatrick ML, et al: Defective gallbladder emptying and cholecystokinin release in celiac disease. Reversal by gluten-free diet. Gastroenterology 88:391, 1985.
61. Inoue K, Yazigi R, Watson LC, et al: Increased release of cholecystokinin after pancreatic duct ligation. Surgery 91:467, 1982.
62. Folsch UR, Schafmayer A, Ebert R, et al: Elevated plasma cholecystokinin concentrations in exocrine pancreatic atrophy in the rat. Digestion 29:60, 1984.
63. Lilja P, Wiener I, Inoue K, et al: Changes in circulating levels of cholecystokinin, gastrin, and pancreatic polypeptide after small bowel resection in dogs. Am J Surg 145:157, 1983.
64. Gornacz GE, Ghatei MA, Al-Mukhtar MYT, et al: Plasma enteroglucagon and CCK levels and cell proliferation in defunctioned small bowel in the rat. Dig Dis Sci 29:1041, 1984.
65. Inoue K, Wiener I, Fried GM, et al: Effect of colectomy on cholecystokinin and gastrin release. Ann Surg 196:691, 1982.
66. Rosenberg L, Duguid WP, Brown RA, et al: The effect of cholecystectomy on plasma CCK and pancreatic growth in the hamster. Gastroenterology 84:1289, 1983.
67. Wiener I, Walker JP, Greeley GH Jr, et al: Increased release of cholecystokinin with intraduodenal fat after cholecystectomy in dogs. Surg Forum 35:196, 1984.
68. Thompson JC, Fried GM, Ogden WD, et al: Correlation between release of cholecystokinin and contraction of the gallbladder in patients with gallstones. Ann Surg 195:670, 1982.
69. Wiener I, Fagan CJ, Newman J, et al: Effect of cholecystectomy on levels of cholecystokinin in man. Surg Forum 34:218, 1983.
70. Gomez G, Lluis F, Guo Y-S, et al: Bile inhibits release of cholecystokinin and neurotensin. Surgery 100:363, 1986.

71. Lilja P, Wiener I, Inoue K, et al: Influence of different anesthetic agents on the release of cholecystokinin in dogs. Surgery 97:415, 1985.
72. Fried GM, Ogden WD, Zhu X-G, et al: Effect of alcohol on the release of cholecystokinin and pancreatic enzyme secretion. Am J Surg 147:53, 1984.
73. Stening GF, Grossman MI: Gastrin-related peptides as stimulants of pancreatic and gastric secretion. Am J Physiol 217:262, 1969.
74. Debas HT, Grossman MI: Pure cholecystokinin: Pancreatic protein and bicarbonate response. Digestion 9:469, 1973.
75. Williams RH, Champagne J: Effects of cholecystokinin, secretin, and pancreatic polypeptide on secretion of gastric inhibitory polypeptide, insulin, and glucagon. Life Sci 25:947, 1979.
76. Hedner P, Persson H, Rorsman G: Effect of cholecystokinin on small intestine. Acta Physiol Scand 70:250, 1967.
77. Lechin DF, van der DiJs B: Physiological effects of endogenous CCK on distal colon motility. Acta Gastroenterol Latinoam 9:195, 1979.
78. Cameron AJ, Phillips SF, Summerskill WHJ: Effect of cholecystokinin on motility of human stomach and gallbladder muscle in vitro. Clin Res 15:416, 1967.
79. Grossman MI: Gastrointestinal hormones: Spectrum of actions and structure-activity relations, in Chey WY, Brooks FP (eds): *Endocrinology of the Gut*. Thorofare, NJ, Charles B Slack, 1974, pp 65—75.
80. Scheurer U, Varga L, Drack E, et al: Mechanism of action of cholecystokinin octapeptide on rat antrum, pylorus, and duodenum. Am J Physiol 244:G266, 1983.
81. Jones RS, Grossman MI: Choleretic effects of cholecystokinin, gastrin II, and caerulein in the dog. Am J Physiol 219:1014, 1970.
82. Burnstein MJ, Vassal KP, Strasberg SM: Results of combined biliary drainage and cholecystokinin cholecystography in 81 patients with normal oral cholecystograms. Ann Surg 196:627, 1982.
83. Shafer RB, Marlette JM, Morley JE: The effects of Lipomul, CCK, and TRH on gallbladder emptying. Clin Nucl Med 8:66, 1983.
84. Stening GF, Grossman MI: Hormonal control of Brunner's glands. Gastroenterology 56:1047, 1969.
85. Bowen JC, Fang W-F, Pawlik W, et al: Gastrointestinal hormones and blood flow, in Thompson JC (ed): *Gastrointestinal Hormones*. Austin, University of Texas Press, 1975, pp 391–400.
86. Konturek SJ, Bilski J, Tasler J, et al: Gut hormones in stimulation of gastroduodenal alkaline secretion in conscious dogs. Am J Physiol 248:G687, 1985.
87. Hersey SJ, May D, Schyberg D: Stimulation of pepsinogen release from isolated gastric glands by cholecystokininlike peptides. Am J Physiol 244:G192, 1983.
88. Lankisch PG: Trophic effects of gastrointestinal hormones. Clinics Gastroenterol 9:773, 1980.
89. Post JA, Hanson KM: Hepatic, vascular and biliary responses to infusion of gastrointestinal hormones and bile salts. Digestion 12:65, 1975.
90. Toouli J, Hogan WJ, Geenen JE, et al: Action of cholecystokinin-octapeptide on sphincter of Oddi basal pressure and phasic wave activity in humans. Surgery 92:497, 1982.
91. Johnson LR, Grossman MI: Analysis of inhibition of acid secretion by cholecystokinin in dogs. Am J Physiol 218:550, 1970.
92. Soll AH, Amirian DA, Park J, et al: Cholecystokinin potently releases somatostatin from canine fundic mucosal cells in short-term culture. Am J Physiol 248:G569, 1985.
93. Shelby HT, Gross LP, Lichty P, et al: Action of cholecystokinin and cholinergic agents on membrane-bound calcium in dispersed pancreatic acinar cells. J Clin Invest 58:1482, 1976.
94. Christophe JP, Frandsen EK, Conlon TP, et al: Action of cholecystokinin, cholinergic agents, and A-23187 on accumulation of guanosine 3′:5′-monophosphte in dispersed guinea pig pancreatic acinar cells. J Biol Chem 251:4640, 1976.
95. Long BW, Gardner JD: Effects of cholecystokinin on adenylate cyclase activity in dispersed pancreatic acinar cells. Gastroenterology 73:1008, 1977.
96. Sakamoto T, Fujimura M, Townsend CM Jr, et al: Differentiation of actions of neurotensin, secretin, and CCK on pancreatic secretions in dogs. Gastroenterology 86:1229, 1984.
97. Khalil T, Fujimura M, Townsend CM Jr, et al: The interaction of neurotensin, secretin, and cholecystokinin-octapeptide on pancreatic secretion in rats. Dig Dis Sci 29:42S, 1984.
98. Sakamoto T, Newman J, Fujimura M, et al: Role of neurotensin in pancreatic secretion. Surgery 96:146, 1984.
99. Sninsky CA, Wolfe MM, McGuigan JE, et al: Alterations in motor function of the small intestine from intravenous and intraluminal cholecystokinin. Am J Physiol 247:G724, 1984.
100. Lilja P, Fagan CJ, Wiener I, et al: Infusion of pure cholecystokinin in humans. Correlation between plasma concentrations of cholecystokinin and gallbladder size. Gastroenterology 83:256, 1982.
101. Watson LC, Townsend CM Jr, Wiener I, et al: Male-female differences in plasma and mucosal cholecystokinin. Gastroenterology 80:1312, 1981.
102. Fried GM, Wiener I, Inoue K, et al: Differences in gallbladder contraction in men and women in response to endogenously-released cholecystokinin. Gastroenterology 82:1062, 1982.
103. Zhu XG, Fried GM, Greeley G, et al: Effect of estrogen and progesterone on cholecystokinin-stimulated gallbladder contraction in vitro. Gastroenterology 82:1218, 1982.
104. Ryan JP: Calcium and gallbladder smooth muscle contraction in the guinea pig: Effect of pregnancy. Gastroenterology 89:1279, 1985.
105. Fried GM, Ogden WD, Greeley G, et al: Cholecystokinin control of the intestinal phase of pancreatic

polypeptide release. Gastroenterology 82:1061, 1982.

106. Lonovics J, Guzman S, Devitt P, et al: Release of pancreatic polypeptide in humans by infusion of cholecystokinin. Gastroenterology 79:817, 1980.
107. Lu Q-H, Greeley GH Jr, Zhu X-G, et al: Intracerebroventricular administration of cholecystokinin-8 elevates plasma pancreatic polypeptide levels in awake dogs. Endocrinology 114:2415, 1984.
108. Gibbs J, Young RC, Smith GP: Cholecystokinin decreases food intake in rats. J Comp Physiol Psychol 84:488, 1973.
109. Smith GP, Gibbs J, Jerome C, et al: The satiety effect of cholecystokinin: A progress report. Peptides 2 (Suppl 2):57, 1981.
110. Pi-Sunyer X, Kissileff HR, Thornton J, et al: C-terminal octapeptide of cholecystokinin decreases food intake in obese men. Physiol Behav 29:627, 1982.
111. Bueno L, Duranton A, Ruckebusch Y: Antagonistic effects of naloxone on CCK-octapeptide induced satiety and rumino-reticular hypomotility in sheep. Life Sci 32:855–863, 1983.
112. Houpt TR: The sites of action of cholecystokinin in decreasing meal size in pigs. Physiol Behav 31:693, 1983.
113. Smith GT, Moran TH, Coyle JT, et al: Anatomic localization of cholecystokinin receptors to the pyloric sphincter. Am J Physiol 246:R127, 1984.
114. Amer MS, McKinney GR: Studies with cholecystokinin *in vitro*. IV. Effects of cholecystokinin and related peptides on phosphodiesterase. J Pharmacol Exp Ther 183:535, 1972.
115. Ondetti MA, Rubin B, Engel SL, et al: Cholecystokinin-pancreozymin: Recent developments. Am J Dig Dis 15:149, 1970.
116. Yau WM, Makhlouf GM, Edwards LE, et al: Mode of action of cholecystokinin and related peptides on gallbladder muscle. Gastroenterology 65:451, 1973.
117. Steigerwalt W, Goldfine ID, Williams JA: Characterization of cholecystokinin receptors on bovine gallbladder membranes. Am J Physiol 247:G709, 1984.
118. Lonovics J, Suddith RL, Guzman S, et al: Actions of VIP, somatostatin, and pancreatic polypeptide on gallbladder tension and CCK-stimulated gallbladder contraction in vitro. Surg Forum 30:407, 1979.
119. Andersson K-E, Andersson R, Hedner P: Cholecystokinetic effect and concentration of cyclic AMP in gall-bladder muscle in vitro. Acta Physiol Scand 85:511, 1972.
120. Peikin SR, Costenbader CL, Gardner JD: Actions of derivatives of cyclic nucleotides on dispersed acini from guinea pig pancreas. J Biol Chem 254:5321, 1979.
121. Barlas N, Jensen RT, Beinfeld MC, et al: Cyclic nucleotide antagonists of cholecystokinin: Structural requirements for interaction with the cholecystokinin receptor. Am J Physiol 242:G161, 1982.
122. Hahne WF, Jensen RT, Lemp GF, et al: Proglumide and benzotript: Members of a different class of cholecystokinin receptor antagonists. Proc Natl Acad Sci USA 78:6304, 1981.
123. Spanarkel M, Martinez J, Briet C, et al: Cholecystokinin-27-32 amide. A member of a new class of cholecystokinin receptor antagonists. J Biol Chem 258:6746, 1983.
124. Jensen RT, Lemp GF, Gardner JD: Interactions of COOH-terminal fragments of cholecystokinin with receptors on dispersed acini from guinea pig pancreas. J Biol Chem 257:5554, 1982.
125. Jensen RT, Jones SW, Gardner JD: COOH-terminal fragments of cholecystokinin. A new class of cholecystokinin receptor antagonists. Biochim Biophys Acta 757:250, 1983.
126. Miller LJ, Reilly WM, Rosenzweig SA, et al: A soluble interaction between dibutyryl cyclic guanosine 3′:5′-monophosphate and cholecystokinin: A possible mechanism for the inhibition of cholecystokinin activity. Gastroenterology 84:1505, 1983.

Section Five

Secretin-Glucagon Family

Chapter 16

Secretin

Howard R. Doyle, M.D., Felix Lluis, M.D., and Phillip L. Rayford, Ph.D.

HISTORY

Bayliss and Starling [1], in 1902, showed that infusion of hydrochloric acid into a denervated loop of small intestine elicited the brisk secretion of pancreatic juice. They reasoned that a substance released from the acidified intestines and carried by the blood to the pancreas was responsible for the stimulation of pancreatic secretion. They named this substance secretin. With the discovery of secretin, the science of endocrinology began, although half a century passed before the impact of endocrinologic studies of gastrointestinal hormones was realized in both health and disease.

In 1965, Mutt et al [2] described the amino acid sequence of secretin, and in the same year, Bodanszky et al [3] synthesized the hormone. Secretin was found to be composed of 27 amino acid residues, 14 of which occupy the same position in secretin as in glucagon [4]. The secretin molecule has a helical configuration and weighs 3055 daltons. The intact secretin molecule is needed for complete biologic activity [5]. A glycine-extended form of secretin, 30 amino acid residues long, has recently been isolated from porcine upper intestinal tissue and found to be as potent as the 27 amino acid classic secretin molecule in stimulating pancreatic secretion of bicarbonate [6].

DISTRIBUTION

Although there are some species variations in all of those studied so far, most of the immunoreactive secretin is localized in the duodenum and jejunum, with a surprisingly high content distal to the proximal duodenum [7–9]. We say surprisingly high because the accepted mechanism of release is acidification, and the requisite pH is not achieved beyond the proximal duodenum.

Secretin-like immunoreactivity and bioactivity have been reported in extracts of antral mucosa of dogs and rats [10]. This finding was correlated with the demonstration of secretin cells by means of immunocytochemistry [10]. At least in dogs, secretin is localized in a special type of endocrine cell. Using the immunogold technique and the electron microscope, Usellini et al [11] identified secretin-containing granules in previously described "K cells," whereas "S cells" lacked secretin immunoreactivity in the dog duodenum. In the cat, pig, and rabbit, secretin was found in "S cells."

Tissue stores of secretin in the gut change under different situations. The microbial flora of the intestine may have some influence on tissue content of secretin. Intestinal extracts from germ-free mice contained higher tissue levels of secretin than those from control animals [12]. Duodenal stores of secretin increase and basal plasma levels decrease after hypophysectomy in the rat [13]. Finally, prolonged fasting modifies the secretin content in the rat small intestine. In the duodenum, 12 hours or more of fasting, and in the jejunum, 24 hours or more of fasting, led to a significant decrease of secretin [14]. In the ileum, secretin levels decreased significantly after 24 hours of fasting and increased after 48 hours or more of fasting [14].

The ontogeny of secretin has been studied in the rat [15] (see Chapter 11). Secretin was not found in acid extracts of the stomach, colon, and brain in 3-day-old rats, whereas the concentration of secretin in the duodenum or ileum was equal to or higher than that found in the adult rat.

Immunoreactive secretin has recently been found in the central nervous system of rats and pigs [16], adding it to the long list of brain-gut peptides. In the rat, the highest concentrations were found in the pineal and pituitary glands, followed by the thalamus and hypothalamus [16]. Preliminary evidence has been provided for the existence of a secretinergic pathway between the brain and neurointermediate lobe of the pituitary [17]; however, the physiologic significance of this finding is not clear.

ASSAY

The bioassay of secretin depends upon its ability to quantitatively stimulate bicarbonate and water secretion by the pancreas [18]. This assay lacks the sensitivity needed to measure concentrations of secretin that exist in small volumes in body fluids, especially plasma. Endogenous release of secretin in the circulation can be detected by the measurement of pancreatic secretion of water and bicarbonate.

Radioimmunoassays (RIA) have been developed by several investigators and have been used to measure levels of secretin in tissues and plasma of humans and of experimental animals [19–23]. Most of these assays are sufficiently sensitive to detect the physiologic release of secretin; however, there is wide variation of values reported by different laboratories [20]. These variations may be due to use of different antisera, standards, methods of labeling radioactive tracer, and other chemical procedures and assay techniques [20,24]. In addition, most plasma samples appear to contain a substance that interferes with the antibody-antigen reaction and thereby hampers the ability of radioimmunoassay to accurately measure secretin [20]. Chemical methods have been used to remove interfering substances in plasma, and this has resulted in lower plasma levels of secretin [20]. It should be noted that use of these extraction procedures has not significantly altered measurements of physiologic release of secretin that have been reported with unextracted plasma.

PHARMACOKINETICS AND CATABOLISM

Over a wide dose range, the disappearance of secretin from blood follows first-order kinetics; the elimination from plasma is strictly exponential. In all species, the plasma half-life is on the order of 2–4 minutes [25,26]. There are studies that show the kidney to be an important site for the catabolism of secretin [27]. In a study in dogs, it was shown that after the kidneys were excluded from the circulation, the disappearance half-life of secretin was doubled, whereas ureteral ligation had no effect [28]. It was concluded that the kidneys extract the hormone through a process that is independent of glomerular filtration. These conclusions have been contested by another investigator who, using a different experimental design, found evidence that secretin is filtered through the glomerular capillary membrane and later reabsorbed by the tubular epithelium [29]. In this study, the calculated plasma threshold, after IV secretin, was about 100 times greater than fasting plasma levels, which may bring the significance of the findings into question. It has also been shown that, besides the kidney, other vascular beds are capable of removing secretin from the circulation in a nonspecific way, in a manner analogous to the removal of gastrin [30,31]. The importance of the kidney in the catabolism of secretin might be due to its greater blood flow. The major mechanism for catabolism appears to be widespread and nonspecific.

RELEASE

Among the various dietary and physicochemical factors studied so far, duodenal acidification with HCl has been the only consistent releasing factor for secretin [21], the secretin response being related to the amount of acid used to irrigate the duodenum (Fig 16-1). Above pH 4.5, secretin is not released in amounts sufficient to stimulate pancreatic secretion, and below pH 3.0, pancreatic output is related to the amount of titratable acid entering the gut [32].

In 1977, Llanos et al [33] used intragastric titration in dogs to study the effects of meals varying in pH on the release of pancreatic bicarbonate and the concentration of plasma secretin. Plasma secretin remained unchanged with a meal at pH 7.0 or 5.0 but increased significantly when the meal was at pH 3.0 (43 percent above basal) and at pH 2.0 (80 percent above basal). Pancreatic bicarbonate output was negligibly increased when the meal was held at pH 7.0 or 5.0 but increased sharply with acidification of a meal; bicarbonate output was near maximal when the gastric content was held at pH 3.0. When the test meal, originally prepared at pH 7.0, was endogenously acidified, plasma secretin level increased when the pH of the gastric contents fell below 4.0 [33]. Schafmayer et al [34] used a surgical preparation in dogs that did not interfere with the normal neutralization of gastric acid in the duodenum and found increased levels of secretin in portal and peripheral blood after a test meal. In a recent study that used an experimental model similar to that of Llanos et al and a more sensitive RIA, the pH threshold for both bicarbonate secretion and secretin release was found to be about 4.5 [35].

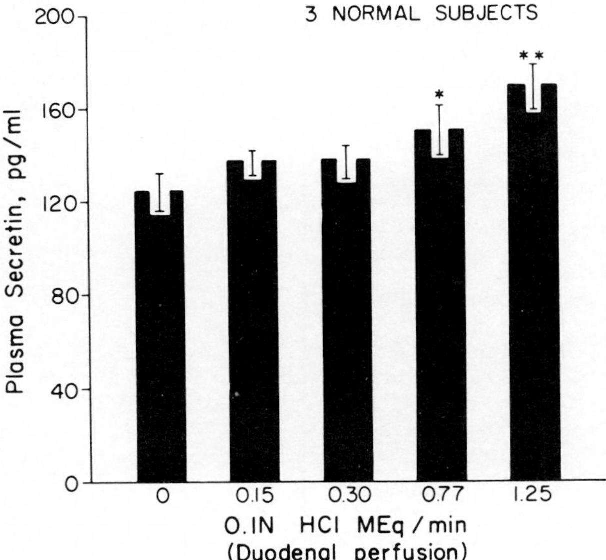

Figure 16-1. Plasma secretin levels in three human subjects before and after intraduodenal infusion of graded quantities (milliequivalents per minute) of 0.1 N HCl. * = significant elevation above basal; ** = significant elevation above basal and all other test periods. (From Rayford et al [21], by permission of the C V Mosby Co.)

In humans, plasma secretin increases postprandially, probably in response to endogenous acid. This release is not sustained, however, but occurs intermittently and is of brief duration. The changes in the levels of immunoreactive secretin appear to coincide with rapid falls in duodenal pH [22,36]. The reported threshold of pH 2.0 seems too low [37]. The intraduodenal (ID) infusion of sodium oleate at a pH of 8.5 has been reported to cause a small but significant rise in circulating immunoreactive secretin. This response was limited to a critical dose range, with the maximal response of plasma secretin and pancreatic bicarbonate occurring at the dose of oleate, 1.0 mmol/15 min. A triglyceride emulsion had no effect [38].

Secretin can also be released from the more distal small intestine in the dog. Perfusion of an isolated segment of jejunum with either HCl or sodium oleate resulted in a significant release of secretin, which closely paralleled pancreatic bicarbonate secretion [39,40]. Acid perfusion of the terminal ileum of the rat increased plasma secretin levels and pancreatic bicarbonate output [41].

There is evidence that immunoreactive secretin in plasma of humans is elevated with ID instillation of bile at a near neutral pH [42–45]. In humans, oral administration of alcohol raised gastrin and secretin levels; however, ID alcohol did not result in a significant release of secretin or gastrin [46] (Fig 16-2). Alcohol probably does not release secretin directly; release probably involves the stomach and may be mediated via the release of gastric acid [46,47].

Another agent that has been reported to release secretin is 1-phenylpentanol, a chemical substance derived from the extract of *Curcuma longa,* which is used as a condiment for Indian curry [48]. The release of secretin is reduced by increasing the osmolality of the duodenal contents [49].

Secretin release seems to be independent of the vagus nerve, plasma levels remaining unchanged after vagal electrical stimulation in dogs [50]. In humans, secretin release is not blocked by atropine [51], and vagotomy does not decrease the release of secretin induced by ID HCl [52].

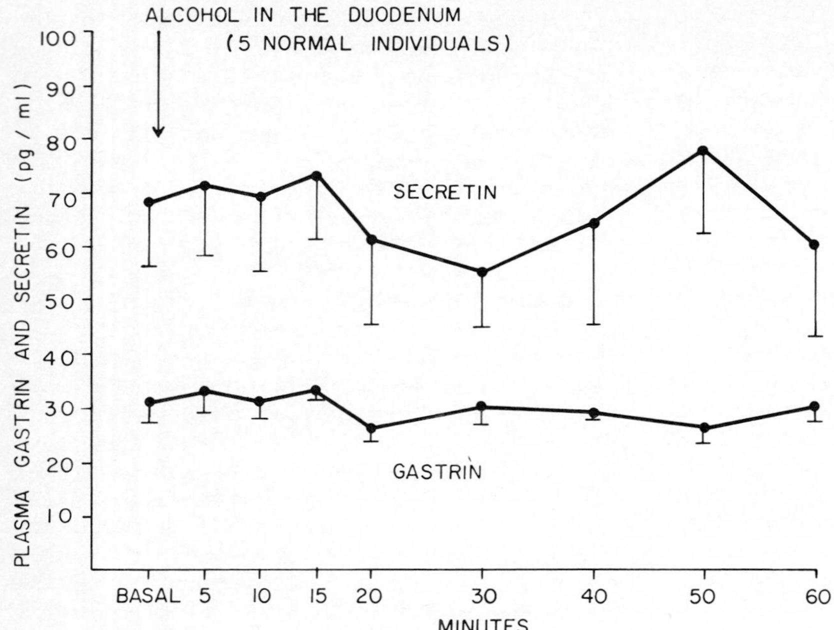

Figure 16-2. Plasma gastrin and secretin levels after the administration of alcohol in the duodenum in five normal subjects. * = significant elevations above basal ($p < 0.05$). (From Llanos et al [46], by permission of the C V Mosby Co.)

Several hormones that have been found to modulate pancreatic bicarbonate secretion have been studied to determine their effects on secretin release. The release of secretin by ID acid is enhanced by bombesin [53,54] and reduced by somatostatin [54,55]. Bombesin alone does not appear to release secretin [23,53,56]. Glucagon and pancreatic polypeptide (PP) do not inhibit secretin release by ID acidification, although pancreatic juice volume and bicarbonate secretion are significantly decreased [57,58]. This suggests that glucagon and PP probably act directly on the pancreas to suppress exocrine secretion. Endogenous release of secretin by ID fat is abolished by somatostatin [59]. The inhibition of pancreatic water and bicarbonate output by prostaglandin E_1 is due, at least in part, to the suppression of plasma secretin release [60]. Neurotensin increases pancreatic protein and bicarbonate secretion, but it appears to act differently from secretin, probably on another set of receptors [61]. Besides being released into the bloodstream, secretin undergoes luminal secretion [62]. The actions of secretin within the bowel lumen are not known.

ACTIONS

Some of the biologic actions of secretin are listed in Table 16-1. Most of these actions are brought about by physiologic concentrations of secretin. The role of secretin in pancreatic bicarbonate secretion is now more firmly established, since it is possible to correlate secretion with circulating levels of the hormone [33,35,36]. The administration of low-dose secretin, leading to plasma levels comparable to those observed postprandially in dogs [35] and humans [63], significantly increases pancreatic water and bicarbonate secretion. Also, the administration of rabbit antise-

Table 16-1. Actions of secretin

Stimulates
- Bicarbonate and water
- Colonic mucin
- Gastrin pepsin secretion
- Gastrin release in ZE syndrome patients
- Pancreatic growth
- Serum parathormone

Inhibits
- Colonic contraction
- Gastric acid
- Gastric emptying
- Gastrin release in duodenal ulcer patients and in normal individuals
- Lower esophageal sphincter tone
- Motility

cretin serum results in a profound decrease in pancreatic flow and the concentration and output of pancreatic bicarbonate. After a meal, the total bicarbonate output was less than 20 percent of that produced during the control experiment using normal rabbit serum [64]. The antisecretin serum also abolished the pancreatic secretion of bicarbonate and protein stimulated by low-dose exogenous secretin [64].

At comparable blood levels, exogenous secretin is less potent than the endogenously released hormone [64], and the final regulation of the pancreatic response to a meal probably involves the interaction of secretin with other released agents, such as cholecystokinin (CCK) and neurotensin [65–67], as well as the presence of an adequate cholinergic tone [51,68]. The presence of noncholinergic, vagal facilitatory pathways has also been suggested [69].

Secretin causes a diminution in the serum gastrin response to food in both humans and dogs [70] (Fig 16-3). Decreased basal gastrin levels in dogs, duodenal ulcer patients [71], normal subjects, and patients with pernicious anemia [71–73] have been found with the administration of secretin. The inhibitory effects of secretin on food-stimulated gastrin release, gastric acid secretion, and emptying are similar in healthy subjects and in duodenal ulcer patients [71,74]. The inhibition of postprandial gastric acid secretion is, of course, only partially mediated by secretin. Infusion of liver extract into the duodenum is a weak but significant stimulant of gastrin release and gastric acid secretion [75]. Acidification of the liver extract meal resulted in a pH-dependent fall in acid output and, at pH 7.0, both gastric acid and gastrin levels fell to basal. Secretin levels increased at the lower pH. Exogenous secretin, however, did not mimic the same effects. When the liver extract meal was kept in the stomach at pH 7.0, exogenous secretin was a weak inhibitor of gastrin release and gastric acid secretion, suggesting that mechanisms other than secretin are involved in the inhibition of gastric acid secretion induced by a meal [75]. Some have postulated that secretin plays no role in the acid-induced inhibition of gastric acid secretion in

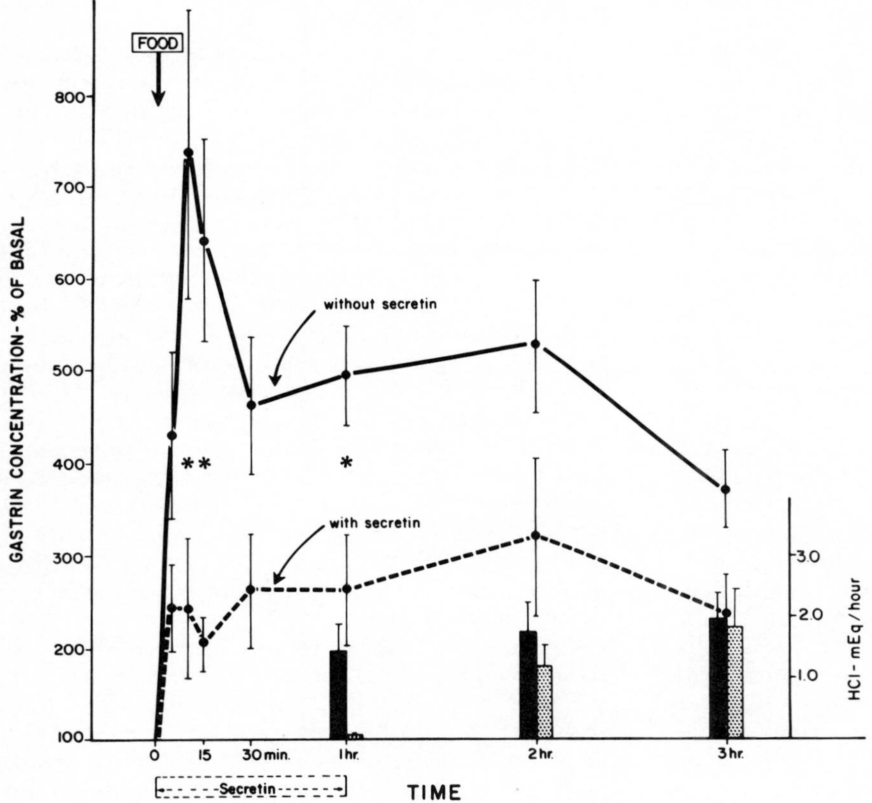

Figure 16-3. Effect of IV secretin on the serum gastrin responses to food in 15 patients and in 8 HP dogs. * = times at which the gastrin responses were significantly diminished by secretin ($p < 0.05$). The bar graph represents hourly HP acid output in response to food in the control studies (solid bars) and in the studies in which secretin was given over the first hour after eating (stippled bars). (From Bunchman HH II et al [70], by permission of the American College of Surgeons.)

humans [76], although the different methods used to stimulate gastric acid secretion may account, at least in part, for this opposite finding.

To further characterize the mechanisms involved in inhibition of gastric acid secretion induced by secretin, in vitro parietal cells were stimulated by histamine, methacholine, and pentagastrin. Secretin had no effect on the secretagogue response, suggesting that it does not act at the parietal cell level [77]. Inhibition of gastric secretion by secretin is accompanied by an increase in somatostatin secretion from the isolated perfused rat stomach [78], although the mechanism involved appears not to be mediated by somatostatin. This is supported by the finding that somatostatin antiserum infused concomitantly with secretin did not prevent inhibition of gastrin release in the perfused rat stomach [79]. In cultured rat antral mucosa, however, this inhibition of gastrin release appears to be mediated, at least in part, through release of antral somatostatin [80]. The inhibitory action of secretin on pentagastrin-stimulated gastric acid secretion in dogs is additive with serotonin [81] and peptide YY [82].

Fat in the duodenum is a potent inhibitor of gastrin release and gastric acid secretion; whether the mechanism involves secretin is not fully clear [83]. The possible role of secretin as an enterogastrone has also been reassessed in the light of our knowledge of the physiologic levels of circulating secretin. It has been shown that, in the dog, the administration of secretin in a physiologic dose can inhibit gastrin-stimulated gastric acid secretion [84]. In the same study, postprandial serum gastrin concentration and acid output were significantly greater following the infusion of antisecretin serum than after the administration of control serum.

In patients with the Zollinger-Ellison (ZE) syndrome, secretin infusion produces significant increases in serum calcium and gastrin levels and in gastric acid secretion [71,85]. The postprandial rise in gastrin concentration observed in some patients with the ZE syndrome after total gastrectomy without tumor excision could be explained by the release of endogenous secretin [71]. The secretin test has been widely used in the biochemical diagnosis of gastrinomas, since it provides an enhanced gastrin release from the tumor and helps to rule out other causes of hypergastrinemia [74]. Furthermore, the secretin test results in improved visualization of gastrinomas during selective angiography [86]. In ZE syndrome patients, the secretin test further increases gastrin levels, whereas there is no increase in duodenal ulcer patients or in control subjects [71,74,87]. The sensitivity of the secretin test remains unchanged or even improves after H_2-blocker treatment [88].

In humans, the infusion of secretin in doses as low as 0.03 U/kg/hr significantly inhibits gastric emptying of a liquid meal [89]. This action of secretin is not potentiated by CCK-8.

Secretin can stimulate the pylorus or inhibit the lower esophageal sphincter; however, the doses needed for these actions are pharmacologic [90,91]. Infusion of secretin at doses that mimic postprandial plasma levels produced relaxation of the sphincter of Oddi in healthy volunteers [92]. Secretin induces HCO_3^- production in gastric mucosa of Heidenhain pouches in dogs [93] as a component of the gastric mucosal barrier. The increases are greater than those achieved with calcium, dibutyryl cGMP, and cimetidine but less than those found with E_2 prostaglandin and carbachol. Secretin stimulates a bicarbonate-rich ductular bile flow in dogs [94–96] and increases bicarbonate secretion from the duodenal Brunner's gland in the rat [97,98]. Pharmacologic doses of secretin induced colonic mucin secretion in dogs [99]. Secretin has been shown to inhibit segmental contractions of the colon [100].

Other effects of secretin include an increase in the levels of serum parathormone in humans; this is dose-dependent and present even at very low doses (0.01 to 2.0 U/kg/hr) [101]. Ingestion of an acid-stimulating test meal in humans resulted in increases in serum parathormone and calcitonin, which were blocked by simultaneous antacid ingestion. Also, there were no meal-induced changes in serum parathormone or calcitonin in achlorhydric patients with pernicious anemia [102]. Endogenous secretin may, therefore, play a physiologic role in modulating the secretion of parathormone and calcitonin.

The effects of secretin on insulin release, although widely studied, appear to be pharmacologic [103]. The administration of 1 U/kg of secretin in a bolus injection produced a rise in the IgM and IgA antibodies specific to cow's milk proteins in the duodenal fluid, in spite of a concomitant decrease in pancreatic enzyme concentrations in the same duodenal aspirate [104].

As for the trophic actions of secretin on the pancreas, there was considerable discrepancy in previous reports [105], and those studies that showed a trophic action used large amounts of exogenous hormone. Recently, however, Johnson [106] has reported that pancreatic growth can be stimulated by continuous intraduodenal perfusion with hydrochloric acid. Secretin infusion was associated with initial duodenal hypertrophy followed by hyperplasia in the rat [107]. In a separate study [108], secretin was found to induce pancreatic hypertrophy in the rat only after 15 days of treatment; pancreatic weight, RNA, and lipase content increased. The trophic effects of a combination of secretin plus caerulein were synergistic in the rat pancreas.

In the hamster, secretin increases pancreatic DNA content, whereas the combination of secretin plus caerulein increases weight and DNA content of pancreatic ductal adenocarcinoma implanted into the cheek pouches of Syrian golden hamsters [109]. The trophic effects of secretin (and CCK) on the intestinal mucosa of rats may be mediated through the stimulation of pancreaticobiliary secretions [110]. Although some of these studies can hardly be considered physiologic, they suggest that endogenous secretin may play a significant role in the regulation of pancreatic growth.

Doses of secretin considered physiologic, or duodenal acidification to a pH of 2.0, does not change pancreatic blood flow in the dog; only higher doses of secretin or a stronger duodenal acidification (pH 1.4) increases pancreatic blood flow [111]. High doses of secretin increase the caliber of the Wirsung duct in humans, thus allowing improved visualization by ultrasonography [112].

PATHOPHYSIOLOGY

Besides in patients with the ZE syndrome, the role of secretin has been studied in some other clinical conditions. Several clinical trials claim secretin is effective in preventing gastric bleeding, although secretin treatment was found less effective than antacids in elevating the intragastric pH. A series of 38 high-risk patients were given either antacids or secretin (0.25 U/kg/hr) for several days in order to prevent gastric stress ulcers. The intragastric pH achieved was higher in the antacid-treated group, and an increase in dosage was necessary in four of the 17 patients under secretin treatment [113]. A more recent study [114] shows that secretin inhibition of stress-induced gastric bleeding in the rat may be mediated through the increase in glycoprotein secretion in the gastric mucosa. Secretin may not be involved in the etiology of ulcers occurring after pancreaticoduodenectomy. Patients with carcinoma of the head of the pancreas were found to have elevated basal levels and diminished secretin response to the oral hydrochloric tolerance test [115]. After pancreaticoduodenectomy and Child's reconstruction, basal secretin levels were within normal range, and the secretin response to the hydrochloric test increased. Plasma secretin response to duodenal acidification is normal in celiac patients after treatment with a gluten-free diet [116]. Postprandial plasma secretin levels after Billroth I and Billroth II anastomosis following subtotal gastrectomy, Roux-en-Y anastomosis and interposed jejunal loop after total gastrectomy, and Child's reconstruction after pancreaticoduodenectomy were measured in patients 2 months after surgery. After subtotal gastrectomy, a diminished secretin response was found after a test meal, the response being lower in the Billroth II than in the Billroth I type of reconstruction. After total gastrectomy, some secretin was measured, suggesting that stimulants other than endogenous acid are capable of releasing secretin [117,118].

REFERENCES

1. Bayliss WM, Starling EH: The mechanism of pancreatic secretion. J Physiol (Lond) 28:325, 1902.
2. Mutt V, Magnusson S, Jorpes JE, et al: Structure of porcine secretin. I. Degradation with trypsin and thrombin. Sequence of the tryptic peptides. The C-terminal residue. Biochemistry 4:2358, 1965.
3. Bodanszky M, Ondetti MA, Levine SD, et al: Synthesis of a heptacosapeptide amide with the hormonal activity of secretin. Chem Indust 42:1757, 1966.
4. Jorpes JE: The isolation and chemistry of secretin and cholecystokinin. Gastroenterology 55:157, 1968.
5. Grossman MI: Structure of secretin. Gastroenterology 57:610, 1969.
6. Gafvelin G, Carlquist M, Mutt V: A proform of secretin with high secretin-like bioactivity. FEBS Lett 184:347, 1985.
7. Curtis PJ, Rayford PL, Thompson JC: Determination of secretin levels in mucosa by radioimmunoassay. Surg Forum 27:428, 1976.
8. Straus E, Yalow RS: Immunoreactive secretin in gastrointestinal mucosa of several mammalian species. Gastroenterology 75:401, 1978.
9. Miller TA, Llanos OL, Swierczek JS, et al: Concentrations of gastrin and secretin in the alimentary tract of the cat. Surgery 83:90, 1978.
10. Chey WY, Chang T-M, Park H-J, et al: Secretin-like immunoreactivity and biological activity in the antral mucosa. Endocrinology 113:651, 1983.
11. Usellini L, Capella C, Frigerio B, et al: Ultrastructural localization of secretin in endocrine cells of the dog duodenum by the immunogold technique.

Comparison with ultrastructurally characterized S cells of various mammals. Histochemistry 80:435, 1984.
12. Pen J, Welling GW: Influence of the microbial flora on the amount of CCK_8- and $secretin_{21-27}$-like immunoreactivity in the intestinal tract of mice. Comp Biochem Physiol 76B:585, 1983.
13. Teichmann RK, Schafmayer A, Hill FLC, et al: Effects of hypophysectomy and hypophysectomy plus growth hormone on secretin release and on concentrations of secretin in the duodenal mucosa. Surg Forum 28:375, 1977.
14. Fujimura M, Sakamoto T, Greeley GH Jr, et al: Effect of fasting on secretin and cholecystokinin levels in the rat small intestine. Fed Proc 43:1072, 1984.
15. Ichihara K, Eng J, Yalow RS: Ontogeny of immunoreactive CCK, VIP and secretin in rat brain and gut. Biochem Biophys Res Commun 112:891, 1983.
16. O'Donohue TL, Charlton CG, Miller RL, et al: Identification, characterization, and distribution of secretin immunoreactivity in rat and pig brain. Proc Natl Acad Sci USA 78:5221, 1981.
17. Charlton CG, O'Donohue TL, Miller RL, et al: Secretin in the rat hypothalamo-pituitary system: Localization, identification and characterization. Peptides 3:565, 1982.
18. Scratcherd T, Case RM, Smith PA: A sensitive method for the biological assay for secretin and substances with "secretin-like" activity in tissues and body fluids. Scand J Gastroenterol 10:821, 1975.
19. Boden G, Chey WY: Preparation and specificity of antiserum to synthetic secretin and its use in a radioimmunoassay (RIA). Endocrinology 92:1617, 1973.
20. Chang T-M, Chey WY: Radioimmunoassay of secretin. A critical review and current status. Dig Dis Sci 25:529, 1980.
21. Rayford PL, Curtis PJ, Fender HR, et al: Plasma levels of secretin in man and dogs: Validation of a secretin radioimmunoassay. Surgery 79:658, 1976.
22. Schaffalitzky de Muckadell OB, Fahrenkrug J: Secretion pattern of secretin in man: Regulation by gastric acid. Gut 19:812, 1978.
23. Hanssen LE, Hanssen KF, Myren J: Inhibition of secretin release and pancreatic bicarbonate secretion by somatostatin infusion in man. Scand J Gastroenterol 12:391, 1977.
24. Straus E: Special problems of the radioimmunoassay for gut hormones. Clinics Gastroenterol 9:555, 1980.
25. Curtis PJ, Fender HR, Rayford PL, et al: Disappearance half-time of endogenous and exogenous secretin in dogs. Gut 17:595, 1976.
26. Hacki WH: Secretin. Clin Gastroenterol 9:609, 1980.
27. Curtis PJ, Fender HR, Rayford PL, et al: Catabolism of secretin by the liver and kidney. Surgery 80:259, 1976.
28. Curtis PJ, Miller TA, Rayford PL, et al: The effect of nephrectomy on the catabolism of secretin. Am J Surg 133:52, 1977.
29. Naruse S: Renal handling of secretin in dogs: Free and stop flow analysis. Metabolism 29:1237, 1980.
30. Thompson JC, Llanos OL, Teichmann RK, et al: Catabolism of gastrin and secretin. World J Surg 3:469, 1979.
31. Thompson JC, Llanos OL, Schafmayer A, et al: Mechanisms of release and catabolism of secretin, in Bloom SR (ed): *Gut Hormones*. New York, Churchill Livingstone, 1978, pp 176–181.
32. Rayford PL, Miller TA, Thompson JC: Secretin, cholecystokinin and newer gastrointestinal hormones. N Engl J Med 295:1093; 1157, 1976.
33. Llanos OL, Konturek SJ, Rayford PL, et al: Pancreatic bicarbonate, serum gastrin, and secretin responses to meals varying in pH. Am J Physiol 233:E41, 1977.
34. Schafmayer A, Teichmann RK, Rayford PL, et al: Physiologic release of secretin measured in peripheral and portal venous blood of dogs. Digestion 17:509, 1978.
35. Chey WY, Konturek SJ: Plasma secretin and pancreatic secretion in response to liver extract meal with varied pH and exogenous secretin in the dog. J Physiol 324:263, 1982.
36. Pelletier MJ, Chayvialle JAP, Minaire Y: Uneven and transient secretin release after a liquid test meal. Gastroenterology 75:1124, 1978.
37. Fahrenkrug J, Schaffalitzky de Muckadell OB, Rune SJ: pH threshold for release of secretin in normal subjects and in patients with duodenal ulcer and patients with chronic pancreatitis. Scand J Gastroenterol 13:177, 1978.
38. Faichney A, Chey WY, Kim YC, et al: Effect of sodium oleate on plasma secretin concentration and pancreatic secretion in dog. Gastroenterology 81:458, 1981.
39. Fujimura M, Sakamoto T, Khalil T, et al: Role of the jejunum and ileum in the release of secretin and cholecystokinin by acid or fat in conscious dogs. Gastroenterology 86:1083, 1984.
40. Fujimura M, Sakamoto T, Khalil T, et al: Role of the small intestine in pancreatic exocrine secretion in dogs: Correlation with secretin and cholecystokinin release by luminal stimulants. Dig Dis Sci 29:28S, 1984.
41. Shinomura Y, Saito R, Himeno S, et al: Effect of acid perfusion of the terminal ileum on plasma immunoreactive secretin and pancreatic secretion in the rat. Horm Metab Res 15:15, 1983.
42. Osnes M, Hanssen LE, Flaten O, et al: Exocrine pancreatic secretion and immunoreactive secretin (IRS) release after intraduodenal instillation of bile in man. Gut 19:180, 1978.
43. Hanssen LE: Pure synthetic bile salts release immunoreactive secretin in man. Scand J Gastroenterol 15:461, 1980.
44. Osnes M, Hanssen LE, Lehnert P, et al: Exocrine

pancreatic secretion and immunoreactive secretin release after repeated intraduodenal infusions of bile in man. Scand J Gastroenterol 15:1033, 1980.

45. Osnes M, Hanssen LE: The influence of intraduodenal administration of pancreatic juice on the bile-induced pancreatic secretion and immunoreactive secretin release in man. Scand J Gastroenterol 15:1041, 1980.
46. Llanos OL, Swierczek JS, Teichmann RK, et al: Effect of alcohol on the release of secretin and pancreatic secretion. Surgery 81:661, 1977.
47. Nishiwaki H, Lee KY, Chey WY: Effect of alcohol on plasma secretin concentration and pancreatic secretion in dogs. Surgery 95:85, 1984.
48. Chey WY, Millikan L, Lee KY, et al: Effect of 1-phenylpentanol on release of secretin and exocrine pancreatic secretion in dogs and humans. Gastroenterology 84:1578, 1983.
49. Teichmann RK, Swierczek JS, Rayford PL, et al: Effect of duodenal osmolality on gastrin and secretin release and on gastric and pancreatic secretion. World J Surg 3:623, 1979.
50. Guzman S, Chayvialle J-A, Banks WA, et al: Effect of vagal stimulation on pancreatic secretion and on blood levels of gastrin, cholecystokinin, secretin, vasoactive intestinal peptide, and somatostatin. Surgery 86:329, 1979.
51. You CH, Rominger JM, Chey WY: Effects of atropine on the action and release of secretin in humans. Am J Physiol 242:G608, 1982.
52. Ward AS, Bloom SR: Effect of vagotomy on secretin release in man. Gut 16:951, 1975.
53. Miyata M, Rayford PL, Thompson JC: Hormonal (gastrin, secretin, cholecystokinin) and secretory effects of bombesin and duodenal acidification in dogs. Surgery 89:209, 1980.
54. Kaminski DL, Deshpande YG: Effect of somatostatin and bombesin on secretin-stimulated ductular bile flow in dogs. Gastroenterology 85:1239, 1983.
55. Boden G, Sivitz MC, Owen OE, et al: Somatostatin suppresses secretin and pancreatic exocrine secretion. Science 190:163, 1975.
56. Miyata M, Guzman SB, Rayford PL, et al: Response of cholecystokinin, secretin, and pancreatic secretion to graded doses of bombesin. Surg Forum 29:390, 1978.
57. Miller TA, Watson LC, Rayford PL, et al: The effect of glucagon on pancreatic secretion and plasma secretin in dogs. World J Surg 1:93, 1977.
58. Lonovics J, Guzman S, Devitt PG, et al: Action of pancreatic polypeptide on exocrine pancreas and on release of cholecystokinin and secretin. Endocrinology 108:1925, 1981.
59. Sakamoto T, Greeley GH Jr, Fujimura M, et al: Effect of fat and somatostatin on release of secretin and cholecystokinin in dogs. Dig Dis Sci 29:72S, 1984.
60. Watson LC, Miller TA, Rayford PL, et al: Effect of prostaglandin E_1 on plasma secretin and pancreatic exocrine function in dogs. Surg Forum 27:426, 1976.
61. Sakamoto T, Fujimura M, Townsend CM, et al: Differentiation of actions of neurotensin, secretin, and CCK on pancreatic secretions in dogs. Gastroenterology 86:1229, 1984.
62. Chang T-M, Chey WY, Kim MS, et al: The release of biologically active secretin-like immunoreactivity into duodenal lumen of dogs. J Physiol 320:393, 1981.
63. Greenberg GR, Domschke S, Domschke W, et al: Effect of low dose secretin and caerulein on pure pancreatic bicarbonate secretion and plasma secretin in man. Acta Hepatogastroenterol 26:478, 1979.
64. Chey WY, Kim MS, Lee KY, et al: Effect of rabbit antisecretin serum on postprandial pancreatic secretion in dogs. Gastroenterology 77:1266, 1979.
65. You CH, Rominger JM, Chey WY: Potentiation effect of cholecystokinin-octapeptide on pancreatic bicarbonate secretion stimulated by a physiologic dose of secretin in humans. Gastroenterology 85:40, 1983.
66. Baca I, Feurle GE, Haas M, et al: Interaction of neurotensin, cholecystokinin, and secretin in the stimulation of the exocrine pancreas in the dog. Gastroenterology 84:556, 1983.
67. Sakamoto T, Newman J, Fujimura M, et al: Role of neurotensin in pancreatic secretion. Surgery 96:146, 1984.
68. Singer MV, Niebel W, Elashoff J, et al: Does basal cholinergic activity potentiate exogenous secretin for stimulation of pancreatic bicarbonate output in dogs? Digestion 24:209, 1982.
69. Grundy D, Hutson D, Scratcherd T: The response of the pancreas of the anaesthetized cat to secretin before, during and after reversible vagal blockade. J Physiol 342:517, 1983.
70. Bunchman HH II, Reeder DD, Thompson JC: Effect of secretin on the serum gastrin response to a meal in man and in dog. Surg Forum 22:303, 1971.
71. Thompson JC, Reeder DD, Bunchman HH, et al: Effect of secretin on circulating gastrin. Ann Surg 176:384, 1972.
72. Hansky J, Soveny C, Korman MG: Effect of secretin on serum gastrin as measured by immunoassay. Gastroenterology 61:62, 1971.
73. Hansky J, Korman MG, Soveny C, et al: Radioimmunoassay of gastrin: Studies in pernicious anaemia. Gut 12:97, 1971.
74. Dalton MD, Eisenstein AM, Walsh JH, et al: Effect of secretin on gastric function in normal subjects and in patients with duodenal ulcer. Gastroenterology 71:24, 1976.
75. Konturek SJ, Rayford PL, Thompson JC: Effect of pH of gastric and intestinal meals on gastric acid and plasma gastrin and secretin responses in the dog. Am J Physiol 233:E537, 1977.
76. Kleibeuker JH, Eysselein VE, Maxwell VE, et al: Role

of endogenous secretin in acid-induced inhibition of human gastric function. J Clin Invest 73:526, 1984.

77. Perez-Reyes E, Payne NA, Gerber JG: Effect of somatostatin, secretin, and glucagon on secretagogue-stimulated aminopyrine uptake in isolated canine parietal cells. Agents Actions 13:265, 1983.
78. Chiba T, Taminato T, Kadowaki S, et al: Effects of glucagon, secretin, and vasoactive intestinal polypeptide on gastric somatostatin and gastrin release from isolated perfused rat stomach. Gastroenterology 79:67, 1980.
79. Saffouri B, DuVal JW, Arimura A, et al: Effects of vasoactive intestinal peptide and secretin on gastrin and somatostatin secretion in the perfused rat stomach. Gastroenterology 86:839, 1984.
80. Wolfe MM, Reel GM, McGuigan JE: Inhibition of gastrin release by secretin is mediated by somatostatin in cultured rat antral mucosa. J Clin Invest 72:1586, 1983.
81. Mate L, Sakamoto T, Greeley GH Jr, et al: Regulation of gastric acid secretion by secretin and serotonin. Am J Surg 149:40, 1985.
82. Lluis F, Fujimura M, Guo Y-S, et al: Regulation of gastric acid secretion by peptide YY, secretin, and neurotensin. Gastroenterology 88:1478, 1985.
83. Rayford PL, Konturek SJ, Thompson JC: Effect of duodenal fat on plasma levels of gastrin and secretin and on gastric acid responses to gastric and intestinal meals in dogs. Gastroenterology 75:773, 1978.
84. Chey WY, Kim MS, Lee KY, et al: Secretin is an enterogastrone in the dog. Am J Physiol 240:G239, 1981.
85. Isenberg JI, Walsh JH, Passaro E Jr, et al: Unusual effect of secretin on serum gastrin, serum calcium, and gastric acid secretion in a patient with suspected Zollinger-Ellison syndrome. Gastroenterology 62:626, 1972.
86. Debas HT, Soon-Shiong P, McKenzie AD, et al: Use of secretin in the roentgenologic and biochemical diagnosis of duodenal gastrinoma. Am J Surg 145:408, 1983.
87. Thompson JC, Lewis BG, Wiener I, et al: The role of surgery in the Zollinger-Ellison syndrome. Ann Surg 197:594, 1983.
88. Quatrini M, Basilisco G, Conte D, et al: Secretin-induced gastrin response in the Zollinger-Ellison syndrome and chronic duodenal ulcer patients before and after cimetidine treatment. Am J Gastroenterol 79:345, 1984.
89. Valenzuela JE, Defilippi C: Inhibition of gastric emptying in humans by secretin, the octapeptide of cholecystokinin, and intraduodenal fat. Gastroenterology 81:898, 1981.
90. Behar J, Field S, Marin C: Effect of glucagon, secretin, and vasoactive intestinal polypeptide on the feline lower esophageal sphincter: Mechanisms of action. Gastroenterology 77:1001, 1979.
91. Phaosawasdi K, Fisher RS: Hormonal effects on the pylorus. Am J Physiol 243:G330, 1982.
92. Carr-Locke DL, Gregg JA, Chey WY: Effects of exogenous secretin on pancreatic and biliary ductal and sphincteric pressures in man demonstrated by endoscopic manometry and correlation with plasma secretin levels. Dig Dis Sci 30:909, 1985.
93. Dayton MT, Schlegel J: The effect of secretin on canine gastric mucosal HCO_3^- production. J Surg Res 35:319, 1983.
94. Wheeler HO, Mancusi-Ungaro PL: Role of bile ducts during secretin choleresis in dogs. Am J Physiol 210:1153, 1966.
95. Nahrwold DL: Secretion by the common duct in response to secretin. Surg Forum 22:386, 1971.
96. Kaminski DL, Deshpande YG: Effect of theophylline on glucagon and secretin stimulated bile flow. Dig Dis Sci 29:261, 1984.
97. Kirkegaard P, Olsen PS, Poulsen SS, et al: Effect of secretin and glucagon on Brunner's gland secretion in the rat. Gut 25:264, 1984.
98. Isenberg JI, Wallin B, Johansson C, et al: Secretin, VIP, and PHI stimulate rat proximal duodenal surface epithelial bicarbonate secretion in vivo. Regul Pept 8:315, 1984.
99. Hattner RS, Margulis AR, Skioldebrand KCG, et al: The effect of secretin on colonic mucin secretion rate in the dog. Eur Surg Res 16:238, 1984.
100. Dinoso VP Jr, Meshkinpour H, Lorber SH, et al: Motor responses of the sigmoid colon and rectum to exogenous cholecystokinin and secretin. Gastroenterology 65:438, 1973.
101. Piubello W, Cominacini L, Vantini I, et al: Effect of graded doses of secretin on parathormone serum levels in man. Digestion 22:321, 1981.
102. Sethi R, Kukreja C, Bowser EN, et al: Effect of meal on serum parathyroid hormone and calcitonin: Possible role of secretin. J Clin Endocrinol Metab 56:549, 1983.
103. Mutt V: Secretin: Isolation, structure, and functions, in Jerzy Glass GB (ed): *Gastrointestinal Hormones.* New York, Raven Press, 1980, pp 85–126.
104. Shah PC, Freier S, Park BH, et al: Pancreozymin and secretin enhance duodenal fluid antibody levels to cow's milk proteins. Gastroenterology 83:916, 1982.
105. Lankisch PG: Trophic effects of gastrointestinal hormones. Clinics Gastroenterol 9:773, 1980.
106. Johnson LR: Effects of gastrointestinal hormones on pancreatic growth. Cancer 47:1640, 1981.
107. Morisset J, Genik P: Effects of acute and chronic administration of secretin and caerulein on rat duodenal and gastric growth. Regul Pept 5:111, 1983.
108. Solomon TE, Petersen H, Elashoff J, et al: Interaction of caerulein and secretin on pancreatic size and composition in rat. Am J Physiol 235:E714, 1978.
109. Townsend CM Jr, Franklin RB, Watson LC, et al:

Stimulation of pancreatic cancer growth by caerulein and secretin. Surg Forum 32:228, 1981.
110. Fine H, Levine GM, Shiau Y-F: Effects of cholecystokinin and secretin on intestinal structure and function. Am J Physiol 245:G358, 1983.
111. Chung RS, Safaie-Shirazi S: The effect of secretin on pancreatic blood flow in the awake and anesthetized dog. Proc Soc Exp Biol Med 173:620, 1983.
112. Bolondi L, Gaiani S, Gullo L, et al: Secretin administration induces a dilatation of main pancreatic duct. Dig Dis Sci 29:802, 1984.
113. Lehmann L, Duesel W, Klaue P, et al: pH-control via secretin or antacid: Prophylaxis of stress ulcers in high-risk surgical patients. Intensive Care Med 10:239, 1984.
114. Murakami M, Fujisaki H, Oketani K, et al: Effect of secretin on stress-induced gastric bleeding in rats. Dig Dis Sci 30:346, 1985.
115. Sudo T, Ishiyama K, Kawamura M, et al: Changes in plasma gastrin and secretin levels after pancreaticoduodenectomy. Surg Gynecol Obstet 158:133, 1984.
116. Kilander AF, Hanssen LE, Gillberg RE: Secretin release in coeliac disease. Plasma secretin concentration and bicarbonate output to the duodenum after intraduodenal acid infusion in coeliac patients before and after treatment. Scand J Gastroenterol 18:765, 1983.
117. Satake K, Nishiwaki H, Umeyama K: Comparative studies of plasma secretin response after reconstructive surgery of the stomach and pancreas. Ann Surg 201:447, 1985.
118. Nishiwaki H, Satake K, Kitamura T, et al: Postprandial plasma secretin response in patients following gastrectomy. Surg Gynecol Obstet 156:69, 1983.

Chapter 17

Glucagon

Anders Alwmark, M.D., Ph.D., and George H. Greeley, Jr., Ph.D.

HISTORY

The pancreatic endocrine peptide, glucagon, was first uncovered by Murlin et al [1,2] in 1923 as a hyperglycemic factor in a crude extract of bovine pancreas. In 1955, Staub et al [3,4] purified and crystallized this factor, which was shown subsequently to have hyperglycemic, glycogenolytic, gluconeogenic, and ketogenic actions. The amino acid sequence of porcine glucagon was determined later by Bromer et al [5] (see Appendix).

Glucagon is a single-chain 29 amino acid peptide with a molecular weight of 3483 daltons. Glucagon is produced in the α cells of the pancreatic islets, and it belongs to a family of structurally related peptides (i.e., secretin, vasoactive intestinal peptide [VIP], gastric inhibitory polypeptide [GIP], peptide histidine isoleucine [PHI], growth hormone-releasing factor [GHRF], and glicentin). Similarities in their primary structures are obvious when they are aligned from the amino-terminal. The amino-terminal region is apparently conserved because of its importance for biologic activity. Unlike many other mammalian peptides, the primary structure of porcine glucagon is identical to that of other mammalian glucagons, with the exception of duck glucagon [6]. Glucagon appears to be widespread phylogenetically [7–17], and the presence of glucagon-like immunoreactive material has been shown in extracts prepared from various insects [18]. The function of this glucagon-like substance in insects, however, is unclear. Although avian and fish glucagons have residue substitutions, they have 29 amino acid residues, suggesting a consistent biosynthetic processing in vertebrates. When present in high concentrations, for example in the α cells of pancreatic islets, glucagon is in the form of an α-helix [19].

There is a heterogeneous group of polypeptides containing glucagon or glucagon-like immunoreactivity (GLI) that has been isolated from the pancreas, stomach, intestine, and brain. These polypeptides are either similar in size to or larger than glucagon 29. They cross-react strongly with the nonspecific antiglucagon sera that are usually directed toward the N-terminal of glucagon, and they cross-react poorly with the glucagon-specific antisera that are directed toward the C-terminal.

There are primarily two enteroglucagon peptides that have been chemically characterized and that contain the glucagon 29 structure plus carboxyl- or amino-terminal extensions. Glucagon 37 consists of glucagon 29 plus a C-terminal extension of a basic octapeptide (MW = 4422). It has been isolated from the intestine and pancreas, and it is also called oxyntomodulin, since it inhibits pentagastrin-induced gastric acid secretion. Glucagon 37 also stimulates adenylate cyclase activity in hepatic membrane preparations and gastric glands of the fundus [20].

The other variant is glucagon 69 (MW = 8137) [21]. It is also called glicentin or proglucagon, and it has an additional N-terminal 32 amino acid extension as well as the C-terminal octapeptide extension. This is the primary form found in intestinal extracts [22]. Other uncharacterized enteroglucagon variants also exist [22].

Sutherland and de Duve [23] reported isolation of a hyperglycemic-glycogenolytic factor in acid-ethanol extracts of canine gastric mucosa. Unger et al [24,25] later found two forms of activity in gastrointestinal extracts of the rat, dog, and human: a large form (MW 12,000–17,000) and a small form (MW 2900–3500). Both forms are distinct from glucagon in terms of their chemical properties. A pure form of gut glucagon was allegedly isolated in 1976 by Sundby et al [26] called glicentin, since it was considered to contain 100 amino acid residues. However, glicentin was later shown to be a 69 amino acid polypeptide by Thim and Moody

[21]. Glicentin-containing cells were then identified as intestinal L cells and pancreatic α cells [27]. Since glicentin was found to contain glucagon 29, glicentin was considered a candidate for proglucagon.

Biosynthetic studies have shown that glucagon is generated from a precursor molecule that is five to six times larger than itself [22,28,29]. Hamster, angler fish, and bovine preproglucagon consists of a polypeptide that includes glucagon plus two glucagon-like peptides [28–30]. Preproglucagon consists of 180 amino acids, a hydrophobic signal peptide followed by glicentin; it terminates with two carboxy glucagon-like peptides. Presumably, the signal peptide is cleaved, and glicentin is processed to a 4500 MW proglucagon peptide and a 3445 MW glicentin-related pancreatic polypeptide (GRPP). The function of these two glucagon-like peptides is unknown.

Based on the molecular weight and immunoreactivity data, the International Glucagon Symposium, held in Dallas, Texas in 1976, proposed a terminology [31] that was further developed by Conlon [32]. All peptides that cross-react with both C- and N-terminal specific antibodies, irrespective of origin, are called immunoreactive glucagon (IRG), and peptides that cross-react only with N-terminal specific antibodies are called glucagon-like immunoreactivity (GLI). The molecular weight is given as a superscript (e.g., IRG^{3500}).

DISTRIBUTION

The distribution of glucagon, like insulin, is not limited to vertebrates or to the endocrine pancreas. As mentioned earlier, glucagon is found in a wide variety of cold- and warm-blooded vertebrates [7–17]. It also exists in the brain [15] and in the retina of various vertebrates [16,17]. Glucagon itself has not been isolated from the distal small bowel as would be anticipated if GLI does serve as a preproglucagon.

In one study, IRG^{9000}, IRG^{3500}, IRG^{2000}, and some smaller degradation products were found in extracts of the canine pancreas and gastric fundus [33], whereas GLI components primarily represent the immunoreactive forms in gut extracts [34], predominantly from the mucosa of the ileum and proximal colon [35]. GLI has also been found by radioimmunoassay studies in mucosal extracts of the stomach and duodenum of rats, dogs, pigs, and humans [24]. By means of immunohistochemical techniques Garaud et al [36] have shown the simultaneous presence of both immunoreactive forms in human α cells and L cells. Recently, GLI components were also found in the central nervous system (CNS) of frogs, tortoises [15], dogs [37], rats [38], and humans [15,39] as well as in the salivary glands [40] and vascular walls [41] of rats.

Gut GLI was first demonstrated in intestinal extracts [24]. Gut GLIs are located in the L cell of the intestinal mucosa [42,43], with the highest concentration of L cells found in the distal small bowel and colon [43]. The gut mucosa has a population of cells that stain with nonspecific antiglucagon or antiglicentin serum but are unstained by specific antiglucagon serum. Nonspecific antiglucagon serum stains pancreatic α cells and gastric endocrine cells, which are similar in many aspects to the pancreatic α cells. Other studies, also using nonspecific antiglucagon serum, demonstrated stained cells in the postduodenal mucosa (called the L cells, which contain GLIs). These immunocytochemical findings agree with the RIA distribution studies of GLI in the gastrointestinal tract and seem to be general features of all species studied [27].

Using immunofluorescence and a specific antiglicentin serum that does not cross-react with glucagon, glicentin-containing cells were found in the islets of Langerhans and in the mucosa of the terminal ileum and colon [27]. These intestinal mucosal cells correspond to the L cells. Interestingly, identical α cells in the pancreatic islets of the rat, pig, dog, and human and in the oxyntic mucosa of the dog contain both glicentin and glucagon. These findings suggest that α and L cells are related ontogenetically and that they synthesize a glicentin-like precursor that is processed to glucagon 29 and glicentin.

Glucagon-like peptides in plasma have also been studied. A reliable value of plasma glucagon (IRG^{3500}) level of a fasting man (100 pg/mL) was not obtained until 1967 [44]. A variety of molecular forms of glucagon (IRG) have been found in the plasma of humans and of laboratory animals [45]. These include forms with molecular weights of >150,000, 9000 to 12,000, 3425, and <2000. A recent study showed that the 150,000 MW form may actually be a plasma protein [45].

Gut GLI is released into the general circulation during a meal in dogs, pigs, and humans, but to date the GLI variants have not been characterized [46]. Plasma GLI concentrations are usually determined by subtracting the concentration of immunoreactivity using a C-terminal antiserum from the concentration of immunoreactivity using an N-terminal antiserum [47]. The rapid enzymatic degradation of glucagon-like peptides in plasma makes it difficult to correlate changes in the level of plasma immunoreactivity with physiologic events [48]. However, this shortcoming can be circumvented by studying glucagon secretion from the isolated perfused pancreas [48,49]. In both dogs and pigs, a single 3500 dalton component has been identified [48,49].

ASSAY

A sensitive radioimmunoassay for glucagon was first described by Unger's group in 1959 [50,51]. A glucagon antiserum called 30K was raised against beef-pork glucagon and was found to cross-react with dog and human glucagon. This antiserum cross-reacts with materials of both enteric and pancreatic origin and is described as "nonspecific" [50]. Apparently, N-terminal antisera cross-react with peptides that have a tertiary structure similar to that of residues 12–15 of porcine glucagon. Later reports [33–35,52] have described specific antibodies, called "C-terminal specific antibodies," which cross-react with pancreatic extracts [32]. It was obvious that a variety of tissue extracts cross-react with this antiglucagon serum. As said earlier, intestinal extracts having glucagon immunoreactivity are called gut glucagon-like immunoreactivity (gut GLIs).

PHARMACOKINETICS AND CATABOLISM

Glucagon 29 loses its biologic activity when it is perfused through the liver or if it is incubated with liver, muscle, or kidney extracts or whole blood. Glucagon fragments resulting from enzymatic degradation fail to demonstrate hyperglycemic action, suggesting that the intact glucagon molecule is obligatory for its biologic activity. In humans, the half-life of glucagon is about 5 minutes [53] and the metabolic clearance rate (MCR) is 13.5 mL/kg/min [54].

Metabolism of glucagon occurs primarily in the liver and kidney [55]. Of the circulating forms of immunoreactive glucagons, IRG^{3500} is metabolized in the liver, whereas the larger variants do not show a gradient across the liver [42]. In healthy rats, the portal-peripheral ratio of IRG is 2.8 and the extraction is 58 percent. IRG^{3500} accounts for most of the IRG portal-peripheral differences [55], since IRG^{3500} is metabolized by the liver. In humans, a fasting portal-peripheral glucagon ratio of 1.7 has been reported [56,57], and in cirrhotic patients with portacaval shunting, the plasma glucagon concentration is elevated 2 to 6-fold [58]. The IRG^{3500} constitutes up to 80 percent of the circulating immunoreactive glucagon in these patients [59]. An explanation for the hyperglucagonemia in liver disease has been discussed. Smith-Laing et al [60] suggested that hepatocellular damage resulted in a relationship between glucagon concentrations and aspartate transaminase levels; Dudley et al [59] found a significant elevation in glucagon levels after portacaval shunting as compared to the glucagon levels before shunting in the same person; Sherwin et al [58] found a normal metabolic clearance rate of glucagon in patients with cirrhosis, although the production rate of glucagon was elevated, and they concluded that hyperglucagonemia during cirrhosis was a consequence of glucagon hypersecretion.

As with gastrin and other small gut peptides, the kidney also plays a role in glucagon catabolism. A high extraction ratio from the kidney and a low urinary clearance rate indicate that glucagon is catabolized by renal tissue [61]. Acute renal artery ligation in dogs leads to a prompt elevation in circulating IRG [62]. Patients with chronic renal failure also show an elevation in their circulating glucagon levels, especially of IRG^{9000} [63]. Nephrectomized and ureteral-ligated rats develop marked hyperglucagonemia (IRG^{9000}), while the IRG level of urine-autoinfused animals is similar to that of control rats [64]. This observation indicates that uremia itself does not account for the hyperglucagonemia.

RELEASE

The release of glucagon from the pancreatic α cells varies little from minute to minute when contrasted with the secretion of pancreatic insulin. A major stimulus for glucagon release is a substantial drop in plasma glucose levels; a rise in glucose causes a fall in glucagon (Fig 17-1). A quick drop in D-glucose or an elevation in L-amino acid levels is a potent stimulus for glucagon secretion. Insulin aids the uptake of the amino acids into muscle, and glucagon protects the CNS from a possible insulin-induced hypoglycemia.

For the most part, control of glucagon sensitivity in the CNS is the reverse of that for insulin. In general, α- and β-adrenergic stimulation causes glucagon release, whether it is exerted by way of agonist infusion, antagonist infusion, or selective

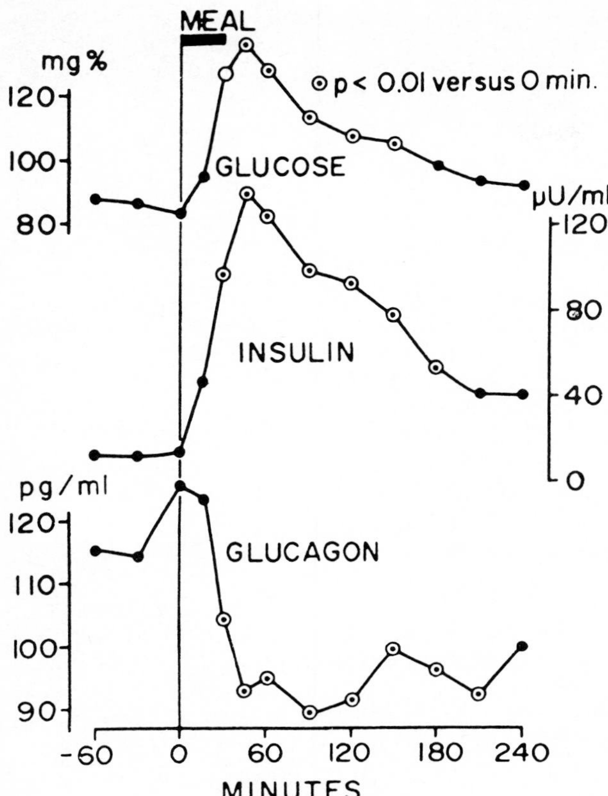

Figure 17-1. Suppression of glucagon by a glucose-containing meal in normal man. (By permission of RH Unger, N Engl J Med 285:443, 1971.)

nerve stimulation [65]. Norepinephrine and acetylcholine cause glucagon release. Norepinephrine causes glucagon release via β_2-adrenergic receptors, although α-adrenergic receptors also participate in a stimulatory fashion. Medullary catecholamines have little effect on glucagon secretion.

Epinephrine, norepinephrine, and acetylcholine, placed into the ventromedial hypothalamus, stimulate glucagon release; however, it is not known whether separate or identical afferent pathways influence the liver and pancreas. Thyrotropin-releasing hormone (TRH), given directly into the CNS, causes glucagon release [66]. Corticotropin-releasing factor, given intracerebroventricularly to dogs or rats, activates the sympathetic nervous system, resulting in a release of norepinephrine, which elevates plasma glucose and glucagon levels [67,68]. 2-Deoxy-D-glucose, given into the lateral cerebral ventricle of dogs and rats, can increase circulating levels of glucagon [69].

Systemic administration of TRH to fasted rabbits causes a dose-dependent elevation in plasma levels of glucagon, insulin, and glucose [70]. VIP also causes a direct release of pancreatic glucagon that is glucose-dependent [71].

The intracellular metabolism of the α cell and certainly also of the L cell is tied intimately to the secretion of glucagon [72]. Thus, elevated intracellular adenosine triphosphate (ATP) concentrations reduce glucagon secretion, whereas a reduction in ATP levels accelerates secretion of glucagon. This may explain the increased glucagon release to hypoxia and hemorrhage in shock and burn patients [73–75] and to the reactive hypoglycemia after exercise [76–78] or ingestion of ethanol [79]. Some of the suppressive effects of insulin on the release of glucagon are probably mediated via increased ATP concentration generated by a stimulated glucose metabolism [72]. Forskolin, a diterpene prepared from the root of an Indian medicinal plant, *Coleus forskohlii,* can stimulate cAMP formation in cells by direct activation of adenylate cyclase [80]. Forskolin can increase cAMP levels in pancreatic cells and can stimulate release of glucagon, somatostatin, and insulin in a dose-responsive manner [89].

A paracrine influence is probably exerted by neighboring cells containing peptide hormones, namely insulin (β cells) and somatostatin (D cells). The existence of gap junctions between cells, the dendrite-like processes, and the capillary arrangements support the concept of an intrinsic interrelationship [81,82]. Further evidence in support of this idea is given in a recent report on the paracrine regulatory process in monolayer cultures of islet cells from neonatal rats [83]. Glucagon can suppress its own secretion [84], and furthermore it can stimulate the secretion of insulin and somatostatin. Somatostatin inhibits the secretion of glucagon and insulin, and insulin inhibits glucagon secretion [85]. Incubation of islets with antisomatostatin serum leads to an elevation of glucagon as well as to release of insulin. This observation provides strong evidence that somatostatin exerts a paracrine inhibitory influence [86,87]. The inhibitory action of somatostatin on glucagon release is thought to be the result of an effect of somatostatin on adenyl cyclase or calcium flux [88].

Endocrine influence on glucagon secretion is stimulated by many of the gastrointestinal hormones [89]. Neurotensin, given intravenously, leads to a rise in plasma glucagon levels in rats [90]. Other studies show that neurotensin can stimulate glucagon release in vitro [91], and neurotensin-induced glucagon release appears to be glucose-dependent [92]. However, in carefully controlled studies, using apparently physiologic concentrations of gut peptides, few peptides are stimulatory [93]. When studied during cholinergic stimulation, glucagon release is augmented by neurotensin and GIP, diminished by somatostatin and glucose, and unchanged by substance P, pancreatic polypeptide, and cholecystokinin [94]. Growth hormone, β-endorphins, and cortisol stimulate secretion of glucagon [95]. At high doses, met-enkephalin also causes release of glucagon from the perfused dog pancreas, and naloxone can reverse the stimulatory action of met-enkephalin and β-endorphin. Interestingly, both met-enkephalin and β-endorphin inhibit glucagon release in an isolated islet model [96]. In sharp contrast to epinephrine, which does not affect glucagon release, circulating norepinephrine promotes release of glucagon [97]. The mechanisms of hormonal stimulation are not yet fully understood, but cAMP and serum calcium have been demonstrated to participate in the stimulus-secretion coupling [98,99]. Parathyroid hormone can enhance arginine-stimulated release of glucagon [100].

Recently, the hypothalamus has drawn great interest as a regulator of circulating levels of glucose. A peptide of 30–31 amino acids, purified from the rat hypothalamus, was shown to stimulate release of glucagon. This glucagon releasing factor may play a role in a presumed hypothalamic-pancreatic neurohormonal link [101].

Extracellular metabolites include above all the prevailing glucose concentration but also free fatty acids, which in surplus depress glucagon secretion. Glucose allegedly acts via insulin, but according to recent studies, it can act directly on the α cell [102,103]. Amino acids, especially L-alanine and L-arginine, are powerful stimulants of glucagon release [104]. Arginine challenge is used to test glucagon secretion in several physiologic and nonphysiologic conditions [105] (Fig 17-2).

Studies in pigs using electrical stimulation of the vagus nerve have demonstrated the importance of the autonomic nervous system in glucagon secretion [106,107]. Pharmacologic manipulations suggest that peptidergic nerves are involved and that VIP is a possible neurotransmitter [108,109]. Similar studies have shown that 1) somatostatin has an inhibitory effect on vagal stimulation of pancreatic secretion [110], 2) splanchnic nerve stimulation results in glucagon secretion, and 3) simultaneous vagal stimulation has an additive effect [111]. Sham feeding increases plasma glucagon levels, an action mediated by a cholinergic mechanism [112]. Stimulation of specific hypothalamic nuclei results in a stimulation of α cells and an inhibition of β cells. Splanchnicectomy can abolish the rise in IRG, indicating a sympathetic input to the endocrine pancreas [113].

The majority of luminal stimuli that cause secretion of gut GLI are related to nutrient absorption. Monosaccharides, especially intraluminal hyperosmolar solutions of glucose, promote GLI release [47]. Intraluminal triglycerides have a similar action, and a mixed meal results in a greater release of GLI [47]. This finding can be explained by passage of the food stimulus farther down the intestine, since a similar enhanced elevation in gut glucagon release was seen after intestinal resection or jejunoileal bypass surgery [114]. Ingestion of a high protein diet may increase the plasma glucagon level for a longer time, as compared to ingestion of glucose and fat [115]. Enteroglucagon secretion is elevated by intraluminal (intestine) administration of lipids and carbohydrates [22]. In contrast to what occurs with GIP, the mere presence of carbohydrates in the lumen and not their transport across the intestinal wall leads to release of enteroglucagon. In fact, the presence of unabsorbed nutrients, as found in patients with jejunoileal bypass, total pancreatectomy, or proximal intestinal resection, results in exaggerated release of enteroglucagon. The same mechanism may operate in triglyceride malabsorption and celiac disease. The L cell appears to be sensitive to hypoglycemia or intravenous arginine.

Physical training appears to influence the α cell response to stimulation by adrenergic and/or glucose plus insulin inhibition [116]. This observation may have relevance for the finding that physical training facilitates glucose homeostasis in rats rendered diabetic by streptozotocin.

ACTIONS

Glucagon is the hormone of energy utilization, as insulin is the hormone of energy storage. In most instances, the actions of glucagon are counter-regulatory to those of insulin. Glucagon causes hyperglycemia and decreases glucose oxidation. In the liver, glucagon promotes glycogenolysis and gluconeogenesis from proteins. Glucagon also stimulates lipolysis in fat, as well as in the liver and, consequently, results in increased gluconeogenesis and ketogenesis. Glucagon cannot influence blood glucose levels after the liver is removed or if circulation through the liver is blocked. Protracted fasting, diabetic acidosis, and

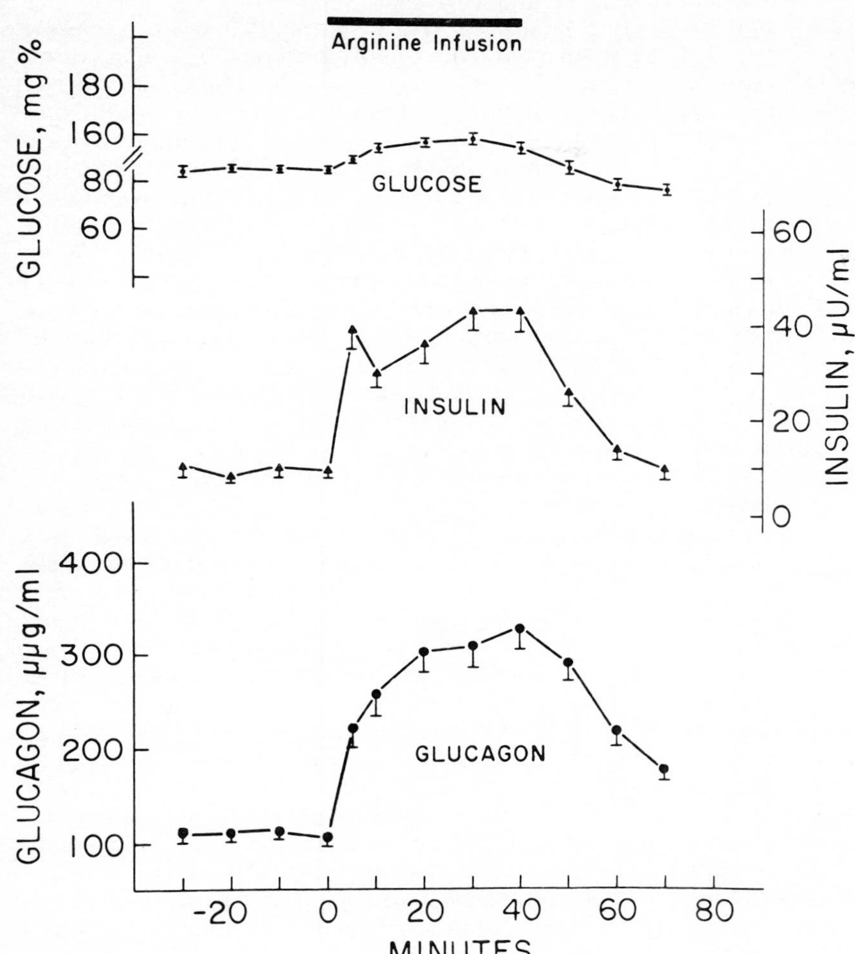

Figure 17-2. Stimulation of glucagon secretion by an arginine infusion in normal man. (By permission of RH Unger, N Engl J Med 285:443, 1971.)

other circumstances that depress liver glycogen stores impair the hyperglycemic action of glucagon. Chronic glucagon treatment leads to elevated nitrogen excretion, a negative nitrogen balance, and a diminished level of amino acids in the circulation.

Glucagon and insulin are the major hormonal regulators of metabolic fuel, storage, and fuel release. Glucagon is well known for its ability to release growth hormone in humans [117]. It is not clear whether glucagon acts directly on the pituitary gland, but many believe that the rise in plasma growth hormone after administration of glucagon is secondary to alterations in plasma glucose levels. The growth hormone-releasing action of glucagon is potentiated by β-receptor blockade, which suggests that glucagon may exert its effect by way of central noradrenergic circuits.

In humans, the principal physiologic actions of glucagon in the liver appear to be limited to stimulation of glycogenolysis, gluconeogenesis, and triglyceride lipolysis. In adipose tissue, glucagon also promotes triglyceride lipolysis and enhanced glycogenolysis. For the "classic action" of glucagon (glycogenolysis), glucagon acts via a specific membrane receptor on the hepatocyte [118]. This process generates cAMP, which starts a cascade, terminating in glycogenolysis via glucose-1-phosphate to glucose. Glucagon acts in the gluconeogenic pathway by means of the activation of a key gluconeogenic enzyme, phosphoenol pyruvate carboxy-kinase [119]. Insulin can inhibit all hepatic actions of glucagon [119].

The inhibitory action of somatostatin on glucagon secretion has been used to study the role of glucagon in glucose homeostasis in vivo. Somatostatin infusion inhibits the basal secretion of insulin and glucagon, accompanied by a fall in blood glucose levels and hepatic glucose output [120]. Infusion of glucagon simultaneously prevents this fall in blood glucose [120,121]. Infusion of insulin results in an augmented and long-lasting decrease in blood glucose levels [121]. Glucagon and insulin have opposing effects on hepatic glucose output. However, an increased glucagon level (via exogenous glucagon) does not significantly affect the blood glucose level, since the acute insulin response is the more important physiologic factor [122]. Acute hypoglycemia results in a rapid rise in glucagon levels which, together with cortisol and catecholamines, promotes a rise in blood glucose levels. These three hormones can act synergistically. Infusion of physiologic doses causes a rise in plasma glucose levels 4-fold greater than the sum of the responses to each hormone alone [123].

The ketogenic and ureogenic properties of glucagon are less clearly defined but can, in part, be studied during prolonged fasting. To maintain hepatic glucose production, glucagon promotes the hepatic uptake of gluconeogenic amino acids [124]. After approximately one week of starvation, the enhanced gluconeogenesis decreases and the organism switches to using ketones, thereby sparing protein [125]. Ketone production from free fatty acids is initiated by an increase in the glucagon:insulin ratio in the presence of increased availability of free fatty acids [126]. A similar mechanism is involved in exercise of long duration. After the utilization of muscle glycogen, circulating glucose and free fatty acids replace glycogen, and finally the free fatty acids become the preferred fuel. Glucagon is involved, but its precise role is unclear [127].

Glucagon also has a variety of effects on gastrointestinal motility. Glucagon can inhibit stomach hunger contractions in humans [128]. It can also diminish food intake [129], gastric emptying [130–134], and motility [131,132,135,136]. In humans and dogs, glucagon can inhibit motility of the colon [136,137]. Glucagon can increase bile secretion, decrease gastric secretion, and diminish gallbladder pressure [138,139]. It also relaxes the sphincter of Oddi in humans [140]. It is worth mentioning that the doses of glucagon used in these studies might be excessive in terms of physiologic amounts.

Only one case of neonatal hyperglycemia attributed to glucagon deficiency has been reported [141]. The child was given glucagon for 3 months, which at first caused improvement but ultimately did not save his life. A congenital autosomal recessive factor was suggested.

Alpha cell tumors causing hyperglucagonemia grow slowly, with a high rate of late metastasis associated with high circulating glucagon levels, causing the glucagonoma syndrome, as reported by Mallinson et al in 1974 [142]. Seven years later, 55 cases were reported with a distinctive clinical syndrome consisting of diabetes, dermatitis termed necrolytic migratory erythema, weight loss, and an increased tendency to thrombosis [143]. The best treatment is surgical excision, which completely reverses all clinical manifestations; in cases with disseminated disease, cytoreductive surgery in combination with chemotherapy is recommended. Further studies of four patients revealed remarkably unaffected glucose homeostasis, normal insulin levels, but low plasma levels of amino acids [144].

Of all the controversies surrounding glucagon, none has stimulated so many debates as the controversy over its role in diabetes mellitus. In 1975, Unger and Orci [145] suggested that the hyperglycemia of diabetes mellitus is caused by a surfeit of glucagon as well as by insulin deficiency. Evidence in favor of this idea was obtained from studies of glucagon infusions to diabetic patients or individuals with somatostatin-suppressed insulin secretion. Glucagon can aggravate the metabolic abnormalities of diabetes [146–148]. In addition, in studies on isolated tissues and organs, glucagon was found to have the property of increasing mobilization of glucose, free fatty acids, and ketone bodies, which are metabolites found in excessive concentrations in the blood of diabetics. This property is inhibited by insulin. Furthermore, plasma glucagon levels are usually elevated in diabetes, the highest values being recorded in uncontrolled diabetes with ketoacidosis [149]. Indirect support for the importance of glucagon in glucose homeostasis was recently given in a report showing that infusion of a glucagon receptor antagonist without addition of exogenous insulin reduced hyperglycemia in diabetic rats [150].

Evidence against the Unger hypothesis has been reported by several groups. Barnes et al [151] found that withholding insulin from diabetics was associated with an abrupt rise in plasma glucagon, blood glucose, and plasma 3-hydroxybutyrate levels. In contrast, the same procedure in pancreatectomized subjects did not significantly increase glucagon and caused only a small increase in blood glucose and 3-hydroxybutyrate. Thus, glucagon is not essential for the development of hyperglycemia and ketoacidosis. In the presence of glucagon, however, both hyperglycemia and ketoacidosis are enhanced. No deterioration has been shown in the diabetic control during several days of infusion of physiologic doses of glucagon to insulin-treated diabetics [122].

Treatment of diabetes with the "artificial pancreas" easily overcomes the effect of a constant rate of glucagon infusion just as was seen in normal β cells when glucagon was infused in nondiabetics [152].

Intramuscular injection of glucagon has a proven effect for treatment of hypoglycemia, in addition to infusion of glucose. Glucagon may be ineffective, however, in cases of hepatic glycogen depletion.

Pharmacologic doses of glucagon have an inotropic cardiac effect. Glucagon has been used in certain cardiac emergency situations and as an antidote to β-blockers [153].

As seen in acute hypovolemic shock in dogs, glucagon infusion can preserve the intestinal perfusion relative to cardiac output [154]. The mechanism seems to be a mesenteric arterial dilatation more than an opening of arteriovenous anastomoses [155]. Glucagon is used infrequently in this situation in humans because there is a risk of cardiovascular collapse in prolonged shock without replacement of a proper part of the lost blood volume [154,155].

Glucagon has a well-known inhibitory action on gastric acid secretion in normal subjects and in patients with gastric ulcers. This action is probably exerted via an inhibition of gastrin release. Normal individuals, as well as patients with duodenal ulcers (Fig 17-3), demonstrate a suppression of gastrin release during glucagon infusion [156]. There is a paradoxic increase in gastrin levels in Zollinger-Ellison patients given glucagon [156]. This finding is the basis for the recognition of the glucagon test in the differential diagnosis of the Zollinger-Ellison syndrome [157]. Reports on the usefulness of glucagon as a treatment for hypersecretive conditions cannot be found.

Glucagon can also act as a satiety factor. When administered to humans and laboratory animals, it

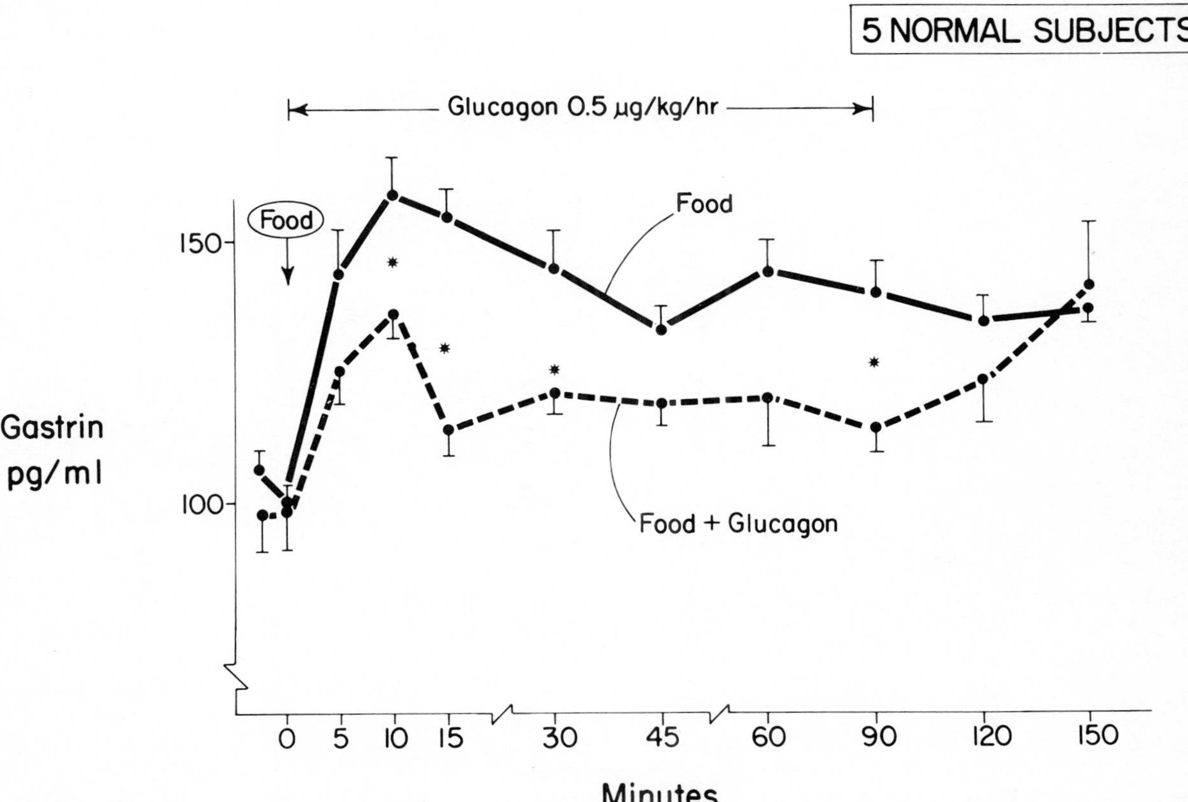

Figure 17-3. Effect of a 90-minute glucagon infusion, low dosage (0.5 μg/kg/hr), on food-stimulated gastrin release in healthy man. * = statistically significant differences between test (food + glucagon) and control studies. (From Becker et al [156], with permission of Williams & Wilkins.)

can inhibit feeding [158,159]. The significance of this action is not clear, since glucagon does not inhibit sham feeding in rats [160].

Glucagon also relaxes and dilates the stomach and duodenum but induces rapid transit through the small intestine [161]. Its paralytic action on the duodenum has encouraged its use in radiographic and endoscopic examinations. A low dose of 0.1 mg has proved adequate to provide duodenal hypotonicity and also to shorten the small bowel follow-through [161]. Glucagon-induced relaxation of the choledochal sphincter [162] has been used to facilitate the introduction of the catheter during ERCP (endoscopic retrograde cholangiopancreaticography), as an aid in expulsion of impacted calculi into the duodenum [163], and to improve the results of operative cholangiography [164].

Glucagon has been shown to suppress exocrine pancreatic secretion in humans [165], and many studies (mostly without controls) have suggested that it can relieve pain and promote clinical improvement in patients with acute pancreatitis [166]. Later studies designed as prospective randomized double-blind studies did not demonstrate the same beneficial effect [167].

Studies from our laboratory have shown that glucagon does suppress the volume (Fig 17-4) and bicarbonate response to duodenal acidification without changing pancreatic enzyme output [168]. Since this effect is achieved without suppression of secretin release, we suggested that glucagon may exert its inhibitory effect by competing with secretin at the pancreatic receptor site.

A combination of insulin and glucagon has been suggested to be the crucial element necessary for hepatic regeneration. The combination has been used in the treatment of severe liver disease and alcoholic hepatitis. The ratio of branched-chain to aromatic amino acids increases [169], and the clinical outcome improves [170].

Glucagon has also been used as a provocative stimulation test for insulin release in the investigation of fasting hypoglycemia, catecholamine release in pheochromocytoma, and growth hor-

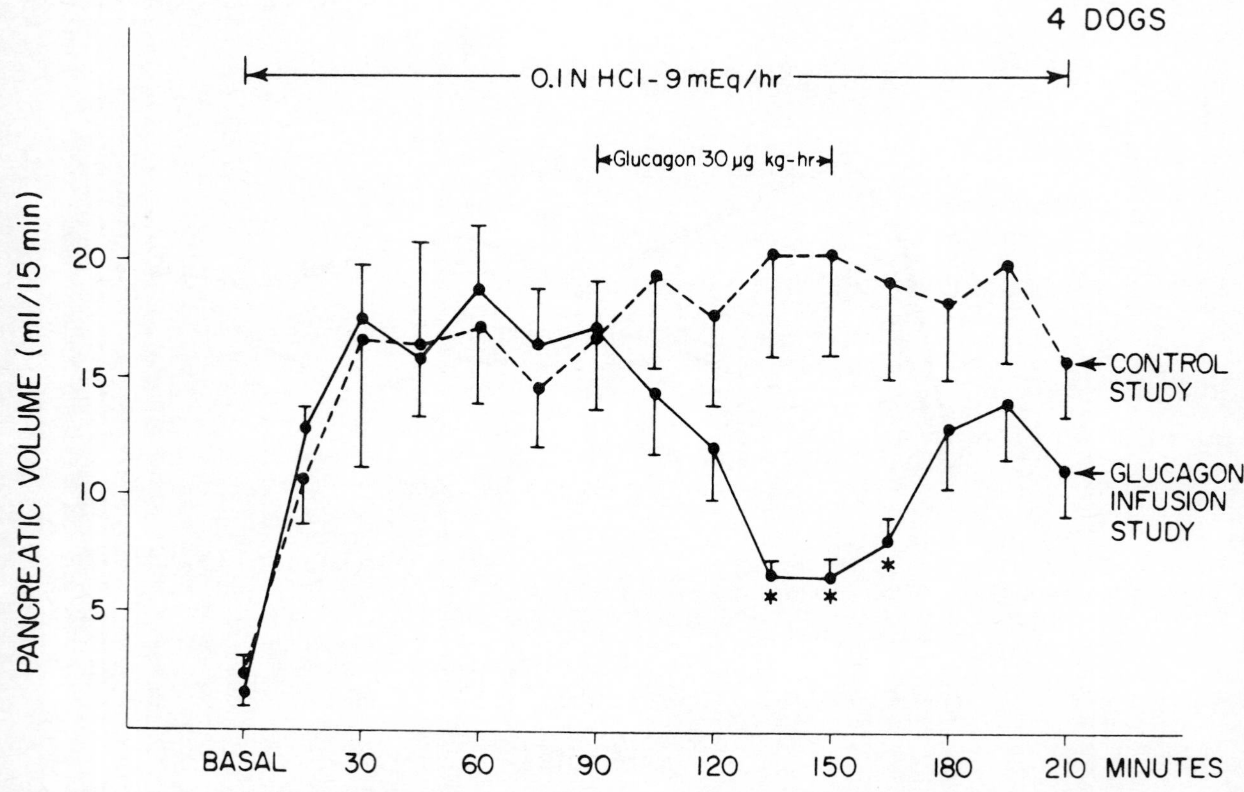

Figure 17-4. Effect of glucagon on pancreatic volume flow. Control animals received only intraduodenal HCl throughout the experiment. Each curve is the mean of experiments performed. * = a significant decrease compared to control studies. (From Miller et al [168], with permission of Springer-Verlag.)

mone release in assessment of anterior pituitary function [171].

REFERENCES

1. Murlin JR, Clough HD, Gibbs CBF et al: Aqueous extracts of pancreas. I. Influence on the carbohydrate metabolism of depancreatized animals. J Biol Chem 56:253, 1923.
2. Kimball CP, Murlin JR: Aqueous extracts of pancreas. III. Some precipitation reactions of insulin. J Biol Chem 58:337, 1923.
3. Staub A, Sinn L, Behrens OK: Purification and crystallization of hyperglycemic glycogenolytic factor (HGF). Science 117:628, 1953.
4. Staub A, Sinn L, Behrens OK: Purification and crystallization of glucagon. J Biol Chem 214:619, 1955.
5. Bromer WW, Staub A, Sinn LG, et al: The amino acid sequence of glucagon. III. The hydrolysis of glucagon by trypsin. J Am Chem Soc 79:2801, 1957.
6. Sundby F: Species variations in the primary structure of glucagon. Metabolism 25(Suppl 1):1319, 1976.
7. Dockray GJ: Molecular evolution of gut hormones: Application of comparative studies on the regulation of digestion. Gastroenterology 72:344, 1977.
8. Kaung H-LC, Elde RP: Distribution and morphometric quantitation of pancreatic endocrine cell types in the frog, *Rana pipiens*. Anat Rec 196:173, 1980.
9. Tomita T, Pollock HG: Four pancreatic endocrine cells in the bullfrog (*Rana catesbeiana*). Gen Comp Endocrinol 45:355, 1981.
10. Fujita T, Yui R, Iwanaga T, et al: Evolutionary aspects of "brain-gut peptides": An immunohistochemical study. Peptides 2 (Suppl 2):123, 1981.
11. El-Salhy M, Abu-Sinna G, Wilander E: The endocrine pancreas of a squamate reptile, the desert lizard (*Chalcides ocellatus*). A histological and immunocytochemical investigation. Histochemistry 78:391, 1983.
12. Buchan AMJ, Lance V, Polak JM: Regulatory peptides in the gastrointestinal tract of *Alligator mississippiensis*. An immunocytochemical study. Cell Tissue Res 231:439, 1983.
13. Rhoten WB: Immunocytochemical localization of four hormones in the pancreas of the garter snake, *Thamnophis sirtalis*. Anat Rec 208:233, 1984.
14. Lance V, Hamilton JW, Rouse JB, et al: Isolation and characterization of reptilian insulin, glucagon, and pancreatic polypeptide: Complete amino acid sequence of alligator (*Alligator mississippiensis*) insulin and pancreatic polypeptide. Gen Comp Endocrinol 55:112, 1984.
15. Dorn A, Bernstein H-G, Rinne A, et al: Insulin- and glucagonlike peptides in the brain. Anat Rec 207:69, 1983.
16. Eldred WD, Karten HJ: Characterization and quantification of peptidergic amacrine cells in the turtle retina: Enkephalin, neurotensin, and glucagon. J Comp Neurol 221:371, 1983.
17. Tornqvist K, Ehinger B: Glucagon immunoreactive neurons in the retina of different species. Graefes Arch Clin Exp Ophthalmol 220:1, 1983.
18. Tager HS, Markese J, Kramer KJ, et al: Glucagon-like and insulin-like hormones of the insect neurosecretory system. Biochem J 156:515, 1976.
19. Carrey EA, Epand RM: Conformational and biological properties of glucagon fragments containing residues 1–17 and 19–29. Int J Pept Protein Res 22:362, 1983.
20. Bataille D, Tatemoto K, Gespach C, et al: Isolation of glucagon-37 (bioactive enteroglucagon/oxyntomodulin) from porcine jejuno-ileum. Characterization of the peptide. FEBS Lett 146:79, 1982.
21. Thim L, Moody AJ: The amino acid sequence of porcine glicentin. Peptides 2 (Suppl 2):37, 1981.
22. Holst JJ: Gut glucagon, enteroglucagon, gut glucagonlike immunoreactivity, glicentin—Current status. Gastroenterology 84:1602, 1983.
23. Sutherland EW, de Duve C: Origin and distribution of the hyperglycemic-glycogenolytic factor of the pancreas. J Biol Chem 175:663, 1948.
24. Unger RH, Ketterer H, Eisentraut AM: Distribution of immuno-assayable glucagon in gastrointestinal tissues. Metabolism 15:865, 1966.
25. Unger RH, Ohneda A, Valverde I, et al: Characterization of the responses of circulating glucagon-like immunoreactivity to intraduodenal and intravenous administration of glucose. J Clin Invest 47:48, 1968.
26. Sundby F, Jacobsen H, Moody AJ: Purification and characterization of a protein from porcine gut with glucagon-like immunoreactivity. Horm Metab Res 8:366, 1976.
27. Ravazzola M, Siperstein A, Moody AJ, et al: Glicentin immunoreactive cells: Their relationship to glucagon-producing cells. Endocrinology 105:499, 1979.
28. Bell GI, Santerre RF, Mullenbach GT: Hamster preproglucagon contains the sequence of glucagon and two related peptides. Nature 302:716, 1983.
29. Lopez LC, Frazier ML, Su C-J, et al: Mammalian pancreatic preproglucagon contains three glucagon-related peptides. Proc Natl Acad Sci USA 80:5485, 1983.
30. Lund PK, Goodman RH, Dee PC, et al: Pancreatic preproglucagon cDNA contains two glucagon-related coding sequences arranged in tandem. Proc Natl Acad Sci USA 79:345, 1982.
31. Unger RH: Report of the nomenclature committee. Metabolism 25 (Suppl 1):ix, 1976.
32. Conlon JM: The glucagon-like polypeptides—Order out of chaos? Diabetologia 18:85, 1980.
33. Srikant CB, McCorkle K, Unger RH: Properties of immunoreactive glucagon fractions of canine stomach and pancreas. J Biol Chem 252:1847, 1977.
34. Tager HS, Markese J: Intestinal and pancreatic glucagon-like peptides. Evidence for identity of higher molecular weight forms. J Biol Chem 254:2229, 1979.
35. Larsson L-I, Holst J, Håkanson R, et al: Distribution and properties of glucagon immunoreactivity in

the digestive tract of various mammals: An immunohistochemical and immunochemical study. Histochemistry 44:281, 1975.

36. Garaud JC, Eloy R, Moody AJ, et al: Glucagon- and glicentin-immunoreactive cells in the human digestive tract. Cell Tissue Res 213:121, 1980.
37. Conlon JM, Samson WK, Dobbs RE, et al: Glucagon-like polypeptides in canine brain. Diabetes 28:700, 1979.
38. Loren I, Alumets J, Håkanson R, et al: Gut-type glucagon immunoreactivity in nerves of the rat brain. Histochemistry 61:335, 1979.
39. Sanders DJ, Zahedi-Asl S, Marr AP: Glucagon and CCK in human brain: Controls and patients with senile dementia of Alzheimer type. Prog Brain Res 55:465, 1982.
40. Lawrence AM, Tan S, Hojvat S, et al: Salivary gland hyperglycemic factor: An extrapancreatic source of glucagon-like material. Science 195:70, 1977.
41. Tanaka J, Shiosaka S, Tsubouchi H, et al: Immunoreactive glucagon in the vascular walls of the rat. Life Sci 33:1599, 1983.
42. Solcia E, Polak JM, Pearse AGE, et al: Lausanne 1977 classification of gastroenteropancreatic endocrine cells, in Bloom SR (ed): *Gut Hormones.* New York, Churchill Livingstone, 1978, pp 40–48.
43. Bloom SR, Polak JM: Gut hormone overview, in Bloom SR (ed): *Gut Hormones.* New York, Churchill Livingstone, 1978, pp 3–18.
44. Sokal JE, Ezdinli EZ, Schiller C, et al: Basal plasma glucagon levels of man. J Clin Invest 46:778, 1967.
45. Soybel D, Jaspan J, Polonsky K, et al: Differential immunoreactivity of plasma glucagon components in man: Studies with different glucagon antibodies. J Clin Endocrinol Metab 56:612, 1983.
46. Jarrousse C, Bataille D, Jeanrenaud B: A pure enteroglucagon, oxyntomodulin (glucagon 37), stimulates insulin release in perfused rat pancreas. Endocrinology 115:102, 1984.
47. Holst JJ: Extrapancreatic glucagons. Digestion 17:168, 1978.
48. Conlon JM, Ipp E, Unger RH: The molecular forms of immunoreactive glucagon secreted by the isolated, perfused dog pancreas. Life Sci 23:1655, 1978.
49. Holst JJ, von Schenck H, Lindkaer S: Gel filtration pattern of immunoreactive glucagon secreted by the isolated, perfused, porcine pancreas. Scand J Clin Lab Invest 39:47, 1979.
50. Unger RH, Eisentraut AM, McCall MS, et al: Glucagon antibodies and an immunoassay for glucagon. J Clin Invest 40:1280, 1961.
51. Unger RH, Eisentraut AM, McCall MS, et al: Glucagon antibodies and their use for immunoassay for glucagon. Proc Soc Exp Biol Med 102:621, 1959.
52. Srikant CB, Unger RH: Evidence for the presence of glucagon-like immunoreactivity (GLI) in the pancreas. Endocrinology 99:1655, 1976.
53. Assan R: In vivo metabolism of glucagon, in Lefebvre PJ, Unger RH (eds): *Glucagon. Molecular Physiology, Clinical and Therapeutic Implications.* New York, Pergamon Press, 1972, pp 47–59.
54. Fisher M, Sherwin RS, Hendler R, et al: Kinetics of glucagon in man: Effects of starvation. Proc Natl Acad Sci USA 73:1735, 1976.
55. Jaspan JB, Huen AH-J, Morley CG, et al: The role of the liver in glucagon metabolism. J Clin Invest 60:421, 1977.
56. Blackard WG, Nelson NC, Andrews SS: Portal and peripheral vein immunoreactive glucagon concentrations after arginine or glucose infusions. Diabetes 23:199, 1974.
57. Dencker H, Hedner P, Holst J, et al: Pancreatic glucagon response to an ordinary meal. Scand J Gastroenterol 10:471, 1975.
58. Sherwin RS, Fisher M, Bessoff J, et al: Hyperglucagonemia in cirrhosis: Altered secretion and sensitivity to glucagon. Gastroenterology 74:1224, 1978.
59. Dudley FJ, Alford FP, Chisholm DJ, et al: Effect of porta-systemic venous shunt surgery on hyperglucagonaemia in cirrhosis: paired studies of pre- and post-shunted subjects. Gut 20:817, 1979.
60. Smith-Laing G, Orskov H, Gore MBR, et al: Hyperglucagonaemia in cirrhosis. Relationship to hepatocellular damage. Diabetologia 19:103, 1980.
61. Lefebvre PJ, Luyckx AS, Nizet AH: Renal handling of endogenous glucagon in the dog: Comparison with insulin. Metabolism 23:753, 1974.
62. Lefebvre PJ, Luyckx AS: Effect of acute kidney exclusion by ligation of renal arteries on peripheral plasma glucagon levels and pancreatic glucagon production in the anesthetized dog. Metabolism 24:1169, 1975.
63. Kuku SF, Jaspan JB, Emmanouel DS, et al: Heterogeneity of plasma glucagon. J Clin Invest 58:742, 1976.
64. Emmanouel DS, Jaspan JB, Kuku SF, et al: Pathogenesis and characterization of hyperglucagonemia in the uremic rat. J Clin Invest 58:1266, 1976.
65. Roy MW, Lee KC, Jones MS, et al: Neural control of pancreatic insulin and somatostatin secretion. Endocrinology 115:770, 1984.
66. Brown MR: Thyrotropin releasing factor: A putative CNS regulator of the autonomic nervous system. Life Sci 28:1789, 1981.
67. Brown MR, Fisher LA, Spiess J, et al: Comparison of the biologic actions of corticotropin-releasing factor and sauvagine. Regul Pept 4:107, 1982.
68. Brown MR, Fisher LA, Spiess J, et al: Corticotropin-releasing factor: Actions on the sympathetic nervous system and metabolism. Endocrinology 111:928, 1982.
69. Yamamoto H, Nagai K, Nakagawa H: Lesions involving the suprachiasmatic nucleus eliminate the glucagon response to intracranial injection of 2-deoxy-D-glucose. Endocrinology 117:468, 1985.
70. Knudtzon J: Thyrotropin-releasing hormone increases plasma levels of glucagon, insulin, glucose and free fatty acids in rabbits. Horm Metab Res 13:371, 1981.
71. Makhlouf GM: Role of VIP in the function of the gut, in Said SI (ed): *Vasoactive Intestinal Peptide.* New York, Raven Press, 1982, pp 425–446.

72. Ostensson C-G, Andersson A, Brolin SE, et al: Effects of insulin on the glucagon release, glucose utilization and ATP content of the pancreatic A cells of the guinea pigs, in Foa PP, Bajaj JS, Foa NL (eds): *Glucagon: Its Role in Physiology and Clinical Medicine.* New York, Springer-Verlag, 1977, pp 243–254.
73. Wood CD, Bentz Y, Martin M, et al: The relationship of glucagon and insulin to sequential changes in metabolic fuel utilization in shock. J Surg Res 28:239, 1980.
74. Lautt WW, Martens ES, Legare DJ: Insulin and glucagon response during hemorrhage induced hyperglycemia. Can J Physiol Pharmacol 60:1624, 1982.
75. Shuck JM, Eaton RP, Shuck LW, et al: Dynamics of insulin and glucagon secretions in severely burned patients. J Trauma 17:706, 1977.
76. Anderson RA, Polansky MM, Bryden NA, et al: Effect of exercise (running) on serum glucose, insulin, glucagon, and chromium excretion. Diabetes 31:212, 1982.
77. Lavine RL, Lowenthal DT, Gellman MD, et al: The effect of long-distance running on plasma immunoreactive glucagon levels. Eur J Appl Physiol 43:41, 1980.
78. Brockman RP: Glucagon responses to exercise in sheep. Aust J Biol Sci 32:215, 1979.
79. Tiengo A, Fedele D, Frasson P, et al: Ethanol effect on glucagon secretion in the pig. Horm Metab Res 6:245, 1974.
80. Hermansen K: Forskolin, an activator of adenylate cyclase, stimulates pancreatic insulin, glucagon, and somatostatin release in the dog: Studies *in vitro*. Endocrinology 116:2251, 1985.
81. Larsson L-I: New aspects on the neural, paracrine and endocrine regulation of islet function. Front Horm Res 7:14, 1980.
82. Asplin CM, Paquette TL, Palmer JP: In vivo inhibition of glucagon secretion by paracrine beta cell activity in man. J Clin Invest 68:314, 1981.
83. Fujimoto WY, Kawazu S, Ikeuchi M, et al: *In vitro* paracrine regulation of islet B-cell function by A and D cells. Life Sci 32:1873, 1983.
84. Kawai K, Unger RH: Inhibition of glucagon secretion by exogenous glucagon in the isolated, perfused dog pancreas. Diabetes 31:512, 1982.
85. Unger RH, Orci L: Glucagon and the A cell. Physiology and pathophysiology (First of Two Parts). N Engl J Med 304:1518, 1981.
86. Gerich JE: Somatostatin and diabetes. Am J Med 70:619, 1981.
87. Miller RE: Pancreatic neuroendocrinology: Peripheral neural mechanisms in the regulation of the islets of Langerhans. Endocr Rev 2:471, 1981.
88. Borgeat P, Labrie F, Drouin J, et al: Inhibition of adenosine 3′,5′-monophosphate accumulation in anterior pituitary gland in vitro by growth hormone-release inhibiting hormone. Biochem Biophys Res Commun 56:1052, 1974.
89. Szecowka J, Lins PE, Efendic S: Effects of cholecystokinin, gastric inhibitory polypeptide, and secretin on insulin and glucagon secretion in rats. Endocrinology 110:1268, 1982.
90. Brown M, Vale W: Effects of neurotensin and substance P on plasma insulin, glucagon and glucose levels. Endocrinology 98:819, 1976.
91. Moltz JH, Dobbs RE, McCann SM, et al: Effects of hypothalamic factors on insulin and glucagon release from the islets of Langerhans. Endocrinology 101:196, 1977.
92. Dolais-Kitabgi J, Kitabgi P, Brazeau P, et al: Effect of neurotensin on insulin, glucagon, and somatostatin release from isolated pancreatic islets. Endocrinology 105:256, 1979.
93. Holst JJ, Jensen SL, Schaffalitzky de Muckadell OB, et al: Secretin and vasoactive intestinal polypeptide in the control of the endocrine pancreas. Front Horm Res 7:119, 1980.
94. Ahren B, Lundquist I: Influences of gastro-intestinal polypeptides and glucose on glucagon secretion induced by cholinergic stimulation. Horm Metab Res 14:529, 1982.
95. Reid RL, Yen SSC: β-endorphin stimulates the secretion of insulin and glucagon in humans. J Clin Endocrinol Metab 52:592, 1981.
96. Kanter RA, Ensinck JW, Fujimoto WY: Disparate effects of enkephalin and morphine upon insulin and glucagon secretion by islet cell cultures. Diabetes 29:84, 1980.
97. Jarhult J, Farnebo L-O, Hamberger B, et al: The relation between catecholamines, glucagon and pancreatic polypeptide during hypoglycaemia in man. Acta Endocrinol 98:402, 1981.
98. Torella R, Giugliano D, Scognamiglio G, et al: Glucagon secretion in patients with hypoparathyroidism: Effect of serum calcium on glucagon release. J Clin Endocrinol Metab 54:229, 1982.
99. Iversen J, Hermansen K: Calcium, glucose and glucagon release. Diabetologia 13:297, 1977.
100. Wingert TD, Martindale RG, Toomey ML, et al: Parathyroid hormone enhances glucagon secretion from the isolated perfused rat pancreas preparation. Endocrinology 116:2469, 1985.
101. Moltz JH, Fawcett CP: Purification of a glucagon releasing factor from the rat hypothalamus. Life Sci 32:1271, 1983.
102. Asplin C, Raghu P, Dornan T, Palmer JP: Glucose regulation of glucagon secretion independent of β cell activity. Metabolism 32:292, 1983.
103. Hollander PM, Asplin CM, Palmer JP: Glucose modulation of insulin and glucagon secretion in nondiabetic and diabetic man. Diabetes 31:489, 1982.
104. Rehfeld JF, Holst JJ, Kuhl C: The effect of gastrin on basal and amino acid-stimulated insulin and glucagon secretion in man. Eur J Clin Invest 8:5, 1978.
105. Palmer JP, Walter RM, Ensinck JW: Arginine-stimulated acute phase of insulin and glucagon secretion. I. In normal man. Diabetes 24:735, 1975.
106. Holst JJ, Grønholt R, Schaffalitzky de Muckadell OB, et al: Nervous control of pancreatic endocrine secretion in pigs. I. Insulin and glucagon responses

to electrical stimulation of the vagus nerves. Acta Physiol Scand 111:1, 1981.
107. Bloom SR, Edwards AV, Hardy RN: The role of the autonomic nervous system in the control of glucagon, insulin and pancreatic polypeptide release from the pancreas. J Physiol 280:9, 1978.
108. Holst JJ, Grønholt R, Schaffalitzky de Muckadell OB, et al: Nervous control of pancreatic endocrine secretion in pigs. II. The effect of pharmacological blocking agents on the response to vagal stimulation. Acta Physiol Scand 111:9, 1981.
109. Ahren B, Lundquist I: Interaction of vasoactive intestinal peptide (VIP) with cholinergic stimulation of glucagon secretion. Experientia 38:405, 1982.
110. Holst JJ, Grønholt R, Schaffalitzky de Muckadell OB, et al: Nervous control of pancreatic endocrine secretion in pigs. IV. The effect of somatostatin on the insulin and glucagon responses to electrical vagal stimulation and intraarterial acetylcholine. Acta Physiol Scand 113:273, 1981.
111. Holst JJ, Grønholt R, Schaffalitzky de Muckadell OB, et al: Nervous control of pancreatic endocrine secretion in pigs. V. Influence of the sympathetic nervous system on the pancreatic secretion of insulin and glucagon, and on the insulin and glucagon response to vagal stimulation. Acta Physiol Scand 113:279, 1981.
112. Nilsson G, Uvnas-Wallensten K: Effect of teasing and sham feeding on plasma glucagon concentration in dogs. Acta Physiol Scand 100:298, 1977.
113. Helman AM, Amira R, Nicolaidis S, et al: Glucagon release induced by ventrolateral hypothalamic stimulation in the rat. Endocrinology 106:1612, 1980.
114. Bloom SR, Polak JM: Plasma hormone concentrations in gastrointestinal disease. Clinics Gastroenterol 9:785, 1980.
115. Ahmed M, Nuttall FQ, Gannon MC, et al: Plasma glucagon and α-amino acid nitrogen response to various diets in normal humans. Am J Clin Nutr 33:1917, 1980.
116. Nadeau A, Rousseau-Migneron S, Tancrede G, et al: Diminished glucagon response to epinephrine in physically trained diabetic rats. Diabetes 34:1278, 1985.
117. Martin JB, Reichlin S, Brown GM: *Clinical Neuroendocrinology.* Philadelphia, FA Davis Co, 1977, p 158.
118. Freychet P: Interactions of polypeptide hormones with cell membrane specific receptors: Studies with insulin and glucagon. Diabetologia 12:83, 1976.
119. Ui M, Claus TH, Exton JH, et al: Studies on the mechanism of action of glucagon on gluconeogenesis. J Biol Chem 248:5344, 1973.
120. Alford FP, Bloom SR, Nabarro JDN, et al: Glucagon control of fasting glucose in man. Lancet 2:974, 1974.
121. Liljenquist JE, Mueller GL, Cherrington AD, et al: Evidence for an important role of glucagon in the regulation of hepatic glucose production in normal man. J Clin Invest 59:369, 1977.
122. Felig P, Wahren J, Sherwin R, et al: Insulin, glucagon, and somatostatin in normal physiology and diabetes mellitus. Diabetes 25:1091, 1976.
123. Eigler N, Sacca L, Sherwin RS: Synergistic interactions of physiologic increments of glucagon, epinephrine, and cortisol in the dog. A model for stress-induced hyperglycemia. J Clin Invest 63:114, 1979.
124. Wahren J, Efendic S, Luft R, et al: Influence of somatostatin on splanchnic glucose metabolism in postabsorptive and 60-hour fasted humans. J Clin Invest 59:299, 1977.
125. Cahill GF Jr: Physiology of insulin in man. Diabetes 20:785, 1971.
126. McGarry JD, Foster DW: Effects of exogenous fatty acid concentration on glucagon-induced changes in hepatic fatty acid metabolism. Diabetes 29:236, 1980.
127. Issekutz B Jr, Vranic M: Role of glucagon in regulation of glucose production in exercising dogs. Am J Physiol 238:E13, 1980.
128. Stunkard AJ, Van Itallie TB, Reis BB: The mechanism of satiety: Effect of glucagon on gastric hunger contractions in man. Proc Soc Exp Biol Med 89:258, 1955.
129. Penick SB, Hinkle LE Jr: Depression of food intake induced in healthy subjects by glucagon. N Engl J Med 264:893, 1961.
130. Miller RE, Chernish SM, Brunelle RL, et al: Double-blind radiographic study of dose response to intravenous glucagon for hypotonic duodenography. Radiology 127:55, 1978.
131. Chernish SM, Miller RE, Rosenak BD, et al: Hypotonic duodenography with the use of glucagon. Gastroenterology 63:392, 1972.
132. Miller RE, Chernish SM, Rosenak BD, et al: Hypotonic duodenography with glucagon. Radiology 108:35, 1973.
133. Miller RE, Chernish SM, Skucas J, et al: Hypotonic roentgenography with glucagon. Am J Roentgenol 121:264, 1974.
134. Ralphs DNL, Bloom SR, Lawson-Smith C, et al: The relationship between gastric emptying rate and plasma enteroglucagon concentration. Gut 16:406, 1975.
135. Johansson H, Segerstrom A: Glucagon and gastrointestinal motility in relation to thyroid-parathyroid function. Ups J Med Sci 77:183, 1972.
136. Paul F: Quantitative studies of the effect of pancreatic glucagon+ and secretin++ on gastrointestinal motility in man recorded by simultaneous electro-manometric registration. Klin Wochenschr 52:983, 1974.
137. Dotevall G, Kock NG: The effect of glucagon on intestinal motility in man. Gastroenterology 45:364, 1963.
138. Lin TM: Action of secretin (S), glucagon (G), cholecystokinin (CCK) and endogenously released S and CCK on gallbladder (GB), choledochus (C) and bile (B) flow in dogs. Fed Proc 33:391, 1974.
139. Lin TM, Spray GF: Effect of pentagastrin, cholecys-

tokinin, caerulein and glucagon on the choledochal resistance and bile flow of conscious dog. Gastroenterology 56:1178, 1969.
140. Nebel OT: Effect of enteric hormones on the human sphincter of Oddi. Gastroenterology 68:962, 1975.
141. Vidnes J, Øyasaetter S: Glucagon deficiency causing severe neonatal hypoglycemia in a patient with normal insulin secretion. Pediatr Res 11:943, 1977.
142. Mallinson CN, Bloom SR, Warin AP, et al: A glucagonoma syndrome. Lancet 2:1, 1974.
143. Prinz RA, Dorsch TR, Lawrence AM: Clinical aspects of glucagon-producing islet cell tumors. Am J Gastroenterol 76:125, 1981.
144. Holst JJ, Helland S, Ingemannson S, et al: Functional studies in patients with the glucagonoma syndrome. Diabetologia 17:151, 1979.
145. Unger RH, Orci L: The essential role of glucagon in the pathogenesis of diabetes mellitus. Lancet 1:14, 1975.
146. Cherrington AD, Lacy WW, Chiasson J-L: Effect of glucagon on glucose production during insulin deficiency in the dog. J Clin Invest 62:664, 1978.
147. Raskin P, Unger RH: Effects of exogenous hyperglucagonemia in insulin-treated diabetics. Diabetes 26:1034, 1977.
148. Simpson RW, Hockaday TDR, Alberti KGMM: Hormonal and metabolic responses to glucagon in diabetes mellitus. Clin Endocrinol 7:203, 1977.
149. Unger RH, Orci L: The role of glucagon in diabetes. Diabetes 8:53, 1982.
150. Johnson DG, Goebel CU, Hruby VJ, et al: Hyperglycemia of diabetic rats decreased by a glucagon receptor antagonist. Science 215:1115, 1982.
151. Barnes AJ, Bloom SR, Alberti KGMM, et al: Ketoacidosis in pancreatectomized man. N Engl J Med 296:1250, 1977.
152. Clarke WL, Santiago JV, Kipnis DM: The effect of hyperglucagonemia on blood glucose concentrations and on insulin requirements in insulin-requiring diabetes mellitus. Diabetes 27:649, 1978.
153. Salzberg MR, Gallagher EJ: Propranolol overdose. Ann Emerg Med 9:26, 1980.
154. Bond JH, Levitt MD: Effect of glucagon on gastrointestinal blood flow of dogs in hypovolemic shock. Am J Physiol 238:G434, 1980.
155. Kazmers A, Wright CD, Whitehouse WM, et al: Glucagon and canine mesenteric hemodynamics: Effects on superior mesenteric arteriovenous and nutrient capillary blood flow. J Surg Res 30:372, 1981.
156. Becker HD, Reeder DD, Thompson JC: The effect of glucagon on circulating gastrin. Gastroenterology 65:28, 1973.
157. Korman MG, Soveny C, Hansky J: The effect of glucagon on serum gastrin. II Studies in pernicious anaemia and the Zollinger-Ellison syndrome. Gut 14:459, 1973.
158. Geary N, Langhans W, Scharrer E: Metabolic concomitants of glucagon-induced suppression of feeding in the rat. Am J Physiol 241:R330, 1981.
159. Smith GP: Satiety effect of gastrointestinal hormones, in Beers RF, Bassett EG (eds): *Polypeptide Hormones*. New York, Raven Press, 1980, pp 413–420.
160. Geary N, Smith GP: Pancreatic glucagon fails to inhibit sham feeding in the rat. Peptides 1:163, 1982.
161. Miller RE, Chernish SM, Greenman GF, et al: Gastrointestinal response to minute doses of glucagon. Radiology 143:317, 1982.
162. Carr-Locke DL, Gregg JA, Aoki TT: Effects of exogenous glucagon on pancreatic and biliary ductal and sphincteric pressures in man demonstrated by endoscopic manometry and correlation with plasma glucagon. Dig Dis Sci 28:312, 1983.
163. Latshaw RF, Kadir S, Witt WS, et al: Glucagon-induced choledochal sphincter relaxation: Aid for expulsion of impacted calculi into the duodenum. AJR 137:614, 1981.
164. Bordley J IV, Olson JE: The use of glucagon in operative cholangiography. Surg Gynecol Obstet 149:583, 1979.
165. Dyck WP, Texter EC Jr, Lasater JM, et al: Influence of glucagon on pancreatic exocrine secretion in man. Gastroenterology 58:532, 1970.
166. Condon JR, Knight M, Day JL: Glucagon therapy in acute pancreatitis. Br J Surg 60:509, 1973.
167. Debas HT, Hancock RJ, Soon-Shiong P, et al: Glucagon therapy in acute pancreatitis: Prospective randomized double-blind study. Can J Surg 23:578, 1980.
168. Miller TA, Watson LC, Rayford PL, et al: The effect of glucagon on pancreatic secretion and plasma secretin in dogs. World J Surg 1:93, 1977.
169. Watanabe A, Higashi T, Hayashi S, et al: Effects of insulin and glucagon on serum amino acid concentrations in liver disease. Acta Med Okayama 36:441, 1982.
170. Baker AL, Jaspan JB, Haines NW, et al: A randomized clinical trial of insulin and glucagon infusion for treatment of alcoholic hepatitis: Progress report in 50 patients. Gastroenterology 80:1410, 1981.
171. Alford FP, Chisholm DJ: Glucagon—New concepts about an "old" hormone. Aust NZ J Med 9:733, 1979.

Chapter 18

Gastric Inhibitory Polypeptide

Talaat Khalil, M.D., Gunnar Alinder, M.D., and Phillip L. Rayford, Ph.D.

HISTORY

In 1930, Kosaka and Lim [1] reported inhibition of gastric acid secretion in dogs, using crude preparations of cholecystokinin-pancreozymin (CCK-PZ). They demonstrated that duodenal extracts, prepared after perfusing the duodenum with olive oil, gave the same effect. Further studies showed that this crude CCK-PZ also possessed an inhibitory activity for acid secretion, stimulated by both exogenous [2] and endogenous [3] gastrin, and for basal and stimulated motor activity of the body of the stomach [4,5]. In 1969, Brown et al [6] and Lucien et al [7] described an enterogastrone, extractable from porcine intestine, which strongly inhibited gastric acid secretion.

In 1970, Brown and Pederson [8] found that further purification of the CCK-PZ activity from this crude material led to a diminution of the acid inhibitory effect. In 1971, Brown and Dryburgh [9,10] purified and sequenced the gastric inhibitory fraction and found it to be a distinct polypeptide. By virtue of its acid inhibitory properties, they named it gastric inhibitory polypeptide (GIP). Further investigations of its actions have shown stimulation of the release of insulin and of elevated glucose levels, and it has been suggested that a more appropriate name for GIP should be "glucose-dependent insulinotropic polypeptide" [11].

GIP is composed of 42 amino acid residues in a single chain with a molecular weight of 4976 daltons [12] (see Appendix for amino acid structure). GIP from human small intestine was found to contain 42 amino acid residues and to differ from porcine GIP only at two residues [13]. GIP exists in more than one molecular form [11,14]; three distinct peaks of immunoreactive GIP have been shown, one with a high molecular weight that could represent a protein peptide complex; one with a high molecular weight that could represent either a big GIP or a pro-GIP, and one with a molecular weight similar to that of pure porcine GIP [14].

Fifteen of the first 26 amino acids occur as they do in glucagon, and nine of the first 26 are in the same position as in secretin. The 17 C-terminal residues are not common to any other intestinal polypeptide. On the basis of these structural homologies, GIP has been placed in the secretin-glucagon-vasoactive intestinal peptide (VIP) family of peptides.

DISTRIBUTION

The availability of suitable antisera to GIP has made it possible to localize the GIP-containing cells by indirect immunofluorescence studies. Polak et al [15] tentatively identified the GIP cell as situated predominantly in the mid-zone of the glands in the duodenum and, less frequently, in the jejunum in both dogs and humans. These cells are most abundant in the villi and upper crypts and have been identified by immunoelectron microscopy and found to contain electron-dense granules with a mean corrected diameter of 444 nm [16]. The site of anti-GIP antiserum activity has been shown to be the K cell [17]. Immunocytochemical studies suggest that the α cells of the pancreas and glucagon-containing cells of the gut may contain GIP-like immunoreactivity [18,19]. Immunoreactive GIP has been detected in the intestine of the fetal rat at the 20th day of gestation, and GIP concentrations in the duodenum and remaining small intestine increased markedly during the first month of life [20]. Immunoreactive GIP (IR-GIP) cells were observed in the pancreas of human fetuses with gestational ages of 18–20 weeks. These cells were located in islet-like cell clusters, at the base of tubular structures, and among the exocrine-like acini [21]. GIP cells were observed in the pancreas of hibernating lizards but not in active ones [22].

ASSAY

Suitable bioassays for measurement of GIP in plasma or tissue extracts have not been reported, but several radioimmunoassays that employ antibodies specific for GIP have been reported [14,23–25]. The first radioimmunoassay for GIP was described by Kuzio et al in 1974 [23]. However, there is disagreement among many of these studies with regard to basal and stimulated serum levels. These discrepancies could be due to several factors, among which are the different affinities of the antisera for each different molecular form of GIP, the poor antigenicity of GIP itself and the need to conjugate it with a larger molecule (which may lead to conformational damage to the molecule), the heterogeneity of GIP antibodies owing to the scant availability of pure preparations of GIP, and the loss of biologic activity during iodination [25]. Recently, a method for iodinating GIP using Iodo-gen tracers as the oxidizing agent resulted in an RIA that detected significantly lower fasting levels of GIP in rats. This may be because of a better preserved immunoreactivity of the Iodo-gen tracer [26]. Levels of GIP measured by radioimmunoassay are usually reported as immunoreactive GIP (IR-GIP).

PHARMACOKINETICS AND CATABOLISM

Exogenously administered GIP has been shown to be cleared relatively slowly from human plasma. Its half-life is around 20 minutes [11,27,28]. Endogenous GIP disappears at the same rate after administration of somatostatin [29]. The apparent space of distribution is 76.8 mL/kg, which is sufficiently close to plasma volume in humans to suggest that GIP does not diffuse freely into all tissue fluids. The calculated metabolic clearance rate is 2.6 mL/kg in humans, which is low, consistent with the long half-life and close to the glomerular filtration rate. The kidney may be an important site for GIP clearance. Basal and food-stimulated serum GIP levels are reported to be elevated in patients with renal insufficiency, and the duration of the food-stimulated response is prolonged [30,31]. Renal arteriovenous gradients also were demonstrated in anesthetized dogs during exogenous GIP infusion, with a maximum gradient of 39 percent [30]. Hanks et al [32] found the hepatic extraction of GIP both in vitro (rats) and in vivo (dogs) to be minimal.

RELEASE

Results obtained with radioimmunoassay suggest that the normal fasting level for IR-GIP in humans is approximately 250 pg/mL. Within 45 minutes of eating a mixed meal, GIP levels rose to 1200 pg/mL and remained elevated above 1000 pg/mL for a period of 3 hours [23]. A high caloric mixed meal almost doubled GIP release compared to a low caloric mixed meal. This difference does not appear to be due to glucose, because blood glucose levels were not significantly changed [33]. GIP was reported to exhibit a circadian variation in humans. GIP levels tend to remain elevated for most of the day until late at night; they peak after each meal [34,35].

GIP is released after ingestion of two major nutrient stimuli, glucose [36] and fat [37], and after the intraduodenal (ID) infusion of solutions containing amino acids [38] or bile [26]. Hydrolysis of triglycerol appears to be important in the release of GIP, and long-chain but not medium-chain fatty acids can stimulate GIP release [39]. Ingestion of proteins produced no significant elevation of GIP [11]. However, recently a prompt elevation in GIP in response to a peptone meal in dogs was shown by means of a highly sensitive GIP radioimmunoassay [40]. GIP can also be released by intravenous (IV) infusion of calcium and by the presence of hypercalcemia [41].

Basal plasma insulin and GIP concentrations are significantly higher in neonatal than in fetal pigs [42,43]. Basal GIP concentrations in the neonatal pigs were also considerably higher than the levels in pregnant sows, or, for that matter, the levels found in adult men [43,44].

The release of GIP by glucose and triglycerides [37] is dose-dependent in dogs and humans [45]. Moreover, McCullough et al [46] recently found that if glucose is administered by constant ID infusion, a constant elevation in GIP could be maintained. The release of GIP from the gut in response to glucose might be regulated by the rate of absorption. It has even been shown that in healthy men fasted for 5 days, a test meal caused an augmented GIP response [47]. GIP release differs between sexes: elderly women have higher GIP levels than elderly men after oral glucose intake [48], but no difference was found between young and old subjects.

The molecular configuration of monosaccharides with the ability to stimulate GIP release has been shown to agree well with the requirements for active transport by the sodium-dependent hexose pathway [49]. Thus, xylitol, which differs in structure from the common actively transported sugars and is thought to be absorbed by passive diffusion, does not stimulate GIP secretion in either humans or dogs [50].

GIP is released by a different group of amino acids than those that cause most pronounced release of gastrin, CCK, and pancreatic polypeptide; ID administration of a mixture of amino acids including arginine, histidine, isoleucine, leucine, lysine, and threonine caused significant release of GIP in humans, whereas administration of a mixture of methionine, phenylalanine, tryptophan, and valine did not [38].

The role of cephalic stimulation in the regulation of GIP is controversial. Insulin-induced hypoglycemia has been shown to release GIP (presumably through stimulation of the vagus) [51], but another study suggested that vagal stimulation inhibited GIP release in order to protect against insulin-induced hypoglycemia [52]. Although truncal vagotomy is associated with an early and exaggerated GIP response to glucose meals, this altered response is thought to reflect early and uncontrolled entry of glucose into the small intestine rather than a direct effect of vagal denervation of the GIP cells [53]. Both physiologic vagal activation by sham feeding and electrical stimulation of the vagus failed to change GIP secretion, but both types of vagal stimulation significantly increased insulin secretion in fasted rats [54]. These findings do not exclude modulatory influences of the central nervous system via the vagus nerve on glucose- or fat-stimulated GIP secretion [54]. Also, sham feeding did not increase basal or meal-stimulated GIP levels in humans, thus failing to demonstrate a cephalic-vagal stimulation of GIP [55].

Isoproterenol (a β-adrenergic agonist) increased fasting levels of both GIP and insulin, which become greater after ingestion of oral glucose. This effect was blocked by propranolol and, therefore, is most likely caused by beta stimulation [56]. The increased blood glucose concentration after beta stimulation is probably of no physiologic importance, since IV infusion of glucose had no effect on GIP concentration [57].

The involvement of the sympathetic nervous system in regulation of GIP release is also controversial. In studies in dogs, GIP response to ID glucose was not affected by IV epinephrine or isoproterenol [58]; in other studies, it was inhibited by both [59]. In humans, the results are also confusing. α-Adrenergic stimulation was demonstrated to have a suppressive effect on GIP response to oral glucose and no effect on fasting levels [60].

Table 18-1 summarizes some of the observations on the effects of the autonomic nervous system on GIP and immunoreactive insulin levels.

Food-stimulated release of GIP may possibly be modulated by other gastrointestinal hormones. In humans, exogenous glucagon depresses fasting serum GIP concentrations and greatly suppresses its response to a test meal [61]. Whether this effect is exerted directly on the GIP-producing cells or indirectly through some mediator such as somatostatin is unknown. In dogs, exogenous gastrin and CCK but not glucagon and secretin significantly increased glucose-stimulated release of GIP [62].

Exogenous insulin inhibits the GIP response to oral fat [11]. Similarly, IV administration of glucose inhibits fat-released GIP [63]. On the other hand, simultaneous infusion of insulin and glucose (to maintain euglycemia) failed to alter the basal concentration of GIP in humans [64]. Perhaps the inhibition of GIP release that has been attributed to insulin under some conditions is actually due to prevention of hyperglycemia rather than to a direct effect of insulin on the GIP cell [65].

Localization studies of the site of GIP release in humans suggested that the proximal small intestine accounts for the major portion of GIP release [66].

Table 18-1. **Effect of autonomic nervous system on release of IR-GIP and insulin**

	IR-GIP	*IRI*
Truncal vagotomy + glucose meal [53]	+	+
Sham feeding (physiologic) [54]	0	+
Electrical stimulation of vagus [54]	0	+
Isoproterenol [56]	+	0
Isoproterenol + oral glucose meal [56]	+	0
Isoproterenol + IV glucose	+	0
α**-Adrenergic** [60]	0	+
α**-Adrenergic + oral glucose** [60]	−	+

0 = no change from normal control; + = higher than normal controls; − = lower than normal controls; IRI = immunoreactive insulin.

ACTIONS

Effects of GIP on the Gastrointestinal Tract

GIP was originally studied as an enterogastrone [1–7]. An enterogastrone can be defined as a substance that is released from the intestinal mucosa by contact with acid, hypertonic solutions, or fat and that acts to inhibit gastric secretion and motility [67].

The role of GIP as an enterogastrone is controversial. A clear relationship between inhibition of acid secretion and GIP release was observed in dogs with denervated fundic pouches. Infusion of porcine GIP to attain circulating levels within the physiologic range inhibited pentagastrin-stimulated acid secretion and, to a lesser extent, histamine-stimulated acid secretion in a dose-dependent manner [68]. Stimulation of endogenous GIP release with intraduodenal fat produced a similar effect, except that the hydrogen ion secretion shortly returned to normal, while GIP levels remained significantly elevated. It was suggested that the triglyceride mixture may release a larger molecular form of GIP that has no enterogastrone activity [69]. Exogenous GIP had only a weak inhibitory effect on meal-stimulated acid secretion in dogs, whereas duodenal perfusion with fat totally abolished the gastric acid response to a meal with only a moderate rise in serum IR-GIP [70]. In addition, perfusion of acid into the duodenum of dogs with denervated pouches inhibited acid secretion without a significant increase in serum GIP [11]. On the other hand, it has been shown that the inhibition of pentagastrin-stimulated acid secretion from denervated pouches of dogs by GIP could be reversed by infusion of urecholine, indicating that parasympathetic mechanisms can interfere with the action of GIP on innervated stomachs [71]. Infusion of acetylcholine or peripheral electrical stimulation of the vagus was also shown to inhibit the release of somatostatin by GIP. The exact interrelationship among GIP, vagal excitation, acetylcholine, and acid secretion is not clear [72]. Recently, Wolfe et al [73], using antibodies to bind endogenous GIP in dogs, demonstrated the capacity of GIP to inhibit meal-stimulated gastric acid secretion.

Table 18-2 summarizes the reported observations on the effect of GIP on acid secretion in dogs.

The role of GIP in the inhibition of acid secretion in humans is even less well understood than in dogs, and reports that conflict with the enterogastrone concept abound. The amount of exogenous GIP required to inhibit acid secretion stimulated by pentagastrin or a peptone meal was reported to be beyond physiologic limits [74]. Studies with graded levels of pentagastrin-stimulated acid secretion have failed to show a convincing enterogastrone effect of exogenous GIP in humans [75]. Furthermore, a report of similar studies on vagotomized patients has also failed to confirm such a role [76]. It was found that the instillation of fat into the jejunum of humans caused dramatic inhibition of gastric acid secretion and a significant increase in circulating plasma levels of GIP, enteroglucagon (GLI), and VIP. The inhibitory effect could not be attributed to any of these peptides alone, and it is possible that GIP is involved with other peptides in the physiologic inhibition of acid secretion [77].

An endocrine-like effect of GIP was reported in dogs with Thiry-Vella loops of the upper jejunum or lower ileum [78]. With the use of a triple-lumen gut perfusion technique in humans, more physiologic doses of GIP also produced a stimulation of intestinal secretion [79]. This effect is unlikely to be mediated by cyclic AMP, since it is caused by doses of GIP that do not seem to stimulate adenylate cy-

Table 18-2. **Relationship between IR-GIP and gastric acid secretion in dogs**

	IR-GIP	*Stimulated acid secretion as compared to control*
Exogenous GIP, HP [68]	+	−
Fat, endogenous GIP, HP [69]	+	−
Exogenous GIP, innervated stomach [70]	+	0
Fat, endogenous GIP, innervated stomach [70]	+	0
Acid, intraduodenal, HP [11]	0	−
Peptone meal + IV GIP antibodies [73]	−	+

0 = no change from normal control; + = higher than normal control; − = lower than normal control. HP = Heidenhain pouch.

clase in either the small intestine [80] or the colon [81].

GIP has an inhibitory effect on motor activity in pouches of the body of the stomach and the antrum [11]; it also lowers both the basal and pentagastrin-stimulated lower esophageal sphincter pressure in cats [82], inhibits pepsin release stimulated by insulin hypoglycemia, and inhibits the movement of sodium from lumen to interstitium in rabbit salivary glands [83]. GIP has been reported to have little or no effect on exocrine pancreatic and biliary secretion and on secretion from pouches of the Brunner's gland area [11].

Effects of GIP on the Endocrine Pancreas

In 1930, La Barre made the suggestion that the duodenum produces a hormone that exerts an effect on the endocrine pancreas. He coined the term "incretin," or insulin-releasing factor [84]. An incretin is an endocrine transmitter produced in the gastrointestinal tract that is released by nutrients, especially carbohydrates, and that stimulates insulin secretion in the presence of glucose [52]. Unger and Eisentraut [85] suggested the term enteroinsular axis to describe the regulatory control exerted by the intestine on the pattern of release of the pancreatic islet hormones. In 1964, McIntyre et al [86] made the classic observation that an oral or intraduodenal glucose load produces a greater insulin response than a similar dose given intravenously.

Early studies with peptides derived from extracts of porcine duodenojejunal mucosa suggested that secretin and CCK-PZ were capable of potentiating the rise in serum insulin in response to hyperglycemia in humans [87]. Studies on insulin secretion in rats showed that the stimulatory effect of 10 percent CCK-PZ was not reproduced with a highly purified preparation [88]. In studies in humans and dogs, GIP isolated from crude CCK-PZ reproduced the stimulation of insulin in the same amounts corresponding to crude CCK-PZ [89]. The insulinotropic action of GIP was also demonstrated in dogs [90], in in vitro perfused isolated rat pancreas preparations [15,91], and in isolated rat islet preparations [92,93].

Infusion of GIP in healthy human volunteers revealed that during basal state glycemia GIP had no insulinotropic effect; in mild hyperglycemia (54 mg/dL above basal) immunoreactive insulin levels were modestly augmented; and in moderate hyperglycemia (143 mg/dL above basal), immunoreactive insulin levels were highly elevated [27]. Induced hormone deficiency through IV injection of GIP-specific antibodies in rats completely eliminated its incretin effect and significantly reduced the insulin response [94,95]. However, a similar study using antibodies against pure GIP reported a limited decrease in insulin output in the first 20 minutes only, suggesting that gut factors other than GIP may act as incretins in the rat and that the incretin effect of GIP is strongest immediately after the glucose load [96]. Studies using isolated, perfused intestine or pancreas have shown that the intestine secretes an insulinotropic factor not chemically related to known hormones [97]. Other known hormones have been suggested as possible incretins [52]. In fact, these gastrointestinal peptides may interfere with insulin secretory mechanisms in a complex manner. For example, CCK-8, which has no effect on glucose-stimulated insulin release, when combined with GIP abolishes the potentiating action of GIP alone [98]. In studies with isolated rat islets, Alwmark et al [99] from our laboratory showed that several peptides (CCK-4, gastrin-releasing peptide, CCK-8, and VIP, for example) have a more potent incretin effect than GIP.

In vitro studies demonstrated that a threshold glucose concentration was necessary for GIP to stimulate insulin release from isolated islets (6–8 nM) [92,93,100] or from the perfused pancreas (5.5 nM) [91]. The observation of a glucose threshold for insulin release by GIP is important as a physiologic mechanism in that fat also releases GIP, which is insulinotropic only in the presence of elevated glucose levels [37,101]. In the euglycemic state, fat-released IR-GIP or exogenously administered porcine GIP within physiologic concentrations is not insulinotropic [91]. Fat-stimulated GIP has insulinotropic activities that are glucose-dependent and are not inhibited by physiologic hyperinsulinemia during euglycemia but are influenced by the ambient glucose level in the presence of hyperinsulinemia [102]. The dependency of the incretin effect upon the glucose levels at physiologic concentrations of the hormone is an important prerequisite of this principle for prevention of hypoglycemia. Thus, an incretin can be released by different intestinal contents, but elevated incretin blood levels stimulate insulin secretion only in the presence of elevated blood glucose levels [52,101].

In the human newborn, the enteroinsulin axis is inactive [103]. Neonatal pigs also lack an enteroinsular response, and in pigs, the lack of an enteroinsular response might be related to a paradoxical decline in plasma GIP after administration of oral glucose [42]. In contrast, adult pigs exhibit a significant enteroinsular axis effect [104]. On the other hand, ID infusion of glucose elicits a substantial rise in plasma GIP in late fetal pigs [42], so that the porcine enteroinsular axis is already developed in late fetal life, but neonatally the axis seems to be blocked by a mechanism as yet unknown. As this reduces the enhancement of plasma insulin levels after a meal, the blocked enteroinsular axis might protect the neonate from insulin-induced hypoglycemic attacks late in the intervals between suckling periods. Moreover, the GIP cell response to an oral triglyceride load is suppressed in late fetal and neonatal pigs [43]. The abolished GIP response to oral triglycerides may play a causal role in the inactivity of the enteroinsular axis, which is seen in both human and animal neonates.

During exercise in humans, plasma levels of GIP are decreased, which would explain the delay in plasma insulin response during exercise [105]. GIP appears to play a minimal role in the hyperinsulinism found in hyperthyroid patients [106].

High levels of GIP (100 μg/mL) stimulate glucagon release from isolated rat pancreas, and with these high concentrations, glucose has no suppressive effect on the secretion [11]. In streptozotocin-treated rats, the elevated GLI levels were further increased by treatment with GIP. In the isolated perfused pancreas, GIP produced a biphasic glucagon release in the presence of 4 mM glucose and also augmented the response to arginine [90,107]. GIP potentiated cholinergically induced glucagon secretion in vivo in rats [108]. A glucagonotropic action for GIP is therefore evident in the rat, although no such action has been described in humans [27]. In normal humans, an IV infusion of porcine GIP (in doses sufficient to raise plasma levels to upper physiologic range) had no effect on plasma glucagon [102,109].

Ipp et al [110] reported that GIP (58 ng/mL) stimulated somatostatin release from the perfused canine pancreas with attached duodenum. High doses of exogenous somatostatin were found to reduce GIP response to a test meal and oral glucose and to inhibit its insulinotropic action in both animals and humans [52,111]. Recently, lower doses of somatostatin were reported to blunt insulin and GIP release after a mixed meal in humans [45,112], which suggested that somatostatin at least partially inhibits GIP release through a direct effect on GIP cells [112].

Metabolic Effect of GIP

GIP may exert some metabolic effects in the absence of insulin. GIP strongly antagonized the lipolytic action of glucagon in isolated fat cells of the rat [113], it enhanced the lipoprotein lipase activity in cultured preadipocytes [114], and it promoted the clearance of chylomicron triglycerides from the circulation in dogs [115].

Pathophysiology of GIP

Table 18-3 summarizes the changes in GIP levels that occur with some diseases.

Diabetes mellitus. There has been much speculation about a possible role of GIP in diabetes mellitus. For example, in maturity onset diabetes, could the enteroinsular axis be operative or even overactive, since diabetes is characterized by a pathologic oral glucose tolerance curve, often with an excessive response [116]?

Measurement of the GIP response to a high caloric meal or oral glucose has been reported to be exaggerated in patients with maturity onset diabetes with high insulin secretion [11,117,118] and normal in juvenile diabetics without insulin reserve [117]. However, in obese subjects, fasting levels of GIP are elevated when compared to nor-

Table 18-3. **Levels of IR-GIP and IRI in some diseases**

	Fasting		*Stimulated*	
	IR-GIP	*IRI*	*IR-GIP*	*IRI*
Diabetes mellitus [115]	0	+	+	+
Obesity [119]	+	+	+	+
Chronic pancreatitis [125]	+	−	+	−
Celiac disease [127]	0	−	−	−
Duodenal ulcer [130]	0	NA	+	NA
Intestinal bypass [133]	+	NA	−	NA

0 = no change from normal controls; + = higher than normal controls; − = lower than normal controls; NA = not available; IRI = immunoreactive insulin.

mals [117,119,120]. Comparing nonobese diabetics to normal subjects revealed no difference between the two groups in basal IR-GIP, but integrated IR-GIP in response to stimulation was higher in diabetics [121].

Insulin has been proposed to exert a negative feedback control on GIP release [11]. The augmented GIP response seen in some diabetic patients could then be explained as the result of a defective insulin feedback mechanism. However, administration of insulin in these patients failed to abolish the elevated levels of GIP [122]. An augmented GIP release has also been reported in some obese patients with hyperinsulinemia and, in these circumstances, the GIP cell may perhaps become insulin-resistant [123]. In normal subjects given infusions of insulin, there is little evidence for negative feedback control [102]. The effect of insulin on GIP release in pathologic circumstances may, however, be quite different. Infusions of GIP into diabetic subjects resulted in a significant rise in levels of serum glucagon. This effect was totally absent in nondiabetics and may represent an indirect action of GIP via glucagon, which is reflected in pathologic glucose tolerance [119].

Obesity. Obesity is accompanied by hyperinsulinemia (both in the fasting state and after stimulation of insulin release [124]) and by resistance to both endogenous and exogenous insulin [57]. Overactivity of the enteroinsular axis and exaggerated release of GIP have been suggested to cause hyperinsulinemia. Insulin responses to glucose and triglycerides were found to be greater in obese subjects than in normals, suggesting a failure of insulin feedback control of GIP in obese subjects [123].

The effect of hyperinsulinemia on stimulating lipogenesis is well established [124]. Recently, the influence of GIP on the incorporation of fatty acid into epididymal adipose tissue in the rat has been studied in vitro, with and without addition of insulin [125]. Without insulin in the medium, GIP induced a slight although significant decrease in fatty acid incorporation. In the presence of insulin (100 μU/mol), GIP significantly enhanced the insulin-induced fatty acid incorporation. GIP action could take place through interactions between receptors that would modify the insulin receptor affinity, but the exact nature of such a mechanism is not known [126].

Chronic Pancreatitis and Cystic Fibrosis (Exocrine Pancreatic Insufficiency). In patients with chronic pancreatitis, the GIP response to glucose or to the ingestion of a test meal was reported to be higher, while immunoreactive insulin was lower when compared to normal subjects [127,128]. Ebert et al [128] further studied this observation and showed that the IR-GIP response is related to the severity of both endocrine and exocrine insufficiencies. GIP levels in these patients increase when they are given pancreatic enzyme supplement [129]. The elevated GIP levels in chronic pancreatitis may be caused by lack of its inhibition by insulin. In this vein, an augmented GIP response to a test meal has been reported following duodenopancreatectomy (Whipple procedure), which could be caused by a reduced feedback inhibition of IR-GIP release [130].

Exocrine pancreatic insufficiency is found in patients with cystic fibrosis. Impaired GIP release after eating a meal of corn oil or milk has been reported [131,132]. This blunted GIP response was corrected by the addition of pancreatic enzymes to the meal [132]. Compared to fasting GIP levels in healthy children, fasting GIP values in children with chronic fibrosis were increased [131] or unchanged [132].

Celiac Disease. Patients with celiac disease were found to have significantly reduced IR-GIP and insulin responses to a test meal. This reduction could be caused by defective absorption of nutrients attributable to the atrophy of intestinal villi that is characteristic of the disease. There was no significant reduction in the absolute number of GIP cells [130].

Duodenal Ulcer. The GIP response to a mixed meal or to a test meal was found to be augmented in patients with duodenal ulcers, and the GIP response to oral glucose was normal or elevated [133]. These findings would rule out any possibility that GIP hyposecretion is a causal factor of duodenal ulcer [134].

Intestinal Bypass. In jejunoileal bypass in humans [15] and rats [135], basal GIP levels were found to be high, while the GIP response to glucose was reduced. The cause of high basal levels could be the result of isolation of GIP cells in the blind loop away from inhibitory factors, while the reduced response could be due to a reduced mass of GIP cells that is exposed to stimulants [135]. Massive small bowel resection in rats reduced GIP levels in response to oral glucose, which supports the second concept [136].

Prolactinoma and Acromegaly. Patients with prolactinoma showed higher GIP levels in response to oral glucose than those with active acromegaly [137]. All of the patients were also hyperinsulinemic. Patients with active acromegaly had lower GIP responses compared to patients with acromegaly in remission and normal controls.

REFERENCES

1. Kosaka T, Lim RKS: Demonstration of the humoral agent in fat inhibition of gastric secretion. Proc Soc Exp Biol Med 27:890, 1930.
2. Gillespie IE, Grossman MI: Inhibitory effect of secretin and cholecystokinin on Heidenhain pouch responses to gastrin extract and histamine. Gut 5:342, 1964.
3. Brown JC, Magee DF: Inhibitory action of cholecystokinin on acid secretion from Heidenhain pouches induced by endogenous gastrin. Gut 8:29, 1967.
4. Brown JC, Johnson LP, Magee DF: The inhibition of induced motor activity in transplanted fundic pouches. J Physiol 188:45, 1967.
5. Johnson LP, Magee DF: Cholecystokinin-pancreozymin extracts and gastric motor inhibition. Surg Gynecol Obstet 121:557, 1965.
6. Brown JC, Pederson RA, Jorpes E, et al: Preparation of highly active enterogastrone. Can J Physiol Pharmacol 47:113, 1969.
7. Lucien HW, Itoh Z, Sun DCH, et al: The purification of enterogastrone from porcine gut. Arch Biochem Biophys 134:180, 1969.
8. Brown JC, Pederson RA: A multiparameter study on the action of preparations containing cholecystokinin-pancreozymin. Scand J Gastroenterol 5:537, 1970.
9. Brown JC: A gastric inhibitory polypeptide. I. The amino acid composition and the tryptic peptides. Can J Biochem 49:255, 1971.
10. Brown JC, Dryburgh JR: A gastric inhibitory polypeptide II: The complete amino acid sequence. Can J Biochem 49:867, 1971.
11. Brown JC, Dryburgh JR, Ross SA, et al: Identification and actions of gastric inhibitory polypeptide. Recent Prog Horm Res 31:487, 1975.
12. Jornvall H, Carlquist M, Kwauk S, et al: Amino acid sequence and heterogeneity of gastric inhibitory polypeptide (GIP). FEBS Lett 123:205, 1981.
13. Moody AJ, Thim L, Valverde I: The isolation and sequencing of human gastric inhibitory peptide (GIP). FEBS Lett 172:142, 1984.
14. Sarson DL, Besterman HS, Bloom SR: Radioimmunoassay of gastric inhibitory polypeptide and its release in morbid obesity and after jejuno-ileal bypass. J Endocrinol 83:155P, 1979.
15. Polak JM, Bloom SR, Kuzio M, et al: Cellular localization of gastric inhibitory polypeptide in the duodenum and jejunum. Gut 14:284, 1973.
16. Buchan AMJ, Polak JM, Capella C, et al: Electroimmunocytochemical evidence for the K cell localization of gastric inhibitory polypeptide (GIP) in man. Histochemistry 56:37, 1978.
17. Buffa R, Polak JM, Pearse AGE, et al: Identification of the intestinal cell storing gastric inhibitory peptide. Histochemistry 43:249, 1975.
18. Alumets J, Håkanson R, O'Dorisio T, et al: Is GIP a glucagon cell constituent? Histochemistry 58:253, 1978.
19. Smith PH, Merchant FW, Johnson DG, et al: Immunocytochemical localization of a gastric inhibitory polypeptide-like material within A-cells of the endocrine pancreas. Am J Anat 149:585, 1977.
20. Gespach C, Bataille D, Jarrousse C, et al: Ontogeny and distribution of immunoreactive gastric inhibitory polypeptide (IR-GIP) in rat small intestine. Acta Endocrinol 90:307, 1979.
21. El-Salhy M, Wilander E, Grimelius L: Immunocytochemical localization of gastric inhibitory peptide (GIP) in the human foetal pancreas. Upsala J Med Sci 87:81, 1982.
22. El-Salhy M, Grimelius L: Immunohistochemical localization of gastrin C-terminus, gastric inhibitory peptide (GIP) and endorphin in the pancreas of lizards with special reference to the hibernation period. Regul Pept 2:97, 1981.
23. Kuzio M, Dryburgh JR, Malloy KM, et al: Radioimmunoassay for gastric inhibitory polypeptide. Gastroenterology 66:357, 1974.
24. Burhol PG, Jorde R, Waldum HL: Radioimmunoassay of plasma gastric inhibitory polypeptide (GIP), release of GIP after a test meal and duodenal infusion of bile, and immunoreactive plasma GIP components in man. Digestion 20:336, 1980.
25. Jorde R, Burhol PG, Schulz TB: Fasting and postprandial plasma GIP values in man measured with seven different antisera. Regul Pept 7:87, 1983.
26. Schulz TB, Jorde R, Waldum HL, et al: Preparation of ^{125}I-labeled gastric inhibitory polypeptide, using water-insoluble 1,3,4,6-tetrachloro-3α,6α-diphenyglycoluril (Iodo-gen) as the oxidizing agent. Scand J Gastroenterol 17:379, 1982.
27. Elahi D, Andersen DK, Brown JC, et al: Pancreatic α- and β-cell responses to GIP infusion in normal man. Am J Physiol 237:E185, 1979.
28. Sarson DL, Hayter RC, Bloom SR: The pharmacokinetics of porcine glucose-dependent insulinotropic polypeptide (GIP) in man. Eur J Clin Invest 12:457, 1982.
29. Sarson DL, Wood SM, Holder D, et al: The effect of glucose-dependent insulinotropic polypeptide infused at physiological concentrations on the release of insulin in man. Diabetologia 22:33, 1982.
30. O'Dorisio TM, Sirinek KR, Mazzaferri EL, et al: Renal effects on serum gastric inhibitory polypeptide (GIP). Metabolism 26:651, 1977.
31. Lauritzen JB, Lauritsen KB, Ege Olsen M, et al: Gastric inhibitory polypeptide (GIP) and insulin release in response to oral and intravenous glucose in uremic patients. Metabolism 31:1096, 1982.
32. Hanks JB, Andersen DK, Wise JE, et al: The hepatic extraction of gastric inhibitory polypeptide and insulin. Endocrinology 115:1011, 1984.
33. Beck B, Villaume C, Chayvialle JA, et al: Influence of caloric intake on gastric inhibitory polypeptide, VIP and gastrin release in man. Peptides 5:403, 1984.
34. Jorde R, Burhol PG, Waldum HL, et al: Diurnal variation of plasma gastric inhibitory polypeptide in man. Scand J Gastroenterol 15:617, 1980.
35. Salera M, Giacomoni P, Pironi L, et al: Circadian

rhythm of gastric inhibitory polypeptide (GIP) in man. Metabolism 32:21, 1983.

36. Cataland S, Crockett SE, Brown JC, et al: Gastric inhibitory polypeptide (GIP) stimulation by oral glucose in man. J Clin Endocrinol Metab 39:223, 1974.
37. Pederson RA, Schubert HE, Brown JC: Gastric inhibitory polypeptide. Its physiologic release and insulinotropic action in the dog. Diabetes 24:1050, 1975.
38. Thomas FB, Sinar D, Mazzaferri EL, et al: Selective release of gastric inhibitory polypeptide by intraduodenal amino acid perfusion in man. Gastroenterology 74:1261, 1978.
39. Ohneda A, Kobayashi T, Nihei J: Response of gastric inhibitory polypeptide to fat ingestion in normal dogs. Regul Pept 8:123, 1984.
40. Wolfe MM, McGuigan JE: Release of gastric inhibitory peptide following a peptone meal in the dog. Gastroenterology 83:864, 1982.
41. Toyota T, Nakanome C, Akai H, et al: Release of gastric inhibitory polypeptide (GIP) during calcium infusion and in hyperparathyroidism. Regul Pept 4:1, 1982.
42. Kuhl C, Hornnes PJ, Lindkaer Jensen S, et al: Gastric inhibitory polypeptide and insulin: Response to intraduodenal and intravenous glucose infusions in fetal and neonatal pigs. Endocrinology 107:1446, 1980.
43. Kuhl C, Hornnes PJ, Lindkaer Jensen S, et al: Effect of intraduodenal and intravenous triglyceride infusions on plasma gastric inhibitory polypeptide and insulin in fetal and neonatal pigs. Diabetologia 23:41, 1982.
44. Hornnes PJ, Kuhl C, Holst JJ, et al: Simultaneous recording of the gastro-entero-pancreatic hormonal peptide response to food in man. Metabolism 29:777, 1980.
45. Flaten O, Tronier B: Dose-dependent increase in concentrations of gastric inhibitory polypeptide and pancreatic polypeptide after small amounts of glucose intraduodenally in man. Scand J Gastroenterol 17:677, 1982.
46. McCullough AJ, Miller LJ, Service FJ, et al: Effect of graded intraduodenal glucose infusions on the release and physiological action of gastric inhibitory polypeptide. J Clin Endocrinol Metab 56:234, 1983.
47. Oektedalen O, Opstad PK, Jorde R: Increased plasma response of gastric inhibitory polypeptide to oral glucose and a liquid meal after prolonged starvation in healthy man. Digestion 26:114, 1983.
48. McConnell JG, Alam MJ, O'Hare MMT, et al: The effect of age and sex on the response of enteropancreatic polypeptides to oral glucose. Age Ageing 12:54, 1983.
49. Sykes S, Morgan LM, English J, et al: Evidence for preferential stimulation of gastric inhibitory polypeptide secretion in the rat by actively transported carbohydrates and their analogues. J Endocrinol 85:201, 1980.
50. Salminen S, Salminen E, Marks V: The effects of xylitol on the secretion of insulin and gastric inhibitory polypeptide in man and rats. Diabetologia 22:480, 1982.
51. Jorde R, Waldum HL, Burhol PG: The effect of insulin-induced hypoglycemia with and without atropine on plasma GIP in man. Scand J Gastroenterol 16:219, 1981.
52. Creutzfeldt W: The incretin concept today. Diabetologia 16:75, 1979.
53. Thomford NR, Sirinek KR, Crockett SE, et al: Gastric inhibitory polypeptide. Response to oral glucose after vagotomy and pyloroplasty. Arch Surg 109:177, 1974.
54. Berthoud HR, Trimble ER, Moody AJ: Lack of gastric inhibitory polypeptide (GIP) response to vagal stimulation in the rat. Peptides 3:907, 1982.
55. Taylor IL, Feldman M: Effect of cephalic-vagal stimulation of insulin, gastric inhibitory polypeptide, and pancreatic polypeptide release in humans. J Clin Endocrinol Metab 55:1114, 1982.
56. Flaten O, Sand T, Myren J: Beta-adrenergic stimulation and blockade of the release of gastric inhibitory polypeptide and insulin in man. Scand J Gastroenterol 17:283, 1982.
57. Rabinowitz D, Zierler KL: Forearm metabolism in obesity and its response to intra-arterial insulin. Characterization of insulin resistance and evidence for adaptive hyperinsulinism. J Clin Invest 41:2173, 1962.
58. Sirinek KR, Cataland S, O'Dorisio T, et al: Sympathetic neuroendocrine regulation of gastric inhibitory polypeptide response to glucose. Surg Forum 28:377, 1977.
59. Williams RH, Biesbroeck J: Gastric inhibitory polypeptide and insulin secretion after infusion of acetylcholine, catecholamines, and gut hormones. Proc Soc Exp Biol Med 163:39, 1980.
60. Salera M, Ebert R, Giacomoni P, et al: Adrenergic modulation of gastric inhibitory polypeptide secretion in man. Dig Dis Sci 27:794, 1982.
61. Ebert R, Arnold R, Creutzfeldt W: Lowering of fasting and food stimulated serum immunoreactive gastric inhibitory polypeptide (GIP) by glucagon. Gut 18:121, 1977.
62. Sirinek KR, Cataland S, O'Dorisio TM, et al: Augmented gastric inhibitory polypeptide response to intraduodenal glucose by exogenous gastrin and cholecystokinin. Surgery 82:438, 1977.
63. Ebert R, Illmer K, Creutzfeldt W: Release of gastric inhibitory polypeptide (GIP) by intraduodenal acidification in rats and humans and abolishment of the incretin effect of acid by GIP-antiserum in rats. Gastroenterology 76:515, 1979.
64. Service FJ, Nelson RL, Rubenstein AH, et al: Direct effect of insulin on secretion of insulin, glucagon, gastric inhibitory polypeptide, and gastrin during maintenance of normoglycemia. J Clin Endocrinol Metab 47:488, 1978.
65. Walsh JH: Gastrointestinal hormones and peptides. Gastric inhibitory polypeptide, in Johnson LR (ed):

Physiology of the Gastrointestinal Tract. New York, Raven Press, 1981, pp 93–99.

66. Thomas FB, Shook DF, O'Dorisio TM, et al: Localization of gastric inhibitory polypeptide release by intestinal glucose perfusion in man. Gastroenterology 72:49, 1977.
67. Gregory RA: Enterogastrone—a reappraisal of the problem, in Shnitka TK, Gilbert JAL, Harrisson RC (eds): *Gastric Secretion.* New York, Pergamon Press, 1967, pp 469–477.
68. Pederson RA, Brown JC: Inhibition of histamine, pentagastrin, and insulin-stimulated canine gastric secretion by pure "gastric inhibitory polypeptide." Gastroenterology 62:393, 1972.
69. Pederson RA, Dryburgh JR, Brown JC: Comparison of the acid inhibitory effect of exogenously administered porcine GIP and endogenously released immunoreactive GIP (IR-GIP) in the dog. Scand J Gastroenterol 13 (Suppl 49):141, 1978.
70. Yamagishi T, Debas HT: Gastric inhibitory polypeptide (GIP) is not the primary mediator of the enterogastrone action of fat in the dog. Gastroenterology 78:931, 1980.
71. Soon-Shiong P, Debas HT, Brown JC: Cholinergic inhibition of gastric inhibitory polypeptide (GIP) action. Gastroenterology 79:867, 1980.
72. McIntosh CHS, Pederson RA, Koop H, et al: Inhibition of GIP stimulated somatostatin-like immunoreactivity (SLI) by acetylcholine and vagal stimulation, in Miyoshi A (ed): *Gut Peptides.* Tokyo, Kodansha Ltd; New York, Elsevier/North-Holland Biomedical Press, 1979, pp 100–104.
73. Wolfe MM, Hocking MP, Maico DG, et al: Effects of antibodies to gastric inhibitory peptide on gastric acid secretion and gastrin release in the dog. Gastroenterology 84:941, 1983.
74. Arnold R, Ebert R, Creutzfeldt W, et al: Inhibition of gastric acid secretion by gastric inhibitory polypeptide (GIP) in man. Scand J Gastroenterol 13 (Suppl 49):11, 1978.
75. Maxwell V, Shulkes A, Brown JC, et al: Effect of gastric inhibitory polypeptide on pentagastrin-stimulated acid secretion in man. Dig Dis Sci 25:113, 1980.
76. Simmons TC, Maxwell VL, Taylor IL, et al: Effect of GIP on gastric acid secretion in vagotomized human subjects. Gastroenterology 78:1260, 1979.
77. Christiansen J, Bech A, Fahrenkrug J, et al: Fat induced jejunal inhibition of gastric acid secretion and release of pancreatic glucagon, enteroglucagon, gastric inhibitory polypeptide and vasoactive intestinal polypeptide in man. Scand J Gastroenterol 13 (Suppl 49):41, 1978.
78. Barbezat GO, Grossman MI: Intestinal secretion: Stimulation by peptides. Science 174:422, 1971.
79. Helman CA, Barbezat GO: The effect of gastric inhibitory polypeptide on human jejunal water and electrolyte transport. Gastroenterology 72:376, 1977.
80. Schwartz CJ, Kimberg DV, Sheerin HE, et al: Vasoactive intestinal peptide stimulation of adenylate cyclase and active electrolyte secretion in intestinal mucosa. J Clin Invest 54:536, 1974.
81. Waldman DB, Gardner JD, Zfass AM, et al: Effects of vasoactive intestinal peptide, secretin, and related peptides on rat colonic transport and adenylate cyclase activity. Gastroenterology 73:518, 1977.
82. Sinar DR, O'Dorisio TM, Mazzaferri EL, et al: Effect of gastric inhibitory polypeptide on lower esophageal sphincter pressure in cats. Gastroenterology 75:263, 1978.
83. Denniss AR, Young JA: Modification of salivary duct electrolyte transport in rat and rabbit by physalaemin, VIP, GIP and other enterohormones. Pflugers Arch 376:73, 1978.
84. La Barre J: Sur les possibilités d'un traitement du diabete par l' incretine. Bull Acad Roy Med Belgique 12:620, 1932.
85. Unger RH, Eisentraut AM: Enteroinsulinar axis. Arch Intern Med 123:261, 1969.
86. McIntyre N, Holdsworth CD, Turner DS: New interpretation of oral glucose tolerance. Lancet 2:20, 1964.
87. Dupre J, Curtis JD, Unger RH, et al: Effects of secretin, pancreozymin, or gastrin on the response of the endocrine pancreas to administration of glucose or arginine in man. J Clin Invest 48:745, 1969.
88. Rabinovitch A, Dupre J: Insulinotropic and glucagonotropic activities in crude preparations of cholecystokinin-pancreozymin. Clin Res 20:945, 1972.
89. Dupre J, Ross SA, Watson D, et al: Stimulation of insulin secretion by gastric inhibitory polypeptide in man. J Clin Endocrinol Metab 37:826, 1973.
90. Pederson RA, Schubert HE, Brown JC: The insulinotropic action of gastric inhibitory polypeptide. Can J Physiol Pharmacol 53:217, 1975.
91. Pederson RA, Brown JC: The insulinotropic action of gastric inhibitory polypeptide in the perfused isolated rat pancreas. Endocrinology 99:780, 1976.
92. Schauder P, Brown JC, Frerichs H, et al: Gastric inhibitory polypeptide: Effect on glucose-induced insulin release from isolated rat pancreatic islets *in vitro.* Diabetologia 11:483, 1975.
93. Schauder P, Schindler B, Panten U, et al: Insulin release from isolated rat pancreatic islets induced by α-ketoisocaproic acid, L-leucine, D-glucose or D-glyceraldehyde: Effect of gastric inhibitory polypeptide or glucagon. Mol Cell Endocrinol 7:115, 1977.
94. Lauritsen KB, Holst JJ, Moody AJ: Depression of insulin release by anti-GIP serum after oral glucose in rats. Scand J Gastroenterol 16:417, 1981.
95. Ebert R, Unger H, Creutzfeldt W: Preservation of incretin activity after removal of GIP from rat gut extracts by immunoabsorption. Diabetologia 21:266, 1981.
96. Ebert R, Creutzfeldt W: Influence of gastric inhibitory polypeptide antiserum on glucose-induced insulin secretion in rats. Endocrinology 111:1601, 1982.
97. Levin SR, Pehlevanian MZ, Lavee AE, et al: Secre-

tion of an insulinotropic factor from isolated, perfused rat intestine. Am J Physiol 236:E710, 1979.

98. Ahren B, Hedner P, Lundquist I: Interaction of gastric inhibitory polypeptide (GIP) and cholecystokinin (CCK-8) with basal and stimulated insulin secretion in mice. Acta Endocrinol 102:96, 1983.

99. Alwmark A, Khalil T, Mate L, et al: Gut hormones as incretin candidates. Surg Forum 35:209, 1984.

100. Fujimoto WY, Ensinck JW, Merchant FW, et al: Stimulation by gastric inhibitory polypeptide of insulin and glucagon secretion by rat islet cultures. Proc Soc Exp Biol Med 157:89, 1978.

101. Andersen DK, Elahi D, Brown JC, et al: Oral glucose augmentation of insulin secretion. Interactions of gastric inhibitory polypeptide with ambient glucose and insulin levels. J Clin Invest 62:152, 1978.

102. Verdonk CA, Rizza RA, Nelson RL, et al: Interaction of fat-stimulated gastric inhibitory polypeptide on pancreatic alpha and beta cell function. J Clin Invest 65:1119, 1980.

103. King KC, Schwartz R, Yamaguchi K, et al: Lack of gastrointestinal enhancement of the insulin response to glucose in newborn infants. J Pediatr 91:783, 1977.

104. Jensen SL, Nielsen OV, Kuhl C: The enteral insulin-stimulation after pancreas transplantation in the pig. Diabetologia 12:617, 1976.

105. Blom PCS, Høstmark AT, Flaten O, et al: Modification by exercise of the plasma gastric inhibitory polypeptide response to glucose ingestion in young men. Acta Physiol Scand 123:367, 1985.

106. Osei K, Falko JM, O'Dorisio TM, et al: Gastric inhibitory polypeptide (GIP) responses after oral glucose ingestion in hyperthyroidism. Diabetes Care 8:436, 1985.

107. Pederson RA, Brown JC: Interaction of gastric inhibitory polypeptide, glucose, and arginine on insulin and glucagon secretion from the perfused rat pancreas. Endocrinology 103:610, 1978.

108. Ahren B, Lundquist I: Influences of gastro-intestinal polypeptides and glucose on glucagon secretion induced by cholinergic stimulation. Horm Metab Res 14:529, 1982.

109. Andersen DK, Elahi D, Brown JC, et al: Insulin and glucagon responses to infusion of gastric inhibitory polypeptide (GIP) in man during controlled glycemia. Scand J Gastroenterol 13 (Suppl 49):7, 1978.

110. Ipp E, Dobbs RE, Harris V, et al: The effects of gastrin, gastric inhibitory polypeptide, secretin, and the octapeptide of cholecystokinin upon immunoreactive somatostatin release by the perfused canine pancreas. J Clin Invest 60:1216, 1977.

111. Pederson RA, Dryburgh JR, Brown JC: The effect of somatostatin on release and insulinotropic action of gastric inhibitory polypeptide. Can J Physiol Pharmacol 53:1200, 1975.

112. Salera M, Pironi L, Giacomoni P, et al: Effect of somatostatin on fasting and glucose-stimulated gastric inhibitory polypeptide release in man. Digestion 24:126, 1982.

113. Dupre J, Greenidge N, McDonald TJ, et al: Inhibition of actions of glucagon in adipocytes by gastric inhibitory polypeptide. Metabolism 25:1197, 1976.

114. Eckel RH, Fujimoto WY, Brunzell JD: Gastric inhibitory polypeptide enhanced lipoprotein lipase activity in cultured preadipocytes. Diabetes 28:1141, 1979.

115. Wasada T, McCorkle K, Harris V, et al: Effect of gastric inhibitory polypeptide on plasma levels of chylomicron triglycerides in dogs. J Clin Invest 68:1106, 1981.

116. Perley MJ, Kipnis DM: Plasma insulin responses to oral and intravenous glucose: Studies in normal and diabetic subjects. J Clin Invest 46:1954, 1967.

117. Ebert R, Frerichs H, Creutzfeldt W: Serum gastric inhibitory polypeptide (GIP) response in patients with maturity onset diabetes and in juvenile diabetics. Diabetologia 12:388, 1976.

118. Crockett SE, Mazzaferri EL, Cataland S: Gastric inhibitory polypeptide (GIP) in maturity-onset diabetes mellitus. Diabetes 25:931, 1976.

119. Bloom SR: Gastric inhibitory peptide, vasoactive intestinal peptide and motilin: Physiological and pathophysiological alterations. J Endocrinol 70:9P, 1976.

120. May JM, Williams RH: The effect of endogenous gastric inhibitory polypeptide on glucose-induced insulin secretion in mild diabetes. Diabetes 27:849, 1978.

121. Ross SA, Brown JC, Dupre J: Hypersecretion of gastric inhibitory polypeptide following oral glucose in diabetes mellitus. Diabetes 26:525, 1977.

122. Lardinois CK, Mazzaferri EL, Starich GH, et al: Increased gastric inhibitory polypeptide is not reduced in patients with noninsulin-dependent diabetes mellitus treated with intense insulin therapy. J Clin Endocrinol Metab 61:1089, 1985.

123. Creutzfeldt W, Ebert R, Willms B, et al: Gastric inhibitory polypeptide (GIP) and insulin in obesity: Increased response to stimulation and defective feedback control of serum levels. Diabetologia 14:15, 1978.

124. Karam JH, Grodsky GM, Forsham PH, et al: Excessive insulin response to glucose in obese subjects as measured by immunochemical assay. Diabetes 12:197, 1963.

125. Loten EG, Rabinovitch A, Jeanrenaud B: In vivo studies on lipogenesis in obese hyperglycaemic (ob/ob) mice: Possible role of hyperinsulinaemia. Diabetologia 10:45, 1974.

126. Beck B, Max J-P: Gastric inhibitory polypeptide enhancement of the insulin effect on fatty acid incorporation into adipose tissue in the rat. Regul Pept 7:3, 1983.

127. Botha JL, Vinik AI, Brown JC: Gastric inhibitory polypeptide (GIP) in chronic pancreatitis. J Clin Endocrinol Metab 42:791, 1976.

128. Ebert R, Creutzfeldt W, Brown JC, et al: Response of gastric inhibitory polypeptide (GIP) to test meal in chronic pancreatitis—Relationship to endocrine and exocrine insufficiency. Diabetologia 12:609, 1976.

129. Ebert R, Creutzfeldt W: Reversal of impaired GIP

and insulin secretion in patients with pancreatogenic steatorrhea following enzyme substitution. Diabetologia 19:198, 1980.

130. Creutzfeldt W, Ebert R, Arnold R, et al: Gastric inhibitory polypeptide (GIP), gastrin and insulin: Response to test meal in coeliac disease and after duodeno-pancreatectomy. Diabetologia 12:279, 1976.

131. Adrian TE, McKiernan J, Johnstone DI, et al: Hormonal abnormalities of the pancreas and gut in cystic fibrosis. Gastroenterology 79:460, 1980.

132. Rogers WA, O'Dorisio TM, Johnson SE, et al: Postprandial release of gastric inhibitory polypeptide (GIP) and pancreatic polypeptide in dogs with pancreatic acinar atrophy. Correction of blunted GIP response by addition of pancreatic enzymes to a meal. Dig Dis Sci 28:345, 1983.

133. Arnold R, Ebert R, Becker HD, et al: Serum gastric inhibitory polypeptide (GIP) response in patients with duodenal ulcer (DU) dependence on glucose tolerance, in Bonfils S, Fromageot P, Rosselin G (eds): *Hormonal Receptors in Digestive Tract Physiology*. New York, North-Holland Publishing Co., 1977, pp 509–510.

134. Griffith GH, Owen GM, Campbell H, et al: Gastric emptying in health and in gastroduodenal disease. Gastroenterology 54:1, 1968.

135. Pederson RA, Buchan AMJ, Zahedi-Asl S, et al: Effect of jejunoileal bypass in the rat on the enteroinsular axis. Regul Pept 5:53, 1982.

136. Buchan AMJ, Pederson RA, Chan CB, et al: The effect of massive small bowel resection (MSBR) and small intestinal bypass (JIB) in the rat on the enteroinsular axis. Regul Pept 7:221, 1983.

137. Cassar J, Ghatei MA, Sarson DL, et al: Enteroglucagon and GIP after oral glucose in patients with prolactinoma and acromegaly. Clin Endocrinol 18:95, 1983.

Chapter 19

Vasoactive Intestinal Peptide

Talaat Khalil, M.D., Gunnar Alinder, M.D., and Phillip L. Rayford, Ph.D.

HISTORY

In 1969, Said and Mutt reported the extraction of a peptide (from normal hog lung) that was capable of causing gradual but prolonged peripheral vasodilatation [1]. In 1970, they described the isolation (from hog intestine) of a potent peripheral and splanchnic vasodilatory peptide, which they named vasoactive intestinal peptide (VIP) [2]. Subsequent purification of VIP allowed determination of its amino acid sequence; it was shown to be a straight-chain polypeptide of 28 amino acid residues, with basic properties due to the predominance of arginine and lysine residues [3]. The peptide tends to adopt a helical structure, as demonstrated by spectroscopic techniques [4]. There is a considerable degree of homology between the amino acids of VIP, secretin, pancreatic glucagon, and gastric inhibitory polypeptide [3].

DISTRIBUTION

In 1974, Polak et al [5], using an immunohistochemical technique, reported the presence of VIP-like immunoreactivity (VIP-IR) in three types of endocrine cells in mammalian and avian gut. VIP immunoreactive neurons and nerve fibers have been found in the gastrointestinal tract [6,7] and in the hypothalamus [7]. We now know that VIP immunoreactive neurons are found all over the central nervous system and are widely distributed in many organ systems, including the gastrointestinal, genitourinary, respiratory, and cardiovascular systems (Table 19-1).

Gastrointestinal Tract

In the gastrointestinal tract, VIP is found throughout the entire length of the gut [6], in the pancreas [8], and in the salivary glands [9]. Largest amounts are found in the colon and ileum, but significant amounts are present in the fundus, duodenum, and jejunum of monkeys [10]. In the rat, VIP is found in especially high concentrations in the jejunoileum (11698 $\pm$ 687 ng/g), duodenum (676 $\pm$ 186 ng/g), and colon (1214 $\pm$ 214 ng/g) [11]. Ontogeny studies in newborn rats have shown that VIP levels can be detected in 3-day-old rats, but at significantly lower levels than in adult rats [12]. There is a continuous increase in VIP concentrations until the age of 28 days, when the rats reach adult levels. The stomach, cecum, and colon attain peak concentrations in rats 14 to 21 days old.

VIP-containing autonomic nerve fibers are seen in all layers of the gut, including muscle, mucosa and submucosa, and around blood vessels [13]. Fibers are most prominent in the lamina propria in close contact with epithelial cells and in the circular muscle layer. They are absent from longitudinal muscle layers, except in the taenia coli [13]. These fibers appear to originate mainly from the intramural ganglion cells, mostly of the submucous plexus, since extrinsic denervation causes little or no change in VIP content or immunostaining [13,14]. Electron microscopic study of the VIP-positive fibers shows that they are characterized by a predominance of small spherical agranular vesicles with a diameter of 40–55 nm and a small percentage of large granular vesicles (100–144 nm) containing labeled dense cores [15]. Abnormal VIP immunoreactivity is seen in diseases that affect the autonomic ganglion cells such as Hirschsprung's disease (a condition characterized by absence of ganglion cells) [16] and Chagas' disease (a condition characterized by degeneration of the ganglion cells) [17]. Conversely, in Crohn's disease, in which neuronal hyperplasia prevails, VIP nerves show a marked increase in immunoreactivity and are highly distorted [18]. These changes are not seen in generalized autonomic nervous system diseases in which there is no gut involvement, such as the Shy-Drager syndrome [17].

VIP-IR autonomic nerve fibers were found in significant amounts in the pancreas (in both the exocrine and endocrine tissue), where they originated from local neuronal cell bodies [8], as well as in the salivary glands and in the acini, ducts, and blood vessels, where they originated from cell bodies that are present in the glandular hilus [9].

Although there is general agreement that VIP can be localized to nerve fibers by immunocytochemistry, there is disagreement about its presence in gut endocrine cells. Polak et al [5] demonstrated (by immunocytochemistry) endocrine cells that cross-reacted with VIP antisera in all parts of the gut of mammals and birds. Buffa et al [19] found VIP-containing cells in both the pancreas and gut of dogs, guinea pigs, and humans. In contrast, Larsson et al [20] reported only occasional endocrine cells with VIP-like immunoreactivity in cat antral mucosa and none in any region of the gut in humans and pigs.

The identity of the VIP immunoreactivity detected in the endocrine cells has been questioned on the grounds that certain potent VIP antibodies detected the peptide only in nerve cells and not in endocrine cells [20]. There is a good deal of indirect evidence to support the contention that authentic octacosapeptide VIP occurred only in nerves and not in endocrine cells of the gastrointestinal tract [21]. Moreover, studies on isolated intestinal epithelial cells showed that they do not have VIP activity, as determined by radioimmunoassay, bioassay, or receptor assay [22]. On the other hand, high levels of VIP were found to be associated with pancreatic tumors accompanying the watery diarrhea, hypokalemia-achlorhydria (WDHA) syndrome [23], which indicated that VIP was not entirely foreign to endocrine cells. Dockray's group has suggested that octacosapeptide VIP may occur in nerve tissue, whereas endocrine cells, as well as nerve tissue, could harbor other VIP-immunoreactive components [21,24].

In the human fetus, VIP was measurable by radioimmunoassay from 10 weeks of gestation. The peptide was distributed in the duodenum, jejunoileum, colon, pancreas, fundus, and antrum [25]. The greatest concentrations were found in the duodenum and jejunoileum. In all tissue extracts, concentrations of VIP were greater in fetuses from 15 to 21 weeks of gestation when compared to those from 9 to 14 weeks of gestation.

A complementary DNA (cDNA) to messenger RNA for the preprohormone of human VIP isolated from pancreatic tumor [26] or neuroblastoma [27] has been characterized. Whether VIP mRNA isolated from normal cells has the same sequence found in these two tumor cells is as yet unknown. The cDNA encodes a protein containing the sequences of both VIP and a PHI-like peptide, PHM-27, a peptide that has an NH_2-terminal histidine and COOH-terminal methionine [28]. The coding sequences for VIP and PHM-27 are located on two adjacent exons in the human genome. Each of these two exons encodes the amino acid residues of both hormones as well as the post-translational processing signal sequences [29]. The cDNA sequence to the mRNA coding for rat VIP precursor from rat cerebral cortex reveals that the precursor contains both rat VIP and PHI-27 [30].

ASSAY

The development of a sensitive and specific radioimmunoassay for VIP has made it possible to measure concentrations of this peptide in plasma and other biologic fluids and in tissue extracts from humans and experimental animals [31,32]. The assays have been necessary for studies on the possible roles of VIP in normal physiology and in disease.

PHARMACOKINETICS AND CATABOLISM

Many tissues, mainly the rat liver [33,34], rat adipose tissue [33], guinea pig exocrine pancreas [35], human gallbladder epithelium [36], rat isolated intestinal epithelium [37], rat pituitary [38] and brain membranes from rat [39] and guinea pig [40], and rat and human lung [41], have been shown to possess VIP receptors. The receptors of VIP were characterized by studying the interaction of radiolabeled VIP with membranes or cells. In some tissues (e.g., intestinal epithelium [37], liver [42], pancreatic acinar cells [35], and lung [40]), two classes of VIP binding sites could be demonstrated: a relatively small number of sites with a high affinity for VIP and a low affinity for secretin, and a relatively large number of sites with a low affinity for VIP and a high affinity for secretin.

The half-life of VIP is very short, averaging only 1–2 minutes in humans and dogs [43,44]. In vivo studies of the role of the liver in removal or inactivation of VIP have not been consistent. Strunz et al [45] reported no significant hepatic inactivation of VIP when its ability to inhibit pentagastrin-stimulated gastric acid secretion was measured during portal and systemic infusion of the peptide. However, VIP elevated levels were reported in patients with hepatic failure [46]. Further, the existence of large portal-systemic concentration gradients of the peptide in vivo [47] and the attenuation of its potency when given by portal vein infusion as compared with systemic infusion [48] are consistent with some inactivation during its passage through the liver. Moreover, the rapid in vivo turnover of VIP suggests that its degrading systems may be widely distributed in body tissues [43,44]. Increased plasma VIP levels have been reported in patients with chronic renal failure (with no associated liver disease), which would indicate a role for the kidney in the metabolism of VIP [50]. Keltz et al [51] demonstrated that the rabbit brain, kidney, and liver contain a protease with a high degree of specificity for VIP. The concentration of VIP-protease in other tissues of the body has not yet been studied.

RELEASE

There is no evidence, to date, of VIP hormonal release during digestion. Several investigators have shown an increase in portal and peripheral levels of VIP after various intraluminal stimuli, including jejunal perfusion with hypertonic saline [52] and intraduodenal perfusion of HCl, ethanol, and fat in humans and in anesthetized pigs (Table 19-2) [53]. Intraduodenal perfusion of amino acids, glucose, hypertonic saline in humans and pigs [53] or of bile in dogs [54] does not increase portal or peripheral VIP levels. A peptone meal in humans [53] or dogs [54,55] did not increase VIP in peripheral plasma, although in dogs there was a significant release of VIP into portal plasma [54,55]. Intragastric instillation of glucose or casein hydrolysate had no effect on VIP release, while instillation of Intralipid increased both portal and peripheral VIP levels. Burhol et al [56] showed a delayed increase in peripheral VIP levels (150–180 min) after ingestion of a test meal in humans.

There is strong evidence for neural release of VIP. High threshold electric stimulation of the vagus and pelvic nerves releases VIP from various regions in the gut [57,58]. This release is blocked by hexamethonium (a nicotinic ganglionic antagonist) but not by atropine [57,58]. VIP release can also be induced by injection of acetylcholine or neostigmine (a cholinesterase inhibitor), which can be blocked by atropine [57,59]. These findings indicate that intramural VIP-containing neurons

Table 19-1. Localization of VIP

Gastrointestinal tract	Central nervous system
Antrum [25]	Amygdala [151–153]
Cecum [12]	Cerebral cortex [151]
Colon [10, 25]	Dentate gyrus [151–153]
Duodenum [10,25]	Hippocampus [151–153]
Fundus [25]	Hypothalamus [151,154]
Ileum [10,25]	Lateral geniculate body [154]
Jejunum [10,25]	Nucleus caudatus [151]
Pancreas [8,19]	Olfactory nucleus [151]
Salivary glands [9]	Spinal cord [151]
Stomach [12]	Stria terminalis [154]
Urogenital tract	Stratum oriens [151–153]
Bladder [156]	Superior colliculus [151]
Cervix [157]	Suprachiasmatic nucleus [151,154,155]
External genitalia (male) [158]	Tractus optici [154]
Prostate [158]	**Other**
Seminal vesicles [158]	Atria [159]
Ureter [156]	Carotid body [160]
Vasa deferentia [158]	Ciliary muscle [161]
	Coronary vasculature [159]
	Retina [161]
	Seromucous gland [162,163]
	Sinoatrial node [159]
	Tracheobronchial wall [164]

are innervated by preganglionic cholinergic excitatory fibers. Electrical stimulation of splanchnic nerves inhibits neural release of VIP via an α-adrenergic mechanism [57]. It is not known whether this effect is produced by presynaptic inhibition of acetylcholine release from preganglionic nerve terminals. The coexistence of fibers containing other amines or peptides and intrinsic VIP-containing neurons is certainly possible but has not yet been demonstrated, as far as we know [17].

VIP is released by intravenous calcium, which results in an increased VIP level within 3 minutes, with a peak at 5 minutes, and a return to normal at 5 minutes [60]. VIP is also released into the portal circulation in dogs in large quantities by experimental intestinal ischemia [49]. VIP is also released by IV injection of apomorphine or bromocriptine in dogs. The effect of apomorphine was blocked by prior injection of haloperidol, which indicates that dopaminergic receptors are involved in the response [61].

VIP was recently shown to be released during prolonged stress in men subjected to prolonged physical exercise, starvation, and sleep deprivation. The plasma concentration returns rapidly to control levels after oral ingestion of a meal or glucose solution [62].

Immunoreactive VIP has been released experimentally from the central nervous system (Table 19-2). Go and Yaksh [63] demonstrated the release of VIP in the resting perfusate from cat and rat spinal cord in vivo. In rats, VIP-IR release could be increased by elevating the potassium concentration in the spinal perfusate. Dorsal rhizotomy resulted in a 70–80 percent depletion of dorsal horn VIP-IR [63]. VIP-IR was released from slices of rat hypothalamus in vitro in response to stimulation with an elevated concentration of potassium [64]. Giachetti et al [65] showed a calcium-dependent release of VIP-IR from nerve endings evoked by high potassium concentrations. The concentration of VIP-IR in hypophyseal portal blood in rats was shown to be almost 20 times that in femoral arteries [65a].

ACTIONS

Vasodilatation

VIP induces vasodilatation in most vascular beds, including the peripheral systemic vessels as well as the splanchnic, coronary, cerebral, extracranial, salivary gland, and pulmonary vessels (vide infra) (Table 19-3).

Effects on Cerebral Circulation. In vitro, VIP has no effect on the tone of resting arteries of the cat, but it produces a dose-related dilatation of vessels that are in a state of active tonic contraction [7].

Table 19-2. Release of VIP

Acetylcholine [57–59]
Exercise [62]
Intrajejunal hypertonic saline [52]
Intraduodenal HCl [53]
Intraduodenal ethanol [53]
Intraduodenal fat [53]
Intravenous apomorphine [61]
Intravenous bromocriptine [61]
Intragastric Intralipid [54]
Neostigmine [57–59]
Potassium [64]
Sleep deprivation [62]
Starvation [62]
Vagal stimulation [57,58]

Table 19-3. Actions of VIP (vasodilatory)

Increases:
Cerebral blood flow [165]
Chloride secretion [81,87,88]
Cyclic AMP [70,166]
Free fatty acid and glucose [92,115,117]
Gallbladder secretion [92,95,100]
Growth hormone release [121,126]
Heart rate [66]
Pancreatic enzyme [72,167]
Pancreatic secretion of water and bicarbonate [90–94,97,98]
Prolactin release [121–123]
Inhibits:
Gastric acid secretion [67–69]
Gastrin release [67,80]
Lower esophageal sphincter tone [103–106]
Pepsin secretion [67–69]
Somatostatin release [125]

Effects on Coronary Circulation and the Cardiovascular System. IV infusion of VIP in dogs causes increased heart rate (see Table 19-3), presumably owing chiefly to reflex changes from vasodilatation. VIP has no intrinsic chronotropic activity on the rate of contraction of cat atrial strips. Blood pressure falls in response to generalized vasodilatation. VIP has a positive inotropic effect that is similar in magnitude to that of glucagon [66].

Effects on the Gastrointestinal Tract

VIP inhibits both acid and pepsin secretion stimulated by food, histamine, and pentagastrin in dogs (see Table 19-3). This inhibition, unlike that caused by secretin, is effective even against histamine-stimulated secretion and is of the competitive type [67–69]. Since VIP inhibits acid secretion in vivo without inhibiting histamine-stimulated cyclic AMP production in isolated fundic glands, it is possible that the inhibitory effect is mediated by release of somatostatin in proximity to the parietal cell; the effect is lost in vitro when parietal and somatostatin cells are uncoupled during isolation of the glands [69]. On the other hand, VIP and secretin stimulate the production of cyclic AMP in isolated glands of the antrum and fundus [70].

In most of the tissues exhibiting specific VIP receptors, VIP was shown to stimulate adenylate cyclase or to increase the cellular cyclic AMP level. In intestinal epithelial cells in rats, the cAMP production was monophasic, of large amplitude, and occurred at VIP concentrations in the range of

10^{-10} to 10^{-7} M [36,71]. In pancreatic acinar cells from guinea pigs, the stimulation occurred in two steps, with a first plateau of low amplitude for low VIP concentrations (10^{-10} to 10^{-7} M) and a second of larger amplitude for higher VIP concentrations [72]. In a human prolactin-secreting pituitary tumor, VIP stimulated adenylate cyclase production with concentrations ranging from 10^{-10} to 10^{-8} M, but higher VIP concentrations had an inhibitory effect [38].

Other gut epithelia (e.g., human colon [73], gallbladder [36], and stomach [74] as well as hamster [75] or guinea pig [76] intestine) possess a production system for cyclic AMP that is comparably VIP-sensitive. However, cyclic AMP levels were not altered by VIP in liver cells [77] and were only slightly elevated with high concentrations of VIP in the brain [78].

VIP and secretin potentiate secretion of pepsinogen from rat fundic mucosa in vitro [79]. These effects are enhanced by either carbachol or CCK-8 and could be reproduced for VIP and secretin by cAMP and for carbachol and CCK-8 by the calcium ionophore A23187, which suggests that pepsinogen secretion is stimulated by two mechanisms, mediated either by cAMP or cellular calcium changes.

VIP inhibits release of gastrin in vivo and in vitro [67,80]. Inhibition in vitro, using an isolated vascularly perfused rat stomach, is accompanied and probably mediated by a reciprocal increase in somatostatin secretion [80], which is thought to regulate gastrin secretion in humans and rats. The concentration of VIP required to inhibit gastric secretion is much too high for a hormonal effect, but this action could be attained if VIP were released from nerve terminals in proximity to somatostatin cells [80].

VIP was demonstrated to be a potent stimulant of intestinal secretion in humans and many mammals. Its secretory efficacy was greater than that of glucagon and secretin [81,82]. VIP potency was 1,000 times that of secretin and was greatly enhanced by subthreshold concentrations of theophylline [82]. Studies in dogs [83,84] and in humans [85] revealed that VIP reversed the normal absorptive process of the small bowel to a net secretion of chloride and bicarbonate (in dogs only) against an electrochemical gradient [81,86]. In vitro studies using rat [87], rabbit [88], or human [88] ileal or colonic mucosa demonstrated a net chloride secretion across the mucosa when VIP was applied to the serosal surface, which may result from inhibition of net sodium absorption and stimulation of chloride secretion. Angiotensin and norepinephrine antagonize the secretory effect of VIP in rat ileum and colon segments in vitro [89].

Effects of VIP on the Pancreas

VIP stimulates pancreatic bicarbonate secretion in many mammals (humans [90], rats [91], dogs [92], cats [93], and pigs [94]) and in birds [91], but is only 1 to 5 percent as effective as secretin [95]. The maximal HCO_3^- response to VIP in dogs is about 17 percent of that of secretin [96].

The influence of neural VIP on pancreatic secretion can probably best be studied in the pig pancreas [80]. Electrical stimulation of the afferent vagus fiber to the pig pancreas elicited a profuse secretion of water and bicarbonate, which was blocked by hexamethonium but not by atropine [97,98]. Blood levels of VIP in the pancreatic venous effluent increased in parallel with pancreatic secretion during vagal stimulation [97]. Furthermore, exogenous infusion of VIP into the vasculature of isolated pig pancreas elicited a profuse secretion equal to that elicited by secretin [94]. The interaction of secretin and VIP showed that VIP is a potent inhibitor of secretin-induced pancreatic secretion in the dog, and the analysis of the dose-response curves to secretin alone and secretin plus VIP showed typical competitive inhibition, which indicates that VIP and secretin share a common receptor site [96].

Effects on Gallbladder and Bile Secretion

VIP increases gallbladder secretion in dogs [92], cats [99], and guinea pigs [100] and in high concentrations that possibly could be achieved by release of VIP from nerve fibers [100]. Secretion appears to consist mainly of bicarbonate [100]. VIP stimulates bile secretion in dogs [101] and in rats [102].

Effects on Gut Smooth Muscle

VIP inhibits the resting tone of the lower esophageal sphincter and antagonizes the contractile effect of pentagastrin in several species (humans [103], monkeys [104], cats [105], and opossums [106]). It is a more potent relaxant than secretin or glucagon, and the minimal dose required to produce this effect causes an unphysiologic increase in plasma levels [103–106]. Esophageal or fundic distention or high-threshold electrical stimulation of the vagus nerve in atropinized cats produced gastric relaxation and a concomitant release of VIP into the gastric venous effluent [58,107].

VIP has a dual effect on intestinal smooth muscle. It relaxes circular muscles of the duodenum and ileum in rats [71] and the colon in guinea pigs [108]. However, at high concentrations, it contracts the longitudinal muscles of the duodenum and ileum in rats [71] and colon in guinea pigs [108], an effect that is blocked by atropine or tetradotoxin and appears to be mediated by an intramural cholinergic neuron [71]. VIP administered both intraluminally and intravenously to an isolated ileal segment in the rabbit produced alterations of migrating action potential complex and repetitive bursts of action potentials [109].

VIP also inhibits the resting tone and CCK-induced contraction of the gallbladder in guinea pigs [110] and opossums [111]. Later studies [112] have shown that VIP has a biphasic effect on the isolated guinea pig gallbladder strip. At low concentrations (10^{-12} to 10^{-10} M) VIP contracted the strip, and at high concentrations (10^{-7} to 10^{-6} M) VIP relaxed the strip. VIP had no effect on the human gallbladder. The physiologic role of VIP as a smooth muscle relaxant should be viewed in the light of a rich VIPergic innervation of the sphincters of the gut. Recent studies suggest that VIP may be an inhibitory neurotransmitter for the internal anal sphincter of the rabbit [113].

Renal Effects of VIP

Recent studies suggest an action of VIP on renal tubular reabsorption. VIP caused a significant increase in urine volume, in fractional excretion of sodium chloride and potassium, and in osmolar clearance in isolated perfused rat kidneys as compared to controls. These effects were not associated with any significant changes in perfusion flow, renal vascular resistance, or insulin clearance [114].

Metabolic Effects of VIP

VIP has a lipolytic effect on adipose cells [115] that leads to liberation of free fatty acids [116]. VIP also stimulates the release of glucose from the liver, probably through glycogenolytic and glucogenic activities. There is no evidence as yet to suggest that VIP has any direct effect on the metabolism of either proteins or amino acids [117–119]. In dogs, continuous IV infusion of VIP elevates plasma glucose [92,117], and in healthy human volunteers it causes a significant increase in plasma glucose and calcium levels and in free fatty acids [116].

VIP has recently been reported to stimulate bone resorption in organ culture [120].

Neuroendocrine Functions

The presence of VIP in the hypothalamic nerve endings of the adenohypophysis and the hypophyseal portal blood [65a] suggests its involvement in the regulation of pituitary secretion.

VIP, administered either intraventricularly or intravenously, caused a significant and dose-related release of prolactin in both anesthetized [121] and conscious ovariectomized rats [122], in a cell line from rat pituitary [122], and in incubated rat hemispheres [123] in vitro. VIP appears to act specifically at the pituitary level on prolactin, and the action is different from and additive to that of thyroliberin (TRH) [38,123]. Both dopamine (10^{-9} to 10^{-6} M) and gamma-aminobutyric acid (GABA) suppressed not only the basal prolactin release from dispersed pituitary cells but also the prolactin response to VIP and thyrotropin-releasing hormone [124]. Moreover, VIP reduces the dopamine inhibition of prolactin release without interacting with dopamine receptors [123]. VIP may well be a new prolactin-releasing factor.

VIP can also increase growth hormone release by inhibiting the action of somatostatin at the hypothalamic and pituitary levels [121]. VIP also, at low concentrations, partially inhibits somatostatin release from mediobasal hypothalamic slices [125]. The presence of an additional site of action at the pituitary level is suggested by the observation that in vitro VIP blocks the inhibition of growth hormone release induced by somatostatin [126].

VIP appears to affect luteinizing hormone (LH) secretion through a central mechanism, since only intraventricular injection of VIP into ovariectomized rats induced a significant increase in plasma LH levels [121]. VIP stimulated the synthesis of cyclic AMP as well as the release of immunoreactive adrenocorticotropic hormone (ACTH) from clonal pituitary tumor cells. This effect was additive with both corticotropin-releasing factor (CRF) and isoproterenol [127]. Moreover, VIP had no effect on LH release from rat hemipituitaries [121,123,128] or purified rat gonadotropic cells [129]. VIP did not affect the release of follicle-stimulating hormone [121,123,129] or thyroid-stimulating hormone [121] in vitro or in vivo.

Effects of VIP on Other Endocrine Organs

VIP increased the release of insulin, glucagon, and somatostatin when infused intrapancreatically in dogs [130,131]. When given as a constant infusion in rats, VIP exerted a direct hypoglycemic effect and modulated the influence of glucose and arginine on insulin and glucagon secretion [132]. The same effect was demonstrated in the perfused pancreas of the rat [133], cat [134], and pig [94] in vitro. The effect of VIP upon the release of insulin and somatostatin is synergistic with glucose [135]; however, the very rapid degradation of VIP by the liver [48] makes it unlikely to act on the endocrine pancreas as an incretin. VIP appears to be a substance that regulates the endocrine pancreas through neuroendocrine pathways [136].

Pathophysiology

High VIP levels have been shown to be associated with the syndrome of watery diarrhea, hypokalemia and achlorhydria (WDHA) [23]. These functioning adenomas or carcinomas arise from various neoplastic lesions, for example, pancreatic endocrine, neuroblastic, pheochromocytoma, and carcinoid tumors [137]. VIP was localized by immunoperoxidase staining in differentiating and mature ganglion cells, ganglioneuroblastomas, and ganglioneurons [138]. Significant amounts of macromolecular VIP were also reported in the plasma of these patients [139].

Abnormalities in Hirschsprung's Disease, Chagas' Disease, and Achalasia

VIP, together with substance P-containing nerves and enteroglucagon and somatostatin-containing cells, was demonstrated to be significantly decreased in areas of bowel affected by Hirschsprung's disease [16]. The VIP content in the diseased specimens was reduced by almost 80 percent [16]. The distribution of VIP in the diseased colon, as studied by immunohistochemical methods, revealed complete absence of VIP neurons and nerve fibers in the aganglionic segment in contrast to the ganglionic and the oligoganglionic segments [140]. Study of rectal biopsies from patients with chronic gastrointestinal Chagas' disease revealed that tissue concentrations of VIP, substance P, enteroglucagon, and somatostatin were all less than half of those of the controls. Immunocytochemistry revealed a considerable reduction in the number of both cells and nerves [14].

In patients with achalasia, the smooth muscles of the lower esophagus contained conspicuously fewer VIP-IR nerve fibers than specimens from control patients. The reduced number of VIP fibers in the achalasic esophagus appears to contribute to incomplete relaxation of the lower esophageal sphincter [141].

The failure of relaxation of the aganglionic segment is thought to be due to the congenital lack of noradrenergic inhibitory neurons [142]. VIP may play a significant role in this relaxation reflex, and the lack of VIP innervation may, therefore, contribute to the nonpropulsive state observed. The possibility is further supported by the observation that impairment of the noradrenergic inhibitory pathway blocks peristaltic activity [143]. Further investigations of the diffuse neuroendocrine system may clarify some of the less well-understood aspects of this condition.

VIP might play a role in the pathophysiology of several other smooth muscle disorders. A significant increase in the intestinal content of VIP, associated with a decrease in intestinal content of substance P, was reported in rats with streptozocin-induced diabetes. This change may contribute to the impaired intestinal motility observed in these rats [144]. The number of VIP-immunoreactive nerves and the concentration of VIP are diminished in the hyperreflexic neuropathic bladder in humans as compared to in the bladder of healthy controls [145]. Neostigmine stimulated a significantly higher plasma level of VIP in patients with irritable bowel syndrome as compared to the level in healthy subjects [146].

Abnormalities in Chronic Inflammatory Bowel Disease

Immunocytochemistry studies of specimens from patients with Crohn's disease revealed thicker and more brightly immunostained fibers in each layer of gut wall. Intensely immunostained fibers filled both the myenteric and submucous plexuses, and there was a clear increase in the number of immunostained ganglion cells in the submucous plexus. Radioimmunoassay of tissue extracts revealed a near doubling of the VIP content in specimens from patients with Crohn's disease in comparison with specimens from controls [18].

O'Morain et al [147] reported a detectable increase in VIP nerves in endoscopic rectal biopsies from patients with Crohn's disease, regardless of whether there was clinical involvement of the rectum. This suggests that evidence for the presence of Crohn's disease can be obtained from biopsies that show no pathologic changes on conventional histologic examination. In contrast to what occurs in Crohn's disease, specimens from patients with ulcerative colitis showed no change from normal in either VIP distribution or tissue content [18,147].

High plasma levels of VIP were found in patients with intestinal ischemia [49], hemorrhagic shock [148], and, recently, with the short bowel syndrome [149]. Deficient VIP innervation of the acini and ducts of sweat glands was reported in patients with cystic fibrosis [150].

REFERENCES

1. Said SI, Mutt V: Long acting vasodilator peptide from lung tissue. Nature 224:699, 1969.
2. Said SI, Mutt V: Polypeptide with broad biological activity: Isolation from small intestine. Science 169:1217, 1970.
3. Said SI, Mutt V: Isolation from porcine-intestinal wall of a vasoactive octacosapeptide related to secretin and to glucagon. Eur J Biochem 28:199, 1972.
4. Fournier A, Saunders JK, St-Pierre S: Solid-phase synthesis conformational studies and biological activities of VIP and related fragments. Regul Pept 6:302, 1983.
5. Polak JM, Pearse AGE, Garaud J-C, et al: Cellular localization of a vasoactive intestinal peptide in the mammalian and avian gastrointestinal tract. Gut 15:720, 1974.
6. Bryant MG, Polak JM, Modlin I, et al: Possible dual role for vasoactive intestinal peptide as gastrointestinal hormone and neurotransmitter substance. Lancet 1:991, 1976.
7. Larsson L-I, Edvinsson L, Fahrenkrug J, et al: Immunohistochemical localization of a vasodilatory polypeptide (VIP) in cerebrovascular nerves. Brain Res 113:400, 1976.
8. Bishop AE, Polak JM, Green IC, et al: The location of VIP in the pancreas of man and rat. Diabetologia 18:73, 1980.
9. Wharton J, Polak JM, Bryant MG, et al: Vasoactive intestinal polypeptide (VIP)-like immunoreactivity in salivary glands. Life Sci 25:273, 1979.
10. Bloom SR, Bryant MG, Polak JM: Distribution of gut hormones. Gut 16:821, 1975.
11. Besson J, Laburthe M, Bataille D, et al: Vasoactive intestinal peptide (VIP): Tissue distribution in the rat as measured by radioimmunoassay and by radioreceptorassay. Acta Endocrinol 87:799, 1978.
12. Ichihara K, Eng J, Yalow RS: Ontogeny of immunoreactive CCK, VIP and secretin in rat brain and gut. Biochem Biophys Res Commun 112:891, 1983.
13. Jessen KR, Saffrey MJ, Van Noorden S, et al: Immunohistochemical studies of the enteric nervous system in tissue culture and *in situ:* Localization of vasoactive intestinal polypeptide (VIP), substance-P and enkephalin immunoreactive nerves in the guinea-pig gut. Neuroscience 5:1717, 1980.
14. Jessen KR, Polak JM, Van Noorden S, et al: Peptide-containing neurones connect the two ganglionated plexuses of the enteric nervous system. Nature 283:391, 1980.
15. Loesch A, Burnstock G: Ultrastructural identification of VIP-containing nerve fibres in the myenteric plexus of the rat ileum. J Neurocytol 14:327, 1985.
16. Bishop AE, Polak JM, Lake BD, et al: Abnormalities of the colonic regulatory peptides in Hirschsprung's disease. Histopathology 5:679, 1981.
17. Long RG, Bishop AE, Barnes AJ, et al: Neural and hormonal peptides in rectal biopsy specimens from patients with Chagas' disease and chronic autonomic failure. Lancet 1:559, 1980.
18. Bishop AE, Polak JM, Bryant MG, et al: Abnormalities of vasoactive intestinal polypeptide-containing nerves in Crohn's disease. Gastroenterology 79:853, 1980.
19. Buffa R, Capella C, Solcia E, et al: Vasoactive intestinal peptide (VIP) cells in the pancreas and gastrointestinal mucosa. Histochemistry 50:217, 1977.
20. Larsson L-I, Fahrenkrug J, Schaffalitzky de Muckadell O, et al: Localization of vasoactive intestinal polypeptide (VIP) to central and peripheral neurons. Proc Natl Acad Sci USA 73:3197, 1976.
21. Dimaline R, Dockray GJ: Multiple immunoreactive forms of vasoactive intestinal peptide in human colonic mucosa. Gastroenterology 75:387, 1978.
22. Gaginella TS, Mekhjian HS, O'Dorisio TM: Vasoactive intestinal peptide: Quantification by radioimmunoassay in isolated cells, mucosa, and muscle of the hamster intestine. Gastroenterology 74:718, 1978.
23. Bloom SR: Vasoactive intestinal peptide, the major mediator of the WDHA (pancreatic cholera) syndrome: Value of measurement in diagnosis and treatment. Am J Dig Dis 23:373, 1978.
24. Dimaline R, Vaillant C, Dockray GJ: The use of region-specific antibodies in the characterization and localization of vasoactive intestinal polypeptide-like substances in the rat gastrointestinal tract. Regul Pept 1:1, 1980.
25. Chayvialle J-A, Paulin C, Descos F, et al: Ontogeny of vasoactive intestinal peptide in the human fetal digestive tract. Regul Pept 5:245, 1983.
26. Bloom SR, Delamarter J, Kawashima E, et al: Diarrhoea in lipoma patients associated with cosecretion of a second active peptide (peptide histidine isoleucine) explained by single coding gene. Lancet 2:1163, 1983.
27. Itoh N, Obata K-I, Yanaihara N, et al: Human preprovasoactive intestinal polypeptide contains a novel PHI-27-like peptide, PMH-27. Nature 304:547, 1983.
28. DeLamarter JF, Buell GN, Kawashima E, et al: Vasoactive intestinal peptide: Expression of the prohormone in bacterial cells. Peptides 6 (Suppl 1):95, 1985.

29. Bodner M, Fridkin M, Gozes I: Coding sequences for vasoactive intestinal peptide and PHM-27 peptide are located on two adjacent exons in the human genome. Proc Natl Acad Sci USA 82:3548, 1985.
30. Nishizawa M, Hayakawa Y, Yanaihara N, et al: Nucleotide sequence divergence and functional constraint in VIP precursor mRNA evolution between human and rat. FEBS Lett 183:55, 1985.
31. Burhol PG, Lygren I, Waldum HL: Radioimmunoassay of vasoactive intestinal polypeptide in plasma. Scand J Gastroenterol 13:807, 1978.
32. Pandian MR, Horvat A, Said SI: Radioimmunoassay of vasoactive intestinal polypeptide in plasma. Scand J Gastroenterol 13:807, 1978.
33. Desbuquois B, Laudat MH, Laudat Ph: Vasoactive intestinal polypeptide and glucagon: Stimulation of adenylate cyclase activity via distinct receptors in liver and fat cell membranes. Biochem Biophys Res Commun 53:1187, 1973.
34. Bataille D, Freychet P, Rosselin G: Interactions of glucagon, gut glucagon, vasoactive intestinal polypeptide and secretin with liver and fat cell plasma membranes: Binding to specific sites and stimulation of adenylate cyclase. Endocrinology 95:713, 1974.
35. Christophe JP, Conlon TP, Gardner JD: Interaction of porcine vasoactive intestinal peptide with dispersed pancreatic acinar cells from the guinea pig. Binding of radioiodinated peptide. J Biol Chem 251:4629, 1976.
36. Dupont C, Broyart J-P, Broer Y, et al: Importance of the vasoactive intestinal peptide receptor in the stimulation of cyclic adenosine 3′,5′-monophosphate in gallbladder epithelial cells of man. Comparison with the guinea pig. J Clin Invest 67:742, 1981.
37. Prieto JC, Laburthe M, Rosselin G: Interaction of vasoactive intestinal peptide with isolated intestinal epithelial cells from rat. 1. Characterization, quantitative aspects and structural requirements of binding sites. Eur J Biochem 96:229, 1979.
38. Gourdji D, Bataille D, Vauclin N, et al: Vasoactive intestinal peptide (VIP) stimulates prolactin (PRL) release and cAMP production in a rat pituitary cell line (GH3/B6). Additive effects of VIP and TRH on PRL release. FEBS Lett 104:165, 1979.
39. Taylor DP, Pert CB: VAsoactive intestinal polypeptide: Specific binding to rat brain membranes. Proc Natl Acad Sci USA 76:660, 1979.
40. Robberecht P, De Neef P, Lammens M, et al: Specific binding of vasoactive intestinal peptide to brain membranes from the guinea pig. Eur J Biochem 90:147, 1978.
41. Christophe J, Chatelain P, Taton G, et al: Comparison of VIP-secretin receptors in rat and human lung. Peptides 2 (Suppl 2):253, 1981.
42. Anuras S, Cooke AR: Effects of some gastrointestinal hormones on two muscle layers of duodenum. Am J Physiol 234:E60, 1978.
43. Domschke S, Domschke W, Bloom SR, et al: Vasoactive intestinal peptide in man: Pharmacokinetics, metabolic and circulatory effects. Gut 19:1049, 1978.
44. Chayvialle JA, Rayford PL, Thompson JC: Radioimmunoassay study of hepatic clearance and disappearance half-time of somatostatin and vasoactive intestinal peptide in dogs. Gut 22:732, 1981.
45. Strunz UT, Walsh JH, Bloom SR, et al: Lack of hepatic inactivation of canine vasoactive intestinal peptide. Gastroenterology 73:768, 1977.
46. Hunt S, Vaamonde CA, Rattassi T, et al: Circulating levels of vasoactive intestinal polypeptide in liver disease. Arch Intern Med 139:994, 1979.
47. Chayvialle JA, Miyata M, Rayford L, et al: Vasoactive intestinal peptide in portal, right heart, and aortic plasma in dogs. Scand J Gastroenterol 13:39, 1978.
48. Kitamura S, Yoshida T, Said SI: Vasoactive intestinal polypeptide: Inactivation in liver and potentiation in lung of anesthetized dogs. Proc Soc Exp Biol Med 148:25, 1975.
49. Modlin IM, Bloom SR, Mitchell S: Plasma vasoactive intestinal polypeptide (VIP) levels and intestinal ischaemia. Experientia 34:535, 1978.
50. Piga M, Altieri P, Floris A, et al: Vasoactive intestinal polypeptide (VIP) plasma levels in chronic renal failure. J Nucl Med Allied Sci 28:77, 1984.
51. Said SI, Straus E, Yalow RS: Degradation of vasoactive intestinal polypeptide by tissue homogenates. Biochem Biophys Res Comm 92:669, 1980.
52. Ebeid AM, Soeters PB, Murray P, et al: Release of vasoactive intestinal peptide (VIP) by intraluminal osmotic stimuli. J Surg Res 23:25, 1977.
53. Schaffalitzky de Muckadell OB, Fahrenkrug J, Holst JJ, et al: Release of vasoactive intestinal polypeptide (VIP) by intraduodenal stimuli. Scand J Gastroenterol 12:793, 1977.
54. Chayvialle J-A, Miyata M, Rayford PL, et al: Effects of test meal, intragastric nutrients, and intraduodenal bile on plasma concentrations of immunoreactive somatostatin and vasoactive intestinal peptide in dogs. Gastroenterology 79:844, 1980.
55. Wolfe MM, Misbin RI, Gardner DF, et al: Enteric release of vasoactive intestinal peptide after a peptone meal in the dog. Regul Pept 5:103, 1983.
56. Burhol PG, Waldum HL, Jorde R, et al: The effect of a test meal on plasma vasoactive intestinal polypeptide (VIP), gastric inhibitory polypeptide (GIP), and secretin in man. Scand J Gastroenterol 14:939, 1979.
57. Fahrenkrug J, Galbo H, Holst JJ, et al: Influence of the autonomic nervous system on the release of vasoactive intestinal polypeptide from the porcine gastrointestinal tract. J Physiol 280:405, 1978.
58. Fahrenkrug J, Haglund U, Jodal M, et al: Nervous release of vasoactive intestinal polypeptide in the gastrointestinal tract of cats: Possible physiological implications. J Physiol 284:291, 1978.
59. Bitar KN, Said SI, Weir GC, et al: Neural release of vasoactive intestinal peptide from the gut. Gastroenterology 79:1288, 1980.

60. Ebeid AM, Murray P, Soeters PB, et al: Release of VIP by calcium stimulation. Am J Surg 133:140, 1977.
61. Uvnas-Moberg K, Goiny M, Posloncec B, et al: Increased levels of VIP (vasoactive intestinal polypeptide)-like immunoreactivity in peripheral venous blood of dogs following injections of apomorphine and bromocriptine. Do dopaminergic agents induce gastric relaxation and hypotension by a release of endogenous VIP? Acta Physiol Scand 115:373, 1982.
62. Oktedalen O, Opstad PK, Fahrenkrug J, et al: Plasma concentration of vasoactive intestinal polypeptide during prolonged physical exercise, calorie supply deficiency, and sleep deprivation. Scand J Gastroenterol 18:1057, 1983.
63. Go VLW, Yaksh TL: Vasoactive intestinal peptide (VIP) and cholecystokinin (CCK8) in cat spinal cord and dorsal root ganglion: Release from cord by peripheral nerve stimulation. Regul Pept Suppl 1:S43, 1980.
64. Johansson O: Localization of vasoactive intestinal polypeptide- and avian pancreatic polypeptide-like immunoreactivity in the Golgi apparatus of peripheral neurons. Brain Res 262:71, 1983.
65. Giachetti A, Said SI, Reynolds RC, et al: Vasoactive intestinal polypeptide in brain: Localization in and release from isolated nerve terminals. Proc Natl Acad Sci USA 74:3424, 1977.
65a. Said SI, Porter JC: Vasoactive intestinal polypeptide: release into hypophyseal portal blood. Life Sci 24:227, 1979.
66. Smitherman TC, Sakio H, Geumei AM, et al: Coronary vasodilator action of VIP, in Said SI (ed): *Vasoactive Intestinal Peptide.* New York, Raven Press, 1982, pp 169–176.
67. Villar HV, Fender HR, Rayford PL, et al: Inhibition of gastrin release and gastric secretion by GIP and VIP, in Thompson JC (ed): *Gastrointestinal Hormones.* Austin, University of Texas Press, 1975, pp 467–474.
68. Konturek SJ, Dembinski A, Thor P, et al: Comparison of vasoactive intestinal peptide (VIP) and secretin in gastric secretion and mucosal blood flow. Pflugers Arch 361:175, 1976.
69. Makhlouf GM, Zfass AM, Said SI, et al: Effects of synthetic vasoactive intestinal peptide (VIP), secretin and their partial sequences on gastric secretion. Proc Soc Exp Biol Med 157:565, 1978.
70. Gespach C, Hoa DHB, Rosselin G: Regulation by vasoactive intestinal peptide, histamine, somatostatin-14 and -28 of cyclic adenosine monophosphate levels in gastric glands isolated from the guinea pig fundus or antrum. Endocrinology 112:1597, 1983.
71. Laburthe M, Prieto JC, Amiranoff B, et al: Interaction of vasoactive intestinal peptide with isolated intestinal epithelial cells from rat. 2. Characterization and structural requirements of the stimulatory effect of vasoactive intestinal peptide on production of adenosine 3′:5′-monophosphate. Eur J Biochem 96:239, 1979.
72. Robberecht P, Conlon TP, Gardner JD: Interaction of porcine vasoactive intestinal peptide with dispersed pancreatic acinar cells from the guinea pig. Structural requirements for effects of vasoactive intestinal peptide and secretin on cellular adenosine 3′:5′-monophosphate. J Biol Chem 251:4635, 1976.
73. Dupont C, Laburthe M, Broyart JP, et al: Cyclic AMP production in isolated colonic epithelial crypts: A highly sensitive model for the evaluation of vasoactive intestinal peptide action in human intestine. Eur J Clin Invest 10:67, 1980.
74. Dupont C, Gespach C, Chenut B, et al: Regulation by vasoactive intestinal peptide of cyclic AMP accumulation in gastric epithelial glands. A characteristic of human stomach. FEBS Lett 113:25, 1980.
75. Gaginella TS, Phillips SF, Dozois RR, et al: Stimulation of adenylate cyclase in homogenates of isolated intestinal epithelial cells from hamsters. Effects of gastrointestinal hormones, prostaglandins, and deoxycholic and ricinoleic acids. Gastroenterology 74:11, 1978.
76. Binder HJ, Lemp GF, Gardner JD: Receptors for vasoactive intestinal peptide and secretin on small intestinal epithelial cells. Am J Physiol 238:G190, 1980.
77. Laburthe M, Bataille D, Rousset M, et al: The expression of cell surface receptors for VIP, secretin, and glucagon in normal and transformed cells of the digestive tract, in Nicholls P et al (eds): *Membrane Protein.* New York, Pergamon Press, 1978, pp 271–290.
78. Borghi C, Nicosia S, Giachetti A, et al: Vasoactive intestinal polypeptide (VIP) stimulates adenylate cyclase in selected areas of rat brain. Life Sci 24:65, 1979.
79. Raufman J-P, Kasbekar DK, Jensen RT, et al: Potentiation of pepsinogen secretion from dispersed glands from rat stomach. Am J Physiol 245:G525, 1983.
80. Chiba T, Taminato T, Kadowaki S, et al: Effects of glucagon, secretin, and vasoactive intestinal polypeptide on gastric somatostatin and gastrin release from isolated perfused rat stomach. Gastroenterology 79:67, 1980.
81. Makhlouf GM: Distinct mechanisms for stimulation of intestinal secretion by vasoactive intestinal peptide (VIP) and glucagon. Gastroenterology 72:368, 1977.
82. Waldman DB, Gardner JD, Zfass AM, et al: Effects of vasoactive intestinal peptide, secretin, and related peptides on rat colonic transport and adenylate cyclase activity. Gastroenterology 73:518, 1977.
83. Makhlouf GM, Said SI: The effect of vasoactive intestinal peptide (VIP) on digestive and hormonal function, in Thompson JC (ed): *Gastrointestinal Hormones.* Austin, University of Texas Press, 1975, pp 599–610.
84. Mailman D: Effects of vasoactive intestinal poly-

peptide on intestinal absorption and blood flow. J Physiol 279:121, 1978.

85. Krejs GJ, Fordtran JS, Bloom SR, et al: Effect of VIP infusion on water and ion transport in the human jejunum. Gastroenterology 78:722, 1980.
86. Krejs GJ, Barkley RM, Read NW, et al: Intestinal secretion induced by vasoactive intestinal polypeptide. A comparison with cholera toxin in the canine jejunum in vivo. J Clin Invest 61:1337, 1978.
87. Racusen LC, Binder HJ: Alteration of large intestinal electrolyte transport by vasoactive intestinal polypeptide in the rat. Gastroenterology 73:790, 1977.
88. Schwartz CJ, Kimberg DV, Sheerin HE, et al: Vasoactive intestinal peptide stimulation of adenylate cyclase and active electrolyte secretion in intestinal mucosa. J Clin Invest 54:536, 1974.
89. Rao MB, O'Dorisio TM, Cataland S, et al: Angiotensin II and norepinephrine antagonize the secretory effect of VIP in rat ileum and colon. Peptides 5:291, 1984.
90. Domschke S, Domschke W, Rosch W, et al: Vasoactive intestinal peptide: A secretin-like partial agonist for pancreatic secretion in man. Gastroenterology 73:478, 1977.
91. Dimaline R, Dockray GJ: Potent stimulation of the avian exocrine pancreas by porcine and chicken vasoactive intestinal peptide. J Physiol 294:153, 1979.
92. Makhlouf GM, Yau WM, Zfass AM, et al: Comparative effects of synthetic and natural vasoactive intestinal peptide on pancreatic and biliary secretion and on glucose and insulin blood levels in the dog. Scand J Gastroenterol 13:759, 1978.
93. Konturek SJ, Domschke S, Domschke W, et al: Comparison of pancreatic responses to portal and systemic secretin and VIP in cats. Am J Physiol 232:E156, 1977.
94. Jensen SL, Fahrenkrug J, Holst JJ, et al: Secretory effects of VIP on isolated perfused porcine pancreas. Am J Physiol 235:E387, 1978.
95. Modlin IM, Mitchell SJ, Bloom SR: The systemic release and pharmacokinetics of VIP, in Bloom SR (ed): *Gut Hormones.* New York, Churchill Livingstone, 1978, pp 470–474.
96. Konturek SJ, Thor P, Dembinski A, et al: Comparison of secretin and vasoactive intestinal peptide on pancreatic secretion in dogs. Gastroenterology 68:1527, 1975.
97. Hickson JCD: The secretion of pancreatic juice in response to stimulation of the vagus nerves in the pig. J Physiol 206:275, 1970.
98. Holst JJ, Schaffalitzky de Muckadell OB, Fahrenkrug J: Nervous control of pancreatic exocrine secretion in pigs. Acta Physiol Scand 105:33, 1979.
99. Adrian TE, Bloom SR, Hermansen K, et al: Pancreatic polypeptide, glucagon and insulin secretion from the isolated perfused canine pancreas. Diabetologia 14:413, 1978.
100. Ipp E, Dobbs RE, Unger RH: Vasoactive intestinal peptide stimulates pancreatic somatostatin release. FEBS Lett 90:76, 1978.
101. Thulin L, Hellgren M: Choleretic effect of vasoactive intestinal peptide. Acta Chir Scand 142:235, 1976.
102. Ricci GL, Fevery J: The action of VIP on bile secretion and bile acid output in the non-anaesthetized rat. Biochem Pharmacol 34:3765, 1985.
103. Domschke W, Lux G, Domschke S, et al: Effects of vasoactive intestinal peptide on resting and pentagastrin-stimulated lower esophageal sphincter pressure. Gastroenterology 75:9, 1978.
104. Siegel SR, Brown FC, Castell DO, et al: Effects of vasoactive intestinal polypeptide (VIP) on lower esophageal sphincter in awake baboons. Comparison with glucagon and secretin. Dig Dis Sci 24:345, 1979.
105. Behar J, Field S, Marin C: Effect of glucagon, secretin, and vasoactive intestinal polypeptide on the feline lower esophageal sphincter: Mechanisms of action. Gastroenterology 77:1001, 1979.
106. Goyal RK, Said S, Rattan S: Influence of VIP antiserum on lower esophageal sphincter relaxation: Possible evidence for VIP as the inhibitory neurotransmitter. Gastroenterology 76:1142, 1979.
107. Chayvialle J-A, Miyata M, Rayford PL, et al: Immunoreactive somatostatin and vasoactive intestinal peptide in the digestive tract of cats. Gastroenterology 79:837, 1980.
108. Bennett A, Bloom SR, Ch'ng J, et al: Is vasoactive intestinal peptide an inhibitory transmitter in the circular but not the longitudinal muscle of guinea-pig colon? J Pharm Pharmacol 36:787, 1984.
109. Sninsky CA, Wolfe MM, Martin JL, et al: Myoelectric effects of vasoactive intestinal peptide on rabbit small intestine. Am J Physiol 244:G46, 1983.
110. Ryan J, Cohen S: Effect of vasoactive intestinal polypeptide on basal and cholecystokinin-induced gallbladder pressure. Gastroenterology 73:870, 1977.
111. Ryan JP, Ryave S: Effect of vasoactive intestinal polypeptide on gallbladder smooth muscle in vitro. Am J Physiol 234:E44, 1978.
112. Feeley TM, Clanachan AS, Scott GW: The effects of vasoactive intestinal polypeptide on the motility of human and guinea pig gallbladder. Can J Physiol Pharmacol 62:356, 1984.
113. Biancani P, Walsh J, Behar J: VIP: A possible inhibitory neurotransmitter for the internal anal sphincter. Regul Pept 6:287, 1983.
114. Rosa RM, Silva P, Stoff JS, et al: Effect of vasoactive intestinal peptide on isolated perfused rat kidney. Am J Physiol 249:E494, 1985.
115. Frandsen EK, Moody AJ: Lipolytic action of a newly isolated vasoactive intestinal polypeptide. Horm Metab Res 5:196, 1973.
116. Domschke S, Domschke W, Bloom SR, et al: Vasoactive intestinal peptide in man: Pharmacokinetics, metabolic and circulatory effects. Gut 19:1049, 1978.
117. Kerins C, Said SI: Hyperglycemic and glycogenolytic effects of vasoactive intestinal polypeptide. Proc Soc Exp Biol Med 142:1014, 1973.

118. Korinek JK, Toft DO, Go VLW, et al: The differential cellular effect of vasoactive intestinal polypeptide (VIP) and glucagon on hepatic glucose release. Gastroenterology 76:1175, 1979.
119. Matsumura M, Akiyoshi H, Saito S, et al: Effects of vasoactive intestinal peptide on glycogenolysis in cultured liver cells. Endocrinol Jpn 26:233, 1979.
120. Hohmann EL, Levine L, Tashjian AH Jr: Vasoactive intestinal peptide stimulates bone resorption via a cyclic adenosine 3′,5′-monophosphate-dependent mechanism. Endocrinology 112:1233, 1983.
121. Vijayan E, Samson WK, Said SI, et al: Vasoactive intestinal peptide: Evidence for a hypothalamic site of action to release growth hormone, luteinizing hormone, and prolactin in conscious ovariectomized rats. Endocrinology 104:53, 1979.
122. Kato Y, Iwasaki Y, Iwasaki J, et al: Prolactin release by vasoactive intestinal polypeptide in rats. Endocrinology 103:554, 1978.
123. Enjalbert A, Arancibia S, Ruberg M, et al: Stimulation of *in vitro* prolactin release by vasoactive intestinal peptide. Neuroendocrinology 31:200, 1980.
124. Matsushita N, Kato Y, Shimatsu A, et al: Effects of VIP, TRH, GABA and dopamine on prolactin release from superfused rat anterior pituitary cells. Life Sci 32:1263, 1983.
125. Epelbaum J, Tapia-Arancibia L, Besson J, et al: Vasoactive intestinal peptide inhibits release of somatostatin from hypothalamus in vitro. Eur J Pharmacol 58:493, 1979.
126. Tapia-Arancibia L, Arancibia S, Bluet-Pajot M-T, et al: Effect of vasoactive intestinal peptide (VIP) on somatostatin inhibition of pituitary growth hormone secretion in vitro. Eur J Pharmacol 63:235, 1980.
127. Reisine T, Heisler S, Hook VYH, et al: Multireceptor-induced release of adrenocorticotropin from anterior pituitary tumor cells. Biochem Biophys Res Commun 108:1251, 1982.
128. Rotsztejn WH, Besson J, Briaud B, et al: Effect of steroids on vasoactive intestinal peptide in discrete brain regions and peripheral tissues. Neuroendocrinology 31:287, 1980.
129. Rotsztejn WH, Benoist L, Besson J, et al: Effect of vasoactive intestinal peptide (VIP) on the release of adenohypophyseal hormones from purified cells obtained by unit gravity sedimentation. Inhibition by dexamethasone of VIP-induced prolactin release. Neuroendocrinology 31:282, 1980.
130. Kaneto A, Kaneko T, Kajinuma H, et al: Effect of vasoactive intestinal polypeptide infused intrapancreatically on glucagon and insulin secretion. Metabolism 26:781, 1977.
131. Ohneda A, Ishii S, Horigome K, et al: Effect of intrapancreatic administration of vasoactive intestinal peptide upon the release of insulin and glucagon in dogs. Horm Metab Res 9:447, 1977.
132. Szecowka J, Lins PE, Tatemoto K, et al: Effects of porcine intestinal heptacosapeptide and vasoactive intestinal polypeptide on insulin and glucagon secretion in rats. Endocrinology 112:1469, 1983.
133. Baitaille D, Javrousse C, Vaulin N, et al: Effect of vasoactive intestinal peptide (VIP) and gastrin inhibitory peptide (GIP) on insulin and glucagon release by perfused rat pancreas, in Foa PP et al (eds): *Glucagon: Its Role in Physiology and Clinical Medicine.* New York, Springer-Verlag, 1977, pp 255–269.
134. Schebalin M, Said SI, Makhlouf GM: Stimulation of insulin and glucagon secretion by vasoactive intestinal peptide. Am J Physiol 232:E197, 1977.
135. Szecowka J, Sandberg E, Efendic S: The interaction of vasoactive intestinal polypeptide (VIP), glucose and arginine on the secretion of insulin, glucagon and somatostatin in the perfused rat pancreas. Diabetologia 19:137, 1980.
136. Larsson L-I, Fahrenkrug J, Holst JJ, et al: Innervation of the pancreas by vasoactive intestinal polypeptide (VIP) immunoreactive nerves. Life Sci 22:773, 1978.
137. Emson PC, Fahrenkrug J, Schaffalitzky de Muckadell OB, et al: Vasoactive intestinal polypeptide (VIP): Vesicular localization and potassium evoked release from rat hypothalamus. Brain Res 143:174, 1978.
138. Mendelsohn G, Eggleston JC, Olson JL, et al: Vasoactive intestinal peptide and its relationship to ganglion cell differentiation in neuroblastic tumors. Lab Invest 41:144, 1979.
139. Yamaguchi K, Abe K: Macromolecular forms of VIP in VIP-secreting tumors, in Said SI (ed): *Vasoactive Intestinal Peptide.* New York, Raven Press, 1982, pp 469–478.
140. Tsuto T, Okamura H, Fukui K, et al: An immunohistochemical investigation of vasoactive intestinal polypeptide in the colon of patients with Hirschsprung's disease. Neurosci Lett 34:57, 1982.
141. Aggestrup S, Uddman R, Sundler F, et al: Lack of vasoactive intestinal polypeptide nerves in esophageal achalasia. Gastroenterology 84:924, 1983.
142. Crema A, del Tacca M, Frigo GM, et al: Presence of a nonadrenergic inhibitory system in the human colon. Gut 9:633, 1968.
143. Crema A, Frigo GM, Lecchini S: A pharmacological analysis of the peristaltic reflex in the isolated colon of the guinea-pig or cat. Br J Pharmacol 39:334, 1970.
144. Ballmann M, Conlon JM: Changes in the somatostatin, substance P and vasoactive intestinal polypeptide content of the gastrointestinal tract following streptozotocin-induced diabetes in the rat. Diabetologia 28:355, 1985.
145. Kinder RB, Restorick JM, Mundy AR: Vasoactive intestinal polypeptide in the hyper-reflexic neuropathic bladder. Br J Urol 57:289, 1985.
146. Shinomura Y, Himeno S, Kurokawa M, et al: Release of vasoactive intestinal peptide by intraduodenal infusion of HCl or fat and intramuscular injection of neostigmine in man. Hepatogastroenterology 32:129, 1985.
147. O'Morain C, Bishop AE, McGregor GP, et al: Vasoactive intestinal peptide concentrations and immunocytochemical studies in rectal biopsies from

patients with inflammatory bowel disease. Gut 25:57, 1984.
148. Clark AJL, Adrian TE, McMichael HB, et al: Vasoactive intestinal peptide in shock and heart failure. Lancet 1:539, 1983.
149. Lezoche E, Carlei F, Vagni V, et al: Elevated plasma levels of vasoactive intestinal polypeptide in short bowel syndrome. Am J Surg 145:369, 1983.
150. Heinz-Erian P, Dey RD, Flux M, et al: Deficient vasoactive intestinal peptide innervation in the sweat glands of cystic fibrosis patients. Science 229:1407, 1985.
151. Loren I, Emson PC, Fahrenkrug J, et al: Distribution of vasoactive intestinal polypeptide in the rat and mouse brain. Neuroscience 4:1953, 1979.
152. Emson PC, Gilbert RFT, Loren I, et al: Development of vasoactive intestinal polypeptide (VIP) containing neurons in the rat brain. Brain Res 177:437, 1979.
153. Sims KB, Hoffman DL, Said SI, et al: Vasoactive intestinal polypeptide (VIP) in mouse and rat brain: An immunocytochemical study. Brain Res 186:165, 1980.
154. Roberts GW, Woodhams PL, Bryant MG, et al: VIP in the rat brain: Evidence for a major pathway linking the amygdala and hypothalamus via the stria terminalis. Histochemistry 65:103, 1980.
155. Edvinsson L, Fahrenkrug J, Hanko J, et al: VIP (vasoactive intestinal polypeptide)-containing nerves of intracranial arteries in mammals. Cell Tissue Res 208:135, 1980.
156. Wharton J, Polak JM, Probert L, et al: Peptide containing nerves in the ureter of the guinea-pig and cat. Neuroscience 6:969, 1981.
157. Lynch EM, Wharton J, Bryant MG, et al: The differential distribution of vasoactive intestinal polypeptide in the normal human female genital tract. Histochemistry 67:169, 1980.
158. Polak JM, Bloom SR: VIP and the genitourinary system of man and animals. Regul Pept 6:322, 1983.
159. Weihe E, Reinecke M, Yanaihara N, et al: Distribution of neural vasoactive intestinal polypeptide in the mammalian heart. Regul Pept 6:334, 1983.
160. Wharton J, Polak JM, Pearse AGE, et al: Enkephalin-, VIP- and substance P-like immunoreactivity in the carotid body. Nature 284:269, 1980.
161. Tornqvist K, Uddman R, Sundler F, et al: Somatostatin and VIP neurons in the retina of different species. Histochemistry 76:137, 1982.
162. Uddman R, Alumets J, Densert O, et al: Occurrence and distribution of VIP nerves in the nasal mucosa and tracheobronchial wall. Acta Otolaryngol 86:443, 1978.
163. Dey RD, Said SI: Immunocytochemical localization of VIP-immunoreactive nerves in bronchial walls and pulmonary vessels. Fed Proc 39:1062, 1980.
164. Uddman R, Malm L, Sundler F: The origin of vasoactive intestinal polypeptide (VIP) nerves in the feline nasal mucosa. Acta Otolaryngol 89:152, 1980.
165. Wilson DA, O'Neill JT, Said SI, et al: Vasoactive intestinal polypeptide and the canine cerebral circulation. Circ Res 48:138, 1981.
166. Kitamura S, Ishihara Y, Said SI: Effect of VIP, phenoxybenzamine and prednisolone on cyclic nucleotide content of isolated guinea-pig lung and trachea. Eur J Pharmacol 67:219, 1980.
167. Fahrenkrug J, Schaffalitzky de Muckadell OB, Holst JJ, et al: Vasoactive intestinal polypeptide in vagally mediated pancreatic secretion of fluid and HCO_3. Am J Physiol 237:E535, 1979.

Section Six

Other Peptides

Chapter 20

Pancreatic Polypeptide

Tsuguo Sakamoto, M.D., Felix Lluis, M.D., and Phillip L. Rayford, Ph.D.

HISTORY

Pancreatic polypeptide (PP) is a 36 straight chain amino acid peptide with a molecular weight of around 4,200 (see Appendix). It was originally isolated from chicken pancreas (avian pancreatic polypeptide, or APP) during the process of purification of insulin [1,2]. Peptides similar to APP have been isolated from the pancreas of several mammalian species, including bovine (BPP), ovine (OPP), porcine (PPP), canine (CPP), and human (HPP) [3]. Bovine, ovine, porcine, and human PP have amino acid sequences that differ in only one to four positions. APP, however, differs from other kinds of PP in more than half of its 36 amino acids. The C-terminal residue, tyrosine amide, has been found to be important for its biologic actions [4,5].

Molecular heterogeneity of PP in human plasma has been described [6]. After gel filtration, the majority of PP immunoreactivity was eluted in the position of PP with 36 amino acids [7]. Large and smaller forms of PP immunoreactivities were also found in normal human plasma [6,8]. However, these forms could not be removed by immunoabsorption or stimulated by insulin hypoglycemia [6,7,9], suggesting that this molecular heterogeneity may be due to nonspecific radioimmunoassay measurements.

In a more recent report [8], at least four different sizes of PP were found in plasma from normal subjects and from patients with chronic renal failure. Their approximate molecular weights were >20,000, 10,000, 4,200, and 2,000 daltons. After a standard breakfast, the concentrations of plasma HPP, with a molecular weight of 10,000, and of HPP, with a molecular weight of 4,200, increased in both normal subjects and renal failure patients, whereas the molecular weights of the other two components did not increase. Further study on the component with a molecular weight of 10,000 revealed that it may correspond to a PP precursor.

It has been shown that PP is synthesized as an N-terminal fragment from a PP precursor, with a molecular weight of 8,000 to 10,000 [10]. The C-terminal coproduct, or pancreatic icosapeptide, is released in equimolar amounts into the plasma [11].

Recently, two new peptides that are structurally similar to PP were isolated from the brain and intestine and designated neuropeptide Y (NPY) [12] and peptide YY (PYY) [13]. These new PP families have biologic activities similar to those of PP (i.e., inhibition of secretin-stimulated pancreatic secretion) [12,13]. PP has been the subject of several excellent reviews [9,14,15].

DISTRIBUTION

PP has been localized in the pancreas of several species by immunochemistry and immunohistochemistry [16–18] (Table 20-1). After total pancreatectomy, plasma PP levels were undetectable in humans, suggesting that, at least in man, the pancreas is the major source of PP [16]. In the dog and opossum, however, PP cells can be found in the stomach [18]. In addition, PP-like immunoreactivity has been found in the central and peripheral nervous systems [19,20]. In a recent study using radioimmunoassay, high performance liquid chromatography, and immunohistochemistry, DiMaggio et al [21] concluded that PP is not present in the rat brain and that the previously identified immunoreactive PP-like material in the rat brain is actually neuropeptide Y. Within the pancreas, most PP cells are found in the juxtaduodenal part in dogs, cats, rats, and mice. Similarly, in the human pancreas, the head and uncinate process are the major places of origin of PP [22]. In most species, PP cells occur both within the islet and scattered about the exocrine acini. In humans, PP cells are found in the periphery of islets, where A and D cells are also located, and in the exocrine pancreatic parenchyma and the epithelia of small and medium-sized ducts [18].

El-Salhy et al [23] found an extrapancreatic source of PP in mucosal cells of the gastrointestinal tract of rats. PP-immunoreactive cells were detected in the colon of a 2-day-old rat; they appeared in the rectum in 7 days; and by the 14th day, these cells appeared transiently in the pylorus. In 21-day-old rats, the number of PP-immunoreactive cells in the colon was greater than in adult rats. In the same study, there was a difference between PYY- and PP-immunoreactive cells concerning distribution, frequency, and ontogeny in the gastrointestinal tract [23]. In the gastrointestinal tract of human fetuses, the PP immunostaining was identified by the tenth week of

Table 20-1. **Distribution of PP cells in the pancreas and gastrointestinal tract of different mammals**

		Pancreas		
		Acinar	*Insular*	*GI Tract*
Mouse	Duodenal lobe	(+)	++	–
	Tail	(+)	+	
Rat	Duodenal lobe	–	+	–
	Tail	–	+	
Hamster	Duodenal lobe	+	++	n.t.
	Tail	(+)	(+)	
Guinea pig		++	++	–
Chinchilla	Duodenal lobe	++	+	n.t.
	Tail	++	+	
Rabbit	Duodenal lobe	+++	(+)	–
	Tail	(+)	(+)	
Opossum	Duodenal lobe	+	++	+(stomach)
	Tail	+	(+)	
Cat	Duodenal lobe	+++	(+)	n.t.
	Tail	++	+	
Dog	Duodenal lobe	+++	(+)	+(stomach)
	Tail	+	+	
Sheep		(+)	+++	n.t.
Cow		(+)	++	n.t.
Horse		++	++	n.t.
Humans		(+)to+	+	n.t.

Key: – = absent or only occasionaly seen; (+) = rare, but regularly seen; + = moderate number; ++ = fairly numerous; +++ = abundant; n.t. = not tested. (From Larsson et al [18].)

gestation in the ileum and by the twelfth week in the oxyntic and colonic mucosa [24].

ASSAY

PP has been measured by a specific radioimmunoassay [25]. Antiserum against HPP and BPP has been raised in rabbits. Both HPP and BPP are used for standards or radiolabeled tracer. In a homologous HPP assay using anti-HPP serum and HPP tracer, the cross-reactivity of BPP, CPP, OPP, and PPP was about 70 percent of the HPP. In a heterologous HPP assay using anti-HPP serum and BPP tracer, the cross-reactivity of CPP, HPP, and PPP was about 70 percent of BPP standard. With anti-BPP serum and BPP tracer, CPP, HPP, and PPP each had less than 50 percent of the potency of BPP standard [25].

R. E. Chance (Lilly Research Laboratories) has generously provided anti-PP serum and purified PP to groups of investigators around the world. In this radioimmunoassay (anti-HPP, anti-BPP), APP, gastric inhibitory polypeptide (GIP), vasoactive intestinal peptide (VIP), gastrin, cholecystokinin (CCK), secretin, glucagon, insulin, porcine proinsulin, and somatostatin do not effectively displace labeled HPP from antibody.

Two region-specific antisera have recently been developed: AbS11 and CTPP, each raised against the C-terminal hexapeptide of PP. By using AbS11, a small amount of PP was found in the rat brain; however, PP concentration in the head of the rat pancreas was 750-fold greater than that measured with the conventional BPP antiserum [26].

A radioimmunoassay with CTPP antiserum measured significant concentrations of PP immunoreactivity in pancreatic extracts of several mammalian and submammalian species; all tissue extracts studied showed parallelism with the PP reference standard (BPP). In addition, CTPP can be used to measure plasma levels of PP in rats, dogs, and humans [27].

PHARMACOKINETICS AND CATABOLISM

In humans, the disappearance half-time of PP is 6.9 minutes, the metabolic clearance rate is 5.0 mL/kg/min, and its volume of distribution is 50 mL/kg [28]. In the dog, the half-time is 5.5 minutes, the metabolic clearance rate is 26 mL/kg/min, and the volume of distribution is 209 mL/kg [29]. In patients with cirrhosis of the liver HPP is apparently extracted by the kidney (18 percent) but not by the liver [30]. In anesthetized pigs, renal and hepatic extraction of PP are 54 and 36 percent, respectively [31], whereas in anesthetized dogs, renal and hepatic extractions of PP are 35 and 2 percent, respectively [32]. In addition, elevated plasma PP concentrations are found in patients with chronic renal failure [33,34]. This mechanism is probably due to increased secretion and decreased metabolism of PP [35].

RELEASE

Plasma PP concentrations measured during interdigestive states fluctuate every 60–90 minutes, associated with cyclic changes in gastric acid and pancreatic exocrine secretions [36,37]. Atropine or a ganglion blocker (pentolinium) abolishes the fluctuation of PP levels [36]. Cyclic changes in vagal cholinergic tone are presumably responsible for the fluctuation of PP release. Plasma concentrations of PP rise after ingestion of protein, fat, and carbohydrates [38,39]. Protein is the most potent stimulant. In dogs, intraduodenal administration of sodium oleate or a mixture of amino acids increases plasma PP concentrations [40]. However, the responses to oleate or amino acids are less than those to a mixed meal [40]. In contrast, IV fat, amino acids, and glucose are ineffective [41,42]. Intravenous glucose inhibits PP release in response to food or gastrointestinal peptides [43–46]. Conversely, PP is sensitive to decreases in blood glucose [41].

Plasma levels of PP in response to food are biphasic (Fig 20-1), namely there is a rapid phase increase occurring within the first few minutes and lasting 30 to 60 minutes, followed by a secondary prolonged phase lasting more than 5 hours [43]. Pancreatic duct ligation in dogs resulted in fibrosis in exocrine parenchyma but not in the islet area [47]. During the initial 60 minutes, the PP release after a meal was diminished significantly by pancreatic duct ligation. The primary rapid phase of PP release, therefore, may be derived chiefly from acinar cells [47]. The exact mechanisms by which food stimulates PP release are unclear. However, it appears that both neural and humoral controls are involved.

Neural Control

An initial rapid phase and a secondary prolonged phase of PP release after a meal are almost

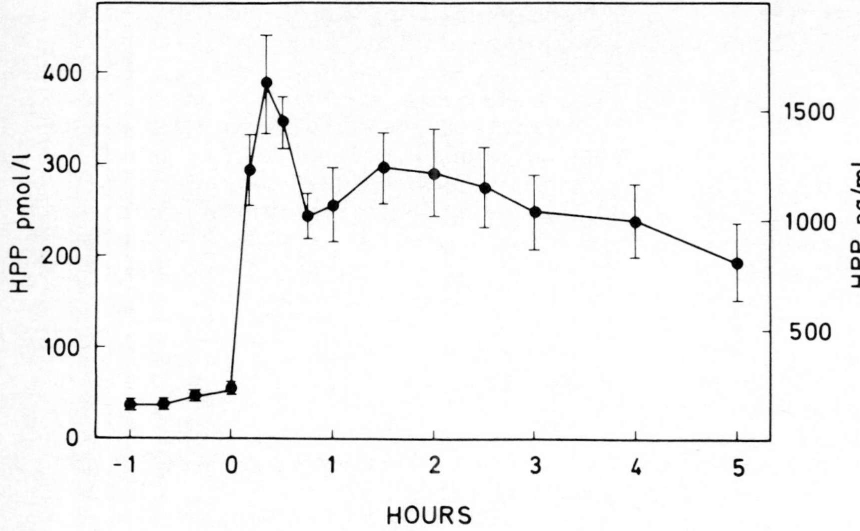

Figure 20-1. Serum HPP (mean ± S.E.M.) in 7 young, normal subjects during a mixed protein-rich meal. (From Schwartz et al [48], by permission of Little, Brown and Co.)

completely abolished by atropine and are greatly reduced by vagotomy [48–50]. Vagal cholinergic mechanisms clearly play the major role in the postprandial release of PP [9]. Sham feeding causes a significant increase in PP release in normal subjects [51,52]. Gastric distention also increases plasma levels of PP in humans [53]. Insulin-induced hypoglycemia is a strong stimulant of PP release [41,42]. Low-frequency electrical stimulation of the vagus in anesthetized pigs causes a significant increase in plasma PP concentrations [7]. Acetylcholine stimulates PP release [7]. The release of PP stimulated by acetylcholine, sham feeding, gastric distention, insulin hypoglycemia, and vagal electrical stimulation is abolished by both atropine and vagotomy [7,53–55].

Atropine and vagotomy act differently on PP release. After truncal vagotomy, the PP response to food was reduced [49], but this residual response was completely abolished by atropine. After vagotomy, the secondary phase of PP response to food reappears postoperatively with time, whereas the rapid phase of PP release does not reappear [56].

An intestinal phase of PP release has been demonstrated in dogs and humans [57–60]. In dogs with upper intestinal Thiry-Vella loops, perfusion of the loops with liver extract causes significant release of PP, which is abolished by atropine [57]. Sodium oleate (C18) appears to be a more potent stimulator of PP release than sodium dodecanoate (C12) [59]. In humans, perfusion of proximal and middle small intestine with amino acids, oleate, or glucose significantly increases plasma concentrations of PP [58] (Fig 20-2). Although it is unclear whether enteropancreatic signals for PP release are neural or humoral, the intestinal phase of PP release is dependent on cholinergic mechanisms [57]. After 75 percent distal small bowel resection in dogs, basal plasma PP levels transiently increased by the third week after resection [61]. This high value did not correlate with plasma CCK values found in the same study, suggesting that a cholinergic reflex may be triggered by bowel resection.

Duodenal stretch (rapid injection of water or saline into the duodenum) resulted in a small and transient release of PP within 2 minutes [62]. In another study [63], dogs in which a pyloric transection had been performed had a significantly reduced PP response to insulin hypoglycemia compared to the preoperative controls. This indicates a close relationship between pancreatic vagal fibers and the pylorus. Enteropancreatic reflex, caused by gastric or duodenal stretch, may play a role in part in food-stimulated PP release. Although PP response to a meal is dependent on cholinergic innervation, food-stimulated PP responses are greater and more prolonged than the responses to gastric distention or sham feeding, suggesting that an additional mechanism, probably hormonal, is involved in the release of PP after a meal. We found close correlation between CCK and PP levels late after a meal and concluded that CCK was physiologically important in the intestinal phase of PP release [60].

Intracerebroventricular (ICV) administration of CCK-8 resulted in a dose-related elevation of

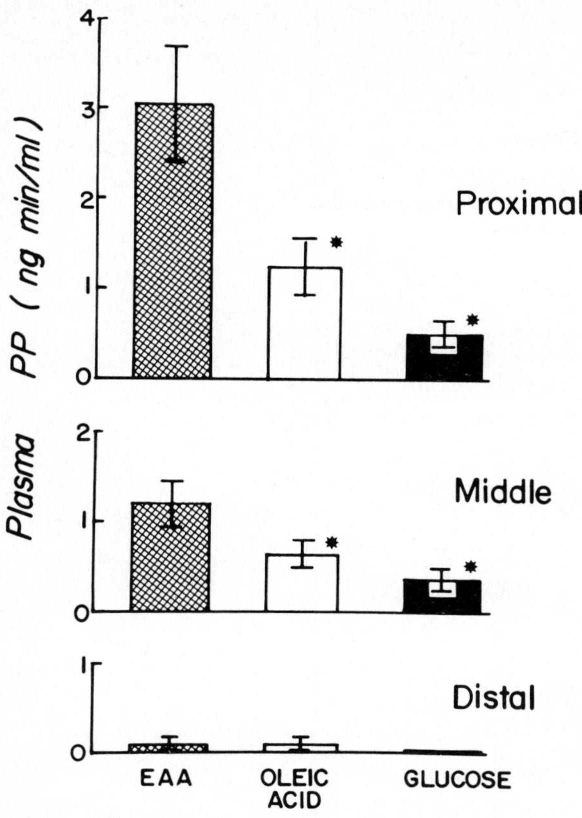

Figure 20-2. Integrated plasma PP response over 60 minutes to perfusion of proximal, middle, and distal small intestine with essential amino acid mixture (EAA), oleic acid, and glucose. (* = significantly less than essential amino acid mixture [$p < 0.05$].) For each individual nutrient, there was a significant reduction in the PP response the more distal the stimulus was placed in the intestine. (From Scarpello et al [58], by permission of Elsevier Science Publishing Co.)

plasma PP levels in conscious dogs [64]. ICV or systemic atropine as well as truncal vagotomy abolished the PP release induced by ICV CCK-8 [64]. In dogs, postprandial PP release is enhanced by β_2-adrenergic mechanisms [65]. Dopaminergic mechanisms may also have a tonic inhibitory effect on HPP secretion in normal subjects [66]. In contrast to cholinergic control, adrenergic control of PP release seems to be of minor importance.

Hormonal Control

Gastrin [67], pentagastrin [41], caerulein [42,68], CCK-33 [67,69], CCK-8 [67], CCK-4 [70], secretin [71], bombesin [72], GIP [73], VIP [73], neurotensin [74], and porcine gastrin-releasing peptide [72,75] have been shown to stimulate PP release in dogs and humans. There are other reports that gastrin [38,76], CCK-8 [77], 99 percent pure CCK [76], and pure secretin [67] failed to stimulate release of PP. These inconsistencies may result, at least in part, from differences in methods. The physiologic significance of these peptide hormones in the stimulation of PP is far from clear.

Using canine pseudoislets in a column-perfusion bioassay system, two secretagogues in canine duodenal mucosa that are larger peptide molecules than those reported previously have been detected, although further studies are needed to identify them [78]. In the isolated perfused pancreas, gastrin, caerulein, secretin, bombesin, CCK, and neurotensin have little or no effect on the release of PP, whereas acetylcholine is a potent stimulus [9,73]. The stimulatory effects of these peptides are influenced by vagal cholinergic tone [9]. Schwartz [9] suggests that the peptides that stimulate PP release probably act via cholinergic pathways rather than directly on the PP cell against the background of a permissive cholinergic tone, and that vagal cholinergic enteropancreatic reflexes are also mainly responsible for the secondary prolonged phase of PP release after a meal. In a study with dogs with completely denervated in situ pancreases, PP did not respond to insulin hypoglycemia, and the PP response to a meal was markedly blunted [79]. In contrast, in the study on the autotransplanted dog pancreas that provided total extrinsic pancreatic denervation, PP responses to a meal were not changed in comparison to those observed before transplantation [80]. Atropine abolished completely the response of PP to food, suggesting that the PP response to a meal is probably mediated not by direct innervation to the pancreas but indirectly through vagal pathways to the stomach or the intestine. Since the vagovagal reflex arch was completely severed in the transplanted pancreas, humoral mediators must be responsible for the gastrointestinal phase of PP release.

Among the candidate peptides for a stimulant of PP, CCK is most likely the important regulator of PP release. Infusion of graded doses of 99 percent pure CCK in dogs resulted in a dose-dependent elevation of PP [67]. Vagotomy decreased but did not abolish the PP response to CCK (Fig 20-3). In humans, pure CCK infusion, which gave plasma CCK levels (50–100 pmol/mL) even lower than those measured after food (180–300 pmol/mL), caused significant release of PP [69] (Fig 20-4). Intraduodenal amino acid or oleate stimulated both CCK and PP [81,82]. These results provide additional evidence that endogenously released CCK may play a role in the prolonged or so-called in-

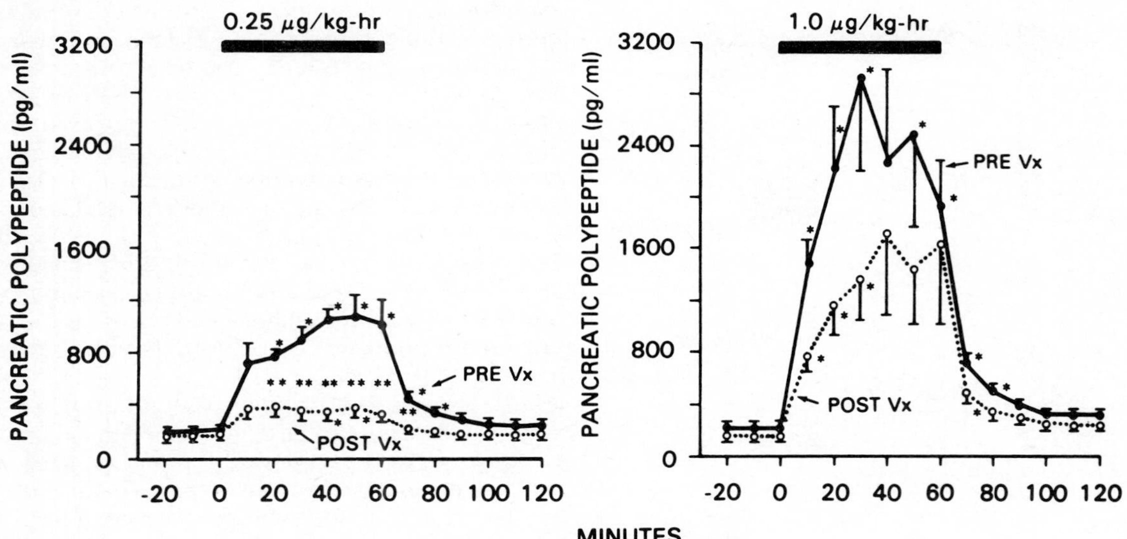

Figure 20-3. Pancreatic polypeptide responses to 99 percent pure cholecystokinin (CCK-99%), 0.25 μg/kg-hr (left), and 1.0 μg/kg-hr (right). Solid line = before vagotomy; broken line = after vagotomy; * = significant difference from basal. (From Guzman et al [67], by permission of The American Physiological Society.)

testinal phase of PP release. The effect of secretin on PP release is controversial. An IV bolus injection of GIH secretin (2 U/kg) increased plasma PP levels in healthy subjects. However, IV infusion of GIH secretin (1.0 U/kg/hr) did not increase plasma PP concentrations in dogs, although plasma secretin levels increased threefold basal [67]. Duodenal acidification did not increase plasma PP or increased it only modestly [83]. It therefore appears that secretin is not a physiologic stimulant for PP.

Bombesin is a stimulant of PP release in dogs [84]. However, in humans, bombesin abolishes meal-stimulated release of PP [85]. Somatostatin suppresses basal levels of PP and release of PP stimulated by food, intraduodenal acidification, pentagastrin, and other gastrointestinal hormones in humans and dogs [83,86,87]. In addition to somatostatin, synthetic enkephalins suppress the PP response to a meal, to sham feeding, and to bombesin [88–91]. Naloxone reverses this inhibitory effect of enkephalins on PP release, suggesting that opiate receptors may participate in modification of PP release [91]. Gastric antrectomy and vagal denervation of the antrum reduce PP response to a meal [92–94], which suggests that PP-releasing factors are present in the antrum. This hypothesis was supported by a study on the autotransplanted pancreas in dogs in which the PP response to a meal with autotransplanted pancreas did not differ from that before transplantation [80]. After subsequent antral vagotomy, postprandial PP response is reduced by 80 percent (Fig 20-5).

ACTIONS

The physiologic role of PP has not been established. Intravenous administration of PP produces a broad spectrum of biologic actions on the gastrointestinal tract. Pharmacologic doses of PP stimulate basal gastric acid secretion and inhibit pentagastrin-stimulated gastric acid secretion [4]. In conscious dogs, depending upon the dose, PP has both stimulatory and inhibitory actions on the motility of the antrum, duodenum, ileum, and colon [95,96]. The most important physiologic action of PP is assumed to be an inhibitory effect on pancreatic exocrine secretion. In dogs, IV infusion of BPP or PPP in a physiologic dose, an amount that is similar to PP levels after a meal, inhibited basal

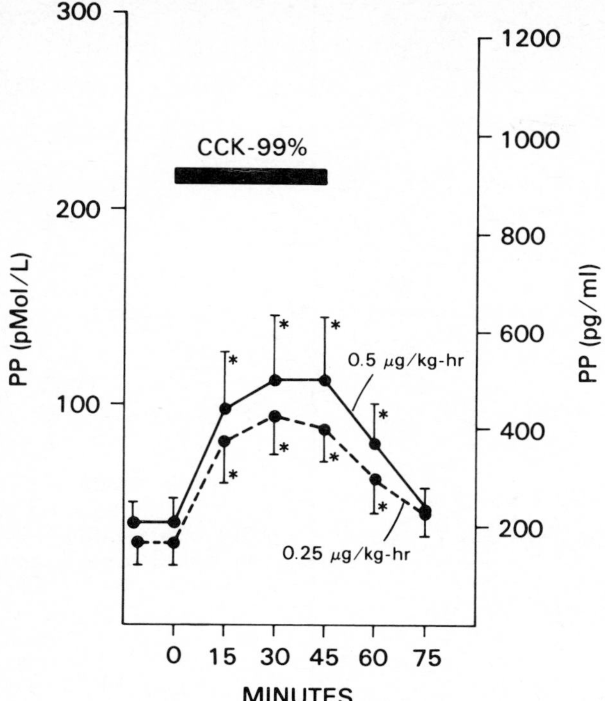

Figure 20-4. PP response to a two-dose infusion of 99 percent pure CCK in six subjects. * = significant elevation above basal values. (From Lonovics et al [69], by permission of Elsevier Science Publishing Co.)

pancreatic secretion and pancreatic secretion stimulated by IV secretin, caerulein, and bethanechol, as well as pancreatic secretion induced by intraduodenal hydrochloric acid, sodium oleate, or amino acids [29,82,97]. PP appears to inhibit pancreatic protein and bicarbonate secretion equally [97].

Exogenous PP did not affect endogenous CCK and secretin release [82]; therefore, the inhibitory effect of PP on pancreatic secretion may be a direct action on the pancreas. The finding that bovine PP inhibits CCK-stimulated pancreatic exocrine secretion in rats in vivo but not in vitro, together with the lack of specific PP binding sites on pancreatic acini, suggests that the inhibitory action of PP on pancreatic secretion is mediated by indirect mechanisms [98]. In humans, IV BPP significantly reduced pancreatic secretion stimulated by secretin or secretin plus caerulein [99,100]. Exogenous BPP, at a physiologic dose, did not change gastric acid and pepsin output in response to pentagastrin or sham feeding but significantly inhibited basal and stimulated pancreatic protein secretion induced by a maximum dose of secretin or CCK-8 [101]. Intraduodenal administration of pancreaticobiliary juice stimulates PP release, which suggests a negative feedback mechanism between pancreatic secretion and PP [102]. However, the physiologic significance of endogenously released PP in the regulation of pancreatic secretion is still uncertain.

Porcine PP, at a physiologic dose, caused a decrease in gallbladder pressure that was dose-dependent in pigs [103]. Bovine PP reduced the intragallbladder pressure and increased choledochal resistance in the dog [95]. PP has no effect on basal or on CCK-induced contraction of human gallbladder strips in vitro [104]. Therefore, it appears that in vivo PP-induced gallbladder relaxation is exerted on a site other than the gallbladder muscle. In humans, a physiologic dose of PP causes apparent reduction in trypsin secretion and almost complete inhibition of bilirubin output into the duodenum [99].

During the interdigestive phase, the cyclic changes in the migrating motor complex are accompanied by a synchronous fluctuation of motilin and PP [105]. The peaks of PP that occur in phase II (late) of the fasting migrating motor complex (MMC) require vagal integrity [106]. This mechanism could be dependent upon direct vagal innervation of the pancreas or associated with the cyclic presence of pancreaticobiliary secretions in the duodenum [107]. The role of PP in the regulation of MMC is incompletely understood. The infusion of physiologic doses of BPP increased the frequency of the migrating myoelectric complex in the whole intestine in dogs and pigs [108]. On the other hand, infusions of PP that mimicked postprandial plasma levels selectively inhibited both phase III of the MMC and the associated increase in plasma motilin in dogs, indicating a possible role for PP in the postprandial inhibition of the MMC [109]. In contrast, physiologic doses of BPP did not induce an active front in humans [110].

PATHOPHYSIOLOGY

The basal plasma levels of PP are significantly elevated with aging, at a rate of about 30 pg/mL per decade [111]. The elevated plasma PP levels are also found in patients with duodenal ulcers [53,112], diabetes mellitus [41], and chronic renal failure [33,34]. The increased PP levels in duodenal ulcer patients was thought to be related to increased vagal activity. Plasma PP measurement in response to an IV bolus injection of bombesin is suggested as a reliable indicator of vagal integrity [113]. Extremely high basal concentrations of PP

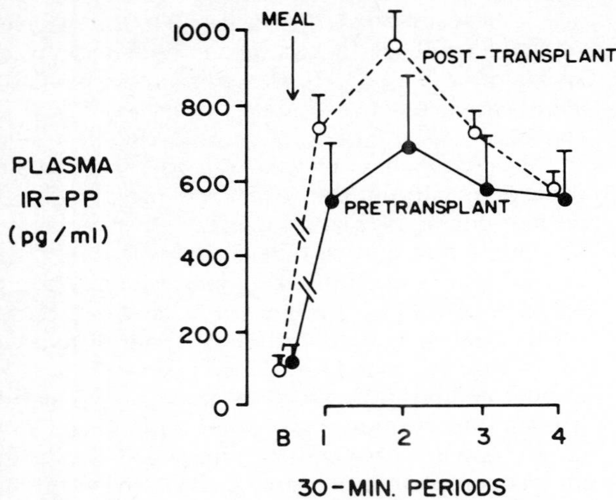

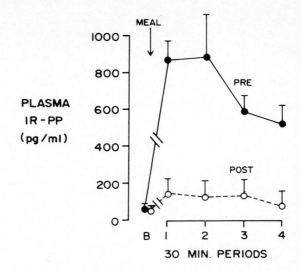

Figure 20-5. Left: Plasma concentration of immunoreactive pancreatic polypeptide (IR-PP) in response to a meal, before and after pancreatic antrotransplantation (denervation). Each point represents the mean (±SE) of one experiment on each of four dogs. Right: Comparison of plasma IR-PP response to a meal in two dogs with pancreatic transplant, before and after antral vagotomy. (From Debas et al [80], by permission of the C V Mosby Co.)

are seen in severe cases of the insulin-dependent maturity-onset type and juvenile-onset type of diabetes mellitus [41]. The basal and meal-stimulated PP responses decrease significantly after dietary plus insulin treatment [114].

Reduced basal and postprandial PP levels are found in patients with severe and moderate chronic pancreatitis. According to one study [115] that included 19 patients with acute pancreatitis, 17 with chronic pancreatitis, 25 with ductal adenocarcinoma of the pancreas, and 27 control subjects, a fasting HPP level of 125 pg/mL or over excludes cancer or chronic pancreatitis with a confidence of 85 to 90 percent. In about 50 percent of patients with chronic pancreatitis, however, HPP remains within normal basal levels [116]. Plasma PP response to meat extract in patients with chronic pancreatitis is reduced significantly, and the amount of PP release in response to a meat extract meal is significantly correlated with total amylase output and maximum amylase concentrations observed during a pancreozymin-secretin test [117]. The plasma PP response to CCK-8 in patients with chronic pancreatitis was significantly reduced [118]. In a comparative study of plasma PP response to food, secretin, and bombesin in normal subjects and in patients with chronic pancreatitis, food stimulated PP release both in normal subjects and in patients with chronic pancreatitis, whereas secretin and bombesin significantly increased plasma PP levels in normal subjects only [119]. The degree of impairment of the PP response varied according to the degree of pancreatic exocrine deficiency. Measurement of plasma PP may be a useful diagnostic tool for assessment of pancreatic exocrine function in chronic pancreatitis.

Plasma PP levels have been measured in several other clinical conditions. Reduced PP response to IV Boots secretin was found in patients with cystic fibrosis who have markedly impaired pancreatic function [120]. In a series of seven patients with achlorhydria, infusion of GIP elicited a significant and sustained release of plasma PP [121]. GIP may possibly participate in the intestinal phase of PP release.

Nine patients with celiac disease underwent a controlled study before and one year after gluten withdrawal. After mucosal regeneration, PP release was unchanged regardless of the degree of regeneration [122], whereas GIP and somatostatin levels increased and gastrin levels decreased. It was concluded that the degree of mucosal impairment does not affect the release of PP in celiac disease.

The release of PP in response to a modified sham feeding test was studied in 13 patients with achalasia, 15 healthy controls, and 10 vagotomized patients [123]. Two different patterns were found in the group of patients with achalasia: six patients had gastric acid secretion and plasma PP levels comparable to the healthy controls, whereas seven patients had neither increased gastric acid secretion nor increased PP release [123]. The latter group was considered to have denervated stomachs in accordance with their abnormal esophageal innervation.

After gastric partitioning operations for morbid obesity in nine patients, postprandial PP release was unchanged, whereas GIP release was significantly increased [124].

Elevated PP levels are found in patients with APUDomas, including insulinoma, gastrinoma, VIPoma, glucagonoma, and carcinoid tumor. The tumors in patients who had high plasma PP levels contained large amounts of PP [125]. Measurement of plasma PP has, therefore, been suggested as a marker for endocrine tumors. We should note, however, that the incidence of elevated PP levels in patients with endocrine tumors varies widely. Adrian et al [126] reported high levels of plasma PP in 18 of 25 patients with VIPoma, five of nine patients with glucagonoma, eight of 31 patients with gastrinoma, and two of nine patients with insulinoma, whereas 53 patients with pancreatic adenocarcinoma had normal PP levels. In another series, 18 of 31 patients with endocrine tumors of the pancreas, gut, and respiratory tract had elevated PP levels [127]. Nine of 12 cases with carcinoid syndrome had elevated PP levels [127].

In a series of 21 patients with pancreatic islet tumors and five patients with intestinal carcinoids, increased PP plasma levels were found in only six patients [128]. Thus, plasma PP levels are not a sensitive marker for endocrine tumors.

PP measurement may be useful in patients with watery diarrhea syndromes because a highly elevated plasma concentration of PP indicates that the causative tumor is in the pancreas [129]. Shulkes et al [130] reported a patient with the watery diarrhea syndrome in whom plasma levels of VIP were sixfold, neurotensin levels were 10-fold, and PP levels were 200-fold greater than those found in normal individuals. The tumor extract from this patient contained high concentrations of these peptides in a ratio similar to those of plasma.

Tumors that produce only PP are rare, perhaps because of the lack of symptoms. Eight patients with PP-producing islet cell tumors and one patient with pseudo-PP-producing tumors have been reported recently [131]. Basal serum PP levels ranged from 394 to 35,100 pg/mL. Two of these patients had multiple endocrine neoplasia syndrome, and two others had diffuse hepatic metastases. However, one patient with a tumor of the stomach was reported to have elevated levels of PP. This tumor was associated with flushing, tachycardia, headache, and lacrimation [132].

Pharmacologic doses of secretin (3 CU/kg/hr) resulted in a significant increase of plasma PP in a series of 28 patients with the ZE syndrome [133]. These high values were not correlated with gastrin levels, gastric acid secretion, or the age of the patient, and the response disappeared after excision of the gastrinoma.

Plasma PP levels have been suggested as a reliable marker for endocrine pancreatic tumors in patients with multiple endocrine neoplasia (MEN) type I [134]. To date, the proportion of patients reported with elevated PP levels in this disease is variable. Friesen et al [135] reported that all of six patients (MEN-I) with pancreatic islet cell tumors showed high concentrations of basal and meal-stimulated PP, whereas only three of 15 nonfamilial patients with sporadic islet cell tumors had high plasma PP levels. Floyd et al [41] reported that four of five patients with pancreatic tumors (MEN-I) had elevated PP levels. Lamers and Diemel [136] reported that only three of eight patients with pancreatic tumors (MEN-I) showed high plasma PP levels. Additional atropine suppression tests [137–139] do not seem to provide clear-cut discrimination for pancreatic endocrine tumors [136].

REFERENCES

1. Kimmel JR, Pollock HG, Hazelwood RL: Isolation and characterization of chicken insulin. Endocrinology 83:1323, 1968.
2. Kimmel JR, Hayden LJ, Pollock HG: Isolation and characterization of a new pancreatic polypeptide hormone. J Biol Chem 250:9369, 1975.
3. Chance RE: US Patent Office, publication X-3097A, 1974 22:3 (842063).
4. Lin T-M, Evans DC, Chance RE, et al: Bovine pancreatic peptide: Action on gastric and pancreatic secretion in dogs. Am J Physiol 232:E311, 1977.
5. Chance RE, Cieszkowski M, Jaworek J, et al: Effect of pancreatic polypeptide and its C-terminal hexapeptide on meal and secretin induced pancreatic secretion in dogs. J Physiol 314:1, 1981.
6. Villanueva ML, Hedo JA, Marco J: Heterogeneity of pancreatic polypeptide immunoreactivity in human plasma. FEBS Lett 80:99, 1977.
7. Schwartz TW, Holst JJ, Fahrenkrug J, et al: Vagal, cholinergic regulation of pancreatic polypeptide secretion. J Clin Invest 61:781, 1978.
8. Garrote FJ, Rovira A, Casado S, et al: Immunoreactive pancreatic polypeptide components in plasma from normal subjects and patients with chronic renal failure in basal and postprandial conditions. Metabolism 33:244, 1984.
9. Schwartz TW: Pancreatic polypeptide: A hormone under vagal control. Gastroenterology 85:1411, 1983.
10. Schwartz TW, Gingerich RL, Tager HS: Biosynthesis of pancreatic polypeptide. Identification of a precursor and a cosynthesized product. J Biol Chem 255:11494, 1980.

11. Schwartz TW, Tager HS: Isolation and biogenesis of a new peptide from pancreatic islets. Nature 294:589, 1981.
12. Tatemoto K, Carlquist M, Mutt V: Neuropeptide Y—a novel brain peptide with structural similarities to peptide YY and pancreatic polypeptide. Nature 296:659, 1982.
13. Tatemoto K: Isolation and characterization of peptide YY (PYY), a candidate gut hormone that inhibits pancreatic exocrine secretion. Proc Natl Acad Sci USA 79:2514, 1982.
14. Lonovics J, Devitt P, Watson LC, et al: Pancreatic polypeptide. A review. Arch Surg 116:1256, 1981.
15. Floyd JC Jr: Pancreatic polypeptide. Clinics Gastroenterol 9:657, 1980.
16. Adrian TE, Bloom SR, Bryant MG, et al: Distribution and release of human pancreatic polypeptide. Gut 17:940, 1976.
17. Baetens D, Rufener C, Orci L: Bovine pancreatic polypeptide (BPP) in the pancreas and in the gastrointestinal tract of the dog. Experientia 32:785, 1976.
18. Larsson L-I, Sundler F, Håkanson R: Pancreatic polypeptide—A postulated new hormone: Identification of its cellular storage site by light and electron microscopic immunocytochemistry. Diabetologia 12:211, 1976.
19. Lundberg JM, Hokfelt T, Anggård A, et al: Coexistence of an avian pancreatic polypeptide (APP) immunoreactive substance and catecholamines in some peripheral and central neurons. Acta Physiol Scand 110:107, 1980.
20. Vincent SR, Johansson O, Hokfelt T, et al: Neuropeptide coexistence in human cortical neurones. Nature 298:65, 1982.
21. DiMaggio DA, Chronwall BM, Buchanan K, et al: Pancreatic polypeptide immunoreactivity in rat brain is actually neuropeptide Y. Neuroscience 15:1149, 1985.
22. Orci L, Malaisse-Lagae F, Baetens D, et al: Pancreatic-polypeptide-rich regions in human pancreas. Lancet 2:1200, 1978.
23. El-Salhy M, Wilander E, Juntti-Berggren L, et al: The distribution and ontogeny of polypeptide YY (PYY)- and pancreatic polypeptide (PP)-immunoreactive cells in the gastrointestinal tract of rat. Histochemistry 78:53, 1983.
24. Leduque P, Paulin C, Dubois PM: Immunocytochemical evidence for a substance related to the bovine pancreatic polypeptide-peptide YY group of peptides in the human fetal gastrointestinal tract. Regul Pept 6:219, 1983.
25. Chance RE, Moon NE, Johnson MG: Human pancreatic polypeptide (HPP) and bovine pancreatic polypeptide (BPP), in Jaffe BM, Behrman HR (eds): *Methods of Hormone Radioimmunoassay*. 2nd Ed. New York, Academic Press, 1979, pp 657–672.
26. Taylor IL, Vaillant CR: Pancreatic polypeptide-like material in nerves and endocrine cells of the rat. Peptides 4:245, 1983.
27. Greeley GH Jr, Trowbridge J, Burdett J, et al: Radioimmunoassay of pancreatic polypeptide in mammalian and submammalian vertebrates using a carboxyl-terminal hexapeptide antiserum. Regul Pept 8:177, 1984.
28. Adrian TE, Greenberg GR, Besterman HS, et al: PP infusion in man: Pharmacokinetics at three dose levels and effects on gastrointestinal and pancreatic hormones. Scand J Gastroenterol 13(Suppl 49):3, 1978.
29. Taylor IL, Solomon TE, Walsh JH, et al: Pancreatic polypeptide. Metabolism and effect on pancreatic secretion in dogs. Gastroenterology 76:524, 1979.
30. Boden G, Master RWP, Owen OE: Hepatic and renal extraction of endogenous human pancreatic polypeptide (HPP). Scand J Gastroenterol 13(Suppl 49):28, 1978.
31. Sive AA, Vinik AI, Hickman-Van Hoorn R, et al: Secretory responses of pancreatic polypeptide in man and pigs. Scand J Gastroenterol 13(Suppl 49):167, 1978.
32. Hagopian W, Lever EG, Cohen D, et al: Predominance of renal and absence of hepatic metabolism of pancreatic polypeptide in the dog. Am J Physiol 245:E171, 1983.
33. Boden G, Master RW, Owen OE, et al: Human pancreatic polypeptide in chronic renal failure and cirrhosis of the liver: Role of kidneys and liver in pancreatic polypeptide metabolism. J Clin Endocrinol Metab 51:573, 1980.
34. Hallgren R, Landelius J, Fjellstrom K-E, et al: Gastric acid secretion in uraemia and circulating levels of gastrin, somatostatin, and pancreatic polypeptide. Gut 20:763, 1979.
35. Lamers CBHW, Diemel CM, van Leer E, et al: Mechanism of elevated serum pancreatic polypeptide concentrations in chronic renal failure. J Clin Endocrinol Metab 55:922, 1982.
36. Schwartz TW, Stenquist B, Olbe L, et al: Synchronous oscillations in the basal secretion of pancreatic-polypeptide and gastric acid. Gastroenterology 76:14, 1979.
37. Chen MH, Joffe SN, Magee DF, et al: Cyclic changes of plasma pancreatic polypeptide and pancreatic secretion in fasting dogs. J Physiol 341:453, 1983.
38. Adrian TE, Bloom SR, Besterman HS, et al: PP—Physiology and pathology, in Bloom SR (ed): *Gut Hormones*. New York, Churchill Livingston, 1978, pp 254–260.
39. Taylor IL, Byrne WJ, Christie DL, et al: Effect of individual L-amino acids on gastric acid secretion and serum gastrin and pancreatic polypeptide release in humans. Gastroenterology 83:273, 1982.
40. Wilson RM, Boden G, Owen OE: Pancreatic polypeptide responses to a meal and to intraduodenal amino acids and sodium oleate. Endocrinology 102:859, 1978.
41. Floyd JC, Fajans SS, Pek S, et al: A newly recognized pancreatic polypeptide; Plasma levels in health and disease. Recent Prog Horm Res 33:519, 1977.
42. Adrian TE, Besterman HS, Cooke TJC, et al: Mechanism of pancreatic polypeptide release in man. Lancet 1:161, 1977.
43. Marco J, Hedo JA, Villanueva ML: Control of pan-

creatic polypeptide secretion by glucose in man. J Clin Endocrinol Metab 46:140, 1978.
44. Sive AA, Vinik AI, van Tonder SV: Pancreatic polypeptide (PP) responses to oral and intravenous glucose in man. Am J Gastroenterol 71:183, 1979.
45. Villanueva ML, Hedo JA, Castillo-Olivares J, et al: Effect of exogenous and endogenous hyperglycaemia on human pancreatic polypeptide (hPP) secretion. Diabetologia 15:278, 1978.
46. Schusdziarra V, Stapelfeldt W, Klier et al: Effect of physiological increments of blood glucose on plasma somatostatin and pancreatic polypeptide levels in dogs. Regul Pept 2:211, 1981.
47. Inoue K, Weiner I, Gourley WK, et al: Reduction of postprandial release of pancreatic polypeptide after development of pancreatic fibrosis. Surg Gynecol Obstet 154:699, 1982.
48. Schwartz TW, Stadil F, Chance RE, et al: Pancreatic-polypeptide response to food in duodenal-ulcer patients before and after vagotomy. Lancet 1:1102, 1976.
49. Taylor IL, Impicciatore M, Carter DC, et al: Effect of atropine and vagotomy on pancreatic polypeptide response to a meal in dogs. Am J Physiol 235:E443, 1978.
50. Glaser B, Floyd JC Jr, Vinik AI: Secretion of pancreatic polypeptide in man in response to beef ingestion is mediated in part by an extravagal cholinergic mechanism. Metabolism 32:57, 1983.
51. Feldman M, Richardson CT, Taylor IL, et al: Effect of atropine on vagal release of gastrin and pancreatic polypeptide. J Clin Invest 63:294, 1979.
52. Taylor IL, Feldman M: Effect of cephalic-vagal stimulation on insulin, gastric inhibitory polypeptide, and pancreatic polypeptide release in humans. J Clin Endocrinol Metab 55:1114, 1982.
53. Schwartz TW, Grotzinger U, Schoon I-M, et al: Vagovagal stimulation of pancreatic-polypeptide secretion by graded distention of the gastric fundus and antrum in man. Digestion 19:307, 1979.
54. Schwartz TW, Rehfeld JH: Mechanism of pancreatic-polypeptide release. Lancet 1:697, 1977.
55. Schwartz TW, Stenquist B, Olbe L: Cephalic phase of pancreatic-polypeptide secretion studied by sham feeding in man. Scand J Gastroenterol 14:313, 1979.
56. Taylor IL, Singer M, Kauffman GL Jr: Time-dependent effects of vagotomy on pancreatic polypeptide release. Dig Dis Sci 27:491, 1982.
57. Modlin IM, Albert D, Crochelt R, et al: Evidence for an intestinal mechanism of pancreatic polypeptide release. Dig Dis Sci 26:587, 1981.
58. Scarpello JH, Vinik AI, Owyang C: The intestinal phase of pancreatic polypeptide release. Gastroenterology 82:406, 1982.
59. Fink AS, Taylor IL, Luxemburg M, et al: Pancreatic polypeptide release by intraluminal fatty acids. Metabolism 30:1063, 1983.
60. Fried GM, Ogden WD, Greeley GH Jr, et al: Physiologic role of cholecystokinin in the intestinal phase of pancreatic polypeptide release. Ann Surg 200:600, 1984.
61. Lilja P, Wiener I, Inoue K, et al: Changes in circulating levels of cholecystokinin, gastrin, and pancreatic polypeptide after small bowel resection in dogs. Am J Surg 145:157, 1983.
62. Fink AS, Floyd JC Jr, Fiddian-Green RG: Release of human pancreatic polypeptide and gastrin in response to intraduodenal stimuli: A case report. Metabolism 28:339, 1979.
63. Poulsen J, Delikaris P, Lovgreen NA, et al: Impaired pancreatic innervation after pyloric transsection in dogs. Reduced pancreatic polypeptide response to insulin hypoglycaemia. Scand J Gastroenterol 18:17, 1983.
64. Lu Q-H, Greeley GH Jr, Zhu X-G, et al: Intracerebroventricular administration of cholecystokinin-8 elevates plasma pancreatic polypeptide levels in awake dogs. Endocrinology 114:2415, 1984.
65. Linnestad P, Guldvog I, Schrumpf E: The effect of alpha- and beta-adrenergic agonists and blockers on postprandial pancreatic polypeptide release in dogs. Scand J Gastroenterol 18:87, 1983.
66. Stern N, Sowers JR, Taylor IL, et al: Dopaminergic modulation of meal-stimulated and circadian secretion of pancreatic polypeptide in man. J Clin Endocrinol Metab 56:300, 1983.
67. Guzman S, Lonovics J, Devitt PG, et al: Hormone-stimulated release of pancreatic polypeptide before and after vagotomy in dogs. Am J Physiol 240:G114, 1981.
68. Tsuda K, Seino Y, Sakurai H, et al: Cerulein-induced pancreatic polypeptide secretion. Its inhibition by atropine and its possible role in regulating gallbladder relaxation. Am J Gastroenterol 74:355, 1980.
69. Lonovics J, Guzman S, Devitt P, et al: Release of pancreatic polypeptide in humans by infusion of cholecystokinin. Gastroenterology 79:817, 1980.
70. Rehfeld JF, Larsson L-I, Goltermann NR, et al: Neural regulation of pancreatic hormone secretion by the C-terminal tetrapeptide of CCK. Nature 284:33, 1980.
71. Glaser B, Vinik AI, Sive AA, et al: Plasma human pancreatic polypeptide responses to administered secretin: Effects of surgical vagotomy, cholinergic blockade, and chronic pancreatitis. J Clin Endocrinol Metab 50:1094, 1980.
72. McDonald TJ, Ghatei MA, Bloom SR, et al: Dose-response comparisons of canine plasma gastroenteropancreatic hormone responses to bombesin and the porcine gastrin-releasing peptide (GRP). Regul Pept 5:125, 1983.
73. Adrian TE, Bloom SR, Hermansen K, et al: Pancreatic polypeptide, glucagon and insulin secretion from the isolated perfused canine pancreas. Diabetologia 14:413, 1978.
74. Blackburn AM, Fletcher DR, Adrian TE, et al: Neurotensin infusion in man: Pharmacokinetics and effect on gastrointestinal and pituitary hormones. J Clin Endocrinol Metab 51:1257, 1980.
75. Inoue K, McKay D, Yajima H, et al: Effect of synthetic porcine gastrin-releasing peptide on plasma levels of immunoreactive cholecystokinin, pan-

creatic polypeptide, and gastrin in dogs. Peptides 4:153, 1983.
76. Taylor IL, Feldman M, Richardson CT, et al: Gastric and cephalic stimulation of human pancreatic polypeptide release. Gastroenterology 75:432, 1978.
77. Regan PT, Go VLW, DiMagno EP: Comparison of the effects of cholecystokinin and cholecystokinin octapeptide on pancreatic secretion, gallbladder contraction, and plasma pancreatic polypeptide in man. J Lab Clin Med 96:743, 1980.
78. Gingerich RL, Kramer JL: Identification of pancreatic polypeptide secretagogues in canine duodenal mucosa. Endocrinology 112:696, 1983.
79. Prinz RA, El Sabbagh H, Adrian TE, et al: Neural regulation of pancreatic polypeptide release. Surgery 94:1011, 1983.
80. Debas HT, Taylor IL, Seal AM, et al: Evidence for vagus-dependent pancreatic polypeptide-releasing factor in the antrum: Studies with the autotransplanted dog pancreas. Surgery 92:309, 1982.
81. Devitt P, Ayalon A, Lonovics J, et al: Pancreatic polypeptide release in response to intestinal fat. Physiologist 22:29, 1979.
82. Lonovics J, Guzman S, Devitt PG, et al: Action of pancreatic polypeptide on exocrine pancreas and on release of cholecystokinin and secretin. Endocrinology 108:1925, 1981.
83. Kayasseh L, Haecki WH, Gyr K, et al: The endogenous release of pancreatic polypeptide by acid and meal in dogs. Effect of somatostatin. Scand J Gastroenterol 13:385, 1978.
84. Taylor IL, Walsh JH, Carter D, et al: Effects of atropine and bethanechol on bombesin-stimulated release of pancreatic polypeptide and gastrin in dog. Gastroenterology 77:714, 1979.
85. Lezoche E, Carlei F, Vagni V, et al: Inhibition of food-stimulated pancreatic polypeptide (PP) by bombesin in man. Gastroenterology 76:1185, 1979.
86. Marco J, Hedo JA, Villanueva ML: Inhibitory effect of somatostatin on human pancreatic polypeptide secretion. Life Sci 21:789, 1977.
87. Feurle GE, Spoleanschi P, Stauder M, et al: Dose-response study of somatostatin on meal-stimulated levels of pancreatic polypeptide and insulin in the dog. Digestion 23:119, 1982.
88. Materia A, Modlin IM, Sank AC, et al: Opiate modulation of pancreatic polypeptide release by a meal in the dog. J Pharmacol Exp Ther 223:355, 1982.
89. Feldman M, Walsh JH, Taylor IL: Effect of naloxone and morphine on gastric acid secretion and on serum gastrin and pancreatic polypeptide concentrations in humans. Gastroenterology 79:294, 1980.
90. Konturek SJ, Kwiecien N, Obtułowicz W, et al: Effect of enkephalin and naloxone on gastric acid and serum gastrin and pancreatic polypeptide concentrations in humans. Gut 24:740, 1983.
91. Materia A, Jaffe BM, Modlin IM, et al: Effect of methionine-enkephalin and naloxone on bombesin-stimulated gastric acid secretion, gastrin, and pancreatic polypeptide release in the dog. Ann Surg 196:48, 1982.
92. Modlin IM, Jaffe BM, Albert D, et al: The role of the antrum in the modulation of plasma pancreatic polypeptide levels. J Surg Res 30:269, 1981.
93. Taylor IL, Kauffman GL Jr, Walsh JH, et al: Role of the small intestine and gastric antrum in pancreatic polypeptide release. Am J Physiol 240:G387, 1981.
94. Lewis BG, Townsend CM Jr, Greeley GH Jr, et al: Effect of antrectomy on gastrin, cholecystokinin, and pancreatic polypeptide release. Surg Forum 34:166, 1983.
95. Lin T-M, Chance RE: Gastrointestinal actions of a new bovine pancreatic peptide (BPP), in Chey WY, Brooks FP (eds): *Endocrinology of the Gut.* Thorofare, NJ, Charles B Slack Inc, 1974, pp 143–145.
96. Lin T-M, Chance RE: Spectrum of gastrointestinal actions of bovine PP, in Bloom SR (ed): *Gut Hormones.* New York, Churchill Livingstone, 1978, pp 242–246.
97. Beglinger C, Taylor IL, Grossman MI, et al: Pancreatic polypeptide inhibits exocrine pancreatic responses to six stimulants. Am J Physiol 246:G286, 1984.
98. Louie DS, Williams JA, Owyang C: Action of pancreatic polypeptide on rat pancreatic secretion: in vivo and in vitro. Am J Physiol 249:G489, 1985.
99. Greenberg GR, Adrian TE, Baron JH, et al: Inhibition of pancreas and gallbladder by pancreatic polypeptide. Lancet 2:1280, 1978.
100. Bloom SR, Adrian TE, Greenberg GR, et al: Effects of pancreatic polypeptide infusion in man. Gastroenterology 74:1012, 1978.
101. Swierczek JS, Konturek SJ, Tasler J, et al: Pancreatic polypeptide and vagal stimulation of gastric and pancreatic secretion in dogs. Hepatogastroenterology 28:206, 1981.
102. Owyang C, Scarpello JH, Vinik AI: Modulation of pancreatic polypeptide secretion by pancreaticobiliary juice. J Clin Endocrinol Metab 54:831, 1982.
103. Adrian TE, Mitchenere P, Sagor G, et al: Effect of pancreatic polypeptide on gallbladder pressure and hepatic bile secretion. Am J Physiol 243:G204, 1982.
104. Pomeranz IS, Davison JS, Shaffer EA: *In vitro* effects of pancreatic polypeptide and motilin on contractility of human gallbladder. Dig Dis Sci 28:539, 1983.
105. Keane FB, DiMagno EP, Dozois RR, et al: Relationships among canine interdigestive exocrine pancreatic and biliary flow, duodenal motor activity, plasma pancreatic polypeptide, and motilin. Gastroenterology 78:310, 1980.
106. Hall KE, Greenberg GR, El-Sharkawy TY, et al: Vagal control of migrating motor complex-related peaks in canine plasma motilin, pancreatic polypeptide, and gastrin. Can J Physiol Pharmacol 61:1289, 1983.
107. Owyang C, Achem-Karam SR, Vinik AI: Pancreatic polypeptide and intestinal migrating motor complex in humans. Gastroenterology 84:10, 1983.
108. Bueno L, Fioramonti J, Rayner V, et al: Effects of motilin, somatostatin, and pancreatic polypeptide on the migrating myoelectric complex in pig and dog. Gastroenterology 82:1395, 1982.
109. Hall KE, Diamant NE, El-Sharkawy TY, et al: Effect

of pancreatic polypeptide on canine migrating motor complex and plasma motilin. Am J Physiol 245:G178, 1983.

110. Janssens J, Hellemans J, Adrian TE, et al: Pancreatic polypeptide is not involved in the regulation of the migrating motor complex in man. Regul Pept 3:41, 1982.
111. Berger D, Crowther R, Floyd JC Jr, et al: Effects of age on fasting levels of pancreatic hormones in healthy subjects. Diabetes 26:381, 1977.
112. Gustavsson S, Adami H-O, Bjorklund O, et al: Fasting blood levels of gastrin, somatostatin, and pancreatic polypeptide in peptic ulcer disease. Scand J Gastroenterol 17:81, 1982.
113. Modlin IM, Albert D, Sank A, et al: Bombesin and insulin-stimulated pancreatic polypeptide release as a discriminator of vagal integrity. Surg Gynecol Obstet 156:729, 1983.
114. Berger D, Floyd JC Jr, Pek S, et al: Effect of insulin treatment on pancreatic polypeptide levels in diabetes mellitus. Clin Res 26:677A, 1978.
115. Koch MB, Go VLW, DiMagno EP: Can plasma human pancreatic polypeptide be used to detect diseases of the exocrine pancreas? Mayo Clin Proc 60:259, 1985.
116. Andersen BN, Hagen C, Klein HC, et al: Correlation between exocrine pancreatic secretion and serum concentration of human pancreatic polypeptide in chronic pancreatitis. Scand J Gastroenterol 15:699, 1980.
117. Yamamura T, Mori K, Tatsumi M, et al: Availability of plasma pancreatic polypeptide measurement in diagnosis of chronic pancreatitis. Scand J Gastroenterol 16:757, 1981.
118. Owyang C, Scarpello JH, Vinik AI: Correlation between pancreatic enzyme secretion and plasma concentration of human pancreatic polypeptide in health and in chronic pancreatitis. Gastroenterology 83:55, 1982.
119. Lamers CBHW, Diemel CM, Jansen JBMJ: Comparative study of plasma pancreatic polypeptide responses to food, secretin, and bombesin in normal subjects and in patients with chronic pancreatitis. Dig Dis Sci 29:102, 1984.
120. Stern A, Davidson GP, Kirubakaran CP, et al: Pancreatic polypeptide secretion. A marker for disturbed pancreatic function in cystic fibrosis. Dig Dis Sci 28:870, 1983.
121. Jorde R, Burhol PG: Release of plasma pancreatic polypeptide in achlorhydric patients after intravenous infusion of gastric inhibitory polypeptide. Digestion 27:239, 1983.
122. Linnestad P, Erichsen A, Fausa O, et al: The release of human pancreatic polypeptide, gastrin, gastric inhibitory polypeptide, and somatostatin in celiac disease related to the histological appearance of jejunal mucosa before and 1 year after gluten withdrawal. Scand J Gastroenterol 18:169, 1983.
123. Dooley CP, Taylor IL, Valenzuela JE: Impaired acid secretion and pancreatic polypeptide release in some patients with achalasia. Gastroenterology 84:809, 1983.
124. Amland PF, Jorde R, Kildebo S, et al: Effects of a gastric partitioning operation for morbid obesity on the secretion of gastric inhibitory polypeptide and pancreatic polypeptide. Scand J Gastroenterol 19:857, 1984.
125. Polak JM, Adrian TE, Bryant MG, et al: Pancreatic polypeptide in insulinomas, gastrinomas, VIPomas, and glucagonomas. Lancet 1:328, 1976.
126. Adrian TE, Bloom SR, Besterman HS, et al: Pancreatic polypeptide in adenocarcinomas and APUDomas including the carcinoid syndrome. Scand J Gastroenterol 13(Suppl 49):2, 1978.
127. Oberg K, Grimelius L, Lundqvist G, et al: Update on pancreatic polypeptide as a specific marker for endocrine tumours of the pancreas and gut. Acta Med Scand 210:145, 1981.
128. Prinz RA, Bermes EW Jr, Kimmel JR, et al: Serum markers for pancreatic islet cell and intestinal carcinoid tumors: A comparison of neuron-specific enolase β-human chorionic gonadotropin and pancreatic polypeptide. Surgery 94:1019, 1983.
129. Schwartz TW: Pancreatic-polypeptide (PP) and endocrine tumours of the pancreas. Scand J Gastroenterol 14(Suppl 53):93, 1979.
130. Shulkes A, Boden R, Cook I, et al: Characterization of a pancreatic tumor containing vasoactive intestinal peptide, neurotensin, and pancreatic polypeptide. J Clin Endocrinol Metab 58:41, 1984.
131. Strodel WE, Vinik AI, Lloyd RV, et al: Pancreatic polypeptide-producing tumors. Silent lesions of the pancreas? Arch Surg 119:508, 1984.
132. Solt J, Kadas I, Polak JM, et al: A pancreatic-polypeptide-producing tumor of the stomach. Cancer 54:1101, 1984.
133. Rigaud D, Accary JP, Mignon M, et al: Abnormal pancreatic polypeptide release by secretin infusion in Zollinger-Ellison syndrome. Dig Dis Sci 29:696, 1984.
134. Friesen S, Kimmel JR, Tomita T: Pancreatic polypeptide as screening marker for pancreatic polypeptide apudomas in multiple endocrinopathies. Am J Surg 139:61, 1980.
135. Friesen SR, Tomita T, Kimmel JR: Pancreatic polypeptide update: Its role in detection of the trait for multiple endocrine adenopathy syndrome, type I and pancreatic polypeptide-secreting tumors. Surgery 94:1028, 1983.
136. Lamers CBHW, Diemel CM: Basal and postatropine serum pancreatic polypeptide concentrations in familial multiple endocrine neoplasia type I. J Clin Endocrinol Metab 55:774, 1982.
137. Schwartz TW: Atropine suppression test for pancreatic polypeptide. Lancet 2:43, 1978.
138. Bloom SR, Adrian TE, Polak JM: Pancreatic polypeptide from pancreatic endocrine tumours. Lancet 2:1026, 1980.
139. Oberg K, Lundqvist G: Meal-stimulated and atropine-inhibited secretion of pancreatic polypeptide in healthy subjects, members of MEA I families and patients with malignant endocrine tumours of the gastrointestinal tract. Regul Pept 5:273, 1983.

Chapter 21

Somatostatin

Jan B. Newman, M.D., Felix Lluis, M.D., Courtney M. Townsend, Jr., M.D.

HISTORY

Somatostatin, a tetradecapeptide, MW 1637, was discovered by Guillemin et al [1] and Schally et al [2] during a search for a growth hormone releasing factor. It has been purified, sequenced, and synthesized [1,3,4]. Somatostatin-28, a 28 amino acid molecule, with somatostatin-14 occupying positions 15 through 28, has been identified in porcine intestine and pig and sheep hypothalamus. Even larger forms have been identified and sequenced [5]. Somatostatin-14 may represent the post-translational form of larger molecules [5]. Thus, somatostatin exhibits molecular heterogeneity in a manner similar to that of other peptide hormones (see Appendix).

Using RNA isolated from a human pancreatic somatostatinoma and recombinant DNA techniques, Shen et al [6] have prepared a cDNA library of human somatostatin. This group had previously cloned and sequenced anglerfish somatostatin. They found two cDNA sequences in the anglerfish; one encoded a 121 amino polypeptide with somatostatin at its COOH-terminus, and the second sequence encoded another somatostatin variant, designated somatostatin II, which differed in two of the 14 amino acids of somatostatin. Somatostatin II selectively inhibited insulin secretion without altering glucagon release. They found only one DNA in a human somatostatinoma. From this cDNA, they derived an mRNA sequence, which contained the preprosomatostatin coding region. This region encodes a 116 amino acid protein containing somatostatin-28 and somatostatin-14 at its C-terminal. These authors [6] note that somatostatin-28 is identical in mammals, and they speculate that after secretion of the preprohormone and removal of the signal peptide thought to be needed for secretion, somatostatin-28 and somatostatin-14 could be generated by processing of the prohormone, which has a molecular weight of 10,348. They suggest three possibilities for the prosomatostatin molecule: 1) the proregion maintains conformation of somatostatin-28 and somatostatin-14 to facilitate processing; 2) it may have its own "somatostatin-like" biologic activity; and 3) the pro-moiety may possess its own biologic activity [6].

Naylor et al [7] have isolated and sequenced the human somatostatin gene. They performed chromosomal mapping of human and rodent somatic cell lines and found the gene to reside on the long arm of human chromosome 3; two polymorphisms occurred. These polymorphisms also occurred among 180 individuals whose blood was screened. These two alleles may be used for gene linkage studies to examine the relation of the human somatostatin gene to disease [7]. According to Low et al [8], proteases that cleave prosomatostatin to somatostatin-28 and somatostatin-14 are not specific to tissues that normally express somatostatin.

In 1982, 10 years after the discovery of somatostatin, three groups of investigators [9–11], working independently at the Salk Institute, isolated and sequenced human growth hormone releasing factor (hpGRF-40) from pancreatic tumors causing acromegaly. One tumor contained only the 40 amino acid peptide; the other contained 44, 40, and 37 amino acids in their sequences [9–11]. These peptide hormones were structurally related to the secretin-glucagon family and have greatest homology with peptide histidine isoleucine-27 [9–11]. The role of hpGRF and its interactions with somatostatin await definition.

Studies of the distribution, pharmacokinetics, and release of somatostatin have given controversial results. The different findings are due in part to differences in antisera, breakdown of tracer, presence of interfering substances in plasma, circulating binding proteins, and rapid degradation of somatostatin (a 50 percent loss of activity in rat blood in 17 minutes at 37°C) [12,13]. These factors result in large discrepancies in values and conflicting data. The conflicts remain unsettled, and few investigators have taken eluted peptides or antibodies and examined bioactivity. Despite these controversies, there are many areas of agreement. We will attempt to delineate the general areas of agreement and point out some of the more glaring controversies.

DISTRIBUTION

Somatostatin has been localized by immunocytochemical and radioimmunoassay techniques. It has been found in the nervous system, in multiple tissues, in body fluids, and in tumors [3,5,14]. In the nervous system, somatostatin has been found in the hypothalamus, pituitary infundibular process, pineal gland, cerebral cortex, cerebellum, spinal cord, and retina. In the peripheral nervous system, it has been found in spinal ganglia and myenteric and submucosal plexus. In the gastrointestinal tract, somatostatin has been found in the antrum, the body and fundus of the stomach, the duodenum, jejunum, ileum, and colon, as well as in the pancreas, with the greatest amount of activity in the stomach and pancreas. In humans, concentrations are equally high in the fundus, antrum, and pancreas [15], whereas in cats, the antral concentration is by far the greatest [16].

Somatostatin cells are of three types, which reflect paracrine, endocrine, and neurocrine functions. Some give off long cytoplasmic processes that end with small bulbous expansions on "effector cells" (see Fig 3-10) and thus could be classified as "paracrine" cells [14,17]. These are most common in the stomach and pancreas. However, Buchan et al [18] used monoclonal antibodies to somatostatin and found no evidence for a close anatomic relationship between somatostatin cells and the other endocrine cells of the intestinal mucosa. Most duodenal somatostatin cells have the appearance of typical gut endocrine cells, but others clearly appear to be nerves in the lamina propria [3,14]. Somatostatin has also been found in the thyroid gland, adrenal medulla, salivary gland, thymus, spleen, lymph nodes, ovary, chorionic villi, decidua of early pregnancy, and the prostate, vas deferens, blood, cerebrospinal fluid, amniotic fluid, and urine [3,5,19,20]. Somatostatin has been found in somatostatinomas of the pancreas, duodenum, jejunum, in medullary carcinoma of the thyroid, and in pheochromocytomas (see Chapter 36) [3,5,20].

Recent studies have sought to define and quantitate somatostatin immunoreactivity in the gastrointestinal tract [21–25]. Ito et al found somatostatin-28 in all cells containing somatostatin-14 in human adult and fetal stomach, intestine, and pancreas [21,22] and in feline and canine stomach [23]. Penman et al [24] utilized radioimmunoassay with gel filtration chromatography and HPLC and immunocytochemistry to localize and quantitate somatostatin in the human stomach, duodenum, pancreas, jejunum, ileum, and colon. They found the highest levels in the duodenum, pancreas, jejunum, and antrum and pylorus of the stomach and lower levels in the body of the stomach, ileum, and colon. The main peak in the antrum, pylorus, duodenum, and pancreas coeluted with somatostatin-14 (approximately 1600 MW), whereas in the body of the stomach, jejunum, ileum, and colon, the highest peak coeluted with somatostatin-28 (approximately 3500 MW). More than 90 percent of the immunoreactivity was in the mucosa and less than 10 percent was in the muscularis. Mucosal somatostatin was located in endocrine-type cells. Muscle layer somatostatin was located in nerves in the myenteric plexus. The authors suggest that different biosynthetic controls may exist in neuronal and endocrine cells [24].

Ravazzola et al [25] developed specific antibodies directed against somatostatin-28 and its N-terminal fragment. Using immunoelectronmicroscopy, they studied the location of somatostatin-28 and its N-terminal cleavage product in human gastrin, pancreatic, and intestinal D cells. Large amounts of somatostatin-28 were found in the Golgi complex of immature secretory granules of pancreatic and gastric D cells, and the cleavage product was found mostly in mature secretory granules. In intestinal D cells, somatostatin-28 was in both mature and immature granules. The cleavage product was in mature granules. In pancreatic and gastric D cells, somatostatin-28 appears to be rapidly converted to somatostatin-14. Somatostatin-14 and its cleavage product are secreted, whereas in the intestine, somatostatin-28 as well as somatostatin-14 is secreted [25]. In the pancreas, somatostatin-14 is the major secretory product [24,25].

ASSAY

The radioimmunoassay of somatostatin has proved difficult because of its rapid degradation in plasma and interference and binding by large molecular weight plasma proteins [12,13]. Wasada et al [26] have been able to measure somatostatin in unextracted plasma, but most investigators [12,13,27–30] have found that acetone, acid, or acid-ethanol extraction is necessary.

Many studies have addressed the problems of

assay of somatostatin in plasma [12,13,31,32]. Polonsky et al [31] found that a large void-volume peak of immunoreactivity in human plasma, which was not altered postprandially, could be eliminated by acid extraction and passage through octadecylsilyl silica cartridges (C-18 Sep-Pak), enabling measurement of postprandial changes. Conlon et al [32] found that high molecular weight globulins in human plasma bind antibody, preventing tracer binding and the reading of high molecular weight forms.

Patel et al [13] found rapid tracer and somatostatin-14 degradation in rat and human plasma. Hilsted and Holst [12] and Patel et al [13] attributed this to tracer breakdown. It appears that acid extraction is necessary in order to eliminate high molecular weight plasma globulins, which either prevent tracer binding or cause tracer breakdown.

The antigenic region of the somatostatin molecule is in the midportion [20,27,33,34], and most antisera are directed toward this region. There is minimal cross-reactivity with other peptide hormones, but binding with larger somatostatin molecules does occur. An N-terminal antibody has been developed that measures only somatostatin-14 [33]. Sacks et al [35] developed three radioimmunoassays that detect different antigenic determinants on the somatostatin molecule; these have been used to measure hepatic clearance. Their three antibodies gave widely divergent results, which they attributed to differences in clearance of different portions of the molecule.

Thus, different antibodies with different antigenic determinants may also cause variation in results. As more investigators use antisera with different specificities to delineate the interaction and roles of somatostatin-14 and somatostatin-28, this issue may be clarified. At present, the reader must critically assess results in light of assay variability. Iodinated-tyrosine-substituted somatostatin, at the 11 or 1 positions, has been used as tracer in an attempt to avoid this problem.

PHARMACOKINETICS AND CATABOLISM

The disappearance half-time of somatostatin is brief. The half-life of somatostatin-14 in the rat has been reported to be as rapid as 0.15 minute (using different antisera this increased to 0.4) [33]. Half-times in dogs, pigs, and humans are 1 to 1.82 [27,34,36,37], 1.9 [12], 1.69 to 1.88 [38], and 3 minutes [39]. Somatostatin-28 has a half-life of 2.8 to 3.64 minutes [36,37]. The metabolic clearance rates (MCR) of somatostatin-14 were 21.9 [37], 63 [34], 95.2 [27], and 157 [36] mL/kg/min in dogs and 27–38 mL/kg/min in pigs [12]. The MCR of somatostatin-28 was 28.1 mL/kg/min in the same dogs in which the clearance of somatostatin-14 was 157 mL/kg/min [36].

Polonsky et al [31] found the MCR in anesthetized dogs to be 9.9 ± 1.4 mL/kg/min for somatostatin-28 and 21.9 ± 6.5 mL/kg/min for somatostatin-14. The reason for the large discrepancy in MCR between the results of Vaysse et al [36] and Polonsky et al [37] is unclear (their plasma halftimes were similar). The volume of distribution for somatostatin-14 in dogs is 114.7 ± 6 mL/kg [27].

Chayvialle et al [27] in our laboratory found no hepatic extraction of somatostatin-14 in awake dogs. Polonsky et al [37] found 43 percent hepatic extraction of somatostatin-14 and 11 percent for somatostatin-28. They also found the kidney to be a major site of extraction, with 82 and 50 percent extraction of somatostatin-14 and somatostatin-28, respectively. Somatostatin-28 was found to be cleared by the rat liver in vivo and in vitro at a rate slower than somatostatin-14. Opposite findings related to the possible conversion from somatostatin-28 to somatostatin-14 in the liver have been reported [40,41]. Results in humans are also conflicting [42]. In patients with end-to-side portacaval shunts, Webb et al [42] found 38 percent hepatic extraction and 45 percent splanchnic extraction. They found no basal portal, hepatic vein, or pulmonary artery gradients.

Sacks et al [35], using an in vitro isolated perfused rat liver system, found a 14 percent extraction of somatostatin-14 with a centrally directed antibody, whereas there was a 35 percent extraction with an N-terminal antibody. Of note in this study is that when a third centrally directed antibody was used, no hepatic degradation was found. There was a 3 to 20 percent degradation in the perfusate used (it contained washed human erythrocytes). They found 19 percent extraction of somatostatin-28 without appreciable conversion to somatostatin-14. The liver probably plays a role in the conversion of somatostatin-14 to intermediates that do not contain the N-terminal fragment.

Patel et al [13] noted a 50 percent in vitro degradation of somatostatin-14 by 17 minutes, when it was incubated at 37°C in rat whole blood. Hilsted and Holst [12] noted that the existence of tracer degrading enzyme in plasma caused rapid degradation. The blood, liver, and kidneys may all contribute to somatostatin metabolism.

Variability of results by different authors may be caused by different antibody specificity. The liver, with its aminopeptidase and endopeptidases, may account for a significant fraction of somatostatin degradation.

RELEASE

Significantly higher peripheral plasma levels of somatostatin are found in newborns and infants during the first 10 months of life, which suggests an active role of somatostatin in nutrient homeostasis [43].

The gastrointestinal tract contains approximately 70 percent of the body's somatostatin [13]; the splanchnic area is the main source of circulating somatostatin. There is a postprandial rise in somatostatin-like immunoreactivity [28,29,44–47]. The release of somatostatin is controlled by numerous metabolic and humoral factors [48] (Table 21-1). In normal dogs, the release of somatostatin into portal and peripheral circulation follows a rhythm with an amplitude ranging from 0.5 to 1.8 hours. In dogs after total pancreatectomy, somatostatin is released in nonperiodic, randomly occurring pulses [49]. Plasma somatostatin, like many peptides, shows meal-related peaks and returns to basal levels between meals [50]. Whether or not these postprandial peaks play a specific role is not known. While some investigators believe that plasma levels are compatible with actions of somatostatin as a circulating hormone, others suggest that somatostatin is only a paracrine agent, the plasma levels representing only a spillover phenomenon. The control by somatostatin of insulin and glucagon release from the islets of Langerhans is probably paracrine [51]. However, Aponte et al [52] provided evidence that suggests an endocrine release of pancreatic somatostatin into islet capillaries. In vivo and in vitro species differences have to be considered.

Somatostatin levels do not increase after sham feeding in humans [53], whereas a significant increase has been found in dogs [54]. Beglinger et al [55] recently demonstrated that during the intestinal phase of a meal (or after the infusion of several gastrointestinal hormones), the pancreatic exocrine response was greater than the increases in plasma levels of somatostatin, which suggests that factors other than intestinal secretagogues contribute to the postprandial release of somatostatin in dogs. Vagal stimulation releases somatostatin into the portal blood [56]. Atropine abolishes plasma somatostatin release after orally ingested and intraduodenally infused nutrients in humans; adrenergic mechanisms do not appear to modulate the postprandial release of somatostatin [57]. Bombesin infusion increases basal and enhances postprandial release of somatostatin [58]. After a meal, there is a gradient whereby portal concentrations of somatostatin are higher than peripheral levels. Somatostatin is, therefore, released from the gastrointestinal tract and might exert physiologic effects on the liver [29]. Antrectomy does not significantly alter the postprandial somatostatin release. Consequently, neither endogenous gastrin nor antral D cells appear to be an essential factor in the meal-induced increase of plasma somatostatin [29]. Bile is a specific releaser of somatostatin from the gastrointestinal tract [29].

Sources other than the stomach and pancreas contribute to increased plasma somatostatin levels. A nutrient release of endogenous somatostatin has been shown from the distal gut [59]. Release of somatostatin from the isolated perfused dog ileum is stimulated by changes in the concentration of calcium, potassium, and arginine, whereas glucose, in contrast to its stimulatory action on pancreatic D cells, has no effect on the ileum [60]. In humans, only supraphysiologic duodenal acidification and not gastric acidification has been found to increase peripheral plasma levels of somatostatin [61]. Insulin-induced hypoglycemia stimulates insulin release. Since insulin with normoglycemia or simultaneous infusion of the H_2 antagonist cimetidine results in no changes in basal levels, a mechanism is proposed whereby insulin hypoglycemia stimulates somatostatin release only through the increase of gastric acid secretion [62]. Vagotomy also prevents insulin-induced hypoglycemia from increasing peripheral somatostatin plasma levels. Guzman et al [63] in our laboratory showed that exogenous gastrin is a potent releaser of somatostatin into portal and systemic plasma in dogs, and this effect is not mediated by acid (Fig 21-1). The release of somatostatin is increased by stimulation of β-adrenergic receptors and is decreased by stimulation of α-adrenergic receptors in dogs [30].

Table 21-1. **Release of somatostatin**

1. **Basal plasma levels are influenced by vagal tone, cholinergic and adrenergic receptors, prostaglandins, fluctuations in the migrating motor complex, and circadian rhythms**
2. **Postprandial plasma levels are stimulated by meals, intraluminal acid, bile, and circulating nutrients; they are modulated by vagal tone, prostaglandins, and cholinergic, adrenergic, histaminergic, and opiate receptors**
3. **Hormones stimulating somatostatin release:**
   In vivo: bombesin, CCK, gastrin-17, GIP, secretin
   Isolated rat pancreas: CCK, gastrin, GIP, secretin, substance P, VIP
   Isolated rat stomach: bombesin, GIP, pentagastrin, secretin

Preparations of the isolated rat pancreas and stomach provide unique models for the study of the mechanisms involved in the release of somatostatin. Many gastrointestinal hormones stimulate the release of somatostatin from both the pancreas and stomach (see Table 21-1). Only substance P and serotonin have a distinctive effect by inhibiting somatostatin release from the isolated perfused rat stomach [64,65]. Interestingly, cysteamine, a drug that induces duodenal ulceration in rats, stimulates gastrin release without any change in the release of somatostatin [66]. A subtype of muscarinic receptors (M_1), selectively sensitive to the antagonist pirenzepine, regulates the release of gastric somatostatin [67].

Endogenous prostaglandins may play a role in the release of gastric somatostatin [68]. PGE_1 and PGE_2 stimulated somatostatin release from the isolated perfused rat pancreas in a glucose dose-dependent manner [69]. In vivo, PGE_2 produced a rise in somatostatin from the canine pancreaticoduodenal artery [70]. When 3-isobutyl-1-methylxanthine was added to the isolated rat pancreas perfused with graded concentrations of glucose in order to facilitate the terminal steps of secretion, somatostatin release was found to be slightly more sensitive to glucose than to insulin release [71].

Immunoreactive and biologically active somatostatin is present in human and sheep's milk; in contrast to plasma, milk contains only somatostatin-14 [72]. Somatostatin is also secreted into the gastric lumen and pancreatic secretions [73]. The role of the intraluminal secreted somatostatin remains controversial. In the absence of pancreatic proteases, intraduodenally administered somatostatin in dogs was capable of inhibiting meal-stimulated pancreatic exocrine secretion. Its potency, however, was eight times less when compared to somatostatin given intravenously [74]. In humans, high intragastric doses of somatostatin had no effect on pentagastrin-stimulated gastric secretion [75]. Abnormally high levels of somatostatin have been found in the pancreatic juice of poorly controlled insulin-dependent diabetic patients, whereas in patients who were well controlled, values did not differ from those found in normal controls [76]. The significance of this finding is not clear. For more details concerning the release of somatostatin, the reader is referred to the excellent review by Schusdziarra [77].

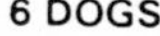

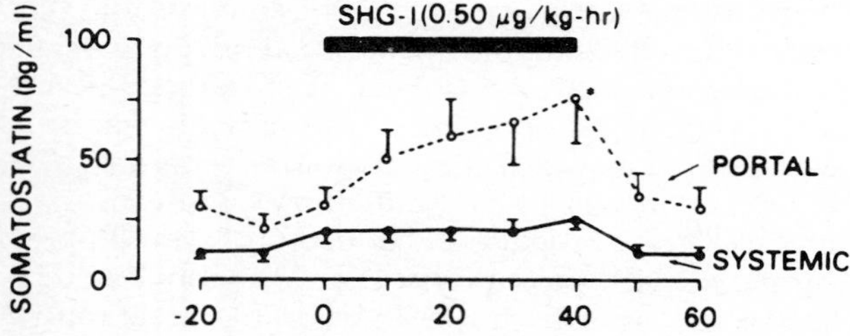

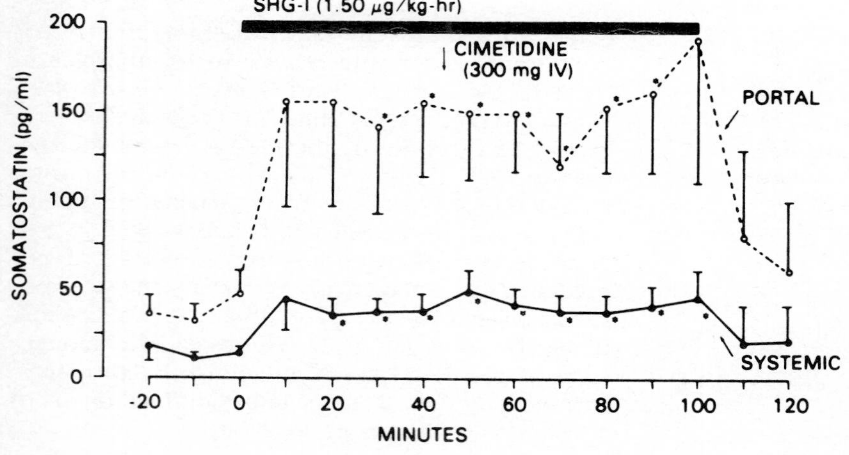

Figure 21-1. Portal (open circles) and systemic (closed circles) plasma concentrations of somatostatin. Upper panel = gastrin infusion of 0.5 μg/kg-hr for 40 minutes. Lower panel = gastrin infusion of 1.5 μg/kg-hr for 100 minutes. (* = $p < 0.05$.) (From Guzman et al [63], by permission of The Endocrine Society.)

ACTIONS

Amino acid residues 7–10 of the somatostatin molecule are essential for biologic activity [39]. We will confine this discussion to the effects of peripherally administered somatostatin. Somatostatin has effects on the gastrointestinal, cardiovascular, endocrine, hematologic, and genitourinary systems. Somatostatin-28 mimics most of the gastrointestinal secretory actions of somatostatin but does not exhibit the intestinal circulatory, metabolic, and motor effects [78].

Actions of somatostatin on the gastrointestinal tract are numerous. Somatostatin inhibits secretion of the salivary gland [79]. It inhibits gastric acid, pepsin, and intrinsic factor secretion [79]. This inhibition is effective against virtually all forms of gastric acid stimulation: pentagastrin, histamine, betazole, insulin, urocholine, carbachol, and meal. The lysyl residue in position 9 is more important than that in position 4 for gastric activity of somatostatin [80]. The reports of lack of inhibition are the exception rather than the rule and occurred with maximal doses of stimulation against low doses of somatostatin [79]. This inhibition is independent of vagal integrity, gastrin, and blood flow [79]. Somatostatin has been found to significantly increase gastric mucus production in humans [81].

Pharmacologic doses of somatostatin inhibit postprandial release of gastrin [82] in normal subjects and in patients with pernicious anemia and the Zollinger-Ellison syndrome. Somatostatin has a direct action on the parietal and peptic cells, inhibiting pentagastrin-stimulated acid and pepsin secretion in cats [83] as well as bethanechol-stimulated pepsin secretion in dogs [84]. Although secretin and somatostatin are released by acid and may account for the bulbogastrone effect (i.e., the inhibition of gastric acid secretion by intraduodenal acidification), the effects of exogenous somatostatin and secretin were not found to be additive on gastric acid output and emptying in a preliminary study in dogs [85].

In humans, low doses of exogenous somatostatin significantly inhibit endogenously stimulated gastric acid secretion [86], and both somatostatin-14 and somatostatin-28 are equally potent on a molar basis as inhibitors of the cephalic and gastric phases of acid and pepsin secretion as well as of the release of pancreatic polypeptide [53]. Based on the concentrations of plasma somatostatin, Konturek et al speculated that somatostatin-28 was a prohormone [53].

The regulation of gastric secretion by somatostatin is a complex and incompletely understood phenomenon. However, there are some valuable pieces of information regarding the feedback control of somatostatin release exerted by gastrin and gastric acid, and the modulatory influences on the tissue content and release of gastric somatostatin (see Table 21-1).

Two classes of binding sites—highly specific for somatostatin and varying in affinity and capacity—have been characterized in the cytosolic fraction of rabbit fundic and antral mucosa [87]. Somatostatin binding sites have been identified in the cytosolic fraction throughout the rabbit intestinal epithelium with similar affinities and different binding capacities, depending on the segment considered [88].

By using the isolated perfused rat stomach and somatostatin antiserum, Saffouri et al [89] concluded that release of both basal and stimulated gastrin is modulated by antral somatostatin. They suggested a functional linkage whereby gastric somatostatin secretion exerts a continuous restraint on basal gastrin secretion, and the stimulation of gastrin secretion may be mediated in part by inhibition of somatostatin secretion. Conversely, Soll et al [90] postulated that cholecystokinin (CCK), a stronger releaser of somatostatin from the fundic mucosa, was in turn weaker than gastrin as a stimulant of the parietal cell. Cysteamine-induced tissue somatostatin deficiency may be mediated through interaction with the somatostatin-14 disulfide bond [91].

The inhibitory action of somatostatin on stimulated gastrin release may be due, at least in part, to the interruption of a cyclic AMP-dependent component of the secretory process of gastrin [92]. Other mechanisms may also be involved.

Prostaglandins have been suggested as the mediators of somatostatin inhibition of gastric acid secretion [93], but recent studies found no evidence to support this hypothesis [94,95]. In humans, endogenous prostaglandins may not be involved in the somatostatin inhibition of gastric acid secretion [96].

Somatostatin inhibits the release of all known gastrointestinal hormones—gastrin, secretin, CCK, GIP, motilin, enteroglucagon, VIP, and PP—as well as both insulin and glucagon [79]. Exogenous somatostatin also decreases the release of thyroid hormones (T_4 and T_3) in humans without affecting basal plasma levels of thyrotropin (TSH) [97]. Somatostatin-14 infused at near physiologic levels (i.e., those obtained postprandially) decreased plasma insulin and glucagon to a smaller degree. Glucose and ketones were increased. These findings support the concept that somatostatin has a true endocrine role [47].

Further support for the role of somatostatin as a circulating hormone is derived from studies in which somatostatin antiserum was infused in vivo, resulting in enhanced postprandial plasma levels of gastrin, insulin, PP, triglycerides [44], parathyroid hormone, and calcitonin [98] as well as increased basal levels of growth hormone and enteroglucagon [51]. Endogenous somatostatin is also a physiologic inhibitor of TSH secretion in rats [99].

Comparative effects of somatostatin-14 and somatostatin-28 on the release of growth hormone, insulin, glucagon, gastrin, and PP and on pancreatic and gastric secretion have been examined [36,100,101]. Klaff et al [100] found that somatostatin-28 suppressed arginine-stimulated insulin release in humans more than somatostatin-14. Suppression of glucagon and PP was equivalent. Marco et al [101] found equal suppression of PP and glucagon in response to meal-stimulated release. Total suppression of insulin release by somatostatin was observed, and no comparison of effects could be made. Somatostatin-14 exhibited longer-lasting effects on suppression of PP and insulin. Vaysse et al [36] summarized the comparative effects of somatostatin-14 and somatostatin-28: somatostatin-28 was more potent than somatostatin-14 (potency ratios 0.11 and 0.13) in the inhibition of pancreatic secretion stimulated by secretin and caerulein in dogs, whereas gastric acid output was suppressed equally by both (potency ratio 0.6), as was gastrin release.

Somatostatin analogues that exhibit differential effects on suppression of growth hormone, glucagon, and insulin are under development [102]. This implies that cell receptors in different organs react with different parts of the molecule, a finding that may be important physiologically as well as pharmacologically. A mechanism whereby insulin secretagogues will induce translocation (recruitment) of somatostatin receptors during insulin exocytosis in the β cell has been proposed by Draznin et al [103] as a part of the paracrine feedback control exerted by somatostatin on the release of insulin.

Conflicting results have been reported on the action of somatostatin on pancreatic exocrine secretion. Early studies in dogs provided evidence that exogenous administration of pharmacologic doses of somatostatin resulted in a competitive inhibition of the action of secretin (but not CCK) on exocrine pancreatic secretion [104]. Somatostatin stimulates pancreatic secretion in rats when given as a bolus (the explanation was that the 5–8 position of the secretin molecule is the same as the 10–13 position of the somatostatin molecule, thus making it a weak agonist) [79]. There are several reports of failure to achieve inhibition of volume, bicarbonate, and/or protein secretion in humans, rats, dogs, and rabbits with secretin, CCK-8, and caerulein stimulation. The majority of studies demonstrate inhibition of protein, bicarbonate, and volume [79]. The effect of prolonged infusion of somatostatin on a patient with a pancreatic fistula of neoplastic origin was studied by Roncoroni et al [105], who found an 80 percent decrease in volume, a 40 percent decrease in bicarbonate, and no change in sodium, potassium, and calcium with an increase in amylase production.

Bile output is reduced by somatostatin [106]. Kaminski and Deshpande [107] found that somatostatin completely inhibited choleresis stimulated by release of endogenous secretin but did not alter the choleretic response to exogenous secretin. In dogs, the major effect of pharmacologic doses of somatostatin on hepatic bile flow is to enhance the ductular reabsorption of fluid and bicarbonate. Although the exact mechanism involved is unknown, somatostatin antagonizes the effect in the bile flow induced by secretin [108]. Somatostatin also had a slight inhibitory effect on taurocholate-stabilized hepatic bile flow, whereas it had no effect on CCK-stimulated bile flow [109]. Somatostatin modifies bile flow mainly by inhibiting the release of choleretic hormones.

Somatostatin selectively modulates peptide-induced smooth muscle contractility [110,111]. Somatostatin inhibited neurotensin- and caerulein-induced contraction of the in vitro guinea pig ileum, whereas it did not modify substance P-induced contraction. The underlying mechanism seems to be, at least in part, related to the release of acetylcholine from the myenteric plexus.

Gallbladder emptying and gastrointestinal motility are altered by somatostatin. Gastric emptying is delayed. Gallbladder emptying is impaired in vivo [79]. Somatostatin does not affect CCK-stimulated gallbladder strip contraction in vitro [112]. In fasting dogs, the frequency of the interdigestive myoelectric complex is doubled, whereas in fed animals, somatostatin caused a pattern similar to that seen in fasting animals [79].

The effects of somatostatin on gastroenteropancreatic functions are summarized in Table 21-2.

The beginning of migratory motor complex activity front in the duodenum of humans was found to correlate with plasma somatostatin peaks. Infusion of somatostatin in doses resulting in plasma levels comparable to those obtained postprandially caused complete inhibition of gastric motility and intestinal phase 2 (the period of irregular contractions) and stimulation of phase 3 (period of rhythmic contractions at maximal frequency). The interval between activity fronts was decreased by over 50 percent [113].

Endogenous somatostatin inhibits both basal and stimulated bicarbonate and epidermal growth factor secretion from the rat duodenal Brunner's gland [114]. Somatostatin inhibits the intestinal transport of ions, resulting in a diminished secretion [115]. Nutrient entry is substantially reduced. Somatostatin reverses the effect of prostaglandin E_1 (inhibition of water absorption) and theophylline (water secretion) in the rat jejunum [116]. The reduction of nutrient entry may be indirect (due to decreased gastric, biliary, or pancreatic secretion and decreased motility and decreased gastrointestinal hormone) or direct (by suppression of carrier mechanisms and function of the mucosal surface) [79]. Somatostatin and insulin might be considered antagonists in the complex process of nutrient intake, whereby insulin inhibits the release of somatostatin and somatostatin has a widespread inhibitory role on hormonal and exocrine secretions and absorption.

Somatostatin decreases splanchnic and portal blood flow selectively in dogs and humans (cirrhotics and normals) without affecting mucosal blood flow. Pharmacologic doses of somatostatin result in a 30 percent reduction of portal blood flow in conscious dogs [117], the organs of the upper gastrointestinal tract being the most suppressed. It slightly increases or has no effect on systemic hemodynamics [79,118,119].

There were early reports of altered hemostasis in baboons receiving somatostatin, but there have been no (or only clinically irrelevant) alterations in hemostasis reported in humans [120]. Somatostatin suppresses endotoxin-induced leukocytosis in humans [121]. Low-dose somatostatin decreases stimulated renin release [122]. In addition, somatostatin antagonizes the effect of ADH, the antidiuretic hormone [123]; the octapeptide analogue is an even more potent diuretic. Receptors for somatostatin have been identified in adrenocortical tissue [124].

Somatostatin has been reported to inhibit cell proliferation in vitro. This is a unique effect of a peptide hormone shared only by ACTH. Somatostatin decreased DNA incorporation of tritiated thymidine (^{3}H) in fundic, antral, duodenal, and jejunal mucosa, and it decreased cell division in antral and fundic mucosa; it also decreased gastrin-stimulated synthesis of DNA in fundic and antral mucosa and gastrin-stimulated cell division in fundic mucosa [125]. Somatostatin blocked epidermal growth factor-stimulated cell growth in gerbil fibroma and HeLa cells. Centrosomal separation was noted to be blocked [126].

In rats treated with secretin and caerulein, an inverse relationship between pancreatic somatostatin content and the degree of pancreatic growth was found, suggesting that pancreatic somatostatin may act locally as an antigrowth factor [127]. Further evidence on the physiologic role of somatostatin in regulating growth stimulation was obtained in lambs immunized against somatostatin at the age of 3 weeks. The rate of weight gain and the final height were greater in the immunized animals [128].

Preliminary data from Chrubasik et al [129] indicate that somatostatin acts as a potent analgesic when injected into the cerebrospinal fluid or epidural space. Somatostatin proved to be as effective as morphine, although its analgesic effect was not blocked by naloxone.

In summary, somatostatin is a molecularly heterogeneous peptide primarily found in the gastrointestinal tract. It has been found in paracrine, endocrine, and nerve cells. It is released postprandially and by a variety of other substances. Inhibition of release may be modulated by the parasympathetic, prostaglandin, or histamine systems. It acts in an entirely inhibitory fashion on multiple organ systems. Whether it functions as a hormone, as a paracrine agent, as a neurotransmitter, or in all of these capacities is uncertain and is a subject of debate.

Table 21-2. **Gastrointestinal and pancreatic functions inhibited by administration of somatostatin**

Organ	*Effect inhibited*
Mouth	Salivary secretion
Stomach	Motility, acid, pepsin, and intrinsic factor secretion
Exocrine pancreas	Bicarbonate and enzyme secretion
Gallbladder	Contraction
Small intestine	Motility, carbohydrate absorption
Splanchnic blood vessels	Blood flow
GI tract endocrine cells	Hormone release: gastrin, CCK, VIP, motilin, GIP, secretin
Endocrine pancreas	Hormone release: glucagon, insulin, PP

Source: Modified from Porte D Jr and Halter JB, in Williams RH (ed), *Textbook of Endocrinology.* 6th Ed. Philadelphia, WB Saunders Co, 1981, p. 751.

CLINICAL TRIALS

Peptic Ulcer Disease

There is much controversy concerning the mechanism by which somatostatin improves the outcome of patients with massive upper gastrointestinal hemorrhage [130]. The inhibitory effect of somatostatin on gastric acid and pepsin secretion appears to be the most likely route. In rats, the inhibitory action of somatostatin on gastric acid secretion is dissociated from its effect on gastric blood flow [131]. In several clinical trials, somatostatin reduced the number of patients needing surgery because of massive upper gastrointestinal bleeding [130,132].

Although depletion of somatostatin is not in itself sufficient to induce ulcer formation in rats, somatostatin tissue concentrations are cytoprotective against the ulcerogenic action of cysteamine [133,134]. Somatostatin may play a role in the pathogenesis of duodenal ulceration. A significant reduction in somatostatin content of the antral mucosa was found in patients with duodenal ulcer [135]. Sakamoto et al [136] found that elevated levels of antral somatostatin may account, at least in part, for the cytoprotective effect of pentagastrin and epidermal growth factor in stress-induced ulcers in rats.

Bleeding Esophageal Varices

Infusion of somatostatin selectively reduces hepatic blood flow and portal pressure in patients with cirrhosis of the liver and severe portal hypertension without altering systemic circulation [119]. The efficacy of somatostatin treatment in the control of acute variceal hemorrhage, although promising, is still a matter of controversy concerning doses and treatment schedules [137].

Pernicious Anemia

Antral content of gastrin and somatostatin was found similar in six controls and in five patients with pernicious anemia. However, fundic gastrin and somatostatin concentrations were higher in pernicious anemia patients, and this finding correlated with an increased number of fundic argyrophilic cells [138]. These patients had high gastrin levels and low somatostatin plasma levels, as expected.

Acute Pancreatitis

Somatostatin and the somatostatin analogue, SS 201-995, have proved useful in preventing some of the changes occurring in experimentally induced pancreatitis in rats, and a significant improvement was observed in rats with established pancreatitis when somatostatin or its analogue was given [139]. The results of somatostatin therapy in patients with pancreatitis are inconclusive [140,141].

Mean basal levels of plasma somatostatin were found to be higher in patients with chronic pancreatitis than in normal individuals and did not increase after insulin hypoglycemia [142]. Pancreatic exocrine and endocrine secretions were found to be less sensitive to the inhibitory action of exogenous somatostatin.

Fistulas

Somatostatin has been used for the treatment of gastrointestinal fistulas; however, a rebound effect after withdrawal has been observed [143]. We have used a somatostatin analogue to good effect in a small number of patients with high-output small bowel fistulas.

Intestinal Absorption

Somatostatin inhibits absorption of glucose and amino acids across the mucosa of the small bowel [144]. The secretory component of water and ions was greatly reduced in a patient with diarrhea caused by malignant carcinoid syndrome [145]. The underlying mechanism appears to be a blockade in cAMP action [116], although different investigators did not observe any change in cAMP or cGMP concentrations [146]. Suppression of diarrhea caused by endocrine tumors appears to be one of the most promising clinical uses of somatostatin.

Dumping Syndrome

Infusion of high doses of somatostatin reduced the symptoms of early dumping syndrome and prevented the hypoglycemia of late dumping syndrome [147,148]. In addition to preventing the secretion of water and electrolytes into the small bowel, somatostatin was found to inhibit plasma levels of neurotensin, VIP, GIP, and enteroglucagon [147].

Treatment of Tumors

Eight patients (one with carcinoid syndrome and seven with peptide-secreting pancreatic tumors) were given the long-acting somatostatin analogue after all conventional measures of treatment had failed. A fall in the increased plasma peptide levels was observed, in addition to an improvement in the patients' tumor-related symptoms [149,150] and a shrinkage of metastases [151].

Somatostatinoma (see Chapter 36)

A recent review of 11 previously reported cases of somatostatinoma [152] indicates that the pancreas was the primary site of a single lesion, ranging in size from 0.5 to 20 cm. The primary site was uncertain in the 12th case [152]. Among other locations, metastasis to the bone, liver, and kidney may occur. Six patients had gallbladder dysfunction, seven had diarrhea or steatorrhea, and diabetes was present in 10 and hypochlorhydria in three. The somatostatinoma is mainly considered as leading to an inhibitory syndrome. However, increased plasma levels of adrenocorticotropic hormone, insulin, and calcitonin are occasionally associated findings. A case of a nonfunctional somatostatinoma of the duodenum has recently been reported [153].

REFERENCES

1. Guillemin R, Gerich JE: Somatostatin: Physiological and clinical significance. Annu Rev Med 27:379, 1976.
2. Schally AV, Dupont A, Arimura A, et al: Isolation and structure of somatostatin from porcine hypothalami. Biochemistry 15:509, 1976.
3. Efendic S, Hokfelt T, Luft R: Somatostatin. Adv Metab Disord 9:367, 1978.
4. Guillemin R: Some thoughts on current research with somatostatin. Metabolism 27(Suppl 1):1453, 1978.
5. Bethge N, Diel F, Usadel KH: Somatostatin—A regulatory peptide of clinical importance. J Clin Chem Clin Biochem 20:603, 1982.
6. Shen L-P, Pictet RL, Rutter WJ: Human somatostatin I: Sequence of the cDNA. Proc Natl Acad Sci USA 79:4575, 1982.
7. Naylor SL, Sakaguchi AY, Shen L-P, et al: Polymorphic human somatostatin gene is located on chromosome 3. Proc Natl Acad Sci USA 80:2686, 1983.
8. Low MJ, Hammer RE, Goodman RH, et al: Tissue-specific post-translational processing of pre-prosomatostatin encoded by a metallothionein-somatostatin fusion gene in transgenic mice. Cell 41:211, 1985.
9. Esch FS, Bohlen P, Ling NC, et al: Primary structures of three human pancreas peptides with growth hormone-releasing activity. J Biol Chem 258:1806, 1983.
10. Guillemin R, Brazeau P, Bohlen P, et al: Growth hormone-releasing factor from a human pancreatic tumor that caused acromegaly. Science 218:585, 1982.
11. Rivier J, Spiess J, Thorner M, et al: Characterization of a growth hormone-releasing factor from a human pancreatic islet tumour. Nature 300:276, 1982.
12. Hilsted L, Holst JJ: On the accuracy of radioimmunological determination of somatostatin in plasma. Regul Pept 4:13, 1982.
13. Patel YC, Zingg HH, Fitz-Patrick D, et al: Somatostatin: Some aspects of its physiology and pathophysiology, in Bloom SR, Polak JM (eds): *Gut Hormones.* 2nd Ed. New York, Churchill Livingstone, 1981, pp 339–349.
14. Larsson L-I: Somatostatin cells, in Bloom SR, Polak JM (eds): *Gut Hormones.* 2nd Ed. New York, Churchill Livingstone, 1981, pp 350–353.
15. McIntosh C, Arnold R, Bothe E, et al: Gastrointestinal somatostatin: Extraction and radioimmunoassay in different species. Gut 19:655, 1978.
16. Chayvialle J-A, Miyata M, Rayford PL, et al: Immunoreactive somatostatin and vasoactive intestinal peptide in the digestive tract of cats. Gastroenterology 79:837, 1980.
17. Larsson LI, Goltermann N, De Magistris L, et al: Somatostatin cell processes as pathways for paracrine secretion. Science 205:1393, 1979.
18. Buchan AMJ, Sikora LKJ, Levy JG, et al: An immunocytochemical investigation with monoclonal antibodies to somatostatin. Histochemistry 83:175, 1985.
19. Gu J, Polak JM, Probert L, et al: Peptidergic innervation of the human male genital tract. J Urol 130:386, 1983.
20. Lundberg JM, Hamberger B, Schultzberg M, et al: Enkephalin- and somatostatin-like immunoreactivities in human adrenal medulla and pheochromocytoma. Proc Natl Acad Sci USA 76:4079, 1979.
21. Ito S, Iwanaga T, Yamada Y, et al: Somatostatin-28 like immunoreactivity in the human gut. Horm Metab Res 14:500, 1982.
22. Ito S, Yamada Y, Iwanaga T, et al: Presence of somatostatin-28 like immunoreactivity in the human pancreas. Life Sci 30:1707, 1982.
23. Ito S, Yamada Y, Suzuki T, et al: Somatostatin-28-like immunoreactivity in the stomach. Tohoku J Exp Med 138:313, 1982.
24. Penman E, Wass JAH, Butler MG, et al: Distribution and characterisation of immunoreactive somatostatin in human gastrointestinal tract. Regul Pept 7:53, 1983.
25. Ravazzola M, Benoit R, Ling N, et al: Immunocytochemical localization of prosomatostatin fragments maturing and mature secretory granules of pancreatic and gastrointestinal D cells. Proc Natl Acad Sci USA 80:215, 1983.
26. Wasada T, Dobbs RE, Harris V, et al: Effect of 2-deoxy-D-glucose on plasma somatostatin levels in conscious dogs. Endocrinology 108:1222, 1981.
27. Chayvialle JA, Rayford PL, Thompson JC: Radioimmunoassay study of hepatic clearance and disappearance half-time of somatostatin and vasoactive intestinal peptide in dogs. Gut 22:732, 1981.
28. Schusdziarra V, Harris V, Conlon JM, et al: Pancreatic and gastric somatostatin release in response

to intragastric and intraduodenal nutrients and HCl in the dog. J Clin Invest 62:509, 1978.
29. Chayvialle J-A, Miyata M, Rayford PL, et al: Effects of test meal, intragastric nutrients, and intraduodenal bile on plasma concentrations of immunoreactive somatostatin and vasoactive intestinal peptide in dogs. Gastroenterology 79:844, 1980.
30. Boden G, Master RW, Sattler MA, et al: Adrenergic control of somatostatin release. Endocrinology 111:1166, 1982.
31. Polonsky KS, Shoelson SE, Docherty HM: Plasma somatostatin 28 increases in response to feeding in man. J Clin Invest 71:1514, 1983.
32. Conlon JM, Bridgeman M, Alberti KGMM: The nature of big plasma somatostatin: Implications for the measurement of somatostatin-like immunoreactivity in human plasma. Anal Biochem 125:243, 1982.
33. Patel YC, Wheatley T: *In vivo* and *in vitro* plasma disappearance and metabolism of somatostatin-28 and somatostatin-14 in the rat. Endocrinology 112:220, 1983.
34. Schusdziarra V, Harris V, Unger RH: Half-life of somatostatin-like immunoreactivity in canine plasma. Endocrinology 104:109, 1979.
35. Sacks HS, Terry LC, Wright RK, et al: Somatostatin metabolism: Differences in clearance of N-terminal and central portions of molecule during perfusion of rat liver. Am J Physiol 246:G226, 1984.
36. Vaysse N, Pradayrol L, Susini C, et al: Somatostatin 28: Biological actions, in Bloom SR, Polak JM (eds): *Gut Hormones.* 2nd Ed. New York, Churchill Livingstone, 1981, pp 358–361.
37. Polonsky K, Jaspan J, Berelowitz M, et al: The *in vivo* metabolism of somatostatin 28: Possible relationship between diminished metabolism and enhanced biological action. Endocrinology 111:1698, 1982.
38. Bethge N, Diel F, Rosick M, et al: Somatostatin half-life: A case report in one healthy volunteer and a three month follow-up. Horm Metab Res 13:709, 1981.
39. Bauer W, Briner U, Doepfner W, et al: SMS 201-995: A very potent and selective octapeptide analogue of somatostatin with prolonged action. Life Sci 31:1133, 1982.
40. Seno M, Seino Y, Takemura Y, et al: Comparison of somatostatin-28 and somatostatin-14 clearance by the perfused rat liver. Can J Physiol Pharmacol 63:62, 1985.
41. Ruggere MD, Patel YC: Hepatic metabolism of somatostatin-14 and somatostatin-28: Immunochemical characterization of the metabolic fragments and comparison of cleavage sites. Endocrinology 117:88, 1985.
42. Webb S, Kravetz D, Bosch J, et al: Splanchnic and hepatic metabolism of somatostatin: A study in cirrhotic patients with a portacaval shunt. Hepatology 3:193, 1983.
43. Koshimizu T, Ohyama Y, Yokota Y, et al: Peripheral plasma concentrations of somatostatin-like immunoreactivity in newborns and infants. J Clin Endocrinol Metab 61:78, 1985.
44. Schusdziarra V, Zyznar E, Rouiller D: Splanchnic somatostatin: A hormonal regulator of nutrient homeostasis. Science 207:530, 1980.
45. Schusdziarra V, Unger RH: Physiology and pathophysiology of circulating somatostatin in dogs, in Bloom SR, Polak JM (eds): *Gut Hormones.* 2nd Ed, New York, Churchill Livingstone, 1981, pp 366–370.
46. Schusdziarra V, Rouiller D, Harris V, et al: Gastric and pancreatic release of somatostatin-like immunoreactivity during the gastric phase of a meal. Effects of truncal vagotomy and atropine in the anesthetized dog. Diabetes 28:658, 1979.
47. Souquet JC, Rambliere R, Riou JP, et al: Hormonal and metabolic effects of near physiological increase of plasma immunoreactive somatostatin 14. J Clin Endocrinol Metab 56:1076, 1983.
48. Beylot M, Chayvialle JA, Riou JP, et al: Regulation of somatostatin secretion in man: Study of the role of free fatty acids and ketone bodies. Metabolism 33:988, 1984.
49. Sirek A, Vaitkus P, Norwich KH, et al: Secretory patterns of glucoregulatory hormones in prehepatic circulation of dogs. Am J Physiol 249:E34, 1985.
50. Jorde R, Burhol PG: Diurnal profiles of gastrointestinal regulatory peptides. Scand J Gastroenterol 20:1, 1985.
51. Schusdziarra V, Rouiller D, Arimura A, et al: Antisomatostatin serum increases levels of hormones from the pituitary and gut, but not from the pancreas. Endocrinology 103:1956, 1978.
52. Aponte G, Gross D, Yamada T: Capillary orientation of rat pancreatic D-cell processes: Evidence for endocrine release of somatostatin. Am J Physiol 249:G599, 1985.
53. Konturek SJ, Kwiecien N, Obtulowicz W, et al: Effects of somatostatin-14 and somatostatin-28 on plasma hormonal and gastric secretory responses to cephalic and gastrointestinal stimulation in man. Scand J Gastroenterol 20:31, 1985.
54. de Graef J, Woussen-Colle MC: Effects of sham feeding, bethanechol, and bombesin on somatostatin release in dogs. Am J Physiol 248:G1, 1985.
55. Beglinger C, Ribes G, Whitehouse I, et al: Effect of exocrine pancreatic secretagogues on circulating somatostatin in dogs. Am J Physiol 250:G15, 1986.
56. Guzman S, Chayvialle J-A, Banks WA, et al: Effect of vagal stimulation on pancreatic secretion and on blood levels of gastrin, cholecystokinin, secretin, vasoactive intestinal peptide, and somatostatin. Surgery 86:329, 1979.
57. Lucey MR, Wass JAH, Fairclough P, et al: Autonomic regulation of postprandial plasma somatostatin, gastrin, and insulin. Gut 26:683, 1985.
58. Schusdziarra V, Rouiller D, Harris V, et al: Effect of bombesin upon plasma somatostatin-like immunoreactivity, insulin and glucagon in normal and chemically sympathectomized dogs. Regul Pept 1:89, 1980.

59. Rouiller D, Schusdziarra V, Conlon JM, et al: Release of somatostatin-like immunoreactivity from the lower gut. Gastroenterology 77:700, 1979.
60. Hermansen K: Somatostatin secretion from the isolated perfused dog ileum. Endocrinology 117:287, 1985.
61. Lucey MR, Wass JAH, Fairclough PD, et al: Does gastric acid release plasma somatostatin in man? Gut 25:1217, 1984.
62. Webb S, Levy I, Wass JAH, et al: Studies on the mechanisms of somatostatin release after insulin induced hypoglycaemia in man. Clin Endocrinol 21:667, 1984.
63. Guzman S, Lonovics J, Chayvialle J-A, et al: Effects of gastrin on circulating levels of somatostatin, pancreatic polypeptide, and vasoactive intestinal peptide in dogs. Endocrinology 107:231, 1980.
64. Kwok YN, McIntosh CHS, Pederson RA, et al: Effect of substance P on somatostatin release from the isolated perfused rat stomach. Gastroenterology 88:90, 1985.
65. Koop H, Arnold R: Serotoninergic control of somatostatin and gastrin release from the isolated rat stomach. Regul Pept 9:101, 1984.
66. McIntosh C, Bakich V, Trotter T, et al: Effect of cysteamine on secretion of gastrin and somatostatin from the rat stomach. Gastroenterology 86:834, 1984.
67. Sue R, Toomey ML, Todisco A, et al: Pirenzepine-sensitive muscarinic receptors regulate gastric somatostatin and gastrin. Am J Physiol 248:G184, 1985.
68. Schusdziarra V, Rouiller D, Jaffe BM, et al: Effect of exogenous and endogenous prostaglandin E upon gastric endocrine function in dogs. Endocrinology 106:1620, 1980.
69. Nishi S, Seino Y, Seino S, et al: Different effects of prostaglandin E_1, E_2 and D_2 on pancreatic somatostatin release. Horm Metab Res 16(Suppl 1):114, 1984.
70. Schusdziarra V, Rouiller D, Harris V, et al: Effect of prostaglandin E_2 upon release of pancreatic somatostatin-like immunoreactivity. Life Sci 28:2099, 1981.
71. Dettori-Gera C, Ronner P, Scarpa A: Difference in dose-response curves for glucose-induced insulin and somatostatin release in rat pancreas. Biochim Biophys Acta 839:281, 1985.
72. Werner H, Amarant T, Millar RP, et al: Immunoreactive and biologically active somatostatin in human and sheep milk. Eur J Biochem 148:353, 1985.
73. Arimura A, Fishback JB: Somatostatin: Regulation of secretion. Neuroendocrinology 33:246, 1981.
74. Konturek S, Tasler J, Cieszkowski M, et al: Studies on the inhibition of pancreatic secretion by luminal somatostatin. Am J Physiol 241:G109, 1981.
75. Limberg B, Kommerell B: Influence of a continuous intragastric and intravenous infusion of somatostatin on stimulated gastric secretion. Res Exp Med 183:153, 1983.
76. Ertan A, Arimura A, Akdamar K, et al: Pancreatic immunoreactive somatostatin and diabetes mellitus. Dig Dis Sci 29:625, 1984.
77. Schusdziarra V: Somatostatin—Physiological and pathophysiological aspects. Scand J Gastroenterol 18(Suppl 83):69, 1983.
78. Konturek SJ, Tasler J, Jaworek J, et al: Gastrointestinal secretory, motor, circulatory, and metabolic effects of prosomatostatin. Proc Natl Acad Sci USA 78:1967, 1981.
79. Arnold R, Lankisch PG: Somatostatin and the gastrointestinal tract. Clinics Gastroenterol 9:733, 1980.
80. Hirst BH, Coy DH: Structure-activity studies with somatostatin: Role of lysine in positions 4 and 9 for gastric activity. Regul Pept 8:267, 1984.
81. Johansson C, Aly A: Stimulation of gastric mucus output by somatostatin in man. Eur J Clin Invest 12:37, 1982.
82. Bloom SR, Mortimer CH, Thorner MO, et al: Inhibition of gastrin and gastric-acid secretion by growth-hormone release-inhibiting hormone. Lancet 2:1106, 1974.
83. Gomez-Pan A, Albinus M, Reed JD, et al: Direct inhibition of gastric acid and pepsin secretion by growth-hormone release-inhibiting hormone in cats. Lancet 1:888, 1975.
84. Ladegaard L, Bech K, Andersen D: Effect of somatostatin on bethanechol-stimulated gastric pepsin secretion in gastric fistula in dogs. Scand J Gastroenterol 20:87, 1985.
85. Lafontaine M, Cadiere G-B, Woussen-Colle M-C, et al: Interactions entre la secretine et la somatostatine sur la secretion acide et la vidange gastrique chez le chien. Gastroenterol Clin Biol 8:343, 1984.
86. Loud FB, Holst JJ, Egense E, et al: Is somatostatin a humoral regulator of the endocrine pancreas and gastric acid secretion in man? Gut 26:445, 1985.
87. Guijarro LG, Arilla E, Lopez-Ruiz MP, et al: Somatostatin binding sites in cytosolic fraction isolated from rabbit antral and fundic gastric mucosa. Regul Pept 10:207, 1985.
88. Lopez-Ruiz MP, Arilla E, Gonzalez-Guijarro L, et al: Somatostatin binding sites in cytosolic fraction of rabbit intestinal mucosa: Distribution throughout the intestinal tract. Comp Biochem Physiol 81B:1041, 1985.
89. Saffouri B, Weir GC, Bitar KN, et al: Gastrin and somatostatin secretion by perfused rat stomach: Functional linkage of antral peptides. Am J Physiol 238:G495, 1980.
90. Soll AH, Amirian DA, Park J, et al: Cholecystokinin potently releases somatostatin from canine fundic mucosal cells in short-term culture. Am J Physiol 248:G569, 1985.
91. Patel YC, Pierzchala I: Cysteamine induces a loss of tissue somatostatin-28 when measured as somatostatin-28(15-28)-like immunoreactivity but not when assessed as somatostatin-28(1-14)-like immunoreactivity: Evidence for the importance of the disulfide bond for cysteamine action. Endocrinology 116:1699, 1985.

92. Harty RF, Maico DG, McGuigan JE: Postreceptor inhibition of antral gastrin release by somatostatin. Gastroenterology 88:675, 1985.
93. Ligumsky M, Goto Y, Debas H, et al: Prostaglandins mediate inhibition of gastric acid secretion by somatostatin in the rat. Science 219:301, 1983.
94. Mogard MH, Kauffman GL Jr, Pehlevanian M, et al: Prostaglandins may not mediate inhibition of gastric acid secretion by somatostatin in the rat. Regul Pept 10:231, 1985.
95. Albinus M, Gomez-Pan A, Hirst BH, et al: Evidence against prostaglandin-mediation of somatostatin-inhibition of gastric secretions. Regul Pept 10:259, 1985.
96. Mogard MH, Maxwell V, Kovacs T, et al: Somatostatin inhibits gastric acid secretion after gastric mucosal prostaglandin synthesis inhibition by indomethacin in man. Gut 26:1189, 1985.
97. Lins PE, Efendic S, Hall K: Effect of 24-hour somatostatin infusion on glucose homeostasis and on the levels of somatomedin A and pancreatic and thyroid hormones in man. Acta Med Scand 206:441, 1979.
98. Williams GA, Hargis GK, Ensinck JW, et al: Role of endogenous somatostatin in the secretion of parathyroid hormone and calcitonin. Metabolism 28:950, 1979.
99. Ferland L, Labrie F, Jobin M, et al: Physiological role of somatostatin in the control of growth hormone and thyrotropin in secretion. Biochem Biophys Res Commun 68:149, 1976.
100. Klaff LJ, Barron JL, Levitt NS, et al: Inhibition of pancreatic hormone secretion by somatostatin-28 and somatostatin-14 in man. Acta Endocrinol 104:91, 1983.
101. Marco J, Correas I, Zulueta MA, et al: Inhibitory effect of somatostatin-28 on pancreatic polypeptide, glucagon and insulin secretion in normal man. Horm Metab Res 15:363, 1983.
102. Wajchenberg BL, Cesar FP, Leme CE, et al: Dissociated effects of somatostatin analogs on arginine-induced insulin, glucagon and growth hormone release in acromegalic patients. Horm Metab Res 15:471, 1983.
103. Draznin B, Leitner JW, Sussman KE: A unique control mechanism in the regulation of insulin secretion. Secretagogue-induced somatostatin receptor recruitment. J Clin Invest 75:1510, 1985.
104. Konturek SJ, Tasler J, Obtułowicz W, et al: Effect of growth hormone-release inhibiting hormone on hormones stimulating exocrine pancreatic secretion. J Clin Invest 58:1, 1976.
105. Roncoroni L, Violi V, Montanari M, et al: Effect of somatostatin on exocrine pancreas evaluated on a total external pancreatic fistula of neoplastic origin. Am J Gastroenterol 78:425, 1983.
106. Holm I, Thulin L, Samnegard H, et al: Anticholeretic effect of somatostatin in anesthetized dogs. Acta Physiol Scand 104:241, 1978.
107. Kaminski DL, Deshpande YG: Effect of somatostatin and bombesin on secretin-stimulated ductular bile flow in dogs. Gastroenterology 85:1239, 1983.
108. Rene E, Danzinger RG, Hofmann AF, et al: Pharmacologic effect of somatostatin on bile formation in the dog. Enhanced ductular reabsorption as the major mechanism of anticholeresis. Gastroenterology 84:120, 1983.
109. Magnusson I, Thulin L, Einarsson K, et al: Effects of substance P and somatostatin on taurocholate-stabilized and CCK- or secretin-induced choleresis in the anesthetized dog. Scand J Gastroenterol 19:1007, 1984.
110. Teitelbaum DH, O'Dorisio TM, Perkins WE, et al: Somatostatin modulation of peptide-induced acetylcholine release in guinea pig ileum. Am J Physiol 246:G509, 1984.
111. Jørgensen KD, Diamant B: Inhibitory effect of aprotinin on gastric acid secretion. Scand J Gastroenterol 19:999, 1984.
112. Lonovics J, Devitt P, Guzman S, et al: Actions of VIP, somatostatin, and pancreatic polypeptide on gallbladder tension and CCK-stimulated gallbladder contraction in vitro. Surg Forum 30:407, 1979.
113. Peeters TL, Janssens J, Vantrappen GR: Somatostatin and the interdigestive migrating motor complex in man. Regul Pept 5:209, 1983.
114. Kirkegaard P, Olsen PS, Nexø E, et al: Effect of vasoactive intestinal polypeptide and somatostatin on secretion of epidermal growth factor and bicarbonate from Brunner's glands. Gut 25:1225, 1984.
115. Donowitz M, Wicks J, Cusolito S, et al: Pharmacotherapy of diarrheal diseases: An approach based on physiologic principles, in Donowitz M, Sharp GWS (eds): *Mechanisms of Intestinal Electrolyte Transport and Regulation by Calcium.* New York, Alan R. Liss, 1984, pp 329–359.
116. Dharmsathaphorn K, Sherwin RS, Dobbins JW: Somatostatin inhibits fluid secretion in the rat jejunum. Gastroenterology 78:1554, 1980.
117. Price BA, Jaffe BM, Zinner MJ: Effect of exogenous somatostatin infusion on gastrointestinal blood flow and hormones in the conscious dog. Gastroenterology 88:80, 1985.
118. Tyden G, Samnegard H, Thulin L, et al: Circulatory effects of somatostatin in anesthetized man. Acta Chir Scand 145:443, 1979.
119. Bosch J, Kravetz D, Rodes J: Effects of somatostatin on hepatic and systemic hemodynamics in patients with cirrhosis of the liver: Comparison with vasopressin. Gastroenterology 80:518, 1981.
120. Mielke CH, Rodvien R: Somatostatin: Influence on hemostasis—A review. Metabolism 27(Suppl 1):1369, 1978.
121. Wagner H, Zierden E, Hauss WH: Effects of synthetic somatostatin on endotoxin-induced changes of growth hormone, cortisol and insulin in plasma, blood sugar and blood leukocytes in man. Klin Wochenschr 53:539, 1975.
122. Izumi Y, Honda M, Hatano M: Effect of somatostatin on plasma renin activity. Endocrinol Jpn 26:389, 1979.
123. Mountokalakis T, Levy M: Effect of a selective octapeptide analogue of somatostatin on renal water excretion in the dog. Metabolism 34:408, 1985.

124. Srikant CB, Patel YC: Somatostatin receptors in the rat adrenal cortex: Characterization and comparison with brain and pituitary receptors. Endocrinology 116:1717, 1985.
125. Lehy T, Dubrasquet M, Bonfils S: Effect of somatostatin on normal and gastric-stimulated cell proliferation in the gastric and intestinal mucosae of the rat. Digestion 19:99, 1979.
126. Mascardo RN, Sherline P: Somatostatin inhibits rapid centrosomal separation and cell proliferation induced by epidermal growth factor. Endocrinology 111:1394, 1982.
127. Sarfati PD, Genik P, Morisset J: Caerulein and secretin induced pancreatic growth: A possible control by endogenous pancreatic somatostatin. Regul Pept 11:263, 1985.
128. Spencer GSG, Garssen GJ, Hart IC: A novel approach to growth promotion using auto-immunisation against somatostatin. I. Effects on growth and hormone levels in lambs. Livestock Prod Sci 10:25, 1983.
129. Chrubasik J, Meynadier J, Blond S, et al: Somatostatin, a potent analgesic. Lancet 2:1208, 1984.
130. Magnusson I, Ihre T, Johansson C, et al: Randomised double blind trial of somatostatin in the treatment of massive upper gastrointestinal haemorrhage. Gut 26:221, 1985.
131. Leung FW, Guth PH: Dissociated effects of somatostatin on gastric acid secretion and mucosal blood flow. Am J Physiol 248:G337, 1985.
132. Kayasseh L, Keller U, Gyr K, et al: Somatostatin and cimetidine in peptic-ulcer haemorrhage. Lancet 1:844, 1980.
133. Szabo S, Reichlin S: Somatostatin depletion of the gut and pancreas induced by cysteamine is not prevented by vagotomy or by dopamine agonists. Regul Pept 6:43, 1983.
134. Szabo S, Usadel KH: Cytoprotection—organoprotection by somatostatin: Gastric and hepatic lesions. Experientia 38:254, 1982.
135. Chayvialle JAP, Descos F, Bernard C, et al: Somatostatin in mucosa of stomach and duodenum in gastroduodenal disease. Gastroenterology 75:13, 1978.
136. Sakamoto T, Swierczek JS, Ogden WD, et al: Cytoprotective effect of pentagastrin and epidermal growth factor on stress ulcer formation. Ann Surg 201:290, 1985.
137. Jenkins SA, Baxter JN, Corbett W, et al: Efficacy of somatostatin and vasopressin in the control of acute variceal hemorrhage. Hepatology 5:344, 1985.
138. Magnusson I, Cho J-W, Ihre T, et al: Gastrin and somatostatin in plasma and gastric biopsy specimens in pernicious anemia. Scand J Gastroenterol 20:623, 1985.
139. Baxter JN, Jenkins SA, Day DW, et al: Effects of somatostatin and a long-acting somatostatin analogue on the prevention and treatment of experimentally induced acute pancreatitis in the rat. Br J Surg 72:382, 1985.
140. Limberg B, Kommerell B: Treatment of acute pancreatitis with somatostatin. N Engl J Med 303:284, 1980.
141. Usadel K-H, Leuschner U, Uberla KK: Treatment of acute pancreatitis with somatostatin: A multicenter double-blind trial. N Engl J Med 303:999, 1980.
142. Czyzyk A, Szadkowski M, Muszynski J: Reduced inhibitory effect of somatostatin on the exocrine function of the pancreas and on serum insulin (IRI) levels in chronic relapsing pancreatitis. Horm Metab Res 16:155, 1984 (Suppl.).
143. Reasbeck PG: Somatostatin treatment of gastrointestinal fistulas: Evidence for a rebound effect on withdrawal. Aust NZ J Surg 54:465, 1984.
144. Krejs GJ, Browne R, Raskin P: Effect of intravenous somatostatin on jejunal absorption of glucose, amino acids, water, and electrolytes. Gastroenterology 78:26, 1980.
145. Davis GR, Camp RC, Raskin P, et al: Effect of somatostatin infusion on jejunal water and electrolyte transport in a patient with secretory diarrhea due to malignant carcinoid syndrome. Gastroenterology 78:346, 1980.
146. Guandalini S, Kachur JF, Smith PL, et al: In vitro effects of somatostatin on ion transport in rabbit intestine. Am J Physiol 238:G67, 1980.
147. Long RG, Adrian TE, Bloom SR: Somatostatin and the dumping syndrome. Br Med J 290:886, 1985.
148. Reasbeck PG, van Rij AM: Somatostatin and the dumping syndrome. Br Med J 290:1147, 1985.
149. Wood SM, Kraenzlin ME, Adrian TE, Bloom SR: Treatment of patients with pancreatic endocrine tumours using a new long-acting somatostatin analogue: Symptomatic and peptide responses. Gut 26:438, 1985.
150. Maton PN, O'Dorisio TM, Howe BA, et al: Effect of a long-acting somatostatin analogue (SMS 201-995) in a patient with pancreatic cholera. N Engl J Med 312:17, 1985.
151. Kraenzlin ME, Ch'ng JLC, Wood SM, et al: Long-term treatment of a VIPoma with somatostatin analogue resulting in remission of symptoms and possible shrinkage of metastases. Gastroenterology 88:185, 1985.
152. Reynolds C, Pratt R, Chan-Yan C, et al: Somatostatinoma—The most recently described pancreatic islet cell tumor. West J Med 142:393, 1985.
153. Chen R, Tang C-K, Lee JY-Y, et al: Duodenal somatostatin-containing tumor with psammoma bodies. Hum Pathol 16:517, 1985.

Chapter 22

Neurotensin

R. Daniel Beauchamp, M.D., and Courtney M. Townsend, Jr., M.D.

HISTORY

Neurotensin (NT) was discovered by Carraway and Leeman in 1973 [1] as a byproduct during purification of substance P from bovine hypothalamus. NT was found to produce vasodilation and hypotension when injected into rats. The amino acid sequence of NT (pGlu-Leu-Tyr-Glu-Asn-Lys-Pro-Arg-Arg-Pro-Tyr-Ile-Leu-OH; molecular weight 1673), its synthesis, and a specific radioimmunoassay were reported shortly thereafter [2–4].

DISTRIBUTION

The distribution of NT has been studied extensively. An immunohistochemically identical substance was subsequently isolated from rat, bovine, and human intestine as well as from a rat cell line of medullary thyroid carcinoma [5]. Intestinal- and tumor-produced NT is indistinguishable from that found in the brain. Over 90 percent of NT occurs outside the central nervous system (CNS), largely in the small intestine [6]. Although there are detectable levels in the esophagus, stomach, duodenum, and colon, the vast majority of NT in rats, dogs [7–11], and in humans [12,13] is found in the small bowel, with the greatest amount in the ileum and somewhat less in the jejunum [6]. NT cells, which appear to be true endocrine cells (called N cells), have been identified in the small intestine of humans and animals by immunohistochemical techniques [10]. NT is stored in large granules concentrated in the basal portion of N cells. The microvilli of N cells may contain receptors which, after contact with contents of the gut lumen, regulate the secretion of NT from N cells [14]. The major stored form of NT is $NT^{1\text{-}13}$ [1,15].

ASSAY

The original assays for NT described by Carraway and Leeman [1] were bioassays that measured the in vivo vascular response to NT injected into rats and the in vitro contractile responses of smooth muscle of rat uterus, duodenum, and guinea pig ileum. The in vivo responses observed included vasodilatation, cyanosis, hypotension, and increased vascular permeability. These characteristic responses were not altered by adrenalectomy, hypophysectomy, or prior administration of atropine, phenoxybenzamine, or propranolol. Smooth muscle responses in vivo demonstrated that NT was as potent as bradykinin in its effects on guinea pig ileum and rat duodenum and only one fifth as potent as bradykinin on rat uterus; again, these effects were not mediated by acetylcholine, serotonin, histamine, or α- or β-adrenergic receptors.

Carraway and Leeman [4] later developed, characterized, and validated a radioimmunoassay that allowed direct measurement of NT extracted from hypothalamic tissue. They used NT diester protein conjugates in order to immunize rabbits. Three antisera were described, two of which were directed exclusively toward the biologically active COOH-terminal, while the third required the intact molecule (with both the NH_2- and COOH-terminals) for binding.

Radioimmunoassay (RIA) and biologic assays [16] and later amino acid sequencing [17] have shown that NT isolated from the mammalian intestinal tract is identical to NT originally isolated from bovine hypothalamus, and that it is also identical to synthetic NT.

Biologic reactivity apparently depends upon the COOH-terminal of the NT molecule [4]. $NT^{2\text{-}13}$

has 100 percent of the biologic activity of NT^{1-13}, whereas NT^{8-13} exhibits only 55 percent as much. NT^{1-9} has less than 0.2 percent activity [4] (Table 22-1).

Neurotensin-like radioimmunoreactivity detected in postprandial plasma has been shown by high pressure liquid chromatography (HPLC) to be composed predominantly of biologically inactive N-terminal fragments 1–8 and 1–11 [18,19]. Therefore, it is important to ensure that a radioimmunoassay specifically detects the biologically active intact NT molecule in plasma before attributing any observed physiologic effects to released hormone detected by RIA. Considerable controversy has arisen regarding the ability of different RIAs to achieve the goal of measuring only biologically active NT.

Shaw and Buchanan [20] have reported detection of intact NT^{1-13} in stomach extracts of human plasma following a meal. Theodorsson-Norheim [21] detected increases in intact NT^{1-13} in unextracted human and rat plasma obtained after fat ingestion by use of a radioimmunoassay with an antiserum specific for the intact NT^{1-13} molecule; the results were verified by ion-exchange chromatography.

Draviam et al [22] in our laboratory have developed an HPLC-RIA method for the separation and quantitation of NT and NT fragments from plasma and tissue extracts. The retention times for authentic NT^{1-13} and NT^{1-8}, NT^{1-11}, NT^{4-13}, and NT^{8-13} were characterized as 19.8, 11.1, 14.3, 16.0, and 16.4 minutes (Figure 22-1). Plasma NT and NT fragments are determined after extraction on C-18 SepPak (Waters Associates, Millipore Corp, Milford, Mass). The SepPaks are prepared by sequential washing with acetonitrile and 0.05 M ammonium acetate (pH 5.5). Plasma is then added and washed out with ammonium acetate. NT is eluted from the SepPak with 3 mL of 1:1 ratio of acetonitrile/ammonium acetate. The extracts are then dried under nitrogen and reconstituted in water. The extracts were subjected to HPLC separation using a stepped gradient of 0.5 percent trifluoroacetic acid (TFA) in water and acetonitrile, and 1 mL fractions were collected. HPLC fractions were quantitated using region-specific NT antisera. A double-antibody radioimmunoassay that uses antineurotensin antiserum raised in rabbits has been developed in our laboratory [23].

PHARMACOKINETICS AND CATABOLISM

Several investigators have examined the clearance of NT in the CNS [24–26] and in the periphery [27,28]. Physiologically inactive, circulating fragments (NT^{1-8}), as well as the active whole molecule (NT^{1-13}), were measured in plasma after ingestion of fat [20,29]. Blackburn et al [30] infused NT into humans and found that the half-life was 3.8 ± 0.02 min, the metabolic clearance rate was 16 ± 1 mL/kg/min, and the space of distribution was 88 ± 6 mL/kg.

In normal humans, after a 75-minute infusion of NT^{1-13}, HPLC analysis has shown that 80 percent of the total immunoreactivity was present as N-ter-

Table 22-1. **Biologic activity of NT and its partial sequence**

Peptide	*Percent biologic activity**
<Glu-Leu-Tyr-Glu-Asn-Lys-Pro-Arg-Arg-Pro-Tyr-Ile-Leu-OH	100
H-Leu-Tyr-Glu-Asn-Lys-Pro-Arg-Arg-Pro-Tyr-Ile-Leu-OH	100
H-Glu-Asn-Lys-Pro-Arg-Arg-Pro-Tyr-Ile-Leu-OH	25
H-Lys-Pro-Arg-Arg-Pro-Tyr-Ile-Leu-OH	20
H-Arg-Arg-Pro-Tyr-Ile-Leu-OH	55
H-Arg-Pro-Tyr-Ile-Leu-OH	1
H-Pro-Tyr-Ile-Leu-OH	<0.1
H-Tyr-Ile-Leu-OH	<0.1
H-Ile-Leu-OH	<0.1
<Glu-Leu-Tyr-Glu-Asn-Lys-Pro-Arg-Arg-Pro-Tyr-Ile-Leu-NH_2	<1
<Glu-Leu-Tyr-Glu-Asn-Lys-Pro-Arg-Pro-OH	<0.2
<Glu-Leu-Tyr-OH	<0.01

* = as determined by the hyperglycemic response in rats. (Modified from Carraway and Leeman [4].)

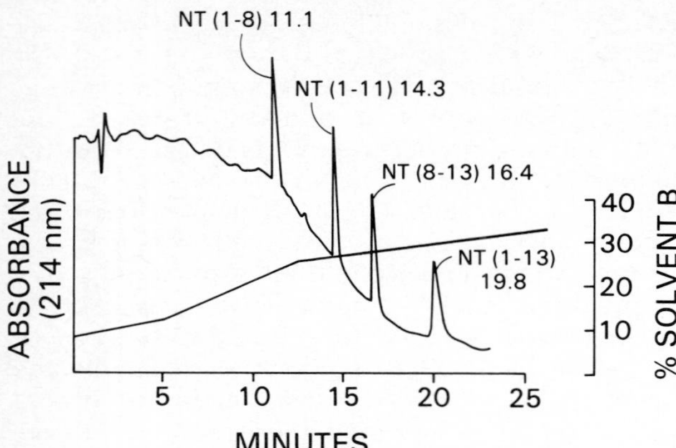

Figure 22-1. HPLC separation of a standard mixture of neurotensin and neurotensin fragments. The solid line extending from the left to the right border represents the HPLC solvent gradient. The peaks represent the UV absorbance of neurotensin and its fragments. Solvent A = 0.05% trifluoroacetic acid in HPLC gradient water; Solvent B = 1:9 Solvent A divided by acetonitrile.) (From Draviam E [22], by permission of The American College of Surgeons.)

minal fragments. In plasma from patients with chronic renal failure, only 40 percent of NT was present as N-terminal fragments; the remainder was $NT^{1\text{-}13}$. In addition, the plasma half-life of the C-terminal immunoreactivity was much longer in patients with chronic renal failure. These findings suggest a role for the kidney in the metabolic clearance of NT; however, in the same report, the authors found that NT was equally degraded in plasma obtained from normal individuals and from patients with chronic renal failure [19,31]. We have detected release of $NT^{1\text{-}13}$ and of fragments of NT by HPLC after ID administration of Lipomul in dogs [22].

RELEASE

In anesthetized dogs, in situ perfusion of the terminal ileum with buffered solution combined with simultaneous collection of blood from the carotid artery, femoral vein, and mesenteric vein draining the terminal ileum [32] produced a positive arteriovenous difference in plasma NT levels. On the other hand, Fujimura et al [33] have found that direct instillation of Lipomul into the isolated ileum does not cause NT release in conscious dogs, whereas infusion into isolated jejunal segments does produce elevated portal vein plasma NT levels. Similar findings have been reported in humans [34]. Ileal infusion of Intralipid significantly delayed small bowel transit time but did not cause significant elevation of peripheral plasma levels of NT. On the other hand, jejunal infusion of Intralipid had no effect on small bowel transit but produced elevations of plasma NT levels. The exact mechanism and source of NT released by ingested fat have not yet been defined.

Walker et al [35] have recently reported that resection of the distal small bowel in dogs abolishes release of NT by both intraduodenal (ID) fat and intravenous (IV) calcium (Fig 22-2).

Oleic acid plus oxbile in micellar form releases NT from the dog ileum [36]. Oleic acid, as well as Intralipid [37], when given ID in humans, is a potent stimulus for NT release.

The most potent stimulus for NT release is fat. This has been confirmed in rats [38], dogs [39], and in humans [40]. In humans, after a mixed fatty meal, NT rose to a peak at 45 minutes after onset of eating and remained elevated, although at lower concentrations, after 2 hours and 45 minutes [41]. Oral glucose or amino acids, however, do not release NT in normal humans [40]. Simultaneous infusion of atropine abolishes the rise in plasma NT levels after ID instillation of fat in dogs [42]. The exact mechanism of meal- or fat-induced NT release is not yet clearly defined. Antral distention does not release NT [43].

Gomez et al [44] from our laboratory have found that bile appears to play a physiologic role in the feedback inhibition of release of NT. They found that ID fat at a low dose (0.5 g/kg/hr) caused no significant release of NT in the presence of normal or excess bile, but bile diversion allowed significant fat-stimulated release of NT.

In patients with the dumping syndrome after gastric surgery for peptic ulcer disease, there is an exaggerated rise in plasma NT levels after oral glucose when compared to patients with similar operations but without symptoms [45]. Infusion of NT, however, does not reproduce the symptoms of the dumping syndrome [45]. Blackburn et al [30] have found exaggerated release of NT after a meal in patients after jejunoileal bypass for morbid obesity. The findings in both groups of patients suggest that rapid transit with direct delivery of glucose or fat into the ileum is responsible for NT release. When NT was infused into humans, no cardiovascular effects were found [30].

An exaggerated release of NT after ingestion of Intralipid or a mixed meal has been reported in patients after jejunoileal bypass [46–48]. There was an apparent delay in the peak release of NT after

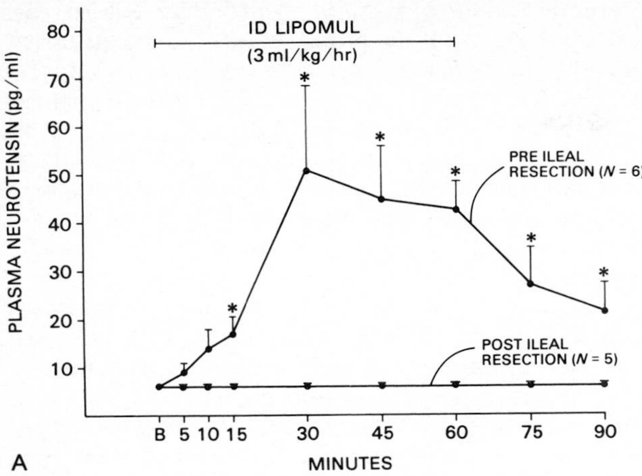

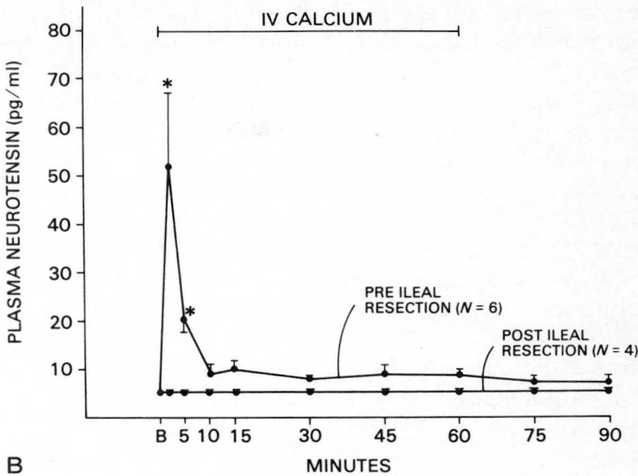

Figure 22-2. A. Release of neurotensin in response to ID infusion of Lipomul, prior to and following distal small bowel resection. (* = $p < 0.05$.) ***B.*** Release of neurotensin in response to IV infusion of calcium ($CaCl_2$, 0.36 mmol/kg, IV bolus followed by 0.36 mmol/kg/hr prior to and following distal small bowel resection. (* = $p < 0.05$.) (From Walker et al [35], by permission of the C V Mosby Co.)

the ingestion of fat, from 30 minutes in normals to 90 minutes in obese patients; plasma NT levels were significantly lower in obese volunteers compared to nonobese normal volunteers [46].

Kihl et al [49] found that both basal and peak NT levels (after 20 mL of ID oleic acid) were significantly lower in duodenal ulcer patients than in control individuals. Proximal gastric vagotomy in duodenal ulcer patients caused no significant difference in the integrated release of NT. In individuals with an intact gastrointestinal tract, glucose is a relatively weak releaser of NT, but after gastrectomy (either partial or total), release of NT by glucose is prompt. Patients with vagotomy and drainage demonstrate a significantly increased release of NT after a test meal compared to control individuals [50].

In patients who have had total gastrectomy, oral glucose releases large amounts of NT, whereas there is no NT release by glucose in normal volunteers [51,52].

Miller and Hendricks [53] have shown that obese Zucker rats (fa/fa) have a significant depression of intestinal NT content compared to lean Zucker rats. In obese animals, NT concentration of the jejunoileum was 2.48 ng/g wet weight compared to 5.45 ng/g wet weight in lean rats. NT caused an increase in levels of plasma cholesterol in rats [54], and infusion of NT into the superior mesenteric artery increased the movement of ^{3}H-oleic acid from the small intestinal lumen into lymph triglyceride [55]. These findings suggest that NT plays a role in intestinal processing of absorbed fat.

Bombesin infusion stimulates the release of NT in humans and dogs [56–60]. Fletcher et al [60] compared the effects of bombesin and gastrin-releasing peptide (GRP) (a mammalian equivalent of bombesin) in equimolar doses and found different responses. Bombesin produced a rise in both NT and pancreatic polypeptide (PP) levels. GRP did not increase plasma NT levels but produced significantly greater elevations of plasma PP. Atropine blocked release of PP during GRP infusion but had no effect on NT or PP released by bombesin. In contrast to meal-stimulated NT release, bombesin-stimulated NT release appears to be cholinergic independent. Despite structural similarities, bombesin and GRP (in the doses tested) do not have similar effects on NT release in humans.

Feurle et al [42] infused atropine (20 μg/kg/hr) into dogs and found a depression of basal and stimulated (ID fat) release of NT. On the other hand, Sakamoto et al [61], from our laboratory, found that, although atropine (0.05 mg/kg bolus plus 0.03 mg/kg/hr infusion) abolished the early peak (15 minutes) of NT release stimulated by ID fat, there was no significant depression of basal levels or of integrated (0–150 minutes) release of NT. Furthermore, vagotomy had no effect on NT release stimulated by ID Lipomul. The discrepancies between these two studies in dogs are not likely to be due to differences in doses of atropine. In contrast to the effects of atropine on meal-stimulated NT release, bombesin-stimulated release of NT is not altered by atropine in humans [60] or by vagotomy in rats [57]. If proximal neural stimuli are important for NT release, vagal-independent, cholinergic mechanisms appear to be involved.

Although the majority of neurotensin is found in the gut, tumors have been found which release neurotensin. The rat medullary thyroid cancer (rMTC6-23) spontaneously releases neurotensin [62]. We [63] have found that bombesin stimulates release of NT from this cell line; somatostatin inhibited release of NT. Furthermore, Collier et al [64] found that five of 20 patients with primary hepatocellular carcinomas had elevated plasma neurotensin levels. Four of these five patients had fibrolamellar hepatomas. Neurotensin may become a useful diagnostic marker for patients with this particular type of hepatoma (which has a better prognosis than other types of hepatomas) and may also be useful to detect subclinical disease after resection.

ACTIONS

Gastrointestinal effects of NT include mesenteric vasodilation [65], inhibition of pentagastrin-stimulated acid secretion with no effect on histamine-stimulated secretion (the inhibition of pentagastrin-stimulated secretion is abolished by vagotomy in dogs [39] and humans [66]), decreased lower esophageal sphincter pressure and inhibition of gastric emptying [66,67] and of small intestinal peristalsis in humans [34]. NT causes a significant decrease in gastric mucosal blood flow as measured by ^{14}C-aminopyrine clearance in humans [68]. Although NT and secretin had an additive inhibitory effect on pentagastrin-stimulated acid secretion, their combined effect on gastric mucosal blood flow was not greater than either peptide alone. In these inhibitory actions, NT is a strong candidate for designation as an enterogastrone, that is, an inhibitor of gastric secretion released from the small bowel by fat.

NT inhibits meal-stimulated gastric acid secretion in humans when infused at a dose of 500 ng/kg/hr [69]. The effects of NT on gastric acid secretion, however, have been considered to require an intact vagal innervation in both dogs and in man [39,70]. IV administration of NT caused a significant inhibition of pentagastrin-stimulated acid secretion in dogs with Pavlov pouches, but in dogs with denervated pouches, there was no effect of NT on pentagastrin-stimulated acid secretion. In patients tested with NT 500 ng/kg/hr before and after parietal cell vagotomy, there was significant inhibition of gastric acid secretion preoperatively, but no effect on pentagastrin-stimulated gastric acid secretion was observed after vagotomy [70]. However, unpublished studies by Mate et al from our laboratory (see below) suggest that failure to secure inhibition postvagotomy may be an artifact induced by diminished sensitivity of the denervated parietal cell.

Histamine-induced gastric acid secretion is not blocked by NT in dogs [39], and intestinally administered oleic acid does not block Histalog-induced gastric acid secretion in man [71], whereas infusion of NT inhibits insulin-induced gastric acid secretion and intestinally administered oleic acid inhibits secretion induced by sham feeding [39,71]. Thus, NT has been considered unique in its actions on gastric secretion among all inhibitors tested; the inhibitory effect of NT appears to require intact vagal innervation. This effect may require further study in light of the results found by Mate et al (below).

There appear to be species differences in the effects of IV NT on pentagastrin- and histamine-stimulated acid secretion in rats, cats, dogs, and man. In rats [72], man [71], and dogs [73], NT does not appear to affect histamine-stimulated acid secretion, whereas it does inhibit pentagastrin-stimulated secretion. In cats, however, there are conflicting data: Hirst et al [74] found that low doses of NT did not inhibit histamine-stimulated acid secretion, but they did not examine doses (20 μg to 40 μg/hr) which produced maximal inhibition of gastrin-stimulated acid secretion; in contrast, Couziqou et al [75] found that IV NT in doses of 3 or 6 μg/kg/30 min inhibited histamine-stimulated acid secretion from both gastric fistulas and Heidenhain pouches in cats.

However, the work of Mate et al (unpublished observation from this laboratory) suggests that this may not be true. They examined the effect of NT on gastric secretion in dogs with gastric fistulas before and 3–5 weeks after vagotomy. IV pentagastrin (1 μg/kg/hr) was infused for 210 minutes, and during the 60–150 minute segment, NT (5.5 μg/kg/hr) was given simultaneously. The sensitivity of the stomach to pentagastrin decreased after vagotomy; therefore, the pentagastrin dose was doubled (2 μg/kg/hr) to achieve a level of gastric secretion similar to that observed before vagotomy, in which case, NT inhibited acid secretion in a manner similar to that achieved prior to vagotomy. These results indicate that vagotomy did not abolish the inhibitory action of NT on pentagastrin-stimulated gastric acid secretion, but that the apparent loss of inhibitory activity was actually due to decreased sensitivity of the parietal cell mass to stimulation by pentagastrin after vagotomy.

The mechanism by which NT achieves its effects is not clear. Recent evidence suggests that prostaglandins mediate some of the NT effects. Rioux et al [76] found that prostaglandin synthetase inhibitors and a phosphatase A_2 inhibitor blocked NT-stimulated contraction of isolated portal vein. Bardon and Ruckebusch [77] found that prostaglandin synthetase inhibitors reduced the magnitude of hypermotility responses of the colon induced by NT. The same inhibitors had a similar effect in reducing meal-induced hypermotility responses. Unpublished studies from our laboratory have shown that treatment with indomethacin (a prostaglandin synthetase inhibitor) abolished the inhibitory effect of NT on pentagastrin-stimulated gastric acid secretion; they have also shown that indomethacin treatment inhibited the NT-stimulated pancreatic output of water, bicarbonate, and protein as well as of PP.

Studies of the molecular basis of NT action have been conducted [78–80]. Goedert et al [78] reported that NT stimulates inositol phospholipid hydrolysis without altering cyclic AMP levels in slices from various regions of the rat brain. Similarly, Canonico et al [79] have shown that NT causes a dose-dependent hydrolysis of polyphosphoinositides when incubated with cultured anterior pituitary cells. This leads to the production of 1,2-diacylglycerol and inositol phosphates. These metabolites may trigger intracellular responses leading to pituitary hormone secretion. Further work by this group [80] has shown that NT causes a dose-dependent increase in arachidonic acid levels from in vitro rat anterior pituitary glands. There is a concomitant increase in prolactin release. Phosphotidylinositol hydrolysis precedes the increase in arachidonate levels and is probably an important cellular source for fatty acid. Specific inhibition of diacylglycerol lipase decreases free arachidonate levels in basal and NT-stimulated conditions and also inhibits prolactin release from the in vitro antrum pituitary glands. This blockade probably occurs after cleavage of inositol phosphates from phosphotidylinositol. When phosphotidylinositol hydrolysis was prevented by the addition of quinacrine to the in vitro pituitary glands, the NT-stimulated arachidonate and prolactin release was similarly inhibited. Indomethacin (a specific cyclo-oxygenase inhibitor) did not alter arachidonate release and even potentiated NT-stimulated prolactin release slightly. This theoretically causes shunting of arachidonic acid from the cyclo-oxygenase-prostaglandin system to the lipo-oxygenase-leukotriene system. Use of BW 755c (an inhibitor of both cyclo-oxygenase and lipo-oxygenase) significantly inhibited both basal and NT-stimulated prolactin release and caused an increase in NT-stimulated arachidonate levels. Thus, release of arachidonate from membrane phospholipids and subsequent metabolism to lipo-oxygenase appear to be an important mechanism of NT action in the pituitary gland, and quite possibly, similar mechanisms are involved in the gastrointestinal tract.

NT inhibits gastric motility in dogs [81] and in humans [66,67]. Pressure of the lower esophageal sphincter is significantly lowered with IV infusion of 12 pmol/kg/min of (Gln^4)-NT [82]. In rats, IV infusion of NT or (Gln^4)-NT was equally effective in abolishing the migrating myoelectric complexes within 2–4 minutes after the onset of infusion. Certain fragments of NT, i.e., $NT^{9\text{-}13}$, $NT^{8\text{-}13}$, $NT^{4\text{-}13}$, $NT^{1\text{-}9}$, and (Gln^4)-$NT^{1\text{-}11}$, have no effect [83]. In man, infusion of (Gln^4)-NT (6 pmol/kg/min) abolished gastric peristalsis [84], and NT itself decreased gastric emptying in humans [66,67] and rats [85].

In conscious dogs, IV NT decreased gastrointestinal motility [81] and intra-arterial administration of a bolus of NT (10 pM) into the small intestine of dogs inhibited α-adrenergic-stimulated, atropine-sensitive contractile responses in the duodenum and ileum [86]. NT may inhibit these gut contractile responses by releasing norepinephrine and, ultimately, acetylcholine.

There is a disparity among reports of smooth muscle responses to NT in vitro. In muscle strips from the rat gastric fundus [87–88] and guinea pig ileum [90–92], NT causes contraction. On the other hand, in the rat duodenum [1,90], ileum [91], and guinea pig colon [93], NT induces relaxation.

However, not all gastrointestinal actions of NT are inhibitory; colonic responses appear to be different. In the dog, systemic infusion of NT induced contractile activity in the colon, which is similar to the meal-stimulated gastrocolic motility response [77]. In humans, IV NT (13.5 pmol/kg/min) stimulates defecation within 2½ hours of receiving a 30-minute infusion [94]. Manometric studies [95] in patients with right-sided double barrel colostomies have shown that there was significantly increased motor activity in the ascending colon during a 30-minute infusion of NT (12 pmol/kg/min). At the end of the infusion, there was also an increase in motility in the rectosigmoid area and discharge of large volumes of loose to watery contents from the colostomy. Healthy volunteers were found to have increased rectosigmoid motility responses and five of seven defecated within one hour after infusion. Furthermore, NT infusion which achieves levels of plasma NT similar to those achieved after a fatty meal, increases ileostomy output and increases the rate of intestinal transit in patients who had previously undergone proctocolectomy for ulcerative colitis [94].

Sakamoto et al [23] and others [96–98] have shown that exogenous infusion of NT stimulates pancreatic secretion directly and augments the action of endogenously released and exogenous cholecystokinin (CCK) and secretin on pancreatic exocrine secretion in dogs. There are differences, however, in that NT combined with hydrochloric acid (which releases secretin) potentiates the effects on pancreatic volume and bicarbonate output, whereas NT and ID amino acids (CCK release) are simply additive with respect to pancreatic enzyme output [23]. NT and CCK have only additive effects on the stimulation of pancreatic protein output [23,97], but others have reported that NT potentiated pancreatic protein secretion when given in combination with secretin and potentiated bicarbonate secretion when given with CCK [98]. Although conflicting results are reported, these findings suggest that NT exerts its actions on receptor systems independent of those for secretin and CCK.

The effects of NT infusion on pancreatic secretion in dogs are not due to the release of other known pancreatic stimulants. We have found that graded doses of NT that stimulate pancreatic secretion in a dose-dependent fashion and release PP do not stimulate release of gastrin, secretin, or CCK, as measured simultaneously in blood by specific radioimmunoassay [23,99].

Intravenous infusion of NT causes release of PP in humans, calves, and dogs [30,99,100]. Significant species differences are reported in the effects of NT infusion on the release of insulin and glucagon. There is no insulin decrease in humans [30], but in calves [100] and rats [101], hyperglycemia is produced by IV administration of NT, which is associated with decreased plasma levels of insulin and increased plasma glucagon. NT released somatostatin from the perfused rat hypothalamus in vitro [102], and caused release of NT into rat hypophyseal blood in vivo [103]. Substance P and NT caused release of somatostatin into portal venous blood in anesthetized rats [104]. On the other hand, infusion of NT into the left gastric artery of the isolated perfused rat stomach caused no release of somatostatin [105]. These studies of hormone-hormone interactions have clearly only touched the surface.

NT affects vascular responses differently in different species and in different areas of the body. In vitro, NT produces contraction of rat coronary arteries [106] and portal veins [107–109]. In dogs, low doses of NT (10–20 pmol/kg/min) decreased blood flow in fat but increased gastrointestinal blood flow without changing heart rate or blood pressure [65]. The vasoactive properties of NT have been evaluated in humans after the infusion of Gln^4-NT in doses resulting in blood levels similar to those measured after a fatty meal [110]. There was reduced blood flow to abdominal fat, and no change in calf muscle blood flow, heart rate, or blood pressure.

Since NT releases PP and since both NT and PP are elevated after fat ingestion, we evaluated the role of NT in regulation of the fat-stimulated intestinal phase of PP release [111]. We found that ID sodium oleate failed to cause NT release, except at 16 mmol/hr dose; however, sodium oleate produced significant release of PP at 4, 8, and 16 mmol/hr. Lipomul (a corn oil emulsification), at 2 g/kg/hr ID, caused release of PP similar to that from 8 and 16 mmol/hr of sodium oleate; however, Lipomul also caused significant release of NT. When IV NT was given to dogs, PP was not released after doses that yielded plasma levels similar to those achieved physiologically by meal stimulation. NT does not appear to have a physiologic role in the release of PP.

In further physiologic studies [112], IV NT was found to cause a dose-related stimulation of pancreatic secretion of water, bicarbonate, and protein in the conscious rat. We have attempted to clarify the role of vagal cholinergic innervation in the release of NT in conscious dogs [61]. Atropine was found to suppress the early release of NT but not the integrated NT response to Lipomul. Vagotomy does not affect fat-induced release of NT. Thus, the release of NT by ID fat appears to be independent of vagal innervation. In the same study, we found that somatostatin inhibited release of NT in response to fat.

Since NT is released by ID fat, it may also play a role in the digestion of fat. Doses of NT that yield physiologic levels in plasma cause a transient contraction of the gallbladder in conscious dogs (CCK-stimulated gallbladder contraction is tonic), as measured by implanted strain-gauge force transducers [113]. NT-stimulated gallbladder contraction is abolished by atropine, and the force and time of onset of gallbladder contraction induced by NT are not dose-related [113].

In another study in which intragallbladder pressure was measured in conscious dogs [114], NT-stimulated gallbladder contraction was found to be dose-dependent, but at about 1/50 the molar potency of CCK-8.

We then studied the effect of IV NT on gallbladder contraction (assessed by ultrasonography) in normal human volunteers [115]. A dose was selected that produced blood levels similar to those obtained after a fatty meal. To our surprise, we found that NT caused gallbladder relaxation in all nine volunteers. The mechanism of this effect is not known. We have found no contractile effect of NT on in vitro strips of rabbit gallbladder that respond normally to CCK-8. NT thus appears to have a varied spectrum of effects on the gallbladder: contraction of dog gallbladder, relaxation of the human gallbladder, and no effect on rabbit gallbladder strips in vitro.

Neurotensin has also been studied for its potential trophic effects. Feurle et al [116] have found that NT treatment stimulates tritiated thymidine uptake and increases DNA content in rat pancreas. The same treatment led to a rise in protein concentration and an increase in gastric antral thickness in the rat. Marx et al [117], on the other hand, found no trophic effects of neurotensin alone or combined with secretin and caerulein on growth of the hamster pancreas. These differences may be explained by species differences and the different doses of neurotensin used in the two studies.

REFERENCES

1. Carraway RE, Leeman SE: The isolation of a new hypotensive peptide, neurotensin, from bovine hypothalami. J Biol Chem 248:6854, 1973.
2. Carraway RE, Leeman SE: The amino acid sequence of a hypothalamic peptide, neurotensin. J Biol Chem 250:1907, 1975.
3. Carraway RE, Leeman SE: The synthesis of neurotensin. J Biol Chem 250:1912, 1975.
4. Carraway RE, Leeman SE: Radioimmunoassay for neurotensin, a hypothalamic peptide. J Biol Chem 251:7035, 1976.
5. Zeytinoglu FN, Gagel RF, Tashjian AH Jr, et al: Characterization of neurotensin production by a line of rat medullary thyroid carcinoma cells. Proc Natl Acad Sci USA 77:3741, 1980.
6. Carraway RE, Leeman SE: Characterization of radioimmunoassayable neurotensin in the rat: Its differential distribution in the central nervous system, small intestine and stomach. J Biol Chem 251:7045, 1976.
7. Doyle H, Greeley GH Jr, Mate L, et al: Distribution of neurotensin in the canine gastrointestinal tract. Surgery 97:337, 1985.
8. Frigerio B, Ravazola M, Ito S, et al: Histochemical and ultrastructural identification of neurotensin cells in the dog ileum. Histochemistry 54:123, 1977.
9. Iwasaki Y, Ito S, Shibata A: Radioimmunoassay of neurotensin and the distribution and concentration of gut neurotensin in rat and dog. Tohoku J Exp Med 130:129, 1980.
10. Orci L, Baetens O, Rufener C, et al: Evidence for immunoreactive neurotensin in dog intestinal mucosa. Life Sci 19:559, 1976.
11. Yanaihara N, Sato H, Inoue A, et al: Comparative study on distribution of bombesin-, neurotensin- and α-endorphin-like immunoreactivities in canine tissues. Adv Exp Med Biol 120A:29, 1979.
12. Helmstaedter V, Feurle GE, Forssmann WG: Ultrastructural identification of a new cell type—the N-cell as the source of neurotensin in the gut mucosa. Cell Tissue Res 184:445, 1977.
13. Polak JM, Bloom SR: Neuropeptides of the gut: A newly discovered major control system. World J Surg 3:393, 1979.
14. Sundler F, Håkanson R, Leander S, et al: Light and electron microscopic localization of neurotensin in the gastrointestinal tract. Ann NY Acad Sci 400:94, 1982.
15. Hammer RA, Leeman SE, Carraway R, et al: Isolation of human intestinal neurotensin. J Biol Chem 255:2476, 1980.
16. Kitabgi P, Carraway R, Leeman SE: Isolation of a tridecapeptide from bovine intestinal tissue and its partial characterization as neurotensin. J Biol Chem 251:7053, 1976.
17. Carraway R, Kitabgi P, Leeman SE: The amino acid sequence of radioimmunoassayable neurotensin from bovine intestine. Identity to neurotensin from hypothalamus. J Biol Chem 253:7996, 1978.
18. Hammer RA, Carraway RE, Leeman SE: Elevation of plasma neurotensinlike immunoreactivity after a meal. Characterization of the elevated components. J Clin Invest 70:74, 1982.
19. Shulkes A, Bijaphala S, Dawborn JK, et al: Metabolism of neurotensin and pancreatic polypeptide in man: Role of the kidney and plasma factors. J Clin Endocrinol Metab 58:873, 1984.
20. Shaw C, Buchanan KD: Intact neurotensin (NT) in human plasma: Response to oral feeding. Regul Pept 7:145, 1983.
21. Theodorsson-Norheim E: Evidence that (Gln^4)-neurotensin is the naturally occurring neurotensin in plasma. Peptides 4:543, 1983.
22. Draviam EJ, Greeley GH Jr, Beauchamp RD, et al: Authentic neurotensin is present in the circulation during fat ingestion in dogs. Surg Forum 36:58, 1985.
23. Sakamoto T, Newman J, Fujimura M, et al: Role of neurotensin in pancreatic secretion. Surgery 96:146, 1984.
24. Dupont A, Merand Y: Enzymic inactivation of

neurotensin by hypothalamic and brain extracts of the rat. Life Sci 22:1623, 1978.

25. Griffiths EC, Linton EA, McDermott JR, et al: The presence of neurotensin-inactivating peptidases in rat brain. J Physiol 324:77P, 1981.
26. McDermott JR, Smith AI, Edwardson JA, et al: Mechanism of neurotensin degradation by rat brain peptidases. Regul Pept 3:397, 1982.
27. Kerouac R, Ruioux F, St-Pierre S, et al: Evidence for the inactivation of neurotensin by guinea pig lungs. Neuropeptides 2:37, 1981.
28. Aronin N, Carraway RE, Ferris CF, et al: The stability and metabolism of intravenously administered neurotensin in the rat. Peptides 3:637, 1982.
29. Theodorsson-Norheim E, Rosell S: Characterization of human plasma neurotensin-like immunoreactivity after fat ingestion. Regul Pept 6:207, 1983.
30. Blackburn AM, Fletcher DR, Adrian TE, et al: Neurotensin infusion in man: Pharmacokinetics and effect on gastrointestinal and pituitary hormones. J Clin Endocrinol Metab 51:1257, 1980.
31. Skidgel RA, Engelbrecht S, Johnson AR, et al: Hydrolysis of substance P and neurotensin by converting enzyme and neutral endopeptidase. Peptides 5:769, 1984.
32. Mashford ML, Nilsson G, Rokaeus Å, et al: Release of neurotensin-like immunoreactivity (NTLI) from the gut in anaesthetized dogs. Acta Physiol Scand 104:375, 1978.
33. Fujimura M, Khalil T, Greeley GH Jr, et al: Release of neurotensin: Effect of selective jejunal or ileal perfusion with sodium oleate in the dog. Gastroenterology 86:1083, 1984.
34. Read NW, McFarlane A, Kinsman RI, et al: Effect of infusion of nutrient solutions into the ileum on gastrointestinal transit and plasma levels of neurotensin and enteroglucagon. Gastroenterology 86:274, 1984.
35. Walker JP, Fujimura M, Sakamoto T, et al: Importance of the ileum in neurotensin release by fat. Surgery 98:224, 1985.
36. Reasbeck PG, Barbezat GO, Shulkes A, et al: Secretion of neurotensin and its effects on the jejunum in the dog. Gastroenterology 86:1552, 1984.
37. Kihl B, Rokaeus A, Rosell S, et al: Inhibition of pentagastrin stimulated gastric acid secretion and rise in the plasma concentration of neurotensin-like immunoreactivity (NTLI) by intraduodenal oleic acid in man. Acta Physiol Scand 110:329, 1980.
38. Rosell S: The role of neurotensin in the uptake and distribution of fat, in Nemeroff CB, Prange AJ Jr (eds): *Neurotensin, A Brain and Gastrointestinal Peptide.* New York, New York Academy of Sciences, 1982, pp 183–197.
39. Andersson S, Chang D, Folkers K, et al: Inhibition of gastric acid secretion in dogs by neurotensin. Life Sci 19:367, 1976.
40. Rosell S, Rokaeus A: The effect of ingestion of amino acids, glucose and fat on circulating neurotensinlike immunoreactivity (NTLI) in man. Acta Physiol Scand 107:263, 1979.
41. Mashford ML, Nilsson G, Rokaeus A, et al: The effect of food ingestion on circulating neurotensin-like immunoreactivity (NTLI) in the human. Acta Physiol Scand 104:244, 1978.
42. Feurle GE, Baca I, Knauf W: Atropine depresses release of neurotensin and its effect on the exocrine pancreas. Regul Pept 4:75, 1982.
43. Schoon I-M, Bloom SR, Olbe L: The effect of antral distension in healthy subjects on betazole-stimulated gastric acid secretion and the plasma concentration of immunoreactive neurotensin. Scand J Gastroenterol 15:277, 1980.
44. Gomez G, Lluis F, Guo Y-S, et al: Bile inhibits release of cholecystokinin and neurotensin. Surgery 100:363, 1986.
45. Blackburn AM, Bloom SR: Neurotensin in man, in Bloom SR, Polak JM (eds): *Gut Hormones.* New York, Churchill Livingstone, 1981, pp 306–311.
46. Wiklund B, Rokaeus A, Hallberg D, et al: Plasma NTLI after administration of fat to obese volunteers and patients operated with jejuno-ileal bypass. Acta Physiol Scand 110:330, 1980.
47. Sarson DL, Scopinaro N, Bloom SR: Gut hormone changes after jejunoileal (JIB) or biliopancreatic (BPB) bypass surgery for morbid obesity. Int J Obes 5:471, 1981.
48. Besterman HS, Sarson DL, Blackburn AM, et al: The gut hormone profile in morbid obesity and following jejuno-ileal bypass. Scand J Gastroenterol 13(Suppl 49):15, 1978.
49. Kihl B, Rokaeus A, Rosell S, et al: Fat inhibition of gastric acid secretion in man and plasma concentrations of neurotensin-like immunoreactivity. Scand J Gastroenterol 16:513, 1981.
50. Shaw C, Watt PCH, Buchanan KD: Post-gastric surgery neurotensin (NT) release: Assessment with two region-specific antisera. Dig Dis Sci 29(Suppl):79S, 1984.
51. Flaten O, Hanssen LE, Kåresen R, et al: Glucose-induced release of neurotensin after gastric surgery. Digestion 24:94, 1982.
52. Ito S, Matsubara Y, Iwasaki Y, et al: Enhanced neurotensin-like immunoreactivity release in total gastrectomized patients after 50 g OGTT. Horm Metab Res 12:551, 1980.
53. Miller JL, Hendricks MS: Gastrointestinal neurotensin-like immunoreactivity (NTLI) in lean and obese Zucker rats. Horm Metab Res 13:506, 1981.
54. Peric-Golia L, Gardner CF, Peric-Golia M: The effect of neurotensin on the plasma cholesterol levels in the rat. Eur J Pharmacol 55:407, 1979.
55. Armstrong MJ, Ferris CF, Leeman SE: Neurotensin increases the translocation of ^{3}H-oleic acid from the intestinal lumen into lymph in rats. Dig Dis Sci 29(Suppl):6S, 1984.
56. Bloom SR, Ghatei MA, Christofides ND, et al: Release of neurotensin, enteroglucagon, motilin and pancreatic polypeptide by bombesin in man. Gut 20:A912, 1979.
57. Rokaeus A, Yanaihara N, McDonald TJ: Increased concentration of neurotensin-like immunoreactiv-

ity (NTLI) in rat plasma after administration of bombesin and bombesin-related peptides (porcine and chicken gastrin-releasing peptides). Acta Physiol Scand 114:605, 1982.

58. McDonald TJ, Ghatei MA, Bloom SR, et al: A qualitative comparison of canine plasma gastroenteropancreatic hormone responses to bombesin and the porcine gastrin-releasing peptide (GRP). Regul Pept 2:293, 1981.
59. Ghatei MA, Jung RT, Stevenson JC, et al: Bombesin: Action on gut hormones and calcium in man. J Clin Endocrinol Metab 54:980, 1982.
60. Fletcher DR, Shulkes A, Bladin PHD, et al: The effect of atropine on bombesin and gastrin releasing peptide stimulated gastrin, pancreatic polypeptide and neurotensin release in man. Regul Pept 7:31, 1983.
61. Sakamoto TS, Fujimura M, Walker JP, et al: Regulation of endogenous release of neurotensin by fat: The effect of atropine, vagotomy and somatostatin. Dig Dis Sci 29:72S, 1984.
62. Zeytinoglu FN, Gagel RF, Tashjian AH Jr, et al: Characterization of neurotensin production by a line of rat medullary thyroid carcinoma cells. Proc Natl Acad Sci USA 77:3741, 1980.
63. Marx M, Seitz PK, Townsend CM Jr, et al: Effects of bombesin and somatostatin on secretion of neurotensin by medullary thyroid carcinoma. Surg Forum 35:207, 1984.
64. Collier NA, Bloom SR, Hodgson HJF, et al: Neurotensin secretion by fibrolamellar carcinoma of the liver. Lancet 1:538, 1984.
65. Rosell S, Burcher E, Chang D, et al: Cardiovascular and metabolic actions of neurotensin and (gln^4)-neurotensin. Acta Physiol Scand 98:484, 1976.
66. Blackburn AM, Bloom SR, Long RG, et al: Effect of neurotensin on gastric function in man. Lancet 1:987, 1980.
67. Rosell S: Enterogastrone candidates among the gastrointestinal polypeptides, in *Proceedings of the International Union of Physiological Sciences.* XXVII International Congress, Budapest, 1980, vol. 14, p. 228.
68. Fletcher DR, Shulkes A, Hardy KJ: The effect of neurotensin and secretin on gastric acid secretion and mucosal blood flow in man. Regul Pept 11:217, 1985.
69. Skov Olsen P, Holst Pedersen J, Kirkegaard P, et al: Neurotensin inhibits meal-stimulated gastric acid secretion in man. Scand J Gastroenterol 18:1073, 1983.
70. Olsen PS, Pedersen JH, Kirkegaard P, et al: Neurotensin induced inhibition of gastric acid secretion in duodenal ulcer patients before and after parietal cell vagotomy. Gut 25:481, 1984.
71. Kihl B, Rokaeus A, Rosell S, et al: The effect of intraduodenal instillation of oleic acid on plasma neurotensin-like immunoreactivity and on gastric acid secretion stimulated by betazole and sham feeding in man. Scand J Gastroenterol 17:633, 1982.
72. El Munshid HA, Håkanson R, Liedberg G, et al: Effects of various gastrointestinal peptides on parietal cells and endocrine cells in the oxyntic mucosa of rat stomach. J Physiol 305:249, 1980.
73. Andersson S, Rosell S, Sjodin L, et al: Inhibition of acid secretion from vagally innervated and denervated gastric pouches by (Gln^4)-neurotensin. Scand J Gastroenterol 15:253, 1980.
74. Hirst BH, Shaw B, Wilson L: Neurotensin inhibition of gastric exocrine secretions in the cat. Regul Pept 3:289, 1982.
75. Couziguo P, Robein MJ, Salmon R, et al: Inhibition by somatostatin and neurotensin of the histamine-stimulated gastric secretion. Gastroenterology 72:A-133/1156, 1977.
76. Rioux F, Quirion R, Leblanc MA, et al: Possible interactions between neurotensin and prostaglandins in the isolated rat portal vein. Life Sci 27:259, 1980.
77. Bardon T, Ruckebusch Y: Neurotensin-induced colonic motor responses in dogs: A mediation by prostaglandins. Regul Pept 10:107, 1985.
78. Goedert M, Pinnock RD, Downes CP, et al: Neurotensin stimulates inositol phospholipid hydrolysis in rat brain slices. Brain Res 323:193, 1984.
79. Canonico PL, Sortino MA, Speciale C, et al: Neurotensin stimulates polyphosphoinositide breakdown and prolactin release in anterior pituitary cells in culture. Mol Cell Endocrinol 42:215, 1985.
80. Canonico PL, Speciale C, Sortino MA, et al: Involvement of arachidonate metabolism in neurotensin-induced prolactin release in vitro. Am J Physiol 249:E257, 1985.
81. Andersson S, Rosell S, Hjelmquist U, et al: Inhibition of gastric and intestinal motor activity in dogs by (Gln^4) neurotensin. Acta Physiol Scand 100:231, 1977.
82. Rosell S, Thor K, Rokaeus A, et al: Plasma concentration of neurotensin-like immunoreactivity (NTLI) and lower esophageal sphincter (LES) pressure in man following infusion of (Gln^4)-neurotensin. Acta Physiol Scand 109:369, 1980.
83. Al-Saffar A, Rosell S: Effects of neurotensin and neurotensin analogues on the migrating myoelectrical complexes in the small intestine of rats. Acta Physiol Scand 112:203, 1981.
84. Thor K, Rosell S, Rokaeus Å, et al: (Gln^4)-neurotensin changes the motility pattern of the duodenum and proximal jejunum from a fasting-type to a fed-type. Gastroenterology 83:569, 1982.
85. Hellstrom PM, Nylander G, Rosell S: Effects of neurotensin on the transit of gastrointestinal contents in the rat. Acta Physiol Scand 115:239, 1982.
86. Daniel EE, Sakai Y, Jury J, et al: Mode of action of neurotensin on gastrointestinal motility, in Wienbeck M (ed): *Motility of the Digestive Tract.* New York, Raven Press, 1982, pp 451–459.
87. Kataoka K, Taniguchi A, Shimizu H, et al: Biological activity of neurotensin and its C-terminal partial sequences. Brain Res Bull 3:555, 1978.
88. Quirion R, Regoli D, Rioux F, et al: The stimulatory effects of neurotensin and related peptides in rat

stomach strips and guinea-pig atria. Br J Pharmacol 68:83, 1980.

89. Quirion R, Regoli D, Rioux F, et al: Structure-activity studies with neurotensin: Analysis of positions 9, 10 and 11. Br J Pharmacol 69:689, 1980.
90. Kitabgi P, Freychet P: Neurotensin contracts the guinea-pig longitudinal ileal smooth muscle by inducing acetylcholine release. Eur J Pharmacol 56:403, 1979.
91. Kitabgi P, Freychet P: Effects of neurotensin on isolated intestinal smooth muscles. Eur J Pharmacol 50:349, 1978.
92. Monier S, Kitabgi P: Effects of β-endorphine, Met-enkephalin and somatostatin on the neurotensin-induced neurogenic contraction in the guinea-pig ileum. Regul Pept 2:31, 1981.
93. Kitabgi P, Vincent J-P: Neurotensin is a potent inhibitor of guinea-pig colon contractile activity. Eur J Pharmacol 74:311, 1981.
94. Calam J, Unwin R, Peart WS: Neurotensin stimulates defaecation. Lancet 1:737, 1983.
95. Thor K, Rosell S: Neurotensin increases colonic motility. Gastroenterology 90:27, 1986.
96. Sakamoto T, Fujimura M, Newman J, et al: Effect of neurotensin on endogenously stimulated pancreatic secretion in dogs. Dig Dis Sci 28:947, 1983.
97. Konturek SJ, Jaworek J, Cieszkowski M, et al: Comparison of effects of neurotensin and fat on pancreatic stimulation in dogs. Am J Physiol 244:G590, 1983.
98. Baca I, Feurle GE, Haas M, et al: Interaction of neurotensin, cholecystokinin, and secretin in the stimulation of the exocrine pancreas in the dog. Gastroenterology 84:556, 1983.
99. Newman J, Townsend CM Jr, Greeley GH Jr, et al: Neurotensin: Effect on pancreatic secretion and release of gastrin, pancreatic polypeptide, and cholecystokinin-33 in dogs. Surg Forum 34:213, 1983.
100. Blackburn AM, Bloom SR, Edwards AV: Pancreatic endocrine responses to exogenous neurotensin in the conscious calf. J Physiol 314:11, 1981.
101. Brown M, Vale W: Effects of neurotensin and substance P on plasma insulin, glucagon, and glucose levels. Endocrinology 98:819, 1976.
102. Shimatsu A, Kato Y, Matsushita N, et al: Effects of glucagon, neurotensin, and vasoactive intestinal polypeptide on somatostatin release from perfused rat hypothalamus. Endocrinology 110:2113, 1982.
103. Abe H, Chihara K, Chiba T, et al: Effect of intraventricular injection of neurotensin and other various bioactive peptides on plasma immunoreactive somatostatin levels in rat hypophysial portal blood. Endocrinology 108:1939, 1981.
104. Saito H, Saito S: Effects of substance P and neurotensin on somatostatin levels in rat portal plasma. Endocrinology 107:1600, 1980.
105. Chiba T, Taminato T, Kadowaki S, et al: Effects of various gastrointestinal peptides on gastric somatostatin release. Endocrinology 106:145, 1980.
106. Quirion R, Rioux F, Regoli D, et al: Neurotensin-induced coronary vessels constriction in perfused rat hearts. Eur J Pharmacol 55:221, 1979.
107. Helle KB, Serck-Hanssen G, Jørgensen G, et al: Neurotensin-induced contractions in venous smooth muscle. J Auton Nerv Syst 2:143, 1980.
108. Rioux F, Quirion R, Leblanc MA, et al: Possible interactions between neurotensin and prostaglandins in the isolated rat portal vein. Life Sci 27:259, 1980.
109. Rioux F, Quirion R, Regoli D, et al: Pharmacological characterization of neurotensin receptors in the rat isolated portal vein using analogues and fragments of neurotensin. Eur J Pharmacol 66:273, 1980.
110. Linde B, Rosell S, Rokaeus A: Blood flow in human adipose tissue after infusion of (Gln^4)-neurotensin. Acta Physiol Scand 115:311, 1982.
111. Sakamoto T, Newman J, Townsend CM Jr, et al: Role of neurotensin in the intestinal phase of pancreatic polypeptide release induced by fat. Gastroenterology 86:1229, 1984.
112. Khalil T, Fujimura M, Greeley GH Jr, et al: Effect of neurotensin on pancreatic secretion in rats. Gastroenterology 86:1133, 1984.
113. Fujimura M, Sakamoto T, Khalil T, et al: Physiologic role of neurotensin in gallbladder contraction in the dog. Surg Forum 35:192, 1984.
114. Sakamoto T, Mate L, Greeley GH Jr, et al: Effect of neurotensin on gallbladder contraction in dogs. Gastroenterology 86:1229, 1984.
115. Walker JP, Khalil T, Wiener I, et al: The role of neurotensin in human gallbladder motility. Ann Surg 201:678, 1985.
116. Feurle GE, Muller B, Ohnheiser G, et al: Action of neurotensin on size, composition, and growth of pancreas and stomach in the rat. Regul Pept 13:53, 1985.
117. Marx M, Glass EJ, Townsend CM Jr, et al: Differential effect of caerulein and neurotensin on pancreatic growth. Dig Dis Sci 29:51S, 1984.

Chapter 23

Motilin

J. Patrick Walker, M.D., and Phillip L. Rayford, Ph.D.

HISTORY

In 1966, John Brown, at the University of British Columbia discovered a property in duodenal extracts that stimulated gastric motor activity [1]. By 1970, he and his colleagues purified, from mucosal extracts of small intestines of hogs (extracts prepared by Mutt at the Karolinska Institute), a polypeptide that possessed this motor-stimulating activity. The peptide was called motilin and was found to be both chemically and physiologically distinct from cholecystokinin-pancreozymin and secretin [2]. In 1971 and 1972, Brown et al determined the amino acid composition [3] and sequence [4] of motilin and found that it had a molecular weight of 2700 daltons. The amino acid sequence is

Phe-Val-Pro-Ile-Phe-Thr-Tyr-Gly-Glu-Leu-Gln-
Arg-Met-Gln-Glu-Lys-Glu-Arg-Asn-Lys-Gly-Gln

Motilin was synthesized by solid-state procedures in 1982 [5].

DISTRIBUTION

In the gastrointestinal tract, motilin immunoreactivity has been found from the esophagus to the colon, including the gallbladder and biliary tree [6–12]. The highest concentrations are located in the duodenum and jejunum [6,12], although in one study, exceptionally high levels of motilin were found in the gallbladder of the monkey [9]. Motilin has been localized to both enterochromaffin cells [6,7] and endocrine nonenterochromaffin cells [10] (Fig 23-1).

Like many (if not most) polypeptide hormones, motilin has been found in the central nervous system. It is present in high concentrations in the pituitary and pineal glands of the dog brain, with lower concentrations in the hypothalamus, corpus striatum, cerebral cortex, and medulla [9].

ASSAY

Motilin can be measured by its ability to stimulate motor activity in isolated rabbit duodenum [13] and in denervated fundic pouches of dogs [14]. These bioassays do not possess the degree of sensitivity needed to quantitate motilin in body fluids of humans and experimental animals.

In 1974, Dryburgh and Brown [14] developed a specific radioimmunoassay and used it to correlate serum levels of motilin with gastric motor activity. Since that time, several investigators [15–17] have reported the development of specific and sensitive radioimmunoassays for motilin.

PHARMACOKINETICS AND CATABOLISM

In studies in humans, the disappearance half-life of exogenously administered motilin and endogenously released motilin was found to be 4.36 and 4.56 minutes, respectively [18]. The space of distribution was calculated to be 5.4 and 4.9 percent of body weight for two different infusion rates, implying distribution mainly in the plasma volume. Metabolic clearance rate was 7.8 $\pm$ 0.5 mL/kg/min [18]. The kidneys appear to play a role in removal of circulating motilin [19].

RELEASE

Motilin release is probably mediated by vagal tone and passage of nutrients through the duode-

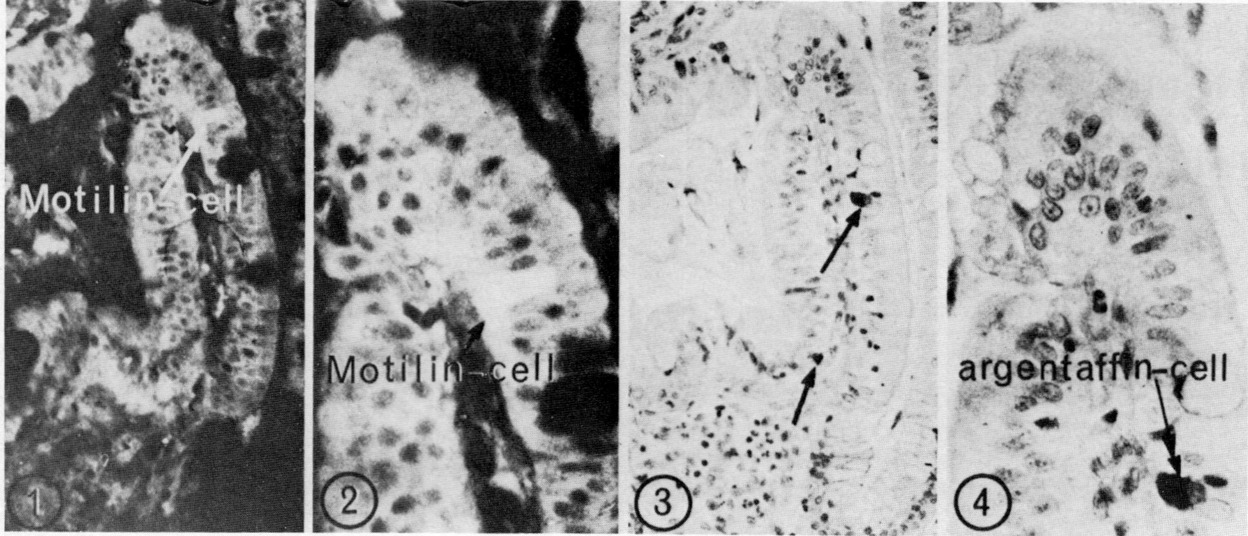

Figure 23-1. (1)Human duodenum stained with the immunofluorescence reaction for the motilin antiserum Erlangen. Two cells of the intestinal villi are stained (×170). (2) Higher magnification of (1) showing one of the motilin cells, with distinct staining and pyramidal shape (×340). (3) Same section and same areas as (1) after subsequent staining with the AA reaction. Two cells different from those in (1) are stained (arrows) (×170). (4) Higher magnification of (3) and the same area as (2). The basal part of the enterochromaffin cell is strongly stained by the reaction (×340). (From Helmstaedter et al [10], by permission of the American Gastroenterological Association.)

num. Bombesin stimulates motilin release in dogs (Fig 23-2) [20], whereas somatostatin inhibits it [21]. Electrical stimulation of the vagus produces a marked rise in motilin levels [22]; however, truncal vagotomy does not produce a change in fasting or stimulated levels of motilin [23]. Intravenous insu-

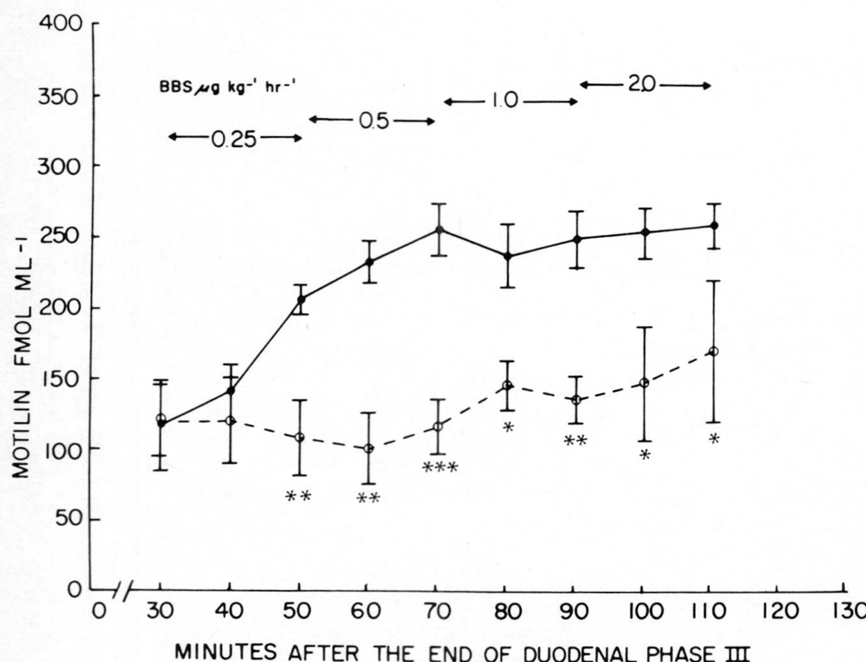

Figure 23-2. Motilin blood levels during bombesin (BBS, closed circles) and saline administration (open circles) beginning at a precise time point of the interdigestive myoelectric complex. (* = $p < 0.05$; ** = $p < 0.025$; *** = $p < 0.01$.) (From Poitras et al [20], by permission of The American Physiological Society.)

lin lowers motilin levels [19]. Mori et al [24] showed a marked decrease in motilin levels by meal-ingestion in the dog with an intact duodenum. When the duodenum was isolated, plasma motilin levels were not suppressed [24].

There is some evidence that motilin release may be modulated, at least in part, by pancreaticobiliary juice. Infusion of pancreaticobiliary juice in the duodenum of patients with chronic pancreatitis restored the previously diminished motilin response [25].

There are controversial reports concerning the control of plasma motilin levels and its function. Itoh et al [16] are strongly in favor of an interdigestive role of motilin, and physiologically this appears to be its primary function. Lee et al [26] agree and have shown that a mixed meal decreases motilin levels and initiates phase II-like myoelectric activity. Collins et al [27] have reported no change of motilin levels in humans following a mixed meal, an increase in motilin with high levels of duodenal acidification, and an increase in motilin levels following fat ingestion but no change following duodenal infusion of fat. Intravenous infusions of glucose and of amino acids have produced decreased motilin levels, while IV fat infusion had no effect on motilin levels [21]. The same study reported that motilin levels were decreased after somatostatin infusion [21]. In humans, however, IV glucose and amino acids suppressed motilin release, with IV lipid increasing plasma motilin levels [28]. Infusion of pancreatic polypeptide (PP) has also been shown to decrease plasma motilin levels [29].

ACTIONS

Functionally, motilin produces contraction of intestinal smooth muscle [13], including the gallbladder [30]. In vitro, intestinal contraction is a direct effect, not influenced by atropine, chlorpheniramine, cimetidine, phentolamine, propranolol, cinanserin, 1-sar-8-ala-angiotensin II, or salicylate [31], but it is decreased by removal of calcium from the medium or by verapamil [31]. The contraction is approximately 100 times stronger than that stimulated by acetylcholine (on a molar basis) and is strongest in the duodenum [31]. In vivo, the effects of motilin appear to be directly on intrinsic excitatory nerves [32]. Motilin increases tone in the spincter of Oddi in the dog [33] and in the opossum [34].

The physiologic role of motilin in the gastrointestinal tract is primarily in the interdigestive period [35], during which motilin produces type III myoelectric activity in the stomach and duodenum that is propagated distally. This activity has been observed in dogs [17] and humans [36]. Motilin may not, according to Sarna et al [37], produce phase III activity but instead may itself be released by migrating myoelectric complexes. Itoh et al [38] have noted that migrating myoelectric complexes associated with motilin do not occur during states of duodenal acidity, even during high levels of plasma motilin. Morphine institutes similar migrating myoelectric complexes; however, these contractions tend to have a greater rate of propagation along the proximal small intestine [39]. Morphine also disrupts further type III cycling. The role of motilin in the control of migrating myoelectric complexes has been supported by studies that show that the administration of antimotilin serum to dogs diminishes the occurrence of migrating myoelectric complexes [40].

Intravenous infusion of motilin produces transient contraction of the gallbladder during the interdigestive period but not during the digestive period [41]. This contraction is *not* dose-dependent and is inhibited by atropine. In comparison, cholecystokinin produces dose-dependent contractility both during digestive and interdigestive periods that is also inhibited by atropine [41]. In isolated human gallbladder muscle strips, no contraction could be elicited with motilin at physiologic or pharmacologic doses [42].

Elevated motilin levels of the type associated with phase III interdigestive patterns have been associated with increased pancreatic bicarbonate output [43], but the role of motilin in exocrine pancreas function is not clear. Konturek et al [44] have shown motilin to produce moderate increases in pancreatic protein, bicarbonate, and volume; however, motilin inhibits secretin-induced bicarbonate flow.

Motilin has been shown to increase gastric emptying of a radioactive meal in humans [45]. In this study, motilin produced elevated insulin levels but had no effect on gastric inhibitory polypeptide, PP, enteroglucagon, pentagastrin, vasoactive intestinal peptide, gastrin, or glucose levels. When selective fat and glucose radioactive-labeled meals are ingested, motilin is seen to increase gastric emptying of the glucose meal but not of the fat meal [46]. Motilin seems to stimulate feeding in fasted rats [47].

Motilin has been shown to produce an inhibitory effect on deiters neurons of the lateral vestibular nucleus in the rat [48] and to produce an excitatory effect on motilin-treated corticospinal neurons of rats [49]. In rat hemipituitaries and dispersed anterior pituitary cells, incubation with motilin released growth hormone but had no effect on luteinizing hormone, thyroid-stimulating hormone, or prolactin release [50].

PATHOPHYSIOLOGY

Fasting plasma motilin levels in children are seen to decrease with advancing age [51]. Clinically, plasma motilin levels have been related to postoperative ileus and recovery from this disorder [52]; levels decreased during ileus and increased immediately on return of gastrointestinal tract function.

In a study from Hiroshima University School of Medicine, elevated levels of serum motilin were seen in patients with irritable colon and in those with dumping syndrome [53]. Motilin levels were higher in the dumping syndrome patients, especially when they were given oral glucose [53]. Plasma levels of motilin were greatly elevated in patients hospitalized with acute diarrhea [54] (Fig 23-3). Plasma motilin response to water taken by mouth is decreased in patients with constipation and megacolon [55].

In patients with gallbladder disease, plasma motilin levels are normal during intercyclical periods (between interdigestive motor complexes) but are reduced during cyclical periods [56]. Wingate and Bloom [57] reported a patient with absent motor and autonomic innervation secondary to acute intermittent porphyria in whom plasma motilin was not detected. They suggested that release of motilin is neurally dependent.

In summary, motilin is a neuropeptide hormone found in the brain and the gut. Its function in the brain is as yet undefined. In the gastrointestinal tract, it appears to be a modulator (probably the chief modulator) of interdigestive motility, performing the housekeeping function of clearing the intestine between meals and preparing it for another nutritional bolus [16,58]. Motilin may be involved in ileus; it may be the factor that, by its absence when its release is disturbed by direct trauma (surgery) or systemic insult (shock) or even by psychogenic (neurogenic?) factors, leads to paralysis of bowel function. The presence of motilin in enterochromaffin cells may serve to remind us of the direct link between gastrointestinal function of the body's maintenance of a neural link with all systems.

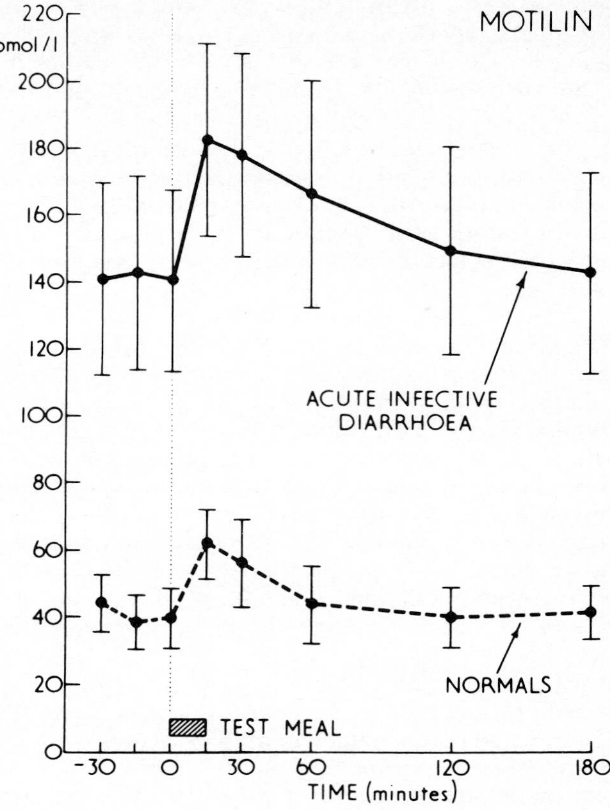

Figure 23-3. Plasma motilin responses to test breakfast in 12 patients with acute diarrhea and 13 healthy controls. (From Besterman et al [54], by permission of the British Medical Association.)

REFERENCES

1. Brown JC: Presence of a gastric motor-stimulating property in duodenal extracts. Gastroenterology 52:225, 1967.
2. Brown JC, Mutt V, Dryburgh JR: The further purification of motilin, a gastric motor activity stimulating polypeptide from the mucosa of the small intestine of hogs. Can J Physiol Pharmacol 49:399, 1971.
3. Brown JC, Cook MA, Dryburgh JR: Motilin, a gastric motor activity-stimulating polypeptide: Final purification, amino acid composition, and C-terminal residues. Gastroenterology 62:401, 1972.
4. Brown JC, Cook MA, Dryburgh JR: Motilin, a gastric motor activity stimulating polypeptide: The complete amino acid sequence. Can J Biochem 51:533, 1973.
5. Coy DH, Coy EJ, Lee K-Y, et al: Solid-phase synthesis and biological activities of gastrointestinal hormones: Secretin and motilin. Peptides 1:137, 1982.
6. Pearse AGE, Polak JM, Bloom SR, et al: Enterochromaffin cells of the mammalian small intestine as the

source of motilin. Virchows Arch [Cell Pathol] 16:111, 1974.
7. Polak JM, Pearse AGE, Heath CM: Complete identification of endocrine cells in the gastrointestinal tract using semithin-thin sections to identify motilin cells in human and animal intestine. Gut 16:225, 1975.
8. Heitz P, Polak JM, Kasper M, et al: Immunoelectron cytochemical localization of motilin and substance P in rabbit bile duct enterochromaffin (EC) cells. Histochemistry 50:319, 1977.
9. Yanaihara C, Sato H, Yanaihara N, et al: Motilin-, substance P- and somatostatin-like immunoreactivities in extracts from dog, tupaia and monkey brain and GI tract. Adv Exp Med Biol 106:269, 1978.
10. Helmstaedter V, Kreppein W, Domschke W, et al: Immunohistochemical localization of motilin in endocrine non-enterochromaffin cells of the small intestine of humans and monkey. Gastroenterology 76:897, 1979.
11. Chey WY, Lee KY: Motilin. Clin Gastroenterol 9:645, 1980.
12. Smith PH, Davis BJ, Seino Y, et al: Localization of motilin-containing cells in the intestinal tract of mammals: A further comparison using region-specific motilin antisera. Gen Comp Endocrinol 44:288, 1981.
13. Strunz U, Domschke W, Mitznegg P, et al: Analysis of the motor effects of 13-norleucine motilin on the rabbit, guinea pig, rat, and human alimentary tract in vitro. Gastroenterology 68:1485, 1975.
14. Dryburgh JR, Brown JC: Radioimmunoassay for motilin. Gastroenterology 68:1169, 1975.
15. Bloom SR, Mitznegg P, Bryant MG: Measurement of human plasma motilin. Scand J Gastroenterol 11(Suppl 39):47, 1976.
16. Itoh Z, Takeuchi S, Aizawa I, et al: Recent advances in motilin research: Its physiological and clinical significance. Adv Exp Med Biol 106:241, 1978.
17. Lee KY, Chey WY, Tai H-H, et al: Radioimmunoassay of motilin. Validation and studies on the relationship between plasma motilin and interdigestive myoelectric activity of the duodenum of dog. Am J Dig Dis 23:789, 1978.
18. Mitznegg P, Bloom SR, Domschke W, et al: Pharmacokinetics of motilin in man. Gastroenterology 72:413, 1977.
19. Jenssen TG, Burhol PG, Jorde R, et al: Radioimmunoassayable plasma motilin in man. Scand J Gastroenterol 19:717, 1984.
20. Poitras P, Tasse D, Laprise P: Stimulation of motilin release by bombesin in dogs. Am J Physiol 245:G249, 1983.
21. Mori K, Seino Y, Itoh Z, et al: Motilin release by intravenous infusion of nutrients and somatostatin in conscious dogs. Regul Pept 1:265, 1981.
22. Lee KY, Chang T, Chey WY: Effect of electrical stimulation of the vagus on plasma motilin concentration in dog. Life Sci 29:1093, 1981.
23. Yoshiya K, Yamamura T, Ishikawa Y, et al: The failure of truncal vagotomy to affect motilin release in dogs. J Surg Res 38:263, 1985.
24. Mori K, Seino Y, Yanaihara N, et al: Role of the duodenum in motilin release. Regul Pept 1:271, 1981.
25. Owyang C, Funakoshi A, Vinik AI: Evidence for modulation of motilin secretion by pancreaticobiliary juice in health and in chronic pancreatitis. J Clin Endocrinol Metab 57:1015, 1983.
26. Lee KY, Kim MS, Chey WY: Effects of a meal and gut hormones on plasma motilin and duodenal motility in dog. Am J Physiol 238:G280, 1980.
27. Collins SM, Lewis TD, Fox J-AET, et al: Changes in plasma motilin concentration in response to manipulation of intragastric and intraduodenal contents in man. Can J Physiol Pharmacol 59:188, 1981.
28. Christofides ND, Bloom SR, Besterman HS, et al: Release of motilin by oral and intravenous nutrients in man. Gut 20:102, 1979.
29. Adrian TE, Greenberg GR, Barnes AJ, et al: Effects of pancreatic polypeptide on motilin and circulating metabolites in man. Eur J Clin Invest 10:235, 1980.
30. Suzuki T, Takahashi I, Itoh Z: Motilin and gallbladder: New dimensions in gastrointestinal physiology. Peptides 2(Suppl 2):229, 1981.
31. Adachi H, Toda N, Hayashi S, et al: Mechanism of the excitatory action of motilin on isolated rabbit intestine. Gastroenterology 80:783, 1981.
32. Fox JET, Daniel EE, Jury J, et al: The mechanism of motilin excitation of the canine small intestine. Life Sci 34:1001, 1983.
33. Neya T, Mizutani M, Takaki M, et al: Effect of motilin on the sphincter of Oddi in the dog. Acta Med Okayama 35:417, 1981.
34. Takahashi I, Honda R, Dodds WJ, et al: Effect of motilin on the opossum upper gastrointestinal tract and sphincter of Oddi. Am J Physiol 245:G476, 1983.
35. Itoh Z, Honda R, Hiwatashi K, et al: Motilin-induced mechanical activity in the canine alimentary tract. Scand J Gastroenterol 11(Suppl 39):93, 1976.
36. You CH, Chey WY, Lee KY: Studies on plasma motilin concentration and interdigestive motility of the duodenum in humans. Gastroenterology 79:62, 1980.
37. Sarna S, Chey WY, Condon RE, et al: Cause-and-effect relationship between motilin and migrating myoelectric complexes. Am J Physiol 245:G277, 1983.
38. Itoh Z, Aizawa I, Honda R, et al: Regular and irregular cycles of interdigestive contractions in the stomach. Am J Physiol 238:G85, 1980.
39. Sarna S, Condon RE, Cowles V: Morphine versus motilin in the initiation of migrating myoelectric complexes. Am J Physiol 245:G217, 1983.
40. Lee KY, Chang T-M, Chey WY: Effect of rabbit antimotilin serum on myoelectric activity and plasma motilin concentration in fasting dog. Am J Physiol 245:G547, 1983.
41. Takahashi I, Suzuki T, Aizawa I, et al: Comparison of gallbladder contractions induced by motilin and

cholecystokinin in dogs. Gastroenterology 82:419, 1982.
42. Pomeranz IS, Davison JS, Shaffer EA: *In vitro* effects of pancreatic polypeptide and motilin on contractility of human gallbladder. Dig Dis Sci 28:539, 1983.
43. Keane FB, DiMagno EP, Dozois RR, et al: Relationships among canine interdigestive exocrine pancreatic and biliary flow, duodenal motor activity, plasma pancreatic polypeptide, and motilin. Gastroenterology 78:310, 1980.
44. Konturek SJ, Krol R, Dembinski A, et al: Effect of motilin on pancreatic secretion. Pflugers Arch 364:297, 1976.
45. Christofides ND, Modlin IM, Fitzpatrick ML, et al: Effect of motilin on the rate of gastric emptying and gut hormone release during breakfast. Gastroenterology 76:903, 1979.
46. Christofides ND, Long RG, Fitzpatrick ML, et al: Effect of motilin on the gastric emptying of glucose and fat in humans. Gastroenterology 80:456, 1981.
47. Garthwaite TL: Peripheral motilin administration stimulates feeding in fasted rats. Peptides 6:41, 1985.
48. Chan-Palay V, Ito M, Tongroach P, et al: Inhibitory effects of motilin, somatostatin, [Leu]enkephalin, [Met]enkephalin, and taurine on neurons of the lateral *sigma*-aminobutyric acid. Proc Natl Acad Sci USA 79:3355, 1982.
49. Phillis JW, Kirkpatrick JR: The actions of motilin, luteinizing hormone releasing hormone, cholecystokinin, somatostatin, vasoactive intestinal peptide, and other peptides on rat cerebral cortical neurons. Can J Physiol Pharmacol 58:612, 1980.
50. Samson WK, Lumpkin MD, McCann SM: Motilin stimulates growth hormone release *in vitro*. Brain Res Bull 8:117, 1982.
51. Janik JS, Track NS, Filler RM: Motilin, human pancreatic polypeptide, gastrin, and insulin plasma concentrations in fasted children. J Pediatr 101:51, 1982.
52. Fujimoto S, Miyazaki M, Ishigami H, et al: Plasma motilin levels in patients with abdominal surgery. Acta Chir Scand 148:33, 1982.
53. Ohe K, Sumii K, Sano K, et al: Serum motilin in gastrointestinal diseases. Endocrinol Jpn 1:167, 1980.
54. Besterman HS, Christofides ND, Welsby PD, et al: Gut hormones in acute diarrhoea. Gut 24:665, 1983.
55. Preston DM, Adrian TE, Christofides ND, et al: Positive correlation between symptoms and circulating motilin, pancreatic polypeptide and gastrin concentrations in functional bowel disorders. Gut 26:1059, 1985.
56. Klapdor R, Hammer E: Interdigestive motilin secretion and gallstone disease. Klin Wochenschr 61:251, 1983.
57. Wingate DL, Bloom SR, Gorchein A: Absent nerves and absent motilin. Scand J Gastroenterol 17(Suppl 71):139, 1982.
58. Itoh Z, Aizawa I, Sekiguchi T: The interdigestive migrating complex and its significance in man. Clinics Gastroenterol 11:497, 1982.

Chapter 24

Substance P

J. Patrick Walker, M.D., and James C. Thompson, M.D.

HISTORY

In 1930, U. S. von Euler was working in the laboratory of H. H. Dole in Hampstead, London, attempting to demonstrate a vagally mediated release of acetylcholine. He discovered a material in intestinal extracts that produced contraction of the rabbit jejunum. He and J. H. Gaddum further investigated the substance, which was found to exist in appreciable quantities in the brain and to produce systemic hypotension on injection. The unknown material was referred to as substance "P," for preparation [1].

In 1966, Leeman and Hammerschlag identified a sialogogic peptide in bovine hypothalamic tissue on gel exclusion chromatography [2]. In the next few years, this peptide was characterized as substance P [3], and its amino acid sequence was determined [4]. Substance P is an endecapeptide:

H-Arg-Pro-Lys-Pro-Gln-Gln-Phe-Phe-Gly-Leu-Met-NH_2

The C-terminal tripeptide (Gly-Leu-Met-NH_2) is a common carboxyl terminal in the class of peptides referred to as tachykinins: physalaemin, eledoisin, kassinin, and phyllomedusin, which are of molluscan and amphibian origin.

DISTRIBUTION

Substance P was the first regulatory peptide described found to be present in both the gut and the brain, and although it is found in the respiratory and genitourinary tracts as well, it has been most thoroughly studied in the nervous system and gastrointestinal tract.

In the central nervous system, highest concentrations are seen in the basal ganglia and, in particular, in the globus pallidus and substantia nigra [5]. The association of substance P with dopamine (5-hydroxytryptamine gamma-aminobutyric acid) in the striatonigral pathways has been firmly established [6,7], but its role is not clear. Iversen [8] postulated that it may act both as a neurotransmitter and as a modulator of behavioral effects.

In the spinal cord, substance P is concentrated in the dorsal horn, particularly in the substantia gelatinosa [9]. Blumenkopf [10] has linked it to pain perception [10] on the basis of its association with enkephalins [11] and of the loss of substance P immunoreactivity in the substantia gelatinosa of patients with familial dysautonomia [12] (Riley-Day syndrome). The modulation of opiate receptors and self-regulation of substance P have been proposed by Lipkowski et al [13].

Substance P-like immunoreactivity is demonstrable along the entire gastrointestinal tract. It is found in highest concentrations in the small bowel, particularly proximally, and in the colon. The lowest concentrations are in the esophagus and the stomach [14] (Table 24-1). Concentrations of substance P in the wall of the gut are greatest in the external muscle layer (including the myenteric plexus) and are minimal in the mucosa [14,15].

ASSAY

Automated solid-phase synthesis of substance P was accomplished in 1974 [16]. Sensitive and specific radioimmunoassays have made possible metabolic studies on substance P [17,18].

PHARMACOKINETICS AND CATABOLISM

Substance P is produced by ribosomes and has an intracellular half-life of 4.4 days [19]. The circulating half-life, space of distribution, and metabolic

Table 24-1. Concentrations of immunoreactive substance P in the gastrointestinal tract of humans

Tissue	*Concentration (pmol/g)*
Duodenum	19.7 ± 3.9
Jejunum	17.5 ± 1.5
Terminal ileum	13.8 ± 3.2
Descending colon	7.1 ± 1.5

(Data from Holzer et al [14].)

clearance rate are not known. A specific enzyme has been identified in neural tissues that appears to be responsible for its degradation [20].

RELEASE

Substance P appears to be released by food challenge, with peak plasma concentrations occurring approximately 15 minutes after a meat meal. Concentrations return to baseline 90 minutes after eating (Fig 24-1) [18].

ACTIONS

The actions of substance P appear to be both direct, mediated by specific receptors, and indirect; they are dependent on acetylcholine. Direct actions include contraction of intestinal smooth muscle [1,21], contraction of the gallbladder, reduction of bile flow, decrease in biliary sodium output, and increase in pancreatic juice output [22].

Vasoactive intestinal peptide- and cholecystokinin-stimulated increases in bile and amylase secretion were reduced to control levels by simultaneous infusion of substance P (Fig 24-2). The mechanism may be one of competition, since CCK inhibits binding of substance P to pancreatic acinar cells [23].

Bathing isolated rat ileum with substance P had several effects on ion transport: 1) chloride transport was changed from absorption to secretion, 2) sodium absorption was decreased, 3) flux of calcium was increased without producing any net change [24].

Similar effects have been demonstrated in dogs. Zinner et al [25] have shown that infusion of substance P into a canine jejunal loop produces secretion of water, sodium, chloride, and potassium. Simultaneous infusion of verapamil reversed this secretion to net absorption, which implies that calcium-channel blockade modulates the effects of substance P.

Stimulation of calcitonin secretion by substance P has been demonstrated in the rat thyroid gland [26]. Interestingly enough, calcitonin gene-related peptide potentially inhibits substance P endopeptidase in cerebral spinal fluid [27]. This prolongs the effects of substance P. Attempts to

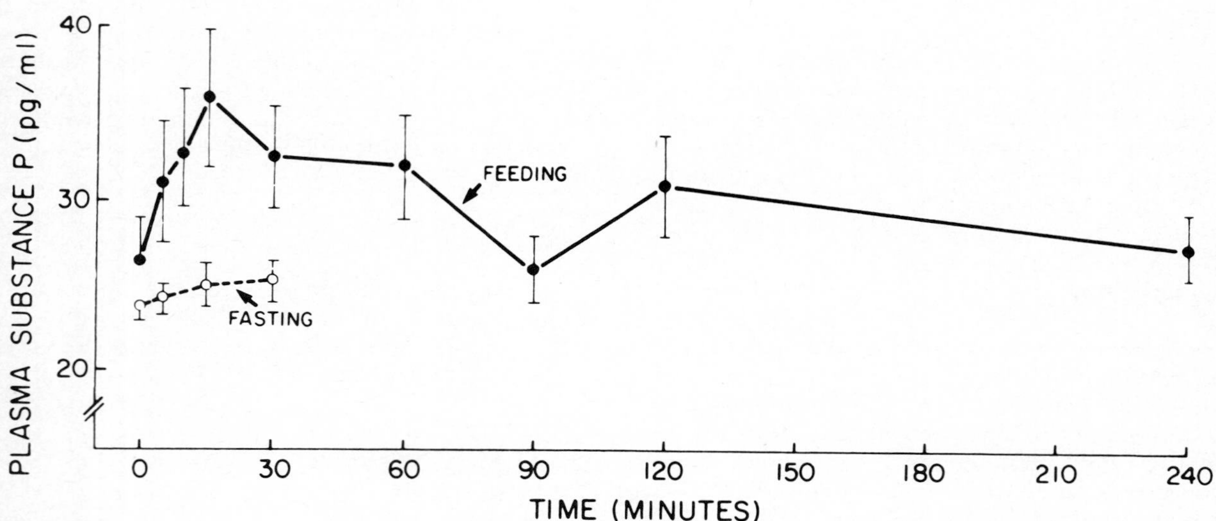

Figure 24-1. The substance P response to a high-protein meal. Data represent the mean ± SEM of values obtained from three dogs (n) in a total of 12 experiments. The control experiments were performed identically, except that the dogs were not fed. (From Akande et al [18], by permission of the C V Mosby Co.)

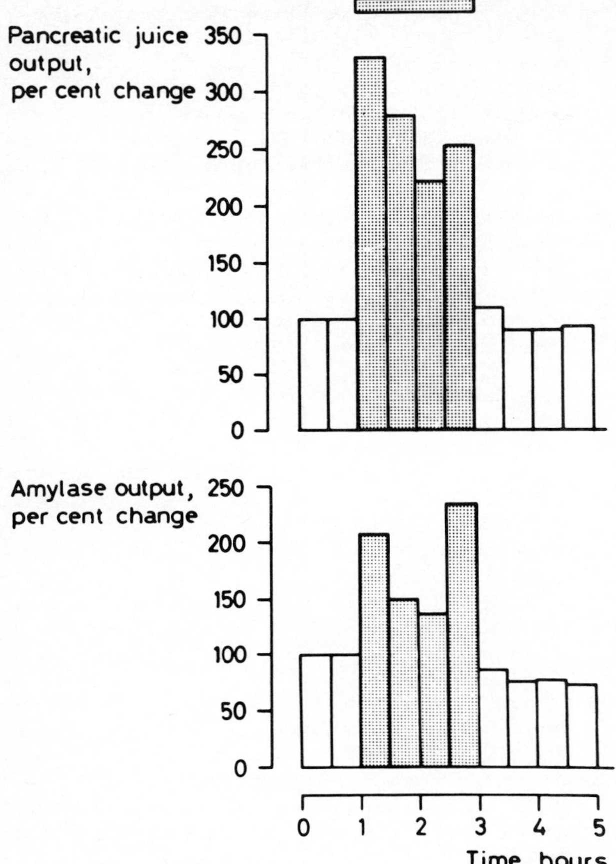

Figure 24-2. Effect of close arterial infusion of substance P (stippled columns) on the output of pancreatic juice. Dosages 20 ng kg^{-1} min^{-1}. (From Thulin and Holm [22], by permission of Raven Press.)

correlate clinical hypermotility (the dumping syndrome) in gastrectomized patients with an increase in serum substance P levels have failed.

Substance P increases proliferation of human T lymphocytes in vitro, as assessed by uptake of tritiated metabolites [28]. It has also been shown that substance P increases production of immunoglobulins (IgA and IgM) and has very little effect on IgG production from immunoglobulin-producing tissue in the gut [29].

The brain-gut link is well demonstrated by the presence of substance P in enterochromaffin cells [30], where it is again associated with 5-hydroxytryptamine [31]. This association is clinically documented by the presence of substance P-like immunoreactivity in intestinal carcinoid tumors as well as in pheochromocytoma [32]. Elevated blood levels of substance P may be associated with symptoms shown by patients with the carcinoid syndrome in whom elevated levels of serotonin are not demonstrated [33]. A recent study by Zinner et al [34] suggests that serotonin as well as substance P may be responsible for some of the manifestations of the dumping syndrome.

Ehrenpreis and Pernow noted in 1953 that substance P was absent in the aganglionic portion of the colon in Hirschsprung's disease [35]. Substance P nerve fibers are not affected by Crohn's disease and remain the same number as in control individuals [36].

Other nongastrointestinal effects have been demonstrated with substance P, i.e., a direct bronchoconstrictor action [37] and a natriuretic effect on the kidney [38]. A paradoxical effect (in humans) is seen with serum levels of substance P, which fell in volunteers placed on a high sodium diet. This same study showed a marked increase in substance P levels in ambulatory individuals compared with those who were supine (from 168 + 31 pmol/L to 401 ± 51 pmol/L) [39]. Substance P is reduced in patients with Huntington's chorea [40].

The diffuse distribution of substance P-like immunoreactivity in the female genital tract, its actions on smooth muscle from the uterus and fallopian tube, and its effects on gonadotropin release have been the stimulus for the birth of the so-called brain-gonad axis [41]. The association between brain substance P and female genital tract substance P is similar to that proposed for the hormones linking the brain-gut axis. Substance P is also found in the male genital tract, where it works presynaptically to modulate tension in the seminal vesicle and vas deferens [42].

In summary, substance P appears to function as a postsynaptic modulatory regulatory peptide in several well-described systems, for example, in dopaminergic/serotonin pathways in the central nervous system, in pain sensory neurons in the spinal cord, and in the role of a neuroendocrine link within viscera, in which it produces diffuse constrictor activity in smooth muscle within the lung, the gut, and the genitourinary tract. Its vasodilatory properties are direct and probably demonstrated clinically in the flushing seen in the carcinoid syndrome. The physiologic role of flushing, however, is unknown.

REFERENCES

1. von Euler US, Gaddum JH: An unidentified depressor substance in certain tissue extracts. J Physiol 72:74, 1931.
2. Leeman SE, Hammerschlag R: Stimulation of salivary secretion by a factor extracted from hypothalamic tissue. Endocrinology 81:803, 1967.

3. Chang MM, Leeman SE: Isolation of a sialogogic peptide from bovine hypothalamic tissue and its characterization as substance P. J Biol Chem 245:4784, 1970.
4. Chang MM, Leeman SE, Niall HD: Amino-acid sequence of substance P. Nature New Biol 232:86, 1971.
5. Cooper PE, Fernstrom MH, Rorstad OP, et al: The regional distribution of somatostatin, substance P and neurotensin in human brain. Brain Res 218:219, 1981.
6. Hokfelt T, Vincent S, Dalsgaard C-J, et al: Distribution of substance P in brain and periphery and its possible role as a co-transmitter, in Porter R, O'Connor M (eds): *Substance P in the Nervous System.* London, Pitman Books Ltd, 1982, pp 84–100.
7. Glowinski J, Torrens Y, Beaujouan JC: The striatonigral substance P pathway and dopaminergic mechanisms, in Porter R, O'Connor M (eds): *Substance P in the Nervous System.* London, Pitman Books Ltd, 1982, pp 281–295.
8. Iversen SD: Behavioural effects of substance P through dopaminergic pathways in the brain, in Porter R, O'Connor M (eds): *Substance P in the Nervous System.* London, Pitman Books Ltd, 1982, pp 307–324.
9. Cuello AC, Priestley JV, Matthews MR: Localization of substance P in neuronal pathways, in Porter R, O'Connor M (eds): *Substance P in the Nervous System.* London, Pitman Books Ltd, 1982, pp 55–83.
10. Blumenkopf MB: Neuropharmacology of the dorsal root entry zone. Neurosurgery 15:900, 1984.
11. LaMotte CC, De Lanerolle NC: Human spinal neurons: Innervation by both substance P and enkephalin. Neuroscience 6:713, 1981.
12. Pearson J, Brandeis L, Cuello AC: Depletion of substance P-containing axons in substantia gelatinosa of patients with diminished pain sensitivity. Nature 295:61, 1982.
13. Lipkowski AW, Osipiak B, Czlonkowski A, et al: An approach to the elucidation of self-regulatory mechanism of substance P action. I. Synthesis and biological properties of pentapeptides related both to the substance P C-terminal fragment and enkephalins. Pol J Pharmacol Pharm 34:63, 1982.
14. Holzer P, Bucsics A, Saria A, et al: A study of the concentrations of substance P and neurotensin in the gastrointestinal tract of various mammals. Neuroscience 7:2919, 1982.
15. Llewellyn-Smith IJ, Furness JB, Murphy R, et al: Substance P-containing nerves in the human small intestine. Distribution, ultrastructure, and characterization of the immunoreactive peptide. Gastroenterology 86:421, 1984.
16. Fisher GH, Humphries J, Folkers K, et al: Synthesis and some biological activities of substance P. J Med Chem 17:843, 1974.
17. Powell D, Leeman S, Tregear GW, et al: Radioimmunoassay for substance P. Nature New Biol 241:252, 1973.
18. Akande B, Reilly P, Modlin IM, et al: Radioimmunoassay measurement of substance P release following a meat meal. Surgery 89:378, 1981.
19. Keen P, Harmar AJ, Spears F, et al: Biosynthesis, axonal transport and turnover of neuronal substance P, in Porter R, O'Connor M (eds): *Substance P in the Nervous System.* London, Pitman Books Ltd, 1982, pp 145–164.
20. Lee C-M: Enzymatic inactivation of substance P in the central nervous system, in Porter R, O'Connor M (eds): *Substance P in the Nervous System.* London, Pitman Books Ltd, 1982, pp 165–185.
21. Rosell S, Bjorkroth U, Chang D, et al: Effects of substance P and analogs on isolated guinea pig ileum, in von Euler US, Pernow B (eds): *Substance P.* New York, Raven Press, 1977, pp 83–88.
22. Thulin L, Holm I: Effect of substance P on the flow of hepatic bile and pancreatic juice, in von Euler US, Pernow B (eds): *Substance P.* New York, Raven Press, 1977, pp 247–251.
23. Sjodin L: Cholecystokinin inhibits binding of substance P to pancreatic acinar cells. Acta Physiol Scand 124:471, 1985.
24. Walling MW, Brasitus TA, Kimberg DV: Effects of calcitonin and substance P on the transport of Ca, Na, and Cl across rat ileum in vitro. Gastroenterology 73:89, 1977.
25. Zinner MJ, Sherlock D, Ferrera A, et al: Verapamil inhibition of the intestinal effects of substance P. Surgery 98:230, 1985.
26. Ahren B, Grunditz T, Ekman R, et al: Neuropeptides in the thyroid gland: Distribution of substance P and gastrin/cholecystokinin and their effects on the secretion of iodothyronine and calcitonin. Endocrinology 113:379, 1983.
27. LeGreves P, Nyberg F, Terenius L, et al: Calcitonin gene-related peptide is a potent inhibitor of substance P degradation. Eur J Pharmacol 115:309, 1985.
28. Payan DG, Brewster DR, Goetzl EJ: Specific stimulation of human T lymphocytes by substance P. J Immunol 131:1613, 1983.
29. Stanisz AM, Befus D, Bienenstock J: Differential effects of vasoactive intestinal peptide, substance P, and somatostatin on immunoglobulin synthesis and proliferations by lymphocytes from Peyer's patches, mesenteric lymph nodes, and spleen. J Immunol 136:152, 1986.
30. Pearse AGE, Polak JM: Immunocytochemical localization of substance P in mammalian intestine. Histochemistry 41:373, 1975.
31. Sundler F, Håkanson R, Larsson L-I, et al: Substance P in the gut: An immunochemical and immunohistochemical study of its distribution and development, in von Euler US, Pernow B (eds): *Substance P.* New York, Raven Press, 1977, pp 59–65.
32. Håkanson R, Bengmark S, Brodin E, et al: Substance P-like immunoreactivity in intestinal carcinoid tumors, in von Euler US, Pernow B (eds): *Substance P.* New York, Raven Press, 1977, pp 55–58.
33. Gamse R, Saria A, Bucsics A, et al: Substance P in

tumors: Pheochromocytoma and carcinoid. Peptides 2(Suppl 2):275, 1981.
34. Zinner MJ, Yeo CJ, Jaffe BM: The effect of carcinoid levels of serotonin and substance P on hemodynamics. Ann Surg 199:197, 1984.
35. Ehrenpreis T, Pernow B: On the occurrence of substance P in the rectosigmoid in Hirschsprung's disease. Acta Physiol Scand 27(Suppl 97):380, 1952.
36. Sjolund K, Schaffalitzky de Muckadell OB, Fahrenkrug J, et al: Peptide-containing nerve fibres in the gut wall in Crohn's disease. Gut 24:724, 1983.
37. Nilsson G, Dahlberg K, Brodin E, et al: Distribution and constrictor effect of substance P in guinea pig tracheobronchial tissue, in von Euler US, Pernow B (eds): *Substance P*. New York, Raven Press, 1977, pp 75–81.
38. Mills IH, Macfarlane NAA, Ward PE: Increase in kallikrein excretion during the natriuresis produced by arterial infusion of substance P. Nature 247:108, 1974.
39. Kramer HJ, Dusing R, Stelkens H, et al: Immunoreactive substance P in human plasma: Response to changes in posture and sodium balance. Clin Sci 59:75, 1980.
40. Sagar SM, Beal MF, Marshall PE, et al: Implications of neuropeptides in neurological diseases. Peptides 5(Suppl 1):255, 1984.
41. Skrabanek P, Powell D: Substance P in obstetrics and gynecology. Obstet Gynecol 61:641, 1983.
42. Stjernquist M, Håkanson R, Leander S, et al: Immunohistochemical localization of substance P, vasoactive intestinal polypeptide and gastrin-releasing peptide in vas deferens and seminal vesicle, and the effect of these and eight other neuropeptides on resting tension and neurally evoked contractile activity. Regul Pept 7:67, 1983.

Chapter 25

Enteric Bombesin-Like Peptides

George H. Greeley, Jr., Ph.D., and Jan Newman, M.D.

HISTORY

Bombesin is a 14 amino acid peptide initially isolated from skin extracts of two European frogs, *Bombina bombina* and *Bombina variegata variegata,* by Erspamer [1]. McDonald et al [2] and Reeve et al [3] later isolated and characterized heptacosapeptides that resembled the C-terminal of bombesin from porcine nonantral gastric and canine intestinal tissue extracts, respectively, with gastrin-releasing activity; these have been named gastrin-releasing peptide (GRP). Orloff et al [4] have described the sequence of a human bombesin-like peptide and the partial structure of a larger form isolated from acid extracts of liver tissue containing a metastatic bronchial carcinoid tumor. McDonald et al [5] have also reported the sequence of a 27-residue chicken proventricular peptide that is structurally homologous to porcine GRP. The C-terminal decapeptide fragment of porcine GRP is identical to the C-terminal decapeptide of bombesin, except for a Gln/His interchange at positions 7 in bombesin and 20 in GRP. The primary structures of each are shown below and their homologous residues are underlined.

Bombesin:

pGlu-Gln-Arg-Leu-Gly-Asn-Gln-
1 2 3 4 5 6 7

Trp-Ala-Val-Gly-His-Leu-Met-NH_2
8 9 10 11 12 13 14

Porcine GRP:

Ala-Pro-Val-Ser-Val-Gly-Gly-Gly-Thr-

Val-Leu-Ala-Lys-Met-Tyr-Pro-Arg-Gly-Asn-
18 19

His-Trp-Ala-Val-Gly-His-Leu-Met-NH_2
20 21 22 23 24 25 26 27

The primary structure of chicken GRP is shown below; the residues homologous to pGRP are underlined:

Ala-Pro-Leu-Gln-Pro-Gly-Gly-Ser-Pro-Ala-
1 6

Leu-Thr-Lys-Ile-Tyr-Pro-Arg-Gly-
11 13 15

Ser-His-Trp-Ala-Val-Gly-His-Leu-Met-NH_2
20 27

More recently, two decapeptides resembling the C-terminal primary structure of bombesin and GRP have been isolated and characterized from porcine canine intestine and spinal cord. These peptides are called GRP-10 (neuromedin C) and neuromedin B [3,6,7]. Reeve et al [3] also described a 23-residue GRP-like peptide that was isolated from canine intestinal extracts.

There are four residue differences between porcine and canine GRP. These *differences* are underlined in the primary structure of canine GRP-27 shown below.

Canine GRP:

Ala-Pro-Val-Pro-Gly-Gly-Gln-Gly-Thr-
4 5 7

Val-Leu-Asp-Lys-Met-Tyr-Pro-Arg-Gly-Asn-
12

His-Trp-Ala-Val-Gly-His-Leu-Met-NH_2

DISTRIBUTION

Bombesin-like immunoreactivity (BLI) has been localized in a wide variety of species and is almost ubiquitous in the body, as determined by radioimmunoassay (RIA) and immunocytochemical methods [8,9]. Bombesin-like immunoreactivity is found in the gill epithelium, myenteric plexus, and stomach of fish; in the gastric antrum and fundus, brain, skin and esophagus of frogs; and in the avian proventricularis and gastrointestinal tract. In these species, bombesin-like immunoreactivity is located in endocrine-like cells.

Detectable levels of BLI are present in rat, rabbit, and human sera [9]; however, whether the bombesin-like immunoreactivity found in blood is authentic bombesin is not clear. Remarkably enough, bombesin-like immunoreactivity has been detected in milk, along with a variety of other peptides [10,11].

BLI has also been found in the stomach, small intestine, and colon of rats and in the gastrointestinal tract of guinea pigs, pigs, rabbits, dogs, monkeys, and humans [12–16]. Localization of BLI has been limited, in large part, to nerve cells, although there is a report of its presence in gut endocrine-type cells [9].

BLI has been detected in rat, guinea pig, and cat lung [8,9,14,17] and in human neonatal and fetal but not adult lungs [18,19]. In the developing human lung, the concentration of BLI increases throughout gestation, plateaus at birth, remains constant during childhood, and then decreases in adulthood to one tenth of adolescent levels. Centers of BLI levels are localized in mucosal neuroendocrine cells of the airway epithelium, mostly in intrapulmonic airways. A marked diminution of bombesin-like immunoreactivity is found in infants who die of acute respiratory distress syndrome. GRP and calcitonin have been identified within the same cell of fetal and adult human lungs [20]. Human small cell carcinomas of the lung have been found to contain bombesin-like immunoreactivity [21–23].

Yamaguchi et al [24] found two immunoreactive variants of GRP in normal human fetal (31–140 ng/g) and adult lungs and in primary lung tumors. One form corresponds to GRP 1-27 and the other elutes behind porcine GRP (14-27) on Sephadex S-50. Some GRP-containing cells are present in bronchial and bronchiolar mucosa of normal adult lungs [25]. GRP-positive cells are also found in significant amounts in medullary carcinomas of the thyroid in humans [26].

In humans, one study indicates that the highest levels of BLI are found in the fundus, antrum, pylorus, and pancreas, with smaller amounts in the duodenum, jejunum, terminal ileum, and colon [16]. BLI is found in both the muscle and mucosal layers of the antrum and colon. Sephadex gel chromatography showed that both GRP- and bombesin-like peptides are present. High pressure liquid chromatography (HPLC) demonstrated that the human GRP peak appears to be closely related to porcine GRP (1-27).

According to Yanaihara et al [27,28], the highest GRP concentration in porcine gut is found in the mucosa of the stomach corpus (2.97 ± 0.89 fmol/mg tissue), whereas the muscle layer (0.64 ± 0.34 fmol/mg) contained about 20 percent of that measured in the mucosa. GRP immunoreactivity was not found in the cardia of the stomach. The antral mucosa contained about 20 percent GRP of that measured in the corpus mucosa. As regards the intestine, the jejunal muscle contained the highest level and the mucosa of the intestine contained very little, if any, GRP. Large amounts of GRP are apparently present in the pancreas (4.21 ± 2.35 fmol/mg). These findings, for the most part, agree with those regarding the distribution of a bombesin-like peptide (which may actually be GRP) in the rat gut [8].

BLI has been found in the central nervous system (CNS) of rats, dogs, and sheep [8,9,13,14]. It was first shown in rat brain by Brown et al [14], and further studies have shown that BLI is found in discrete brain nuclei [29] and in the spinal cord [30]. Using sequence-specific antisera, Roth et al [31] suggested that authentic bombesin is not present in the rat or guinea pig brain. In the guinea pig brain, peptides that resemble porcine GRP (18-27), GRP (1-27), and GRP (1-16) were found, whereas in the rat CNS, peptides resembling GRP (18-27) and GRP (1-16) were observed. Roth et al suggested that the GRP (18-27) of guinea pig CNS extracts was identified as bombesin in earlier studies. Furthermore, the rat and guinea pig peptides are not identical, since they behave differently on HPLC and are not identically recognized by different antisera.

Mammalian tissue stores of GRP- or bombesin-like immunoreactivity can be separated chromatographically into at least three variants. Two major peaks of GRP-like immunoreactivity have been described for the pig stomach, pancreas, and duodenum [27]. One peak co-elutes with authentic porcine GRP (1-27) and another co-elutes with porcine GRP (14-27) on gel chromatograpy. Subsequent chromatography on CM Sephadex of the smaller variant results in two separate immunoreactive peaks. McDonald et al [32] have also found at least two forms of GRP immunoreactivity in porcine gut extracts. Apparently, a β-aspartyl shift is present in the Asn-His sequence of a form of GRP.

Immunohistochemical studies show specific GRP immunoreactivity (bombesin absorbed antisera) in nerve fibers and in neurons of the rat and guinea pig gastrointestinal wall, whereas specific GRP immunoreactivity is absent in the endocrine/paracrine cells of the chicken proventriculus. The close proximity of GRP/bombesin-containing nerves to gut muscles and myenteric ganglion cells suggests their possible role in regulating gastrointestinal motility [33]. More recently, Moghimzadeh et al [34] reported that immunoreactive GRP is contained in neuronal elements of the pig pancreas and alimentary canal of numerous mammals. GRP-containing fibers appear to be intramural, since GRP-containing nerve bodies are found in the myenteric ganglia all along the gut. Thus, GRP may function to regulate intramural neural activity, smooth muscle tone, gut secretion, and absorption. Panula et al [35] have shown bombesin/GRP-like immunoreactivity in rat sensory ganglion and spinal cord. These observations coincide with the idea that there is a bombesin/GRP-containing primary sensory pathway that runs from the sensory ganglia to the spinal cord.

Dockray et al [36] have found two molecular forms of bombesin-like activity in their extracts of the rat stomach.

Yanaihara et al [27] reported the presence of GRP immunoreactive nerve fibers in the myenteric nerve plexus of the porcine duodenum and in the intrapancreatic ganglion, but GRP-positive cells were not seen in the endocrine cells of the porcine stomach and intestinal mucosa. Dockray et al [36] gave immunohistochemical evidence for bombesin-like peptides in the mucosa of the rat stomach but not in the intestine. Polak et al [37] have reported immunochemical localization of bombesin in human mucosal endocrine cells. These differences might be attributed to technical or intraspecies differences. In any case, these data suggest that a family of small peptides with a COOH-terminal identical to that of bombesin and GRP exists in the mammalian alimentary canal. The amount of GRP variants and their relative concentrations may vary among species. Whether GRP variants exist predominantly in the mucosa or muscle layer of the gut also seems to vary among species. More recently, Spindel et al [38] have isolated and cloned cDNAs corresponding to mRNAs encoding for the precursor of human GRP.

ASSAY

Several RIAs have been developed to measure bombesin-like peptides [8,16,27,39]. Many of these antibodies are directed to the C-terminal and are generated against the C-terminal nonapeptide or lysine substituted bombesin, which is conjugated to bovine serum albumin (BSA), or human α-globulin, etc. Tyr-4 or Tyr-10 bombesin is radioiodinated and used as a trace. Most of these antibodies show a high specificity for bombesin and GRP, with minimal cross-reactivity with substance P, vasoactive intestinal peptide, ranatensin, and litorin [8,14,17]. Tissues require acid extraction [8,14,17] before they are subjected to assay.

PHARMACOKINETICS AND CATABOLISM

In humans, the disappearance half-time of bombesin is 3.1 ± 0.6 min and the metabolic clearance rate (MCR) is 34.3 ± 5.8 mL/kg/min [40]. The apparent volume of distribution is 146 mL/kg. In the pig, the disappearance of GRP from the plasma is characterized by slow and fast components ($T\frac{1}{2}$ = 1.4, 6.6 min) [39]. The MCRs are 37 ± 8 and 76 ± 23 mL/kg min at the high and low levels of GRP concentration during the infusion.

RELEASE

The exact mechanism of bombesin release is unknown. Postprandial elevations have not been found, except by Erspamer and Melchiorri [41]. Many aspects of the location, mechanism of release, and physiologic functions of bombesin are unexplored. In conscious adrenalectomized calves, splanchnic nerve stimulation resulted in release of bombesin-like immunoreactivity, suggesting that the pancreatic endocrine responses (insulin, glucagon) are mediated in part by bombesin-like immunoreactivity [42]. Release of BLI is stimulated from the isolated perfused rat stomach [43,44] by acetylcholine. Electrical stimulation of the vagus nerves results in an hexamethonium-blockable elevation of the release of GRP from the isolated pancreas and a concurrent increase in pancreatic exocrine secretion [45]. Gastric inhibitory polypeptide (GIP) can inhibit BLI release, which is dependent on intraluminal pH. Blockade of muscarinic and nicotinic cholinergic receptors abolished the effect of acetylcholine [43]. In pigs, electrical stimulation of the vagi leads to release of GRP from the fundus and antrum, whereas splanchnic stimulation is ineffective [39].

ACTIONS

Bombesin exhibits direct and indirect effects on the gastrointestinal system, including release of hormones, motility, and pancreatic gastric and intestinal secretion [46]. Bombesin stimulates release of gastrin [40,46,47], pancreatic polypeptide (PP) [40], cholecystokinin (CCK) [47,48], motilin, neurotensin, enteroglucagon [40], pancreatic glucagon, and insulin in humans and dogs and release of fasting and postprandial somatostatin in dogs [40,49]. In humans, bombesin administration (2.4 pmol/kg/min) also caused elevation in serum calcium, a reduction in plasma parathyroid hormone and glucose levels, and a late rise in calcitonin [40]. We were unable to release secretin in dogs with bombesin infusion [48].

There is a report [50] that GRP cannot release neurotensin in humans and that atropine can enhance the gastrin-releasing action of GRP but not of bombesin. Atropine also blocked the rise in GRP-induced PP release but not in bombesin-induced PP release. Apparently, in contrast to meal-stimulated neurotensin release, bombesin-stimulated neurotensin release is cholinergic-independent. More interesting, the peptide-releasing activities of bombesin and GRP are different despite structural homologues. In humans, GRP infusion (0.7 and 2.9 pmol/min/kg) causes gastrin, CCK, and neurotensin release and potentiates glucose-induced insulin secretion [51]. Vagotomy is reported to increase bombesin-stimulated release of gastrin [52], to either decrease [53] or have no effect on bombesin-stimulated release of PP [54], and to have no effect on bombesin-stimulated release of CCK [52]. Atropine can inhibit bombesin-induced PP release but is without effect on release of gastrin, whereas bethanechol decreases gastrin release but is ineffective on PP release [55]. Met-enkephalin can suppress bombesin-stimulated PP release, which can be reversed by naloxone [56]. Larson et al [57] found that bombesin-induced tachyphylaxis of gastrin release caused by prolonged bombesin infusion significantly enhanced meal-stimulated gastrin release. Tachyphylaxis also occurred with PP release, but meal-stimulated enhancement of PP did not occur. In the dog, bombesin does not mediate food-stimulated release of gastrin.

In rats, vagotomy has no effect on bombesin-stimulated release of neurotensin [58]. Similar patterns of neurotensin release are caused by bombesin, synthetic porcine GRP, and natural porcine and chicken GRP in rats [58]. In the dog, bombesin and synthetic porcine GRP exhibit equimolar potency in stimulation of gastrin, PP, glucagon, enteroglucagon, and insulin [59]. Bombesin can stimulate motilin release, yet it inhibits the action of motilin (peristalsis as measured by the interdigestive migratory motor complex) [60]. Hence, bombesin probably does not act physiologicaly as an endocrine regulator of motilin release, although it might act as a paracrine or neuroendocrine stimulator of motilin release.

Bombesin apparently can stimulate gastric secretion directly or via release of gastrin [48]. It also stimulates pancreatic secretion directly and via release of CCK [47,48,61]. Like CCK, bombesin and GRP can cause residual stimulation of isolated pancreatic acini [62]. Bombesin can also inhibit absorption of water, sodium, and chloride from the jejunum [63].

In vivo administration of bombesin causes gallbladder contraction [9,64,65]; however, such contraction may be due to CCK release. Bombesin can increase spontaneous activity and pacesetter potentials and cause contraction in the stomach and small intestine in many species [9,33,64–66]. This bombesin-induced increase in pacesetter potential results in a decrease in peristalsis because of a loss of normal propagation and lack of coordinated activity. In smooth muscle preparations, GRP-27 is less potent than bombesin-14 [67]. Chronic administration of bombesin causes hyperplasia of antral gastrin cells in the rat [68].

Both central and peripheral administration of bombesin induce satiety in rats [9,69,70]; and in combination with CCK, the bombesin effect is additive [69] and apparently not mediated by the vagus [70]. Centrally administered bombesin can decrease gastric and pancreatic secretion in rats [71–73]. In rats, intracerebroventricular (ICV) administration of bombesin causes them to respond to changes in environmental temperature in a poikilothermic manner. Goats maintained at 20°C become hypothermic [9]. These effects are also observed with anterior hypothalamic injection of bombesin but not with injection into other brain areas or intracisternal injection [9].

Tache et al [74] have investigated the effect of administration of GRP into the brain on gastric acid secretion of rats. Intracisternal administration of GRP resulted in an elevation of serum gastrin levels 2 hours later, whereas systemic injection of GRP caused immediate gastrin release. Interestingly, intracisternal injection of GRP inhibited gastric secretion (both volume and acidity) in a dose-dependent manner, whereas intravenous GRP was ineffective. Intracisternal GRP can also block the stimulatory action of intracisternally administered thyrotropin-releasing hormone, 2-deoxyglucose, or subcutaneous histamine on gastric acid secretion. These data suggest that GRP may exert a central neural inhibitory action on gastric secretion. Furthermore, this unique action of GRP in the CNS is independent of gastrin release. Lesion and knife-cut studies indicate that the gastrin-releasing effect of ICV bombesin is dependent upon axons traversing the posterior, lateral, and medial borders of the lateral hypothalamus and is independent of gastric pH changes [75]. The lateral hypothalamic area is not necessary for the acid-stimulatory action of bombesin in rats.

In dogs, ICV administration of bombesin results in elevated serum gastrin levels, whereas peripheral blood levels of PP and CCK are unaffected [76]. Vagotomy does not influence this release of gastrin induced by ICV injection of bombesin [76]. This ICV bombesin-induced release of gastrin may be a result of the reduction in acid secretion, since Pappas et al [77] have shown that bombesin, given centrally, can inhibit pentagastrin-induced acid secretion in the innervated and vagally denervated canine stomach. They have also shown [77] that bombesin, given centrally, inhibits meal-induced acid secretion.

Other central effects of bombesin include release of somatostatin into the hypothalamohypophyseal blood of rats [9], excess grooming and locomotor activity, and inhibition of the avoidance response. Bombesin also potentiates sedation and impairment of the aerial righting reflex caused by ethanol [9]. GRP can inhibit growth hormone secretion in part by causing release of hypothalamic somatostatin [78,79].

Administration of GRP or bombesin results in qualitatively similar secretory patterns of gastrin, PP, enteroglucagon, GIP, and pancreatic glucagon in dogs [80]. In dogs, bombesin and GRP cause a transient rise in insulin secretion. In rats, GRP causes a delayed transient release of insulin and an immediate prolonged release of gastrin [81]. In rats, however, the elevation in insulin is preceded or coincides with an elevated serum GIP level, indicating that bombesin and GRP can exert their insulinotropic action via GIP release as well as directly [82]. McDonald et al [80] report that release of GIP occurs after insulin release. In dogs, GRP can release CCK, PP, and gastrin [83]. Both GRP and bombesin cause dose-dependent elevations in gastric acid output and elevations in circulating PP and gastrin levels in dogs. At 1,140 pmol/kg/hr, both GRP and bombesin inhibit gastric acid output and serum gastrin secretion. This study indicates that these peptides are equipotent [84]. In humans [51], GRP infused intravenously (0.7 and 2.9 pmol/min/kg) causes release of gastrin, CCK, and neurotensin, and GRP potentiates the insulin-releasing action of glucose. Bombesin can elevate plasma somatostatin levels in dogs, which is under vagal-cholinergic control [85].

GRP exhibits a variety of actions that are reminiscent of bombesin. Although it is 5–10 times less potent [67], central administration of GRP results in a dose-dependent hypothermia and hyperglycemia in rats [86]. The hyperglycemic action of GRP is probably mediated via the CNS-adreno-medullary-pancreatic axis. Central administration of GRP, like bombesin, causes a rise in plasma epinephrine. GRP also causes a stereotypic scratching of the neck and face. On a molar basis, GRP is approximately 30 percent less potent than bombesin in inhibiting food intake in rats [87]. GRP, given centrally in rats, can inhibit prolactin secretion induced by a met-enkephalin analogue [88] and can also blunt domperidone-induced prolactin release. GRP was ineffective on prolactin release in an in vitro pituitary model, suggesting that it exerts its action via central dopaminergic systems. In rats, IV GRP does not influence serum growth hormone or follicle-stimulating hormone levels, but it stimulates leutinizing hormone release and inhibits thyroid-stimulating hormone release [89].

Reeve et al [3] reported that 27- and 10-residue bombesin-like peptides isolated from the dog gut are quantitatively similar in potency to bombesin and pGRP on gastric secretion in rats and stimulation of gastric smooth muscle contraction in dogs. Interestingly, a synthetic carboxy-terminal decapeptide of pGRP, which is identical to canine bombesin decapeptide, is 30 times less potent in comparison to synthetic pGRP with regard to its CNS action. In conscious dogs, bombesin and GRP-27 were more potent than GRP-23 and GRP-10 in terms of gastrin release [90].

In studies with isolated mouse acini, pGRP and bombesin exerted a stimulatory effect on amylase release and on 2-DG uptake and an inhibitory effect on the uptake of α-aminoisobutyric acid [91]. CCK-8 and carbachol exerted similar effects, but the effects of pGRP were not blocked by dibutyryl cyclic guanosine-3′,5′-monophosphate or atropine, in contrast to the inhibitory action of the dibutyryl cyclic guanosine-3′,5′-monophosphate on CCK and atropine on carbachol. These findings suggest that pGRP actions in mouse acini are mediated by its own receptor.

REFERENCES

1. Anastasi A, Erspamer V, Bucci M: Isolation and structure of bombesin and alytesin, two analogous active peptides from the skin of the European amphibians *Bombina* and *Alytes*. Experientia 27:166, 1971.
2. McDonald TJ, Jornvall H, Nilsson G, et al: Characterization of a gastrin releasing peptide from porcine non-antral gastric tissue. Biochem Biophys Res Commun 90:227, 1979.

3. Reeve JR Jr, Walsh JH, Chew P, et al: Amino acid sequences of three bombesin-like peptides from canine intestine extracts. J Biol Chem 258:5582, 1983.
4. Orloff MS, Reeve JR Jr, Ben-Avram CM, et al: Isolation and sequence analysis of human bombesin-like peptides. Peptides 5:865, 1984.
5. McDonald TJ, Jornvall H, Ghatei M, et al: Characterization of an avian gastric (proventricular) peptide having sequence homology with the porcine gastrin-releasing peptide and the amphibian peptides bombesin and alytesin. FEBS Lett 122:45, 1980.
6. Minamino N, Kangawa K, Matsuo H: Neuromedin B: A novel bombesin-like peptide identified in porcine spinal cord. Biochem Biophys Res Commun 114:541, 1983.
7. Minamino N, Kangawa K, Matsuo H: Neuromedin C: A bombesin-like peptide identified in porcine spinal cord. Biochem Biophys Res Commun 119:14, 1984.
8. Walsh JH, Wong HC, Dockray GJ: Bombesin-like peptides in mammals. Fed Proc 38:2315, 1979.
9. Nemeroff CB, Luttinger D, Prange AJ Jr: Neurotensin and bombesin, in Iversen LL, Iverson SD, Snyder SH (eds): *The Handbook of Psychopharmacology.* New York, Plenum Press, 1983, pp 363–466.
10. Jahnke GD, Lazarus LH: A bombesin immunoreactive peptide in milk. Proc Natl Acad Sci USA 81:578, 1984.
11. Ekman R, Ivarsson S, Jansson L: Bombesin, neurotensin and pro-*sigma*-melanotropin immunoreactants in human milk. Regul Pept 10:99, 1985.
12. McDonald TJ: Non-amphibian bombesin-like peptides, in Bloom SR, Polak JM (eds): *Gut Hormones.* New York, Churchill Livingstone, 1981, pp 407–412.
13. Walsh JH, Reeve JR Jr, Vigna SR: Distribution and molecular forms of mammalian bombesin, in Bloom SR, Polak JM (eds): *Gut Hormones.* New York, Churchill Livingstone, 1981, pp 413–418.
14. Brown M, Allen R, Villarreal J, et al: Bombesin-like activity: Radioimmunologic assessment in biological tissues. Life Sci 23:2721, 1978.
15. Greeley GH Jr, Spannagel A, Burdett JB, et al: Distribution of gastrin-releasing peptide and bombesin-like peptides in the alimentary canal of rats, rabbits, dogs and humans. Gastroenterology 86:1097, 1984.
16. Price J, Penman E, Wass JAH, et al: Bombesin-like immunoreactivity in human gastrointestinal tract. Regul Pept 9:1, 1984.
17. Ghatei MA, Sheppard MN, O'Shaughnessy DJ, et al: Regulatory peptides in the mammalian respiratory tract. Endocrinology 111:1248, 1982.
18. Wharton J, Polak JM, Bloom SR, et al: Bombesin-like immunoreactivity in the lung. Nature 273:769, 1978.
19. Ghatei MA, Sheppard MN, Henzen-Logman S, et al: Bombesin and vasoactive intestinal polypeptide in the developing lung: Marked changes in acute respiratory distress syndrome. J Clin Endocrinol Metab 57:1226, 1983.
20. Tsutsumi Y, Osamura RY, Watanabe K, et al: Simultaneous immunohistochemical localization of gastrin releasing peptide (GRP) and calcitonin (CT) in human bronchial endocrine-type cells. Virchows Arch [A] 400:163, 1983.
21. Sorenson GD, Bloom SR, Ghatei MA, et al: Bombesin production by human small cell carcinoma of the lung. Regul Pept 4:59, 1982.
22. Erisman MD, Linnoila RI, Hernandez O, et al: Human lung small-cell carcinoma contains bombesin. Proc Natl Acad Sci USA 79:2379, 1982.
23. Moody TW, Russell EK, O'Donohue TL, et al: Bombesin-like peptides in small cell lung cancer: Biochemical characterization and secretion from a cell line. Life Sci 32:487, 1983.
24. Yamaguchi K, Abe K, Kameya T, et al: Production and molecular size heterogeneity of immunoreactive gastrin-releasing peptide in fetal and adult lungs and primary lung tumors. Cancer Res 43:3932, 1983.
25. Tsutsumi Y, Osamura RY, Watanabe K, et al: Immunohistochemical studies on gastrin-releasing peptide- and adrenocorticotropic hormone-containing cells in the human lung. Lab Invest 48:623, 1983.
26. Kameya T, Bessho T, Tsumuraya M, et al: Production of gastrin releasing peptide by medullary carcinoma of the thyroid. An immunohistochemical study. Virchows Arch [A] 401:99, 1983.
27. Yanaihara N, Yanaihara C, Mochizuki T, et al: Immunoreactive GRP. Peptides 2(Suppl 2):185, 1981.
28. Yanaihara C, Inoue A, Mochizuki T, et al: Bombesin-like immunoreactivity in mammalian tissues. Biomed Res 1:96, 1980.
29. Moody TW, O'Donohue TL, Jacobowitz DM: Biochemical localization and characterization of bombesin-like peptides in discrete regions of rat brain. Peptides 2:75, 1981.
30. O'Donohue TL, Massari VJ, Pazoles CJ, et al: A role for bombesin in sensory processing in the spinal cord. J Neurosci 4:2956, 1984.
31. Roth KA, Evans CJ, Lorenz RG, et al: Identification of gastrin releasing peptide-related substances in guinea pig and rat brain. Biochem Biophys Res Commun 112:528, 1983.
32. McDonald TJ, Jornvall H, Tatemoto K, et al: Identification and characterization of variant forms of the gastrin-releasing peptide (GRP). FEBS Lett 156:349, 1983.
33. Caprilli R, Melchiorri P, Improta G, et al: Effects of bombesin and bombesin-like peptides on gastrointestinal myoelectric activity. Gastroenterology 68:1228, 1975.
34. Moghimzadeh E, Ekman R, Håkanson R, et al: Neuronal gastrin-releasing peptide in the mammalian gut and pancreas. Neuroscience 10:553, 1983.
35. Panula P, Hadjiconstantinou M, Yang H-YT, et al: Immunohistochemical localization of bombesin/gastrin-releasing peptide and substance P in primary sensory neurons. J Neurosci 3:2021, 1983.
36. Dockray GJ, Vaillant C, Walsh JH: The neuronal origin of bombesin-like immunoreactivity in the rat gastrointestinal tract. Neuroscience 4:1561, 1979.
37. Polak JM, Hobbs S, Bloom SR, et al: Distribution of a bombesin-like peptide in human gastrointestinal tract. Lancet 1:1109, 1976.

38. Spindel ER, Chin WW, Price J, et al: Cloning and characterization of cDNAs encoding human gastrin-releasing peptide. Proc Natl Acad Sci USA 81:5699, 1984.
39. Knuhtsen S, Holst JJ, Knigge U, et al: Radioimmunoassay, pharmacokinetics, and neuronal release of gastrin-releasing peptide in anesthetized pigs. Gastroenterology 87:372, 1984.
40. Ghatei MA, Jung RT, Stevenson JC, et al: Bombesin: Action on gut hormones and calcium in man. J Clin Endocrin Metab 54:980, 1982.
41. Erspamer V, Melchiorri P: Growth hormone release inhibitory hormone, substance P, neurotransmitters, skin hormones: Amphibian skin polypeptides active on the gut. J Endocrinol 70:12p, 1976.
42. Bloom SR, Edwards AV: Characteristics of the neuroendocrine responses to stimulation of the splanchnic nerves in bursts in the conscious calf. J Physiol 346:533, 1984.
43. Schusdziarra V, Bender H, Pfeffer A, et al: Modulation of acetylcholine-induced secretion of gastric bombesin-like immunoreactivity by cholinergic and histamine H_2-receptor, somatostatin and intragastric pH. Regul Pept 8:189, 1984.
44. Schusdziarra V, Bender H, Pfeiffer EF: Release of bombesin-like immunoreactivity from the isolated perfused rat stomach. Regul Pept 7:21, 1983.
45. Knuhtsen S, Holst JJ, Jensen SL, et al: Gastrin-releasing peptide: Effect on exocrine secretion and release from isolated perfused porcine pancreas. Am J Physiol 248:G281, 1985.
46. Erspamer V, Melchiorri P: Actions of bombesin on secretions and motility of the gastrointestinal tract, in Thompson JC (ed): *Gastrointestinal Hormones.* Austin, University of Texas Press, 1975, pp 575–589.
47. Fender HR, Curtis PJ, Rayford PL, et al: Effect of bombesin on serum gastrin and cholecystokinin in dogs. Surg Forum 27:414, 1976.
48. Miyata M, Rayford PL, Thompson JC: Hormonal (gastrin, secretin, cholecystokinin) and secretory effects of bombesin and duodenal acidification in dogs. Surgery 87:209, 1980.
49. Schusdziarra V, Rouiller D, Harris V, et al: Effect of bombesin upon plasma somatostatin-like immunoreactivity, insulin and glucagon in normal and chemically sympathectomized dogs. Regul Pept 1:89, 1980.
50. Fletcher DR, Shulkes A, Bladin PHD, et al: The effect of atropine on bombesin and gastrin releasing peptide stimulated gastrin, pancreatic polypeptide and neurotensin release in man. Regul Pept 7:31, 1983.
51. Wood SM, Jung RT, Webster JD, et al: The effect of the mammalian neuropeptide, gastrin-releasing peptide (GRP), on gastrointestinal and pancreatic hormone secretion in man. Clin Sci 65:365, 1983.
52. Rayford PL, Guzman S, Hill FLC, et al: The effects of vagotomy on bombesin-stimulated release of gastrin and cholecystokinin in dogs. Physiologist 21:97, 1978.
53. Modlin IM, Lamers CB, Jaffe BM: Evidence for cholinergic dependence of pancreatic polypeptide release by bombesin—a possible application. Surgery 88:75, 1980.
54. Singer MV, Niebel W, Lamers C, et al: Effects of truncal vagotomy and antrectomy on bombesin-stimulated pancreatic secretion, release of gastrin, and pancreatic polypeptide in the anesthetized dog. Dig Dis Sci 26:871, 1981.
55. Taylor IL, Walsh JH, Carter D, et al: Effects of atropine and bethanechol on bombesin-stimulated release of pancreatic polypeptide and gastrin in dog. Gastroenterology 77:714, 1979.
56. Materia A, Jaffe BM, Modlin IM, et al: Effect of methionine-enkephalin and naloxone on bombesin-stimulated gastric acid secretion, gastrin, and pancreatic polypeptide release in the dog. Ann Surg 196:48, 1982.
57. Larson T, Sanchez J, Taylor IL: Bombesin-induced tachyphylaxis markedly enhances gastrin response to a meal. Am J Physiol 244:G652, 1983.
58. Rokaeus A, Yanaihara N, McDonald TJ: Increased concentration of neurotensin-like immunoreactivity (NTLI) in rat plasma after administration of bombesin and bombesin-related peptides (porcine and chicken gastrin-releasing peptides). Acta Physiol Scand 114:605, 1982.
59. McDonald TJ, Ghatei MA, Bloom SR, et al: Dose-response comparisons of canine plasma gastroenteropancreatic hormone responses to bombesin and the porcine gastrin-releasing peptide (GRP). Regul Pept 5:125, 1983.
60. Poitras P, Tasse D, Laprise P: Stimulation of motilin release by bombesin in dogs. Am J Physiol 245:G249, 1983.
61. Deschodt-Lanckman M, Robberecht P, De Neef P, et al: In vitro action of bombesin and bombesin-like peptides on amylase secretion, calcium efflux, and adenylate cyclase activity in the rat pancreas. A comparison with other secretagogues. J Clin Invest 58:891, 1976.
62. Howard JM, Jensen RT, Gardner JD: Bombesin-induced residual stimulation of amylase release from mouse pancreatic acini. Am J Physiol 248:G196, 1985.
63. Barbezat GO, Reasbeck PG: Effects of bombesin, calcitonin, and enkephalin on canine jejunal water and electrolyte transport. Dig Dis Sci 28:273, 1983.
64. Endean R, Erspamer V, Erspamer GF, et al: Parallel bioassay of bombesin and litorin, a bombesin-like peptide from the skin of *Litoria aurea.* Br J Pharmacol 55:213, 1975.
65. Erspamer V, Erspamer GF, Inselvini M, et al: Occurrence of bombesin and alytesin in extracts of the skin of three European discoglossid frogs and pharmacological actions of bombesin on extravascular smooth muscle. Br J Pharmacol 45:333, 1972.
66. Kowalewski K, Kolodej A: Effect of bombesin, a natural tetradecapeptide, on myoelectrical and mechanical activity of isolated, *ex vivo* perfused, canine stomach. Pharmacology 14:8, 1976.
67. Mazzanti G, Erspamer GF, Piccinelli D: Relative potencies of porcine bombesin-like heptacosapeptide

(PB-27), amphibian bombesin (B-14) and litorin, and bombesin C-terminal nonapeptide (B-9) on in vitro and in vivo smooth muscle preparations. J Pharm Pharmacol 34:120, 1982.
68. Lehy T, Accary JP, Labeille D, et al: Chronic administration of bombesin stimulates antral gastrin cell proliferation in the rat. Gastroenterology 84:914, 1983.
69. Morley JE, Levine AS, Kneip J, et al: The effect of vagotomy on the satiety effects of neuropeptides and naloxone. Life Sci 30:1943, 1982.
70. Stein LJ, Woods SC: Cholecystokinin and bombesin act independently to decrease food intake in the rat. Peptides 2:431, 1981.
71. Morley JE, Levine AS, Silvis SE: Central regulation of gastric acid secretion: The role of neuropeptides. Life Sci 31:399, 1982.
72. Tache Y: Bombesin: Central nervous system action to increase gastric mucus in rats. Gastroenterology 83:75, 1982.
73. Dubrasquet M, Roze C, Ling N, et al: Inhibition of gastric and pancreatic secretions by cerebroventricular injections of gastrin-releasing peptide and bombesin in rats. Regul Pept 3:105, 1982.
74. Tache T, Marki W, Rivier J, et al: Central nervous system inhibition of gastric secretion in the rat by gastrin-releasing peptide, a mammalian bombesin. Gastroenterology 81:298, 1981.
75. Tache Y, Grijalva CV, Gunion MW, et al: Lateral hypothalamic mediation of hypergastrinemia induced by intracisternal bombesin. Neuroendocrinology 39:114, 1984.
76. Swierczek SJ, Lu Q-H, Zhu X-G, et al: Effects of vagotomy on the release of gastrointestinal hormones induced by peripheral and central administration of bombesin in dogs. Gastroenterology 84:1328, 1983.
77. Pappas T, Hamel D, Debas H, et al: Cerebroventricular bombesin inhibits gastric acid secretion in dogs. Gastroenterology 89:43, 1985.
78. Kabayama Y, Kato Y, Shimatsu A, et al: Inhibition by gastrin-releasing peptide of growth hormone (GH) secretion induced by human pancreatic GH-releasing factor in rats. Endocrinology 115:649, 1984.
79. Kentroti S, McCann SM: The effect of gastrin-releasing peptide on growth hormone secretion in the rat. Endocrinology 117:1363, 1985.
80. McDonald TJ, Ghatei MA, Bloom SR, et al: A qualitative comparison of canine plasma gastroenteropancreatic hormone responses to bombesin and the porcine gastrin-releasing peptide (GRP). Regul Pept 2:293, 1981.
81. Greeley GH Jr, Thompson JC: Effect of gastrin-releasing peptide on serum insulin levels in adult male rats. Proc Soc Exp Biol Med 172:271, 1983.
82. Greeley GH Jr, Burdett JB, Hill FLC, et al: Bombesin-(BBS), gastrin-releasing peptide-(GRP), and neuromedin-induced release of gastric inhibitory polypeptide (GIP) and insulin in rats. Dig Dis Sci 29:31S, 1984.
83. Inoue K, McKay D, Yajima H, et al: Effect of synthetic porcine gastrin-releasing peptide on plasma levels of immunoreactive cholecystokinin pancreatic polypeptide and gastrin in dogs. Peptides 4:153, 1983.
84. Lambert JR, Hansky J, Soveny C, et al: Comparative effects of bombesin and porcine gastrin-releasing peptide in the dog. Dig Dis Sci 29:1036, 1984.
85. De Graef J, Woussen-Colle MC: Effects of sham feeding, bethanechol, and bombesin on somatostatin release in dogs. Am J Physiol 248:G1, 1985.
86. Brown M, Marki W, Rivier J: Is gastrin releasing peptide mammalian bombesin? Life Sci 27:125, 1980.
87. Stein LJ, Woods SC: Gastrin releasing peptide reduces meal size in rats. Peptides 3:833, 1982.
88. Matsushita N, Kato Y, Katakami H, et al: Inhibition of prolactin secretion by gastrin releasing peptide (GRP) in the rat. Proc Soc Exp Biol Med 172:118, 1983.
89. Gullner H-G, Owen WW, Yajima H: Effect of porcine gastrin releasing peptide on anterior pituitary hormone release. Biochem Biophys Res Commun 106:831, 1982.
90. Orloff MS, Melendez RL, Rivier J, et al: Serum gastrin and gastric acid output in response to infusion of bombesin and three gastrin releasing peptides in conscious dogs. Gastroenterology 86:1202, 1984.
91. Iwamoto Y, Nakamura R, Akanuma Y: Effects of porcine gastrin-releasing peptide on amylase release, 2-deoxyglucose uptake, and α-aminoisobutyric acid uptake in mouse pancreatic acini. Endocrinology 113:2106, 1983.

Chapter 26

Candidate Agents

James C. Thompson, M.D., and others

For many years, the only universally recognized gastrointestinal hormones were gastrin, cholecystokinin, and secretin. Criteria for acceptance as a full-fledged member varied. Even today, experts would disagree if attempts were made to compile a list of absolutely accepted gastrointestinal hormones. Grossman [1] gave this problem careful thought and suggested that peptides that satisfy the following criteria are likely to function as hormones: 1) they should be present in endocrine cells; 2) they should be released by feeding or some other physiologic stimulus, and in the process of release they should increase their plasma concentrations and produce their characteristic biologic effects; and 3) they should mimic, by infusion of exogenous peptide, the plasma concentration which, when observed with endogenous release, reproduces the biologic effect. There may be some problems with the last part of that definition. We have recently studied a group of inhibitors of pancreatic secretion that produce no effect when infused individually in amounts that achieve postprandial plasma concentrations but that do achieve inhibition when infused together in the same amounts. Stimulation of pancreatic secretion by interaction of secretin and cholecystokinin may be another example of this phenomenon.

Most classifications are arbitrary, and the division of agents into those that are physiologic and those that are not probably requires a series of arbitrary choices. The problem is not unimportant. Vast efforts were expended in the study of the effect of gastrin on the lower esophageal sphincter before a consensus was achieved that the effect was present only with supraphysiologic concentrations of gastrin in serum. When Grossman and others [2] described 19 candidate hormones of the gut in 1974, only gastrin, secretin, and cholecystokinin were recognized. Most would agree now that gastric inhibitory polypeptide and probably the enteric forms of glucagon are gut hormones. Motilin also appears likely to satisfy the test of time. I suspect that many of the agents discussed in Chaps. 20–25 qualify, although the significance of the activities of pancreatic polypeptide is not yet clear. VIP is a neurotransmitter and not a hormone.

The agents to be discussed in this chapter (the intestinal phase hormone, analogues of pancreatic polypeptide, epidermal growth factor/urogastrone, and peptide histidine isoleucine) are clear examples of arbitrary choices. Each agent is in a different stage of study. The intestinal phase hormone has been postulated on physiologic evidence since the 1920s, but there is, as yet, scant chemical confirmation. Peptide YY may be the most active ingredient in Harper's pancreotone [3].

REFERENCES

1. Grossman MI: Physiological effects of gastrointestinal hormones. Fed Proc 36:1930, 1977.
2. Grossman MI, Brown JC, Said S, et al: Candidate hormones of the gut. Gastroenterology 67:730, 1974.
3. Harper AA, Hood AJC, Mushens J, et al: Pancreotone, an inhibitor of pancreatic secretion in extracts of ileal and colonic mucosa. J Physiol 292:455, 1979.

INTESTINAL PHASE HORMONE

Anders Alwmark, M.D., Ph.D., and James C. Thompson, M.D.

In 1902 Pavlov noticed a stimulation of the acid secretion from his dog's stomach when food passed the small intestine [1]. About 20 years later, Ivy and coworkers found an increased acid secretion even though a gastric pouch was denervated [2], and furthermore, they proposed the existence of an intestinal phase of gastric secretion. In 1941,

Ivy and Gregory transplanted a stomach pouch subcutaneously and found stimulation of the acid secretion from an intestinal meal, thus giving evidence for a positive humoral stimulus [3]. Evidence in regard to this stimulus has been previously reviewed [4–7].

Stimulation of acid secretion by distention of the small intestine, first demonstrated by Sircus [4] and later confirmed [8,9], was to become the strongest evidence in favor of a humoral stimulus for the intestinal phase as opposed to the concept that absorption of amino acids was actually responsible for the stimulation of acid secretion during the latter phases of digestion [10,11].

Most work in favor of the existence of a distinct hormone, called *entero-oxyntin* by Grossman et al [12], has been done by Orloff et al [7] starting from the well-demonstrated phenomenon of acid hypersecretion found in both animals and humans after portacaval shunting [6]. Orloff et al have further demonstrated that an extract of hog jejunal mucosa had a stimulatory effect on gastric secretion [13]. This was confirmed in a study which reported that a peptide fraction from the proximal intestine of pigs had some of the characteristics of entero-oxyntin [14].

The concept that amino acids serve as the mediator of the so-called intestinal phase of secretion has its most persuasive advocates in Landor et al [10], who have found many properties shared by amino acids and the putative intestinal phase hormone [11]. They have recently modified their concept to suggest that the intestinal phase of secretion results from the combined effect of absorbed amino acids and hormonal influences [15].

One obvious question is whether this so-called intestinal phase of gastric secretion is separate from the other known stimulants of gastric secretion—gastrin, histamine, and vagal acetylcholine. Histamine is nearly completely extracted on a single hepatic transit [16] and is therefore not a candidate. Gastrin levels are not elevated after stimulation of the intestinal phase of secretion [17–20]. The vagus does have a possible modulatory role in intestinal phase secretion [21,22], whereas the sympathetic nervous system does not seem to

Table 26-1. **A specific intestinal phase hormone**

Evidence in favor of

Instillation of proteins, peptides, or amino acids into the small intestine stimulates acid secretion from the stomach (even from a denervated pouch) [3,22,23].
Bypassing the jejunum diminishes the secretion [24].
An intestinal meal potentiates other physiologic stimuli (gastrin, histamine, cholecystokinin, pentagastrin) [22,25].
Intestinal distention causes increased acid secretion [4,8].
The supposed hormone should be metabolized in the liver, as seen from the portacaval shunt-related hypersecretion [26,27].
The supposed hormone should originate mainly from the proximal part of the jejunum, as seen from food stimulation of different parts of the intestine [28].
Recent studies show that protein given intraintestinally produced greater gastric secretion than did amino acids given intravenously [15].
Extracts from hog intestinal mucosa (HIME) have effects on acid secretion in accordance with a proposed hormone [13].
Promising results from fractionation and characterization [7,14,29].

Evidence against

The hormone is not yet isolated or characterized.
Amino acids given enterally or parenterally give an equally high and rapid response in gastric acid secretion [30].*
Amino acids potentiate the effect of histamine and pentagastrin [11].*
The effect of amino acid infusion diminishes if given intraportally [11].*
The effect of amino acids given intestinally or in the portal vein in shunted dogs was increased compared to when it was given in nonshunted dogs [10].*

* Points advanced by Landor and colleagues in support of their contention that the actions of the so-called intestinal phase hormone or entero-oxyntin are actually caused by absorbed amino acids.

control the release or the action of a putative intestinal phase hormone [19].

The evidence for and against the existence of a specific intestinal phase hormone, collected from pertinent studies, is presented in Table 26-1.

REFERENCES

1. Pavlov JP: *The Work of the Digestive Glands.* Thompson WH (translator): London, Charles Griffin & Company, Ltd., 1902, pp 1–189.
2. Ivy AC, Lim RKS, McCarthy JE: Contributions to the physiology of gastric secretion. II. The intestinal phase of gastric secretion. Q J Exp Physiol 15:55, 1925.
3. Gregory RA, Ivy AC: The humoral stimulation of gastric secretion. Q J Exp Physiol 31:111, 1941.
4. Sircus W: The intestinal phase of gastric secretion. Q J Exp Physiol 38:91, 1953.
5. Thompson JC, Peskin GW: The intestinal phase of gastric secretion. Am J Med Sci 241:159, 1961.
6. Thompson JC: Alterations in gastric secretion after portacaval shunting. Am J Surg 117:854, 1969.
7. Orloff MJ, Hyde PVB, Kosta LD, et al: The intestinal phase hormone. World J Surg 3:523, 1979.
8. Nagano K, Johnson AN Jr, Cobo A, et al: The effect of distension of the duodenum on gastric secretion. Surg Forum 10:152, 1959.
9. Thompson JC, Tramontana JA, Lerner HJ, et al: Physiologic scope of the antral inhibitory hormone. Ann Surg 156:550, 1962.
10. Landor JH, Gough AL, Rai VS, et al: Amino acids as possible mediators of the intestinal phase of gastric secretion. Surg Gynecol Obstet 150:203, 1980.
11. Mariano EC, Beloni A, Landor JH: Some properties shared by amino acids and entero-oxyntin. Ann Surg 188:181, 1978.
12. Grossman MI and others: Candidate hormones of the gut. Gastroenterology 67:730, 1974.
13. Orloff MJ, Charters AC, Nakaji NT: Further evidence for an intestinal phase hormone that stimulates gastric acid secretion. Surgery 80:145, 1976.
14. Vagne M, Mutt V: Entero-oxyntin: A stimulant of gastric acid secretion extracted from porcine intestine. Scand J Gastroenterol 15:17, 1980.
15. Mariano EC, Deak S, Reddell MT, et al: Mechanisms of protein activation of the intestinal phase of gastric secretion. Surgery 95:492, 1984.
16. Thompson JC, Reeder DD, Davidson WD, et al: Effect of hepatic transit of gastrin, pentagastrin, and histamine measured by gastric secretion and by assay of hepatic vein blood. Ann Surg 170:493, 1969.
17. Wheeler MH, Bhattacherjee S, Psaila JV, et al: Studies on the release of extra-antral gastrin. Evidence of vagal inhibition in the dog. World J Surg 1:639, 1977.
18. Kauffman GL Jr, Grossman MI: Serum gastrin during intestinal phase of acid secretion in dogs. Gastroenterology 77:26, 1979.
19. Grabner P, Donahue PE, Grabner ET, et al: The lack of effect of propranolol on the intestinal-phase secretion in the dog. Scand J Gastroenterol 16:65, 1981.
20. Grabner P, Donahue PE, Grabner T, et al: Non-gastrin, intestinal-phase secretion. Experimental confirmation in the dog. Scand J Gastroenterol 15:165, 1980.
21. Konturek SJ, Llanos OL, Rayford PL, et al: Vagal influence on gastrin and gastric acid responses to gastric and intestinal meals. Am J Physiol 232:E542, 1977.
22. Way LW, Cairns DW, Deveney CW: A pharmacological profile of entero-oxyntin. Surgery 77:841, 1975.
23. Kelly KA, Nyhus LM, Harkins HN: A reappraisal of the intestinal phase of gastric secretion. Am J Surg 109:1, 1965.
24. Hesselfeldt P, Christiansen J, Rehfeld JF, et al: Meal-stimulated gastric acid and gastrin secretion before and after jejuno-ileal shunt operation in obese patients. A preliminary report. Scand J Gastroenterol 14:13, 1979.
25. Debas HT, Slaff GF, Grossman MI: Intestinal phase of gastric acid secretion: Augmentation of maximal response of Heidenhain pouch to gastrin and histamine. Gastroenterology 68:691, 1975.
26. Orloff MJ, Windsor CWO: Effect of portacaval shunt on gastric acid secretion in dogs with liver disease, portal hypertension and massive ascites. Ann Surg 164:69, 1966.
27. Orloff MJ, Villar-Valdes H, Rosen H, et al: Humoral mediation of the intestinal phase of gastric secretion and of acid hypersecretion associated with portacaval shunts. Surgery 66:118, 1969.
28. Orloff MJ, Villar-Valdes H, Abbott AG, et al: Site of origin of the hormone responsible for gastric hypersecretion associated with portacaval shunt. Surgery 68:202, 1970.
29. Orloff MJ, Charters AC, Nakaji NT: Isolation of the hormone responsible for the intestinal phase of gastric secretion. Gastroenterology 70:A-132/990, 1976.
30. Landor JH, Ipapo VS: Gastric secretory effect of amino acids given enterally and parenterally in dogs. Gastroenterology 73:781, 1977.

PANCREATIC POLYPEPTIDE ANALOGUES: PEPTIDE YY AND NEUROPEPTIDE Y

Tsuguo Sakamoto, M.D., and
George H. Greeley, Jr., Ph.D.

History

Recently, two novel peptides, peptide YY (PYY) and neuropeptide Y (NPY), which are structurally similar to pancreatic polypeptide (PP), have been isolated and characterized from porcine brain and intestinal extracts [1–3]. Another 37-residue peptide, isolated and characterized by Andrews et al [4] from the endocrine pancreas of the angler fish, is also structurally related to PYY and NPY. NPY and PYY, like PP, consist of a linear chain of 36 amino acids, with a COOH-terminal tyrosine amide [5,6]. PYY and NPY were isolated using a novel biochemical method, which detects a carboxy-terminal α-amide group. Primary structures of PYY (porcine) and NPY (porcine) and of P-PP, B-PP, and A-PP follow.

NPY:
Tyr-Pro-Ser-Lys-Pro-Asp-Asn-Pro-Gly-Gly-Asp-
Ala-Pro-Ala-Glu-Asp-Leu-Ala-Arg-Tyr-
Tyr-Ser-Ala-Leu-Arg-His-Tyr-Ile-Asn-
Leu-Ile-Thr-Arg-Gln-Arg-Tyr-NH_2

PYY:
Tyr-Pro-Ala-Lys-Pro-Glu-Ala-Pro-Gly-Glu-Asp-
Ala-Ser-Pro-Glu-Glu-Leu-Ser-Arg-Tyr-
Tyr-Ala-Ser-Leu-Arg-His-Tyr-Leu-Asn-
Leu-Val-Thr-Arg-Gln-Arg-Tyr-NH_2

P-PP:
Ala-Pro-Leu-Glu-Pro-Val-Tyr-Pro-Gly-Asp-Asp-
Ala-Thr-Pro-Glu-Gln-Met-Ala-Gln-Tyr-
Ala-Ala-Glu-Leu-Arg-Arg-Tyr-Ile-Asn-
Met-Leu-Thr-Arg-Pro-Arg-Tyr-NH_2

B-PP:
Ala-Pro-Leu-Glu-Pro-Glu-Tyr-Pro-Gly-Asp-Asn-
Ala-Thr-Pro-Glu-Gln-Met-Ala-Gln-Tyr-
Ala-Ala-Glu-Leu-Arg-Arg-Tyr-Ile-Asn-
Met-Leu-Thr-Arg-Pro-Arg-Tyr-NH_2

A-PP:
Gly-Pro-Ser-Gln-Pro-Thr-Tyr-Pro-Gly-Asp-Asp-
Ala-Pro-Val-Glu-Asp-Leu-Ile-Arg-Phe-
Tyr-Asp-Asn-Leu-Gln-Gln-Tyr-Leu-
Asn-Val-Val-Thr-Arg-His-Arg-Tyr-NH_2

NPY has a high degree of sequence homology with PYY (70 percent) and avian-PP (55 percent), since there are identical residues in the 25 and 20 positions, respectively [5]. There is slightly less primary structural homology between NPY and human, porcine, and bovine PP. In addition, these peptides exhibit biologic activity similar to that of PP (i.e., inhibition of pancreatic exocrine secretion) [1,2,5,6]. Hence, these peptides, which are structurally and biologically similar, belong to a novel family of brain-gut peptides [3].

Distribution

NPY is found widely distributed in the mammalian peripheral and central nervous systems [7–23]. In the human brain [7,18], NPY exists in large amounts in the hippocampus, amygdala, limbic system, septal nuclei, hypothalamus, nucleus accumbens, caudate, putamen, and Brodmann's area 4. NPY appears to be the most abundant neuropeptide in both human and rat brain, even exceeding the levels of cholecystokinin-8 (CCK-8) and somatostatin [15]. In the rat, NPY is found in catecholamine neurons of the lower medulla oblongata [8], in the spinal cord [11], in the juxtaglomerular apparatus [12], in the respiratory tract and middle ear [14,24], and in the innervation of the heart [10]. NPY is also found in peripheral noradrenergic neurons (e.g., cervical, stellate, and celiac ganglia) of various mammals, including humans [19]. Immunoreactive NPY-containing cells are also found colocalized with choline acetyltransferase in the submucous neurons of the small intestine of the guinea pig [20]. In the guinea pig, NPY is found in the gallbladder, cystic duct, and common bile duct [13]. NPY-containing nerves are especially dense in the guinea pig myenteric and mucosa plexuses. Blood vessels in many organs, including the nasal mucosa, submandibular gland, heart, lung, pancreas, uterus, and urinary bladder, are surrounded by NPY-containing nerves [25,26].

Although NPY-containing neuronal elements have been demonstrated in the gut and pancreas [27], NPY-containing endocrine cells in the gut and pancreas have not been detected [9]. NPY-containing fibers are found in all layers of the gut wall; hence NPY may have multiple functions, such as regulation of intramural neuronal activity, smooth muscle tone, and local blood flow [27]. NPY has been isolated from acid extracts of adrenal medullary pheochromocytoma tissue [28,29] and from the normal adrenal gland of several mammalian species [21]. NPY may well be the peptide that was previously thought to be PP in the central nervous system [9].

PYY-containing cells have been found in the alimentary canal of several mammalian species [1,2,5,6,9,30–35]. In the human gastrointestinal tract [31], PYY-IR cells are identified in the distal ileum, the colon, and the rectum. PYY-containing cells are of the open type [9], and PYY immunoreactivity does not occur in the same endocrine cell as does PP [32]. In the gastrointestinal tract of the rat [30,32], PYY-containing cells are present mainly in the pylorus, ileum, and colon and in the periphery of the pancreatic islets. PYY appears to be colocalized with glucagon in the endocrine cells of the gut and pancreas [36]. PYY immunoreactivity is not found in the brain or proximal small intestine, and PYY is apparently undetectable in rat plasma [30]. The inability to detect PYY in the circulation of the rat may actually reflect a lack of an appropriate radioimmunoassay (RIA) for plasma PYY. PYY-containing cells have been found in rectal carcinoid tumor specimens [37].

Radioimmunoassay

Various specific antisera and RIAs for PYY and NPY have been described [33–35,38–41]. Circulating levels of PYY in humans have been reported [39] with a mean value of 49 pg/mL.

An antiserum for NPY was raised against natural porcine NPY. This antiserum does not cross-react with P-PP, PYY, or A-PP [7].

Actions

Centrally administered NPY causes hypotension and bradypnea in anesthetized rats [42]. Since NPY immunoreactivity is found in central adrenergic nerve cell bodies [8], this finding suggests a possible role of NPY as a comodulator in the central adrenergic system. NPY causes a dose-dependent inhibition of electrically stimulated contractions of uterine cervical smooth muscle preparations of estrogen-primed rats [43]. Because the contractile response to electrical stimulation is abolished by atropine or tetrodotoxin, NPY may act on prejunctional pathways of cholinergic nerves. The contractile response of the rat vas deferens to electrical stimulation is inhibited by B-PP, H-PP, A-PP, and NPY in a dose-dependent manner. The inhibitory action of NPY on the vas deferens is not altered by α-adrenergic blockade. Hence, NPY may be involved in presynaptic inhibitory mechanisms [44].

In a perfused, isolated, spontaneously beating rabbit heart preparation, a dose-dependent negative inotropic effect is observed in response to NPY [45]. In the same studies, coronary perfusion rates are reduced by NPY. Local intra-arterial infusion of NPY causes a slowly developing vasoconstriction of long duration in the cat submandibular gland [46]. Simultaneous infusion of norepinephrine and NPY can mimic electrically stimulated vasoconstriction, whereas norepinephrine alone does not. These findings suggest that PP-related transmitters such as NPY, in conjunction with norepinephrine, may account for the vascular effects of sympathetic stimulation. Systemic administration of NPY causes a long-lasting increase in systemic arterial blood pressure [19]. The large amounts of NPY contained in nerve cell bodies of the basal ganglia suggest that NPY participates in the central neural control of motor function in humans [7].

NPY, given intracerebroventricularly, can result in release of luteinizing hormone in the rat [47], which suggests that it may play a role in the central neural regulation of gonadotropin secretion in the rat. NPY also stimulates feeding in the rat [48] and enhanced isoprenaline, thyroid-stimulating hormone, and vasoactive intestinal peptide-induced iodothyronine secretion in mice [49].

Taylor [33] has shown that a meal results in a release of PYY and Fink et al [50] have shown that selective perfusion of the distal gut has the same effect. In contrast to its effect on PP release, vagal stimulation is not effective in releasing PYY [33].

PYY can inhibit pancreatic bicarbonate and protein secretion stimulated by secretin alone or together with CCK in the anesthetized cat [6] and conscious dog [40,51,52]. PYY inhibition of secretin-induced bicarbonate secretion is independent of cholinergic pathways [51]. P-PP, at similar doses, did not affect pancreatic secretion in the same study [6]. Local intra-arterial infusion of PYY results in a slowly developing vasoconstriction with a long duration in the cat submandibular salivary gland [53], and the vasoconstrictor effect of PYY persists during α-adrenergic blockade. Intra-arterial administration of PYY into the superior mesenteric artery in cats causes vasoconstriction and an inhibition of jejunal and colonic motility [30]. These effects of PYY also persist in the face of adrenergic blockade. During interdigestive states, an intravenous bolus of PYY can inhibit, in a transient fashion, the interdigestive migrating contractions (IMC) in the innervated main stomach, but PYY does not influence Heidenhain pouch contractions, suggesting that PYY inhibits the IMC in the stomach, probably through extrinsic nerves [54]. PYY can also inhibit bile flow and pancreatic secretions by a direct action of the sphincter of Oddi [55]. Both NPY and PYY appear to inhibit cholinergic transmission in the myenteric plexus of the guinea pig colon, which is mediated via α_2-adrenoreceptors [56]. This results in the relaxation of colonic longitudinal muscle. There is some indication that PYY may actually be pancreatone or one of its constituents [57,58], since PYY inhibits meal-stimulated pancreatic exocrine and gastric secretion in dogs [40]. However, PYY has not yet been shown to inhibit CCK-induced gallbladder contraction [59]. With regard to the action of PYY on the endocrine pancreas, in fed anesthetized rats PYY (100 pmol/kg/min) can inhibit arginine-induced insulin and glucagon secretion but is ineffective on basal secretion of insulin and glucagon and on glucose-induced insulin secretion [60].

Both Lluis [51,52] and Pappas [40,61] and their colleagues have shown that PYY can inhibit gastric acid secretion in the dog. PYY appears to be less potent than secretin but more potent than neurotensin [52]. Pappas et al [61] have reported evidence that PYY is a specific inhibitor of the cephalic phase of gastric acid secretion. Guo et al [62] have reported that PYY can inhibit pentagastrin-induced but is ineffective on histamine-induced acid secretion. Pappas has also suggested that PYY is the putative mediator of the ileal brake [63], whereas NPY was ineffective. Adrian et al [64] have reported that levels of plasma PYY were increased in response to an oral glucose load in patients with the dumping syndrome in comparison to what occurred in normal volunteers. Peptide YY levels were also elevated in patients with steatorrhea due to mucosal atrophy of the small bowel (tropical sprue), chronic destructive pancreatitis, inflammatory bowel disease, and acute infective diarrhea [65]. Based on these new studies, PYY and NPY appear to be two exceptionally interesting peptides.

REFERENCES

1. Tatemoto K, Carlquist M, Mutt V: Neuropeptide Y—A novel brain peptide with structural similarities to peptide YY and pancreatic polypeptide. Nature 296:659, 1982.
2. Tatemoto K, Mutt V: Isolation of two novel candidate hormones using a chemical method for finding naturally occurring polypeptides. Nature 285:417, 1980.
3. Solomon TE: Pancreatic polypeptide, peptide YY, and neuropeptide Y family of regulatory peptides. Gastroenterology 88:838, 1985.
4. Andrews PC, Hawke D, Shively JE, et al: A nonamidated peptide homologous to porcine peptide YY and neuropeptide YY. Endocrinology 116:2677, 1985.
5. Tatemoto K: Neuropeptide Y: Complete amino acid sequence of the brain peptide. Proc Natl Acad Sci USA 79:5485, 1982.
6. Tatemoto K: Isolation and characterization of peptide YY (PYY), a candidate gut hormone that inhibits pancreatic exocrine secretion. Proc Natl Acad Sci USA 79:2514, 1982.
7. Adrian TE, Allen JM, Bloom SR, et al: Neuropeptide Y distribution in human brain. Nature 306:584, 1983.
8. Hokfelt T, Lundberg JM, Tatemoto K, et al: Neuropeptide Y (NPY)- and FMRFamide neuropeptide-like immunoreactivities in catecholamine neurons of the rat medulla oblongata. Acta Physiol Scand 117:315, 1983.
9. Lundberg JM, Terenius L, Hokfelt T, et al: Comparative immunohistochemical and biochemical analysis of pancreatic polypeptide-like peptides with special reference to presence of neuropeptide N in central and peripheral neurons. J Neurosci 4:2376, 1984.
10. Gu J, Polak JM, Allen JM, et al: High concentrations of a novel peptide, neuropeptide Y, in the innervation of mouse and rat heart. J Histochem Cytochem 32:467, 1984.
11. Gibson SJ, Polak JM, Allen JM, et al: The distribution and origin of a novel brain peptide, neuropeptide Y, in the spinal cord of several mammals. J Comp Neurol 227:78, 1984.
12. Ballesta J, Polak JM, Allen JM, et al: The nerves of the juxtaglomerular apparatus of man and other mammals contain the potent peptide NPY. Histochemistry 80:483, 1984.
13. Allen JM, Gu J, Adrian TE, et al: Neuropeptide Y in the guinea-pig biliary tract. Experientia 40:765, 1984.
14. Uddman R, Sundler F, Emson P: Occurrence and distribution of neuropeptide-Y-immunoreactive nerves in the respiratory tract and middle ear. Cell Tissue Res 237:321, 1984.
15. Allen YS, Adrian TE, Allen JM, et al: Neuropeptide Y distribution in the rat brain. Science 221:877, 1983.
16. Allen JM, McGregor GP, Woodhams PL, et al: Ontogeny of a novel peptide, neuropeptide Y (NPY) in rat brain. Brain Res 303:197, 1984.
17. Mantyh PW, Kemp JA: The distribution of putative neurotransmitters in the lateral geniculate nucleus of the rat. Brain Res 288:344, 1983.
18. Dawbarn D, Hunt SP, Emson PC: Neuropeptide Y: Regional distribution, chromatographic characterization and immunohistochemical demonstration in post-mortem human brain. Brain Res 296:168, 1984.
19. Lundberg JM, Terenius L, Hokfelt T, et al: High levels of neuropeptide Y in peripheral noradrenergic neurons in various mammals including man. Neurosci Lett 42:167, 1983.
20. Furness JB, Costa M, Keast JR: Choline acetyltransferase- and peptide immunoreactivity of submucous neurons in the small intestine of the guinea-pig. Cell Tissue Res 237:329, 1984.
21. Varndell IM, Polak JM, Allen JM, et al: Neuropeptide tyrosine (NPY) immunoreactivity in norepinephrine-containing cells and nerves of the mammalian adrenal gland. Endocrinology 114:1460, 1984.
22. Ekblad E, Ekelund M, Graffner H, et al: Peptide-containing nerve fibers in the stomach wall of rat and mouse. Gastroenterology 89:73, 1985.
23. Lee Y, Shiosaka S, Emson PC, et al: Neuropeptide Y-like immunoreactive structures in the rat stomach with special reference to the noradrenalin neuron system. Gastroenterology 89:118, 1985.
24. Sheppard MN, Polak JM, Allen JM, et al: Neuropeptide tyrosine (NPY): A newly discovered peptide is present in the mammalian respiratory tract. Thorax 39:326, 1984.
25. Lundberg JM, Terenius L, Hokfelt T, et al: Neuropeptide Y (NPY)-like immunoreactivity in peripheral noradrenergic neurons and effects of NPY on sympathetic function. Acta Physiol Scand 116:477, 1982.
26. Ekblad E, Edvinsson L, Wahlestedt C, et al: Neuropeptide Y co-exists and co-operates with noradrenalin in perivascular nerve fibers. Regul Pept 8:225, 1984.
27. Sundler F, Moghimzadeh E, Håkanson R, et al: Nerve

fibers in the gut and pancreas of the rat displaying neuropeptide-Y immunoreactivity. Intrinsic and extrinsic origin. Cell Tissue Res 230:487, 1983.

28. Corder R, Emson PC, Lowry PJ: Purification and characterization of human neuropeptide Y from adrenal-medullary phaeochromocytoma tissue. Biochem J 219:699, 1984.
29. Adrian TE, Terenghi G, Brown MJ, et al: Neuropeptide Y in phaeochromocytomas and ganglioneuroblastomas. Lancet 2:540, 1983.
30. Lundberg JM, Tatemoto K, Terenius L, et al: Localization of peptide YY (PYY) in gastrointestinal endocrine cells and effects on intestinal blood flow and motility. Proc Natl Acad Sci USA 79:4471, 1982.
31. El-Salhy M, Grimelius L, Wilander E, et al: Immunocytochemical identification of polypeptide YY (PYY) cells in the human gastrointestinal tract. Histochemistry 77:15, 1983.
32. El-Salhy M, Wilander E, Juntti-Berggren L, et al: The distribution and ontogeny of polypeptide YY (PYY)- and pancreatic polypeptide (PP)-immunoreactive cells in the gastrointestinal tract of rat. Histochemistry 78:53, 1983.
33. Taylor IL: Distribution and release of peptide YY in dog measured by specific radioimmunoassay. Gastroenterology 88:731, 1985.
34. Greeley GH Jr, Partin M, Hill FLC, et al: Distribution of peptide YY in the canine alimentary canal. Gastroenterology 88:1403, 1985.
35. Roddy DR, Koch TR, Reilly WA, et al: Distribution of immunoreactive peptide YY (PYY) in normal human gut. Gastroenterology 88:1557, 1985.
36. Ali-Rachedi A, Varndell IM, Adrian TE, et al: Peptide YY (PYY) immunoreactivity is co-stored with glucagon-related immunoreactants in endocrine cells of the gut and pancreas. Histochemistry 80:487, 1984.
37. Wilander E, El-Salhy M, Lundqvist M, et al: Polypeptide YY (PYY) and pancreatic polypeptide (PP) in rectal carcinoids. An immunocytochemical study. Virchows Arch [A] 401:67, 1983.
38. O'Hare MMT, Chen M-H, Tatemoto K, et al: Lack of cross reactivity of peptide YY (PYY) and neuropeptide Y (NPY) with antibodies to pancreatic polypeptide (PP) in radioimmunoassay. Clin Chem 29:1553, 1983.
39. Chen M-H, Balasubramanian A, Murphy RF, et al: Sensitive radioimmunoassay for measurement of circulating peptide YY. Gastroenterology 87:1332, 1984.
40. Pappas TN, Debas HT, Goto Y, et al: Peptide YY inhibits meal-stimulated pancreatic and gastric secretion. Am J Physiol 248:G118, 1985.
41. Adrian TE, Ferri G-L, Bacarese-Hamilton AJ, et al: Human distribution and release of a putative new gut hormone, peptide YY. Gastroenterology 89:1070, 1985.
42. Fuxe K, Agnati LF, Harfstrand A, et al: Central administration of neuropeptide Y induces hypotension bradypnea and EEG synchronization in the rat. Acta Physiol Scand 118:189, 1983.
43. Stjernquist M, Emson P, Owman C, et al: Neuropeptide Y in the female reproductive tract of the rat. Distribution of nerve fibres and motor effects. Neurosci Lett 39:279, 1983.
44. Ohhashi T, Jacobowitz DM: The effects of pancreatic polypeptides and neuropeptide Y on the rat vas deferens. Peptides 4:381, 1983.
45. Allen JM, Bircham PMM, Edwards AV, et al: Neuropeptide Y (NPY) reduces myocardial perfusion and inhibits the force of contraction of the isolated perfused rabbit heart. Regul Pept 6:247, 1983.
46. Lundberg JM, Tatemoto K: Pancreatic polypeptide family (APP, BPP, NPY and PYY) in relation to sympathetic vasoconstriction resistant to α-adrenoceptor blockade. Acta Physiol Scand 116:393, 1982.
47. Kalra SP, Crowley WR: Norepinephrine-like effects of neuropeptide Y on LH release in the rat. Life Sci 35:1173, 1984.
48. Clark JT, Kalra PS, Crowley WR, et al: Neuropeptide Y and human pancreatic polypeptide stimulate feeding behavior in rats. Endocrinology 115:427, 1984.
49. Grunditz T, Håkanson R, Rerup C, et al: Neuropeptide Y in the thyroid gland: Neuronal localization and enhancement of stimulated thyroid hormone secretion. Endocrinology 115:1537, 1984.
50. Fink AS, Meyer JH, Savage K, et al: Peptide YY release by regionally perfused fatty acids in dog. Gastroenterology 88:1383, 1985.
51. Lluis F, Fujimura M, Guo Y-S, et al: Peptide YY pancreatic action is independent of cholinergic pathways. Gastroenterology 88:1478, 1985.
52. Lluis F, Fujimura M, Guo Y-S, et al: Regulation of gastric acid secretion by peptide YY, secretin, and neurotensin. Gastroenterology 88:1478, 1985.
53. Lundberg JM, Tatemoto K: Vascular effects of the peptides PYY and PHI: Comparison with APP and VIP. Eur J Pharmacol 83:143, 1982.
54. Suzuki T, Nakaya M, Itoh Z, et al: Inhibition of interdigestive contractile activity in the stomach by peptide YY in Heidenhain pouch dogs. Gastroenterology 85:114, 1983.
55. Grace PA, Muller El, Conter RL, et al: Peptide YY inhibits sphincter of Oddi phasic wave activity in the prairie dog. Gastroenterology 88:1402, 1985.
56. Wiley J, Owyang C: Neuropeptide Y and peptide YY inhibit cholinergic transmission in the isolated guinea pig colon: Mediation through α adrenoreceptors. Gastroenterology 88:1632, 1985.
57. Harper AA, Hood AJC, Mushens J, et al: Inhibition of external pancreatic secretion by intracolonic and intraileal infusions in the cat. J Physiol 292:445, 1979.
58. Harper AA, Hood AJC, Mushens J, et al: Pancreotone, an inhibitor of pancreatic secretion in extracts of ileal and colonic mucosa. J Physiol 292:455, 1979.
59. Lluis F, Fujimura M, Guo Y-S, et al: Peptide YY and gallbladder contraction. Gastroenterology 88:1479, 1985.
60. Szecowka J, Tatemoto K, Rajamaki G, et al: Effects of

PYY and PP on endocrine pancreas. Acta Physiol Scand 119:123, 1983.
61. Pappas TN, Debas HT, Taylor IL: Specific inhibition of the cephalic phase of acid secretion by peptide YY (PYY). Gastroenterology 88:1530, 1985.
62. Guo Y-S, Fujimura M, Lluis F, et al: Peptide YY: A physiologic role in the regulation of gastric secretion. Gastroenterology 88:1408, 1985.
63. Pappas TN, Chang AM, Debas HT, et al: Does peptide YY (PYY) mediate the ileal brake? Gastroenterology 88:1529, 1985.
64. Adrian TE, Long RG, Fuessl HS, et al: Plasma peptide YY (PYY) in dumping syndrome. Dig Dis Sci 30:1145, 1985.
65. Adrian TE, Savage AP, Bacarese-Hamilton AJ, et al: Peptide YY abnormalities in gastrointestinal diseases. Gastroenterology 90:379, 1986.

EPIDERMAL GROWTH FACTOR/UROGASTRONE

J. Patrick Walker, M.D., and
Courtney M. Townsend, Jr., M.D.

History

In the late 1930s, Sandweiss et al [1] observed that peptic ulcer disease was particularly unusual during pregnancy. They injected Mann-Williamson dogs (a peptic ulcer model in dogs prepared with an anastomosis between the stomach and distal small bowel) with an extract from urine of pregnant rats, which prevented formation of ulcers. In 1939, Gray et al [2] reported inhibition of gastric secretion by extracts of normal male urine. At about this same time, Friedman et al [3] reported inhibition of histamine-stimulated gastric secretion by urinary extracts. Gray et al [4] called this substance urogastrone because of its putative similarities to enterogastrone. Initial properties and extraction procedures for urogastrone were described in 1942 [5], and further steps toward purification and delineation of physiologic properties were reported by Gregory [6] in 1955. A chromatographic technique for preparation of large quantities of urogastrone was described in 1962 [7], and in the same year, studies that related structure to activity were described by Rosenoer [8].

Also in 1962, Cohen [9], who was studying a nerve growth-promoting protein in the mouse salivary gland, noticed that injection of partially purified extracts of the gland into newborn mice produced precocious eruption of teeth as well as accelerated eyelid opening. He purified this compound, established its biologic properties, and determined the amino acid composition. Cohen and Elliott [10] later reported the stimulation of epidermal keratinization by this protein.

In 1965, Cohen [11] published studies involving the effects of this substance, which he called epidermal growth factor (EGF), on skin from chick embryos in tissue culture. He noted stimulation of epidermis as well as increased thymidine uptake in the basal cell layers. A rapid isolation procedure for EGF was developed in 1972, which allowed further characterization of its chemical properties [12] as well as the elucidation of its primary structure [13]. Carrea et al [14] purified a glycoprotein in humans that possessed gastric antisecretory activities similar to those attributed to urogastrone. EGF was identified in human urine in 1975 [15], and it was isolated and its chemical and biologic properties were determined later the same year [16].

By September 1975, the structure of urogastrone had been described and its relationship to epidermal growth factor noted [17,18]. Of the 53 amino acids of urogastrone and mouse EGF, 37 are common to both peptides, and Gregory concluded ". . . it is probable that urogastrone and human EGF are one and the same" [17].

Human urogastrone was known to exist in two forms, beta and alpha, which differ by a single arginine residue. Human beta urogastrone contains 53 amino acids in comparison to human EGF, which has 49 amino acids. Mouse EGF also has 53 amino acids. They all possess similar properties: they stimulate fibroblast proliferation, they inhibit gastric acid secretion, and they act as powerful mitogens causing epithelial proliferation and keratinization of squamous epithelial cells. They share common receptors in human fibroblasts [19]. They have few, if any, differing properties, and they are found in the same tissues and secretions.

Distribution

EGF was originally described in the mouse submaxillary glands [9–11], and urogastrone has additionally been localized in the human submandibular gland [20–22]. Urogastrone is present in Brunner's glands in human duodenum [21,22], and EGF/urogastrone is present in the submandibular gland, thyroid, pancreas, duodenum, jejunum, and kidney of humans [23]. Concentrations in nonsalivary tissues are, however, only a fraction of those found in the submandibular gland.

Urogastrone has been found in human serum, saliva, and gastric juice [24] as well as in human pancreatic juice [25]. Serum concentrations of EGF appear to be elevated during pregnancy [26]. EGF is found in human milk [27] and appears to have diurnal variation during lactation [28]. Recently, EGF/urogastrone has been associated with blood platelets in human plasma and is released during coagulation [29].

EGF receptors have been demonstrated in mouse duodenum, jejunum, and ileum, with slightly higher concentrations in the mouse jejunum [30], as well as in rat small intestine [31].

Assay

Solid-phase, specific radioimmunoassay for mouse EGF has been developed by Byyny et al [32,33]. Before its availability, bioassay based on precocious eye-opening in immature mice was used for detection of EGF. A heterologous RIA for human EGF/urogastrone was reported in 1977 [34] and a homologous radioimmunoassay [35] in 1978.

Pharmacokinetics and Catabolism

Once release is accomplished, EGF is bound to specific receptors on target cells, which contain a protein kinase activity specific for tyrosine residues [36]. EGF, after binding to the surface receptor, appears to be internalized within the cell and then rapidly degraded. This degradation is blocked by inhibotors of metabolic energy production [37]. The gene for the human EGF receptor has been assigned to chromosome 7 [38].

The amount of EGF present in the submandibular gland appears to be dependent upon the presence of androgens, since administration of exogenous androgens increases extractable EGF [39]. In mice with muscular dystrophy in which there is a reduced level of salivary gland EGF, treatment with thyroxine elevated EGF levels to those of normal mice, but androgens were ineffective [40].

Release

As noted previously, EGF exists as a single polypeptide chain with a molecular weight of approximately 6000 daltons. However, within the salivary gland itself, EGF occurs as part of a 74,000 dalton complex, which has been named high-molecular-weight EGF [41]. This high-molecular-weight EGF appears to be composed of two molecules of EGF and two copies of a molecule with arginine esterase properties. Following secretion, the four units that are noncovalently bound are dissociated, with release of EGF of low molecular weight [42]. The stimulus for secretion seems to be primarily mediated to activation of α-adrenergic receptors [39]. This seems to be somewhat dependent upon calcium, but it is independent of cyclic AMP [43]. Cyclocytidine, an antitumor agent, has been shown to produce degranulation of the granular convoluted tubule, the location of immunoreactive EGF in the submandibular gland. This degranulation is abolished by the administration of phenoxybenzamine hydrochloride but not by propranolol, indicating that the secretory effect is mediated by α-adrenergic receptors [44]. Kirkegaard et al [45] have shown that the release of EGF from Brunner's glands in the duodenum is stimulated by acetylcholine and that this stimulation is augmented by vasoactive intestinal peptide (VIP). There was no effect, however, when VIP was given alone.

Actions

Since EGF produces precocious opening of the eyelids and eruption of the incisors in newborn mice, this growth factor has been considered at times to be a potent mitogen. The carcinogenicity of topically applied methylcholanthrene was found to be enhanced by parenteral administration of EGF in 1965 [46]. Many studies on the effect of EGF on tumor growth followed; some of these are reviewed below. Hoober and Cohen [47,48] showed that epidermal cultures from chick embryos treated with EGF were more than twice as active in incorporating labeled amino acids and in stimulating the net accumulation of protein and RNA when compared to controls. There was no detectable net accumulation of DNA. EGF produces a marked increase in activity of ornithine decarboxylase, an enzyme necessary for biosynthesis of polyamines [49,50]. Although EGF caused no change in ornithine decarboxylase activity, it did bring about increased activity of histidine decarboxylase [51].

The addition of EGF to human fibroblasts in tissue culture induces proliferation that is associated with increased thymidine uptake [52,53], which has been related to increased DNA synthesis [54]. Addition of EGF to cultures of human fibroblasts is associated with an increase in glycolysis [55] as well as an increase in possible phosphofructokinase activity [56]. Control of the cell-surface protein fibronectin also seems to be associated with EGF [57]. Human fibroblasts in culture appear to be able to modulate their EGF receptor, depending upon concentrations of EGF in the culture medium. Addition of EGF to culture media decreases EGF receptors by down-regulation, and removal of EGF increases the receptors available [58]. The increase in cell growth stimulated by EGF in tissue culture is inhibited by somatostatin [59].

EGF has been shown to increase cellular growth in organ cultures of many tissues, including rat ureter, vas deferens, trachea, uterus, vagina, prostate glands, submandibular and parotid salivary glands, kidney, and lung [60]. EGF also increased liver growth in vitro and in vivo [61,62] and stimulated in vitro growth of thyroid [63] and mammary glands [64,65]. EGF not only stimulates this apparently nonspecific proliferation of mammary tissue but also appears to inhibit functional differentiation of the breast.

EGF may be trophic for the gut, at least in young mice and rats. Hiramatsu et al [66] increased glucosamine-6-phosphate synthetase activity in the colon with both single and daily administration of EGF 2–4 μg/g body weight. Dembinski and Johnson [67] showed increased gastric weight and acid secretion in weanling rats given EGF for 5 days. Majumdar [68] administered EGF to nutritionally deprived weanling rats and promoted gastrointestinal as well as body growth.

EGF stimulates prostaglandin biosynthesis by canine kidney cells in vitro [69]. Induction of cleft palate in the mouse by cortisone is potentiated by EGF [70]. Chronic administration of EGF to neonatal animals produces induction of fatty liver [71].

The effects of EGF on gastrointestinal function have been studied in vivo and in vitro. Longsdon and Williams [72] noted that the basal and cholecystokinin (CCK)-8-stimulated release of amylase from isolated mouse pancreatic acini is increased by EGF, as is the incorporation of tritiated leucine into protein. Others found no change in canine pancreatic function in response to EGF, either basal or stimulated by secretin or CCK, but EGF inhibited gastric secretion [73]. Since EGF applied topically to gastric mucosa diminished histamine-stimulated acid secretion to near basal levels, the inhibition of gastric secretion appears to be a direct effect of EGF on fundic mucosa [74]. Elder et al [75] found that urogastrone in humans inhibited pentagastrin- and histamine-stimulated acid secretion but had less effect on gastric pepsin output. Infusion of urogastrone in duodenal ulcer patients diminished basal acid secretion as well as the output of pepsin and intrinsic factor [76]. Urogastrone has been successful in inhibition of gastric secretion in Zollinger-Ellison patients, in whom the pattern of inhibition is compatible with a competitive action against gastrin for receptor sites on the oxyntic cells [77,78]. Sakamoto et al [79], from our laboratory, have linked the cytoprotective effects of EGF in rats with stress ulcers to a restoration of stress-diminished levels of somatostatin.

The effects of EGF on tumor growth have been carefully studied in several tumors. The most widely studied tumor in humans and animals has been breast cancer. EGF may stimulate or inhibit tumor growth. The binding of EGF to human breast cancer cells has been demonstrated [80] as has an association with intracellular calcium during the process of binding [80,81]. The addition of EGF to cells of human benign and malignant breast tumors in culture caused an increased rate of growth [82–85]. Imai et al [86] have correlated the growth of mammary epithelial cells from human breast cancer to the presence of EGF receptors and have noted that increased activity was associated with increased EGF receptors. However, Pathak et al [87] noticed no correlation between EGF receptors and the ability of EGF to stimulate growth of various tumors in culture.

The effects of EGF on tumor growth may be related to influence on other hormones. Reproductive hormones, long known to influence growth of tumors, are influenced by EGF. Specifically, Shaw et al [88] have shown EGF to inhibit follicular estradiol production.

In addition to breast cancer, other tumors have the ability to bind EGF with resultant stimulation of growth. Addition of EGF to serum-free media stimulates the in vitro growth of human colon cancer [89]. Differentiation of malignant hepatoma and neuroblastoma cells from the tissue of origin has been shown to change both EGF receptors and their ability to bind EGF [90,91].

Recently, tumor cells have been associated with another growth factor, designated transforming growth factor. This peptide has an amino acid sequence that is similar to the sequence of EGF [92], and transforming growth factor and EGF may well interact through a similar, or possibly the same, receptor. Murine sarcoma cells that have had their colony-forming activity increased by transforming growth factor also can have this activity enhanced by EGF [93].

Cohen [94] has noted that DNA tumor viruses that induce sarcomas in mice and cats lose the ability to bind to EGF, whereas RNA tumor viruses, when inducing sarcomas, do not cause loss of EGF receptors. This may be a differential action in transformation of malignant cells between DNA and RNA tumor viruses. Although EGF generally increases tumor growth in most neoplastic cell lines tested, in the human epidermoid carcinoma, A-431, there is inhibition of growth by EGF [95,96], an inhibition associated with reduction of cellular levels of adenosine triphosphate [97].

REFERENCES

1. Sandweiss DJ, Saltzstein HC, Farbman A: The prevention or healing of experimental peptic ulcer in Mann-Williamson dogs with the anterior pituitary-like hormone (antuitrin-S). A preliminary report. Am J Dig Dis 5:24, 1938.
2. Gray JS, Wieczorowski E, Ivy AC: Inhibition of gastric secretion by extracts of normal male urine. Science 89:489, 1939.
3. Friedman MHF, Recknagel RO, Sandweiss DJ, et al: Inhibitory effect of urine extracts on gastric secretion. Proc Soc Exp Biol Med 41:5093, 1939.
4. Gray JS, Culmer CU, Wieczorowski E, et al: Preparation of pyrogen-free urogastrone. Proc Soc Exp Biol Med 43:2258, 1940.
5. Gray JS, Wieczorowski E, Wells JA, et al: The preparation and properties of urogastrone. Endocrinology 30:129, 1942.
6. Gregory RA: A new method for the preparation of urogastrone. J Physiol 129:528, 1955.
7. Mongar JL, Rosenoer VM: The preparation of urogastrone. J Physiol 162:163, 1962.
8. Rosenoer VM: The relation of peptide bonds, disulphide bonds and sulphydryl groups to urogastrone activity. J Physiol 162:173, 1962.
9. Cohen S: Isolation of a mouse submaxillary gland protein accelerating incisor eruption and eyelid opening in the newborn animal. J Biol Chem 237:1555, 1962.
10. Cohen S, Elliott GA: The stimulation of epidermal keratinization by a protein isolated from the submaxillary gland of the mouse. J Invest Dermatol 40:1, 1963.
11. Cohen S: The stimulation of epidermal proliferation by a specific protein (EGF). Develop Biol 12:394, 1965.
12. Savage CR Jr, Cohen S: Epidermal growth factor and a new derivative. J Biol Chem 247:7609, 1972.
13. Savage CR Jr, Inagami T, Cohen S: The primary structure of epidermal growth factor. J Biol Chem 247:7612, 1972.
14. Carrea G, Casellato MM, Manera E, et al: Purification of a human urinary glycoprotein with gastric antisecretory activity. Biochim Biophys Acta 295:274, 1973.
15. Starkey RH, Cohen S, Orth DN: Epidermal growth factor: Identification of a new hormone in human urine. Science 189:800, 1979.
16. Cohen S, Carpenter G: Human epidermal growth factor: Isolation and chemical and biological properties. Proc Natl Acad Sci USA 72:1317, 1975.
17. Gregory H: Isolation and structure of urogastrone and its relationship to epidermal growth factor. Nature 257:325, 1975.
18. Gregory H, Preston BM: The primary structure of human urogastrone. Int J Pept Protein Res 9:107, 1977.
19. Hollenberg MD, Gregory H: Human urogastrone and mouse epidermal growth factor share a common receptor site in cultured human fibroblasts. Life Sci 20:267, 1976.
20. Elder JB, Williams G, Gregory H: Cellular localization of urogastrone by an immunofluorescent technique. Br J Surg 63:657, 1976.
21. Elder JB, Williams G, Lacey E, et al: Cellular localisation of human urogastrone/epidermal growth factor. Nature 271:466, 1978.
22. Heitz PU, Kasper M, van Noorden S, et al: Immunohistochemical localisation of urogastrone to human duodenal and submandibular glands. Gut 19:408, 1978.
23. Hirata Y, Orth DN: Epidermal growth factor (urogastrone) in human tissues. J Clin Endocrinol Metab 48:667, 1979.
24. Gregory H, Walsh S, Hopkins CR: The identification of urogastrone in serum, saliva, and gastric juice. Gastroenterology 77:313, 1979.
25. Hirata Y, Uchihashi M, Nakajima M, et al: Immunoreactive human epidermal growth factor in human pancreatic juice. J Clin Endocrinol Metab 54:1242, 1982.
26. Ances IG: Serum concentrations of epidermal growth factor in human pregnancy. Am J Obstet Gynecol 115:357, 1973.
27. Carpenter G: Epidermal growth factor is a major growth-promoting agent in human milk. Science 210:198, 1980.
28. Moran JR, Courtney ME, Orth DN, et al: Epidermal growth factor in human milk: Daily production and diurnal variation during early lactation in mothers delivering at term and at premature gestation. J Pediatr 103:402, 1983.
29. Oka Y, Orth DN: Human plasma epidermal growth factor/β-urogastrone is associated with blood platelets. J Clin Invest 72:249, 1983.
30. Gallo-Payet N, Hugon JS: Epidermal growth factor receptors in isolated adult mouse intestinal cells: Studies *in vivo* and in organ culture. Endocrinology 116:194, 1985.
31. Blay J, Brown KD: Functional receptors for epidermal growth factor in an epithelial-cell line derived from the rat small intestine. Biochem J 225:85, 1985.
32. Byyny RL, Orth DN, Cohen S, et al: Solid phase radioimmunoassay (RIA) for epidermal growth factor (EGF). Clin Res 19:29, 1971.
33. Byyny RL, Orth DN, Cohen S: Radioimmunoassay of epidermal growth factor. Endocrinology 90:1261, 1972.
34. Starkey RH, Orth DN: Radioimmunoassay of human epidermal growth factor (urogastrone). J Clin Endocrinol Metab 45:1144, 1977.
35. Dailey GE, Kraus JW, Orth DN: Homologous radioimmunoassay for human epidermal growth factor (urogastrone). J Clin Endocrinol Metab 46:929, 1978.
36. Cohen S, Fava RA, Sawyer ST: Purification and characterization of epidermal growth factor receptor/protein kinase from normal mouse liver. Proc Natl Acad Sci USA 79:6237, 1982.

37. Carpenter G, Cohen S: ^{125}I-labeled human epidermal growth factor. Binding, internalization, and degradation in human fibroblasts. J Cell Biol 71:159, 1976.
38. Davies RL, Grosse VA, Kucherlapati R, et al: Genetic analysis of epidermal growth factor action: Assignment of human epidermal growth factor receptor gene to chromosome 7. Proc Natl Acad Sci USA 77:4188, 1980.
39. Byyny RL, Orth DN, Cohen S, et al: Epidermal growth factor: Effects of androgens and adrenergic agents. Endocrinology 95:776, 1974.
40. Watson AY, Radie K, McCarthy M, et al: Thyroxine reverses deficits of nerve growth factor and epidermal growth factor in submandibular glands of mice with muscular dystrophy. Endocrinology 110:1392, 1982.
41. Taylor JM, Cohen S, Mitchell WM: Epidermal growth factor: High and low molecular weight forms. Proc Natl Acad Sci 67:164, 1970.
42. Server AC, Shooter EM: Comparison of the arginine estero-peptidases associated with the nerve and epidermal growth factors. J Biol Chem 251:165, 1976.
43. Roberts ML: Secretion of epidermal growth factor. The role of calcium in stimulus-secretion coupling and structural modification of the growth factor molecule during secretion. Biochim Biophys Acta 540:246, 1978.
44. Barka T, Gresik EW, van der Noen H: Stimulation of secretion of epidermal growth factor and amylase by cyclocytidine. Cell Tissue Res 186:269, 1978.
45. Kirkegaard P, Olsen PS, Poulsen SS, et al: Exocrine secretion of epidermal growth factor from Brunner's glands. Stimulation of VIP and acetylcholine. Regul Pept 7:367, 1983.
46. Reynolds VH, Boehm FH, Cohen S: Enhancement of chemical carcinogenesis by an epidermal growth factor. Surg Forum 16:108, 1965.
47. Hoober JK, Cohen S: Epidermal growth factor. I. The stimulation of protein and ribonucleic acid synthesis in chick embryo epidermis. Biochim Biophys Acta 138:347, 1967.
48. Hoober JK, Cohen S: Epidermal growth factor. II. Increased activity of ribosomes from chick embryo epidermis for cell-free protein synthesis. Biochim Biophys Acta 138:357, 1967.
49. Stastny M, Cohen S: The stimulation of ornithine decarboxylase activity in testes of the neonatal mouse. Biochim Biophys Acta 261:177, 1972.
50. Stastny M, Cohen S: Epidermal growth factor. IV. The induction of ornithine decarboxylase. Biochim Biophys Acta 204:578, 1970.
51. Blosse PT, Fenton EL, Henningsson S, et al: Activities of decarboxylases of histidine and ornithine in young mice after injection of epidermal growth factor. Experientia 30:22, 1974.
52. Carpenter G, Cohen S: Human epidermal growth factor and the proliferation of human fibroblasts. J Cell Physiol 88:227, 1976.
53. Rose SP, Pruss RM, Herschman HR: Initiation of 3T3 fibroblast cell division by epidermal growth factor. J Cell Physiol 86:593, 1975.
54. Hollenberg MD, Cuatrecasas P: Insulin and epidermal growth factor. Human fibroblast receptors related to deoxyribonucleic acid synthesis and amino acid uptake. J Biol Chem 250:3845, 1975.
55. Diamond I, Legg A, Schneider JA, et al: Glycolysis in quiescent cultures of 3T3 cells. Stimulation by serum, epidermal growth factor, and insulin in intact cells and persistence of the stimulation after cell homogenization. J Biol Chem 253:866, 1978.
56. Schneider JA, Diamond I, Rozengurt E: Glycolysis in quiescent cultures of 3T3 cells. Addition of serum epidermal growth factor and insulin increases the activity of phosphofructokinase in a protein synthesis-independent manner. J Biol Chem 253:872, 1978.
57. Chen LB, Gudor RC, Sun T-T, et al: Control of a cell surface major glycoprotein by epidermal growth factor. Science 197:776, 1977.
58. Aharonov A, Pruss RM, Herschman HR: Epidermal growth factor. Relationship between receptor regulation and mitogenesis in 3T3 cells. J Biol Chem 253:3970, 1978.
59. Mascardo RN, Sherline P: Somatostatin inhibits rapid centrosomal separation and cell proliferation induced by epidermal growth factor. Endocrinology 111:1394, 1982.
60. Jones RO: The *in vitro* effect of epithelial growth factor on rat organ cultures. Exp Cell Res 43:645, 1966.
61. Bucher NLR, Patel U, Cohen S: Hormonal factors and liver growth. Adv Enzyme Regul 16:205, 1978.
62. McGowan JA, Strain AJ, Bucher NLR: DNA synthesis in primary cultures of adult rat hepatocytes in a defined medium: Effects of epidermal growth factor, insulin, glucagon, and cyclic-AMP. J Cell Physiol 108:353, 1981.
63. Westermark K, Karlsson FA, Westermark B: Epidermal growth factor modulates thyroid growth and function in culture. Endocrinology 112:1680, 1983.
64. Taketani F, Oka T: Epidermal growth factor stimulates cell proliferation and inhibits functional differentiation of mouse mammary epithelial cells in culture. Endocrinology 113:871, 1983.
65. Turkington RW: The role of epithelial growth factor in mammary gland development in vitro. Exp Cell Res 57:79, 1969.
66. Hiramatsu M, Kashimata M, Minami N, et al: Effect of epidermal growth factor on glucosamine-6-phosphate synthetase activity in the colon of neonatal mice. J Endocrinol 105:197, 1985.
67. Dembinski AB, Johnson LR: Effect of epidermal growth factor on the development of rat gastric mucosa. Endocrinology 116:90, 1985.
68. Majumdar APN: Postnatal undernutrition: Effect of epidermal growth factor on growth and function of the gastrointestinal tract in rats. J Pediatr Gastroenterol Nutr 3:618, 1984.
69. Levine L, Hassid A: Epidermal growth factor stimulates prostaglandin biosynthesis by canine kidney (MDCK) cells. Biochem Biophys Res Commun 76:1181, 1977.
70. Bedrick AD, Ladda RL: Epidermal growth factor po-

tentiates cortisone-induced cleft palate in the mouse. Teratology 17:13, 1978.
71. Heimberg M, Weinstein I, LeQuire VS, et al: The induction of fatty liver in neonatal animals by a purified protein (EGF) from mouse submaxillary gland. Life Sci 4:1625, 1965.
72. Logsdon CD, Williams JA: Epidermal growth factor binding and biologic effects on mouse pancreatic acini. Gastroenterology 85:339, 1983.
73. Konturek SJ, Cieszkowski M, Jaworek J, et al: Effects of epidermal growth factor on gastrointestinal secretions. Am J Physiol 246:G580, 1984.
74. Fink U, Rutten M, Murphy RA, et al: Effects of epidermal growth factor on acid secretion from guinea pig gastric mucosa: In vitro analysis. Gastroenterology 88:1175, 1985.
75. Elder JB, Ganguli PC, Gillespie IE, et al: Effect of urogastrone on gastric secretion and plasma gastrin levels in normal subjects. Gut 16:887, 1975.
76. Koffman CG, Elder JB, Ganguli PC, et al: Effect of urogastrone on gastric secretion and serum gastrin concentration in patients with duodenal ulceration. Gut 23:951, 1982.
77. Elder JB, Ganguli PC, Gillespie IE, et al: Effect of urogastrone in Zollinger-Ellison syndrome. Br J Surg 61:916, 1974.
78. Elder JB, Ganguli PC, Gillespie IE, et al: Effect of urogastrone in the Zollinger-Ellison syndrome. Gut 15:840, 1974.
79. Sakamoto T, Swierczek JS, Ogden WD, et al: Cytoprotective effect of pentagastrin and epidermal growth factor on stress ulcer formation. Ann Surg 201:290, 1985.
80. Osborne CK, Hamilton B, Nover M: Receptor binding and processing of epidermal growth factor by human breast cancer cells. J Clin Endocrinol Metab 55:86, 1982.
81. Findlay DM, Ng KW, Niall M, et al: Processing of calcitonin and epidermal growth factor after binding to receptors in human breast cancer cells (T 47D). Biochem J 206:343, 1982.
82. Osborne CK, Hamilton B, Titus G, et al: Epidermal growth factor stimulation of human breast cancer cells in culture. Cancer Res 40:2361, 1980.
83. Taylor-Papadimitriou J, Shearer M, Stoker MGP: Growth requirements of human mammary epithelial cells in culture. Int J Cancer 20:903, 1977.
84. Turkington RW: Stimulation of mammary carcinoma cell proliferation by epithelial growth factor *in vitro*. Cancer Res 29:1457, 1969.
85. Stoker MGP, Pigott D, Taylor-Papadimitriou J: Response to epidermal growth factors of cultured human mammary epithelial cells from benign tumours. Nature 264:764, 1976.
86. Imai Y, Leung CKH, Friesen HG, et al: Epidermal growth factor receptors and effect of epidermal growth factor on growth of human breast cancer cells in long-term tissue culture. Cancer Res 42:4394, 1982.
87. Pathak MA, Matrisian LM, Magun BE, et al: Effect of epidermal growth factor on clonogenic growth of primary human tumor cells. Int J Cancer 30:745, 1982.
88. Shaw G, Jorgensen GI, Tweedale R, et al: Effect of epidermal growth factor on reproductive function of ewes. J Endocrinol 107:429, 1985.
89. Murakami H, Masui H: Hormonal control of human colon carcinoma cell growth in serum-free medium. Proc Natl Acad Sci USA 77:3464, 1980.
90. Costrini NV, Beck R: Epidermal growth factor-urogastrone receptors in normal human liver and primary hepatoma. Cancer 51:2191, 1983.
91. Mummery CL, van der Saag PT, de Laat SW: Loss of EGF binding and cation transport response during differentiation of mouse neuroblastoma cells. J Cell Biochem 21:63, 1983.
92. Marquardt H, Hunkapiller MW, Hood LE, et al: Transforming growth factors produced by retrovirus-transformed rodent fibroblasts and human melanoma cells: Amino acid sequence homology with epidermal growth factor. Proc Natl Acad Sci USA 80:4684, 1983.
93. Roberts AB, Anzano MA, Lamb LC, et al: Isolation from murine sarcoma cells of novel transforming growth factors potentiated by EGF. Nature 295:417, 1982.
94. Todaro GJ, De Larco JE, Cohen S: Transformation by murine and feline sarcoma viruses specifically blocks binding of epidermal growth factor to cells. Nature 264:26, 1976.
95. Barnes DW: Epidermal growth factor inhibits growth of A431 human epidermoid carcinoma in serum-free cell culture. J Cell Biol 93:1, 1982.
96. Haigler H, Ash JF, Singer SJ, et al: Visualization by fluorescence of the binding and internalization of epidermal growth factor in human carcinoma cells A-431. Proc Natl Acad Sci USA 75:3317, 1978.
97. Melner MH, Sawyer ST, Evanochko WT, et al: Phosphorus-31 nuclear magnetic resonance analysis of epidermal growth factor action in A-431 human epidermoid carcinoma cells and SV-40 virus transformed mouse fibroblasts. Biochemistry 22:2039, 1983.

PEPTIDE HISTIDINE ISOLEUCINE

Talaat Khalil, M.D., and
Courtney M. Townsend, Jr., M.D.

History

Peptide histidine isoleucine (PHI), a polypeptide containing C-terminal histidine and N-terminal isoleucine, was discovered and isolated by Tatemoto and Mutt in 1978. They isolated PHI from porcine upper intestinal tissue by using a novel method for detection of peptide hormones and active peptides [1]. The method is based on chemical detection of peptides that possess the COOH-terminal α-amide structure; this is an unusual chemical feature found in some peptide hormones and other peptides. Porcine PHI was identified in intestinal extracts by the presence of its COOH-terminal isoleucine amide structure [2].

PHI consists of 27 amino acid residues and has the following amino acid sequence:

His-Ala-Asp-Gly-Val-Phe-Thr-Ser-Asp-
Phe-Ser-Arg-Leu-Leu-Gly-Gln-Leu-Ser-
Ala-Lys-Lys-Tyr-Leu-Glu-Ser-Leu-Ile-NH_2

The remarkable homology in amino acid sequence of PHI to vasoactive intestinal peptide (VIP), secretin, glucagon, and gastric inhibitory polypeptide (see Appendix) places this peptide as a member of the glucagon-secretin family. In fact, several biologic activities of PHI are qualitatively similar to those of VIP and secretin [3].

Two different forms of PHI were recently isolated from human [4] and bovine [5] intestine. Like porcine PHI, both of these peptides are composed of 27 amino acid residues. Porcine and human PHI differ only at positions 12 and 27, exchanging arginine for lysine and isoleucine for methionine [4]. Porcine and bovine PHI differ at only one position: the phenylalanine at position 10 in the former is exchanged for a tyrosine residue in bovine PHI [5].

Chromatography of human ileal or colonic tissue extracts using both gel and ion exchange methods revealed the presence of only one major molecular form of PHI [6].

Distribution

PHI-immunoreactivity is found in the human and porcine small and large intestine, mainly in the ileum and colon [6,7]. The highest concentrations are in the lamina propria, with smaller concentrations in the submucosa and muscularis. No PHI is detectable in the epithelium. More than 99 percent of PHI is confined to the nonepithelial layers of the gut wall, suggesting that it may be more likely to behave as a neurotransmitter or neuromodulator than as a gut hormone [6]. PHI has been detected in the pancreas of humans, guinea pigs, dogs, and rats [8].

PHI is present in rat brain, particularly in the median eminence [9,10]. It is also present in the respiratory tract of the cat, rat, and guinea pig, with the highest concentrations in the trachea and bronchus and the lowest in the lung parenchyma and nasal mucosa [11]. It is also present in the urinary bladder, erectile tissue of the penis, the uterus of humans and cats, and in other peripheral tissues, including skin, eyes, and cardiovascular system in rats, guinea pigs, cats, and humans [12,13].

Immunocytochemical studies show that PHI-containing ganglion cells occur in the gastrointestinal, respiratory, and genitourinary tract in the rat, guinea pig, cat, and human. Comparative studies in these species indicate that PHI and VIP are co-stored in the same neurons and are identically distributed, which suggests the existence of a common precursor [14].

Assay

There is no published standard bioassay for PHI. Specific radioimmunoassays for PHI for measurement of concentrations in tissue extracts and in plasma have been reported [6,15]. The lowest human plasma concentration of PHI is 3.0 pmol/L, measured with an antibody that recognizes the sequence 3-8 of the 27 amino acid peptide. The mean fasting plasma concentration in humans is 14.2 pmol/L, with no sex-related differences noted [15]. Considerable species differences in PHI-like immunoreactivity were reported in various mammalian intestinal extracts (rat, guinea pig, cat, and human) fractioned by gel filtration and high performance liquid chromatography [16]. In humans, pigs, cats, and rats, PHI immunoreactivity from gastric extracts eluted at two different peaks. PHI immunoreactivity from ileal extracts eluted at one peak [7].

Pharmacokinetics and Catabolism

PHI is extremely effective in inhibiting the binding of ^{125}I VIP to its receptors on cell membranes of either liver of intestinal epithelial cells [17]. However, these membranes do not contain specific receptors for PHI, and its binding to these membranes may be entirely accounted for by its affinity for the VIP receptors. The apparent affinity of PHI for VIP receptors is much higher than that of secretin [17].

PHI stimulates the production of cyclic AMP in intestinal epithelial and fat cell membranes [17], in lung membranes from humans, rats, mice, and guinea pigs [18], and in heart membranes from humans [19]. PHI also increases the intracellular accumulation of cyclic AMP in the exocrine pancreas of guinea pigs [20]. The potency of PHI is 30–40 percent of that of VIP. However, in isolated gastric glands from rats in which the cyclic AMP system is highly sensitive to secretin and 200 times less sensitive to VIP, PHI is 2–5 percent as potent as secretin and 5–10 times more potent than VIP. In isolated fat cell preparations of rats, which contain both VIP and secretin receptors that are equally sensitive to VIP and secretin, PHI was 10–25 percent as potent as VIP or secretin [17].

In AtT-20 cells (derived from mouse pituitary tumors), PHI rapidly promotes secretion of ACTH in a concentration-dependent manner. Its ED_{50}, however, is about sixfold higher than that observed for VIP in these tumor cells [21,22]. PHI, however, does not stimulate ACTH secretion of normal corticotropins, even at concentrations of 1 mM [22]. The ability of PHI to stimulate ACTH release appears to require a prior increase in the formation of cyclic AMP [22,23]. Somatostatin [21,24] and oxotremorine [22,24], both of which block cyclic AMP synthesis and ACTH secretion in response to VIP, also antagonize PHI action on AtT-20 cells. Similarly, dexamethasone [21–23] and nifedipine [22] also reduce PHI-stimulated ACTH release.

We know of no published information on the half-life, catabolism, or volume of distribution of PHI.

Actions

PHI appears to be an intestinal secretagogue that induces a reversible net secretion of fluid and electrolytes in the jejunum and ileum and has lesser effects in the colon in pigs [25], rats [26], and humans [27,28].

PHI also relaxes gallbladder smooth muscles [29] and inhibits gallbladder fluid reabsorption [30] in the guinea pig.

PHI is a potent stimulant of flow of pancreatic juice in anesthetized turkeys and is about half as active as chicken VIP [31]. However, in anesthetized rats, PHI, similar to VIP, is a weak stimulant of the pancreatic juice [31]. In vitro, PHI inhibited the binding of ^{125}I VIP, increased cellular AMP, and stimulated amylase secretion from dispersed acini from guinea pig pancreas [20].

When given as a constant infusion in rats, both PHI and VIP exert a direct hypoglycemic effect and enhance the influences of glucose and arginine on insulin and glucagon secretion [32]. In vitro, PHI at a concentration of 3 ng/mL induced insulin release from the isolated perfused rat pancreas at basal and increased glucose levels. Furthermore, it enhanced arginine-stimulated glucagon secretion but did not affect arginine-stimulated insulin release [33]. Alwmark et al [34] from our laboratory recently found that PHI stimulates insulin release from isolated pancreatic islets from rats.

PHI releases prolactin in rats both in vivo and in vitro, with a potency similar to that of VIP or thyrotropin-releasing hormone; PHI may be a candidate for the role of prolactin-releasing factor [35]. Endogenous PHI in rats is involved at least in the mechanism of 5-hydroxytryptophan-induced prolactin release, in which the dopaminergic control may also be involved [36].

PHI relaxes the isolated tracheal smooth muscle from guinea pigs in a dose-dependent manner; it is 200 times more potent than epinephrine but 2–3 times less potent than VIP [11]. Intra-arterial infusions of PHI caused an atropine-resistant vasodilatation in the submandibular salivary gland of the cat. On the other hand, parasympathetic nerve stimulation of these glands caused salivary secretion, vasodilatation, and a co-release of VIP and PHI [37]. On a molar basis, PHI was, however, almost 1000-fold less potent than VIP as a vasodilatory agent [38]. PHI stimulated intracellular accumulation of cAMP in Molt 4b lymphoblast cell culture [39]. PHI-mediated protein phosphorylation in these cultures was demonstrated. PHI may be involved in the modulation of lymphocyte function.

REFERENCES

1. Tatemoto K, Mutt, V: Chemical determination of gastrointestinal hormones. Scand J Gastroenterol Suppl 49:181, 1978.
2. Tatemoto K, Mutt V: Isolation of two novel candidate hormones using a chemical method for finding naturally occurring polypeptides. Nature 285:417, 1980.
3. Tatemoto K, Mutt V: Isolation and characterization of the intestinal peptide porcine PHI (PHI-27), a new member of the glucagon-secretin family. Proc Natl Acad Sci USA 78:6603, 1981.
4. Itoh N, Obata K-I, Yanaihara N, et al: Human preprovasoactive intestinal peptide contains a novel PHI-27-like peptide, PHM-27. Nature 304:547, 1983.
5. Carlquist M, Kaiser R, Tatemoto K, et al: A novel form of the polypeptide PHI isolated in high yield from bovine upper intestine. Relationships to other peptides of the glucagon-secretin family. Eur J Biochem 144:243, 1984.
6. Christofides ND, Yiangou Y, Aarons E, et al: Radioimmunoassay and intramural distribution of PHI-IR in human intestine. Dig Dis Sci 28:507, 1983.
7. Yiangou Y, Christofides ND, Blank MA, et al: Molecular forms of peptide histidine isoleucine-like immunoreactivity in the gastrointestinal tract. Gastroenterology 89:516, 1985.
8. Yiangou Y, Christofides ND, Evans JE, et al: The presence of peptide histidine-isoleucine in human, dog, guinea-pig and rat pancreas. Diabetologia 25:125, 1983.
9. Hokfelt T, Fahrenkrug J, Tatemoto K, et al: PHI, a VIP-like peptide, is present in the rat median eminence. Acta Physiol Scand 116:469, 1982.

10. Christofides ND, Yiangou Y, McGregor GP, et al: Distribution of PHI in the rat brain. Biomed Res 3:573, 1982.
11. Christofides ND, Yiangou Y, Piper PJ, et al: Distribution of peptide histidine isoleucine in the mammalian respiratory tract and some aspects of its pharmacology. Endocrinology 115:1958, 1984.
12. Christofides ND, Yiangou Y, Blank MA, et al: Are peptide histidine isoleucine and vasoactive intestinal peptide co-synthesised in the same pro-hormone? Lancet 2:1398, 1982.
13. Gu J, Blank MA, Huang WM, et al: Peptide-containing nerves in human urinary bladder. Urology 24:353, 1984.
14. Polak JM, Bloom SR: Regulatory peptides—The distribution of two newly discovered peptides: PHI and NPY. Peptides 5(Suppl 1):79, 1984.
15. Fahrenkrug J, Pedersen JH: Development and validation of a specific radioimmunoassay for PHI in plasma. Clin Chim Acta 143:183, 1984.
16. Christofides ND, Yiangou Y, Tatemoto K, et al: Characterization of peptide histidine isoleucine-like immunoreactivity in the rat, human, guinea-pig and cat gastrointestinal tracts—Evidence of species differences. Digestion 30:165, 1984.
17. Bataille D, Gespach C, Laburthe M, et al: Porcine peptide having N-terminal histidine and C-terminal isoleucine amide (PHI). FEBS Lett 114:240, 1980.
18. Robberecht P, Tatemoto K, Chatelain P, et al: Effects of PHI on vasoactive intestinal peptide receptors and adenylate cyclase activity in lung membranes. A comparison in man, rat, mouse and guinea pig. Regul Pept 4:241, 1982.
19. Taton G, Chatelain P, Delhaye M, et al: Vasoactive intestinal peptide (VIP) and peptide having N-terminal histidine and C-terminal isoleucine amide (PHI) stimulate adenylate cyclase activity in human heart membranes. Peptides 3:897, 1982.
20. Jensen RT, Tatemoto K, Mutt V, et al: Actions of a newly isolated intestinal peptide PHI on pancreatic acini. Am J Physiol 241:G498, 1981.
21. Westendorf JM, Phillips MA, Schonbrunn A: Vasoactive intestinal peptide stimulates hormone release from corticotropic cells in culture. Endocrinology 112:550, 1983.
22. Heisler S, Veilleux R, Labrie F: PHI stimulates ACTH release from pituitary tumor cells. Mol Cell Endocrinol 35:183, 1984.
23. Reisine T, Heisler S, Hook VYH, et al: Multireceptor-induced release of adrenocorticotropin from anterior pituitary tumor cells. Biochem Biophys Res Commun 108:1251, 1982.
24. Heisler S, Reisine TD, Hook VYH, et al: Somatostatin inhibits multireceptor stimulation of cyclic AMP formation and corticotropin secretion in mouse pituitary tumor cells. Proc Natl Acad Sci USA 79:6502, 1982.
25. Anagnostides AA, Manolas K, Christofides ND, et al: Peptide histidine isoleucine (PHI). A secretagogue in porcine intestine. Dig Dis Sci 28:893, 1983.
26. Ghiglione M, Christofides ND, Uttenthal LO, et al: Effect of the intestinal peptide PHI on net intestinal fluid transport in the rat. Gut 23:A913, 1982.
27. Moriarty KJ, Hegarty JE, Tatemoto K, et al: Effect of peptide histidine isoleucine on water and electrolyte transport in the human jejunum. Gut 25:624, 1984.
28. Anagnostides AA, Christofides ND, Tatemoto K, et al: Peptide histidine isoleucine: A secretagogue in human jejunum. Gut 25:381, 1984.
29. Brennan LJ, McLoughlin TA, Mutt V, et al: Effects of PHI, a newly isolated peptide, on gall-bladder function in the guinea-pig. J Physiol (Lond) 329:71P, 1982.
30. Wood JR, Brennan LJ, McLoughlin TA, et al: Comparison of the effects of natural and synthetic PHI on gallbladder fluid transport. Regul Pept 4:383, 1982.
31. Dimaline R, Dockray GJ: Actions of a new peptide from porcine intestine (PHI) on pancreatic secretion in the rat and turkey. Life Sci 27:1947, 1980.
32. Szecowka J, Lins PE, Tatemoto K, et al: Effects of porcine intestinal heptacosapeptide and vasoactive intestinal polypeptide on insulin and glucagon secretion in rats. Endocrinology 112:1469, 1983.
33. Szecowka J, Tatemoto K, Mutt V, et al: Interaction of a newly isolated intestinal polypeptide (PHI) with glucose and arginine to effect the secretion of insulin and glucagon. Life Sci 26:435, 1980.
34. Alwmark A, Khalil T, Mate L, et al: Gut hormones as incretin candidates. Surg Forum 35:209, 1984.
35. Kaji H, Chihara K, Abe H, et al: Stimulatory effect of peptide histidine isoleucine amide 1-27 on prolactin release in the rat. Life Sci 35:641, 1984.
36. Kaji H, Chihara K, Abe H, et al: Effect of passive immunization with antisera to vasoactive intestinal polypeptide and peptide histidine isoleucine amide on 5-hydroxy-L-tryptophan-induced prolactin release in rats. Endocrinology 117:1914, 1985.
37. Lundberg JM, Fahrenkrug J, Larsson O, et al: Corelease of vasoactive intestinal polypeptide and peptide histidine isoleucine in relation to atropine-resistant vasodilation in cat submandibular salivary gland. Neurosci Lett 52:37, 1984.
38. Lunberg JM, Tatemoto K: Vascular effects of the peptides PYY and PHI: Comparison with APP and VIP. Eur J Pharmacol 83:143, 1982.
39. O'Dorisio MS, Wood CL, Wenger GD, et al: Cyclic AMP-dependent protein kinsase in Molt 4b lymphoblasts: Identification by photoaffinity labeling and activation in intact cells by vasoactive intestinal polypeptide (VIP) and peptide histidine isoleucine (PHI). J Immunol 134:4078, 1985.

Chapter 27

Opioid Peptides (Endorphins and Enkephalins)

Laszlo Mate, M.D., and George H. Greeley, Jr., Ph.D.

HISTORY

Opioid alkaloids have been used to treat a variety of clinical maladies, and they have also been used as recreational drugs for several thousand years. In addition to their euphoric effect, opioids are particularly important because of their ability to relieve pain and diarrhea. Their action on the central nervous system (CNS) is well documented.

In 1972, opiate receptors in the brain were first described [1,2], but the endogenous ligands for these receptors were not found until 1975, when peptides with morphine-like properties were isolated from the porcine CNS. Chemical characterization of these two pentapeptides showed that the C-terminal amino acid was either a methionine or a leucine residue. Hence, the peptides were named methionine-enkephalin (met-enkephalin) and leucine-enkephalin (leu-enkephalin), respectively [3]. A number of other peptides with opioid properties (that is, opiate-receptor binding and analgesic activity) were described subsequently. These peptides have an N-terminal pentapeptide structure in common that is either met- or leu-enkephalin. In addition, their biologic activity is partially antagonized at the receptor level by naloxone [4,5]. The structure and terminology of opioid peptides have been reviewed [6].

The larger opioid peptides or endorphins were subsequently isolated and their amino acid sequence discovered [7]. Their primary structure is identical to a fragment of β-lipotropin [8,9], a peptide consisting of 91 amino acids that was isolated from the pituitary and characterized in 1964 [10] but to which no biologic activity was attributed. Later, a 31,000-dalton peptide was found in the pituitary that contained both adrenocorticotropic hormone (ACTH) and melanophore-stimulating hormone (MSH), in addition to β-lipotropin. It was therefore named pro-opiomelanocortin, or pro-opiocortin [11–13].

Besides pro-opiomelanocortin, proenkephalin A and proenkephalin B (prodynorphin) are known precursor molecules of the opioid peptides. The name enkephalin was introduced for peptides with opioid activity; it replaced the previously used name, endorphin, which is now used only for a special group of opioid peptides that contain the 61–76 amino acid sequence of β-lipotropin (α-endorphin). The longest, the most important, and the best studied of the endorphins is β-endorphin, which contains the 61–91 fragment of β-lipotropin.

According to their precursor molecule, opioid peptides can be classified into three groups. All of them have one of the enkephalins at their N-terminal. The first group takes its origin from a 31,000-dalton molecule [13] called pro-opiomelanocortin. It also contains ACTH and MSH, besides β-lipotropin [12]. These peptides are present in the highest concentration in the anterior pituitary [14], but low amounts are detected in the sympathetic trunk, celiac ganglion, gastric mucosa, pancreas, and thyroid gland. Unlike the anterior pituitary, where β-lipotropin occurs in quantities greater than those of β-endorphin, the human gastric mucosa contains only negligible amounts of β-lipotropin, while β-endorphin occurs in larger amounts [15]. Although the peptides of this first group contain met-enkephalin, the information so far available does not support the notion that met-enkephalin is produced from endorphins, since the tissue distribution of enkephalins is different, and even in the pituitary gland, where both are localized, they are present in different cells [16].

A second group of opioid peptides originates from proenkephalin A, a large molecule containing four met-enkephalin fragments and one each of leu-enkephalin, met-enkephalin Arg^6Phe^7, and met-enkephalin $Arg^6Gly^7Leu^8$ [17]. The ratio of these peptides is 4:1:1:1 in peripheral tissues, which corresponds well to their ratio in the parent molecule. Apparently, the two extended met-enkephalin molecules (with Arg^6Phe^7 and $Arg^6Gly^7Leu^8$ extensions) are not broken down to met-enkephalin but are biologically active in these forms [15]. These peptides bind to Δ and μ receptors [19].

A third group of opioid peptides is derived from proenkephalin B (prodynorphin). Dynorphin, a heptadecapeptide, is a typical example. The peptides of this group have in common a leu-enkephalin sequence at their N-terminal. In the cow, the highest concentration is in the neurointermediate lobe of the pituitary; however, dynorphin and neoendorphin are also detected in the alimentary canal of humans and cows [15,19]. In the CNS, these two peptides are localized in the same cells and have a distribution pattern different from that of enkephalins [20]. The peptides of this group are specific ligands for κ-receptors [21].

DISTRIBUTION

Opioid peptides are distributed in numerous tissues and in a variety of animal species. The tissues best studied are the pituitary gland and the CNS.

The highest concentration of enkephalins is found in the CNS, where the striatum, limbic system, and the preoptic nuclei of the hypothalamus have the highest content. In the spinal cord, the highest concentration of enkephalins is found in the Rexed I and II layers, where nociceptive stimuli are mediated [22]. Little opioid activity is detected in the cerebellum and in the cerebral cortex [23].

In the peripheral nervous system, the vagus, as well as the splanchnic and sciatic nerves, contain met-enkephalin, among several other peptides [24]. A high opioid content is detected in the adrenal medulla, where it is stored and released, together with catecholamines from the intracellular vesicles [25,26].

The gut has a significantly lower content of opioids when compared to the CNS. The highest concentration of enkephalins is found in the stomach and in the proximal small intestine. Smaller amounts of opioid peptides are found in the gallbladder and in the pancreas [27,28].

Within the gut wall, the greatest amount of enkephalin immunoreactivity is detected in the neuronal elements, both in the cell bodies and axons of the myenteric plexus. Some endocrine cells contain a small amount of opioid peptides [29,30]. Met-enkephalin is present in the highest concentration in the guinea pig ileum (820 ± 90 pmol/g), while leu-enkephalin is detected in much smaller amounts [31]. In the guinea pig small intestine, leu-enkephalin immunoreactivity is absent in the submucous plexus in contrast to the myenteric plexus, where 25 percent of all nerves contain this peptide [32]. Enkephalin-containing nerves are a separate system of enteric nerves, which can be distinguished from other peptide-containing nerves by morphologic analysis [33].

Met-enkephalin-like immunoreactivity is found in gastric cells in several species [34], and the same cells were shown to contain ACTH [35], suggesting that pro-opiocortin may be present. Besides met-enkephalin, met-enkephalin-Arg^6Phe^7 is found in the myenteric plexus, in the circular smooth muscle, and in gastric cells [36].

The mucosa and the muscularis of the human stomach contain higher levels of leu- than met-enkephalin [28]. Enkephalin-like immunoreactivity has been detected also in rat [37] and chicken embryos [38].

The occurrence of the other opioid peptides in the gut has not been thoroughly studied. Dynorphin and β-endorphin have been isolated in small quantities (one tenth the concentration of met-enkephalin) [19]. Radioimmunoassay (RIA) studies indicate that β-endorphin and ACTH are present in the human gastric mucosa [15] and pancreas [39] and in the gut of rats [40].

ASSAY

A quantitative measurement for both types of enkephalins, endorphins, and dynorphin is possible with radioimmunoassays [41,42].

Bioassays are still useful, since they can distinguish the different types of receptors and can differentiate biologically active from inactive forms. The most common bioassays are preparations of guinea pig ileum and of the isolated mouse vas deferens [43–45]. Analgesic action is quantitated easily with the hot plate test or the mouse tail flick test. A common and effective test is the receptor binding assay using ^{3}H-naloxone as the competitive ligand [46]. These tests were originally developed for opiate alkaloids and generally have a preference for the different types of receptors. It is important that the activities of new substances be tested in several assay systems. By comparing their relative potencies, their receptor preference can be determined. High pressure liquid chromatography (HPLC) is a useful tool in the separation and measurement of opioid peptides, since it allows the separation of structurally related compounds [47].

PHARMACOKINETICS AND CATABOLISM

As mentioned earlier, the existence of opiate receptors was established years before the actual opioid peptides were discovered. After the discovery of the opioid peptides and the synthesis of several different analogues, the potencies of the natural and synthetic analogues were found to be unequal in the various bioassay systems. The ability of naloxone to antagonize these analogues varied considerably from one system to another, suggesting that different types of receptors are involved in these systems [48]. Further studies revealed several classes of receptors [49,50].

Receptors were first described for opiate drugs; we now know that the endogenous ligands are peptides chemically unrelated to opiate drugs. The receptors are, therefore, better known as "opioid" [6]. Four types of opioid receptors have been described: μ (mu), δ or Δ (delta), κ (kappa), and σ (sigma). A fifth type, ϵ (epsilon), has been mentioned but is not well understood. The classification of receptors is related to the drugs that bind preferentially with each class [6].

The classic morphine-like drugs interact in all systems with μ-receptors. The μ-receptors mediate the analgesic activity of these substances. Dynorphine and the related peptides preferentially bind to κ-receptors, which have subclasses [51,52], together with the synthetic benzomorphans. Met- and leu-enkephalins exert their action via Δ- and μ-receptors. The morphine antagonist naloxone preferentially binds to μ-receptors, and its affinity for Δ-receptors is lower [53]. The morphine-like drugs interact with σ-receptors, suggesting a common mechanism with nonopioid substances, since ketamine and phencyclidine can also bind to these receptors [54]. The existence of ϵ-receptors is suggested, since β-endorphin shows an extremely high potency in the rat vas deferens preparation in comparison to other assay systems and to other peptides [55].

In the guinea pig ileum, μ-receptors are dominant, but a small number of κ-receptors is also present. Delta receptors predominate in the mouse vas deferens. In CNS homogenates, all receptor types are found, but their proportions are species-related [56–59]. So far, only one system, the rabbit vas deferens, has been reported, in which only one receptor type (κ) exists [60].

The distribution of μ- and Δ-receptors in the central and peripheral nervous systems shows separate patterns [51,61], while the distribution of κ-receptors is still unclear.

Interestingly enough, the C-terminal, unsulfated heptapeptide of cholecystokinin (CCK), interacts with the opioid receptors in the brain and peripheral tissues [62]. The significance of this observation is unclear, since, although CCK and opioid receptors occur in the CNS, it is not known whether unsulfated CCK-27-33 actually occurs there.

At present, two enzymes appear to be involved in the catabolism of enkephalins, an aminopeptidase and an enkephalinase. Both enzymes are exceptionally active, but they are apparently not specific for enkephalins [63].

The first event in enkephalin inactivation is the cleavage of the 1-2 peptide bond, as measured by the use of ^{3}H-tyrosine-labeled enkephalin [64]. The aminopeptidases capable of this cleavage have been isolated from blood and CNS [65–67]. Substitution of D-Ala in the second position of the enkephalins blocks this catabolic pathway, which probably explains why the D-Ala^2 enkephalin analogues are more potent.

A second cleavage site occurs at the 3-4 peptide bond [68]. Enkephalinase acts at this site. Enkephalinase is membrane-bound, and its distribution in the CNS appears to parallel that of opioid receptors [69]. Enkephalinase may be the major catabolic enzyme at the synapse, whereas aminopeptidase acts primarily in the systemic circulation. Both met- and leu-enkephalin are rapidly degraded in tissues or in the circulation [70] and upon hepatic transit [71]. Catecholamines antagonize the degradation of met-enkephalin [72]. The pathways involved in the inactivation of the other opioid peptides are not known.

The half-lives of β-endorphin and β-lipotropin are longer than 30 minutes in humans [73,74]. In the canine small intestine, β-endorphin is processed into several fragments that remain capable of stimulating gut motility [75].

RELEASE

In rat brain slices, potassium-induced release of both met- and leu-enkephalins is calcium-dependent [76]. A similar release mechanism for endorphins is observed for mouse pituitary tumor cells [77].

In humans, β-endorphin, measured by RIA, is released into plasma after a meal or after duodenal acidification [78]. In rats, the β-endorphin and ACTH contents of the gut decrease after feeding, implying a simultaneous release of these peptides after intake of food [40]. A similar, concomitant release of the two peptides from the pituitary was measured after stimulation [79,80] and after electrical shock [81]. Whether these peptides are released in their active circulating form or as proopiomelanocortin (which is then metabolized to ACTH, β-lipotropin, and MSH) is unclear. Intravenous morphine released leu-enkephalin in dogs, as measured in the portal, jugular, and femoral veins [82].

Recently, the release of a substance that binds to opioid receptors in the brain was detected after in vitro perfusion of rat small intestine as well as after calcium and tolbutamide stimulation, but this large molecule did not react with met-enkephalin, β-endorphin, or dynorphin antibodies [83]; therefore, the exact identity of this substance is not known.

Electrical stimulation of isolated strips of guinea pig ileum causes release of opioids into the bathing fluid [84], and the phenomenon of fading contractions in response to electrical stimulation is prevented by naloxone. This implies the participation of opioids in the contraction [85]. Similar results were obtained from the cat pylorus [86]. Electrical stimulation of canine splanchnic nerves caused an increase in met-enkephalin immunoreactivity in the adrenal vein [87].

ACTIONS

Opioid peptides have, in part, a range of actions on the alimentary canal that is similar to that of morphine. In humans, naloxone reduces both basal and meal-stimulated acid secretion, which suggests an endogenous background of opioid stimulation on basal gastric secretion. In another study, however, naloxone was found to be ineffective [88].

Konturek et al [89] found that morphine and met-enkephalin produced a dose-dependent elevation in histamine or pentagastrin-induced gastric acid and pepsin secretion. Kostritsky-Pereira et al [90] reported that enkephalins inhibit meal-induced acid secretion. Enkephalin can stimulate gastric mucosal blood flow alone, without affecting basal acid secretion. Enkephalin also enhanced the stimulatory effect of other secretagogues in dogs [71]; met-enkephalin, on the other hand, inhibited the increase in bombesin- or vagal-induced gastric secretion, unlike morphine, which enhances further gastric secretion in dogs [91,92]. Morphine as well as met- and leu-enkephalin can diminish the rate of fractional gastric emptying in dogs [90].

In humans, a met-enkephalin analogue diminished vagal- and pentagastrin- but not histamine-stimulated gastric acid secretion and pancreatic polypeptide release, with a concurrent elevation in the serum gastrin levels [93].

In rats, met-enkephalin did not affect serum gastrin levels, but it decreased somatostatin release in vitro [94]. In dogs, enkephalins and morphine inhibited gastrin release [90]; leu-enkephalin was less effective than met-enkephalin. Vagal stimulation inhibited somatostatin release, and this effect was blocked by naloxone [95]. In fact, the stimulatory effect of met-enkephalin can be blocked not only by naloxone but also by atropine and H_2 blockers, which suggests a complex mode of interaction among stimulants. Central administration of opioid peptides inhibited gastric acid secretion. Morphine and an enkephalin analogue are effective in the prevention of stress ulcers in rats after peripheral or direct administration into the CNS. Besides a reduction in gastric acid output, an increase in prostaglandin synthesis was found [96].

With regard to pancreatic exocrine secretion, morphine and enkephalins have an inhibitory action on secretin- and CCK-stimulated pancreatic exocrine secretion. This inhibition by morphine and enkephalins appears to be, at least in part, a direct effect on the exocrine pancreas. In addition, the release of secretin, and probably of CCK, is also reduced in dogs [97].

Naloxone alone had no effect on basal pancreatic secretion in humans [88]. Met-enkephalin decreased meal-stimulated release of pancreatic polypeptide [98]. ICV administration of β-endorphin (0.8 to 25 μg) inhibited basal gastric and pancreatic secretions in a dose-dependent manner [99].

In the isolated dog pancreas, β-endorphin as well as morphine suppressed somatostatin release and increased the stimulated release of insulin and glucagon [100,101]. In normal humans, both insulin and glucagon were released after a bolus injection of β-endorphin, whereas in diabetics, only glucagon levels increased [101]. In isolated rat islets, a synthetic met-enkephalin analogue enhanced release of insulin [102].

Both morphine and enkephalin blocked the effect of secretagogues on the small intestine [103,104]. Enkephalin stimulated the absorption of water, sodium, and chloride from the small intestine in several species [105–107], which may be one of the mechanisms by which opiates relieve diarrhea. This effect is mediated by way of the Δ-receptor [108].

Substances with opioid activity block the electrically evoked contraction of the guinea pig ileum in vitro. This inhibitory effect is partly due to the blocking effects of opiates on acetylcholine release, which is reversible with naloxone [109,110]. Tetrodotoxin pretreatment of the preparation prevented the effect of opiates, suggesting the involvement of neural pathways [111]. The release or actions of other humoral agents may be blocked by opiates in a manner similar to the actions of opioids on substance P [112,113].

Opioids block not only the electrically stimulated motility of the guinea pig ileum but also contractions evoked by other stimulants such as neurotensin [114], caerulein [115], histamine [116], prostaglandin E_1 [117], and bombesin [118], as well as morphine; and enkephalin does not block substance P-induced contractions [119]. Dynorphin also antagonized neurotensin-induced contractions [120], and recent data suggest that dynorphin may be a physiologic inhibitor of such intestinal motility [121].

Although enkephalins inhibit the stimulated contractions in the guinea pig ileum, enkephalins alone cause contraction of the intestine in dogs, humans, and other species. In cats, met-enkephalin increases the basal intestinal tone without affecting peristalsis [122]. In the dog ileum, it stimulated both tonic and phasic contractions [123]. Similar contractions are observed in a rat colon preparation, where both atropine and tetrodotoxin potentiate the effects [124]. In another study, however, tetrodotoxin abolished this effect and a serotonin antagonist, methysergide, diminished it significantly, which suggests the involvement of serotonin [125]. Although these findings would suggest a mediator, morphine, enkephalins, and dynorphin have been shown to be capable of stimulating the contraction of isolated guinea pig stomach muscle cells, which implies a direct effect [126]. β-Endorphin stimulated dog small intestinal motility, where it was metabolized to several biologically active fragments [127].

Opiates can also stimulate alkaline secretion in the duodenum by an apparent activation of the Cl^-/HCO_3^- exchange. The influence of opiates on secretion of alkali is probably mediated by a local neural component [128,129], which is interesting since morphine is known to prevent stress ulceration in laboratory animals [129].

Met-enkephalin caused a decrease in the frequency of interdigestive myoelectric complex and prolonged the time required for this complex to traverse the small bowel [130].

Met-enkephalin has been demonstrated in the biliary system [131]. Morphine is a well known constrictor of the sphincter of Oddi, where it acts to increase the biliary pressure and to inhibit the passage of bile into the duodenum. The basal activity of the sphincter of Oddi in the cat was inhibited by naloxone, which suggests an endogenous opioid tone [132].

In humans, naloxone alone is without effect on gallbladder volume, whereas morphine and a synthetic met-enkephalin analogue inhibit CCK-induced evacuation of the gallbladder [133]. Met-enkephalin, applied in vitro, was a stimulant of the guinea pig circular gallbladder muscle, and in the same study, naloxone caused a partial inhibition of CCK-stimulated contraction, which suggests that the mediation of contraction is opioid dependent [134].

REFERENCES

1. Pert CB, Snyder SH: Opiate receptor: Demonstration in nervous tissue. Science 179:1011, 1973.
2. Kuhar MJ, Pert CB, Snyder SH: Regional distribution of opiate receptor binding in monkey and human brain. Nature 245:447, 1973.
3. Hughes J, Smith TW, Kosterlitz HW, et al: Identification of two related pentapeptides from the brain with potent opiate agonist activity. Nature 258:577, 1975.
4. Martin WR: Opioid antagonists. Pharmacol Rev 19:463, 1967.
5. Fuxe K, Andersson K, Hokfelt T, et al: Localization and possible function of peptidergic neurons and their interactions with central catecholamine neurons, and the central actions of gut hormones. Fed Proc 38:2333, 1979.
6. Cox BM: Endogenous opioid peptones: A guide to structures and terminology. Life Sci 31:1645, 1982.
7. Ling N, Burgus R, Guillemin R: Isolation, primary structure, and synthesis of α-endorphin and γ-endorphin, two peptides of hypothalamic-hypophysial origin with morphinomimetic activity. Proc Natl Acad Sci USA 73:3942, 1976.
8. Lazarus LH, Ling N, Guillemin R: β-Lipotropin as a prohormone for the morphinomimetic peptides

endorphins and enkephalins. Proc Natl Acad Sci USA 73:2156, 1976.
9. Li CH, Chung D: Isolation and structure of an untriakontapeptide with opiate activity from camel pituitary glands. Proc Natl Acad Sci USA 73:1145, 1976.
10. Li CH: Lipotropin, a new active peptide from pituitary glands. Nature 201:924, 1964.
11. Mains RE, Eipper BA, Ling N: Common precursor to corticotropins and endorphins. Proc Natl Acad Sci USA 74:3014, 1977.
12. Cox BM, Opheim KE, Teschemacher H, et al: A peptide-like substance from pituitary that acts like morphine. 2. Purification and properties. Life Sci 16:1777, 1975.
13. Nakanishi S, Inoue A, Kita T, et al: Nucleotide sequence of cloned cDNA for bovine corticotropin-β-lipotropin precursor. Nature 278:423, 1979.
14. Bloom F, Battenberg E, Rossier J, et al: Endorphins are located in the intermediate and anterior lobes of the pituitary gland, not in the neurohypophysis. Life Sci 20:43, 1977.
15. Imura H, Nakai Y, Nakao K, et al: Biosynthesis and distribution of opioid peptides. J Endocrinol Invest 6:139, 1983.
16. Bloom F, Battenberg E, Rossier J, et al: Neurons containing β-endorphin in rat brain exist separately from those containing enkephalin: Immunocytochemical studies. Proc Natl Acad Sci USA 75:1591, 1978.
17. Noda M, Furutani Y, Takahashi H, et al: Cloning and sequence analysis of cDNA for bovine adrenal preproenkephalin. Nature 295:202, 1982.
18. Magnan J, Paterson SJ, Kosterlitz HW: The interaction of [met^5]enkephalin and [leu^5]enkephalin sequences, extended at the C-terminus, with the μ-, γ- and κ-binding sites in the guinea-pig brain. Life Sci 31:1359, 1982.
19. Tachibana S, Araki K, Ohya S, et al: Isolation and structure of dynorphin, an opioid peptide, from porcine duodenum. Nature 295:339, 1982.
20. Weber E, Roth KA, Barchas JD: Immunohistochemical distribution of α-neo-endorphin/dynorphin neuronal systems in rat brain: Evidence for colocalization. Proc Natl Acad Sci USA 79:3062, 1982.
21. Corbett AD, Paterson SJ, McKnight AT, et al: Dynorphin$_{1-8}$ and dynorphin$_{1-9}$ are ligands for the κ-subtype of opiate receptor. Nature 299:79, 1982.
22. Hokfelt T, Ljungdahl A, Terenius L, et al: Immunohistochemical analysis of peptide pathways possibly related to pain and analgesia: Enkephalin and substance P. Proc Natl Acad Sci USA 74:3081, 1977.
23. Hughes J, Kosterlitz HW, Smith TW: The distribution of methionine-enkephalin and leucine-enkephalin in the brain and peripheral tissues. Br J Pharmacol 61:639, 1977.
24. Lundberg JM, Hokfelt T, Nilsson G, et al: Peptide neurons in the vagus, splanchnic and sciatic nerves. Acta Physiol Scand 104:499, 1978.
25. Schultzberg M, Lundberg JM, Hokfelt T, et al: Enkephalin-like immunoreactivity in gland cells and nerve terminals of the adrenal medulla. Neuroscience 3:1169, 1978.
26. Lundberg JM, Hamberger B, Schultzberg M, et al: Enkephalin- and somatostatin-like immunoreactivities in human adrenal medulla and pheochromocytoma. Proc Natl Acad Sci USA 76:4079, 1979.
27. Polak JM, Bloom SR, Sullivan SN, et al: Enkephalin-like immunoreactivity in the human gastrointestinal tract. Lancet 1:972, 1977.
28. Feurle GE, Helmstaedter V, Weber U: Met- and leu-enkephalin immuno- and bio-reactivity in human stomach and pancreas. Life Sci 31:2961, 1982.
29. Alumets J, Håkanson R, Sundler F, et al: Leu-enkephalin-like material in nerves and enterochromaffin cells in the gut. An immunohistochemical study. Histochemistry 56:187, 1978.
30. Linnoila RI, DiAugustine RP, Miller RJ, et al: An immunohistochemical and radioimmunological study of the distribution of [met^5]- and [leu^5]-enkephalin in the gastrointestinal tract. Neuroscience 3:1187, 1978.
31. Furness JB, Costa M, Murphy R, et al: Detection and characterisation of neurotransmitters, particularly peptides, in the gastrointestinal tract. Scand J Gastroenterol 17(Suppl 71):61, 1982.
32. Furness JB, Costa M, Franco R, et al: Neuronal peptides in the intestine: Distribution and possible functions, in Costa E, Trabucchi M (eds): *Neural Peptides and Neuronal Communication.* New York, Raven Press, 1980, pp 601–617.
33. Probert L, De Mey J, Polak JM: Ultrastructural localization of four different neuropeptides within separate populations of p-type nerves in the guinea pig colon. Gastroenterology 85:1094, 1983.
34. Larsson L-I, Stengaard-Pedersen K: Enkephalin/endorphin-related peptides in antropyloric gastrin cells. J Histochem Cytochem 29:1088, 1981.
35. Larsson L-I: ACTH-like immunoreactivity in the gastrin cell. Independent changes in gastrin and ACTH-like immunoreactivity during ontogeny. Histochemistry 56:245, 1978.
36. Bu'lock AJ, Vaillant C, Dockray GJ: Immunohistochemical studies on the gastrointestinal tract using antisera to met-enkephalin and met-enkephalin arg^{6}phe^7. J Histochem Cytochem 31:1356, 1983.
37. Dahl JL, Epstein ML, Silva BL, et al: Multiple immunoreactive forms of met- and leu-enkephalin in fetal and neonatal rat brain and in rat gut. Life Sci 31:1853, 1982.
38. Saffrey MJ, Polak JM, Burnstock G: Distribution of vaso-active intestinal polypeptide-, substance P-, enkephalin- and neurotensin-like immunoreactive nerves in the chicken gut during development. Neuroscience 7:279, 1982.
39. Larsson L-I: Corticotropin-like peptides in central

nerves and in endocrine cells of gut and pancreas. Lancet 2:1321, 1977.
40. Orwoll ES, Kendall JW: β-endorphin and adrenocorticotropin in extrapituitary sites: Gastrointestinal tract. Endocrinology 107:438, 1980.
41. Rossier J, Bayon A, Vargo TM, et al: Radioimmunoassay of brain peptides: Evaluation of a methodology for the assay of β-endorphin and enkephalin. Life Sci 21:847, 1977.
42. Simantov R, Childers SR, Snyder SH: Opioid peptides: Differentiation by radioimmunoassay and radioreceptor assay. Brain Res 135:358, 1977.
43. Gyang EA, Kosterlitz HW: Agonist and antagonist actions of morphine-like drugs on the guinea-pig isolated ileum. Br J Pharmacol Chemother 27:514, 1966.
44. Henderson G, Hughes J, Kosterlitz HW: A new example of a morphine-sensitive neuro-effector junction: Adrenergic transmission in the mouse vas deferens. Br J Pharmacol 46:764, 1972.
45. Hughes J, Kosterlitz HW, Leslie FM: Effect of morphine on adrenergic transmission in the mouse vas deferens. Assessment of agonist and antagonist potencies of narcotic analgesics. Br J Pharmacol 53:371, 1975.
46. Pasternak GW, Wilson HA, Snyder SH: Differential effects of protein-modifying reagents on receptor binding of opiate agonists and antagonists. Molec Pharmacol 11:340, 1975.
47. Meek JL, Bohan TP: Use of high pressure liquid chromatography (HPLC) to study enkephalins. Adv Biochem Psychopharmacol 18:141, 1978.
48. Wuster M, Schulz R, Herz A: Multiple opiate receptors in peripheral tissue preparations. Biochem Pharmacol 30:1883, 1981.
49. Chang K-J, Cooper BR, Hazum E, et al: Multiple opiate receptors: Different regional distribution in the brain and differential binding of opiates and opioid peptides. Molec Pharmacol 16:91, 1979.
50. Pfeiffer A, Herz A: Different types of opiate agonists interact distinguishably with mu, delta and kappa opiate binding sites. Life Sci 31:1355, 1982.
51. Wolozin BL, Pasternak GW: Classification of multiple morphine and enkephalin binding sites in the central nervous system. Proc Natl Acad Sci USA 78:6181, 1981.
52. Pfeiffer A, Pasi A, Mehraein P, et al: A subclassification of κ-sites in human brain by use of dynorphin 1–17. Neuropeptides 2:89, 1981.
53. Chang K-J, Hazum E, Cuatrecasas P: Possible role of distinct morphine and enkephalin receptors in mediating actions of benzomorphan drugs (putative κ and σ agonists). Proc Natl Acad Sci USA 77:4469, 1980.
54. Herling S, Woods JH: IV. Discriminative stimulus effects of narcotics: Evidence for multiple receptor-mediated actions. Life Sci 28:1571, 1981.
55. Wuster M, Schulz R, Herz A: Specificity of opioids towards the μ-, γ- and ϵ-opiate receptors. Neurosci Lett 15:193, 1978.
56. Lord JAH, Waterfield AA, Hughes J, et al: Endogenous opioid peptides: Multiple agonists and receptors. Nature 267:495, 1977.
57. Lemaire S, Berube A, Derome G, et al: Synthesis and biological activity of β-endorphin and analogues. Additional evidence for multiple opiate receptors. J Med Chem 21:1232, 1978.
58. Chavkin C, Goldstein A: Demonstration of a specific dynorphin receptor in guinea pig ileum myenteric plexus. Nature 291:591, 1981.
59. Gillan MGC, Kosterlitz HW: Spectrum of the μ-, γ- and κ-binding sites in homogenates of rat brain. Br J Pharmacol 77:461, 1982.
60. Oka T, Negishi K, Suda M, et al: Rabbit vas deferens: A specific bioassay for opioid κ-receptor agonists. Eur J Pharmacol 73:235, 1980.
61. Leslie FM, Chavkin C, Cox BM: Opioid binding properties of brain and peripheral tissues: Evidence for heterogeneity in opioid ligand binding sites. J Pharmacol Exp Ther 214:395, 1980.
62. Schiller PW, Lipton A, Horrobin DF, et al: Unsulfated C-terminal 7-peptide of cholecystokinin: A new ligand of the opiate receptor. Biochem Biophys Res Commun 85:1332, 1978.
63. Hughes J: Biogenesis, release and inactivation of enkephalins and dynorphins. Br Med Bull 39:17, 1983.
64. Craviso GL, Musacchio JM: Inhibition of enkephalin degradation in the guinea pig ileum. Life Sci 23:2019, 1978.
65. Hambrook JM, Morgan BA, Rance MJ, et al: Mode of deactivation of the enkephalins by rat and human plasma and rat brain homogenates. Nature 262:782, 1976.
66. Coletti-Previero M-A, Mattras H, Descomps B, et al: Purification and substrate characterization of a human enkephalin-degrading aminopeptidase. Biochim Biophys Acta 657:122, 1981.
67. Hersh LB: Solubilization and characterization of two rat brain membrane-bound aminopeptidases active on met-enkephalin. Biochemistry 20:2345, 1981.
68. Sullivan S, Akil H, Barchas JD: *In vitro* degradation of enkephalin: Evidence for cleavage at the gly-phe bond. Commun Psychopharm 2:525, 1979.
69. Schwartz J-C, Malfroy B, de la Baume S: Biological inactivation of enkephalins and the role of enkephalin-dipeptidyl-carboxypeptidase ("enkephalinase") as neuropeptidase. Life Sci 29:1715, 1981.
70. Dupont A, Cusan L, Garon M, et al: Extremely rapid degradation of [^{3}H] methionine-enkephalin by various rat tissues *in vivo* and *in vitro*. Life Sci 21:907, 1977.
71. Walus KM, Pawlik W, Konturek SJ, et al: Effect of met-enkephalin and morphine on gastric secretion and blood flow. Acta Physiol Pol 32:383, 1981.
72. Caffrey JL, Hodges DH: Inhibition of the enzymatic degradation of met-enkephalin by catecholamines. Endocrinology 110:291, 1982.
73. Foley KM, Kourides IA, Inturrisi CE, et al: β-endor-

phin: Analgesic and hormonal effects in humans. Proc Natl Acad Sci USA 76:5377, 1979.
74. Liotta AS, Li CH, Schussler GC, et al: Comparative metabolic clearance rate, volume of distribution and plasma half-life of human β-lipotropin and ACTH. Life Sci 23:2323, 1978.
75. Hynes MR, Culling AJ, Galligan JJ, et al: Processing of β-endorphin in the dog intestine: Regional specificity. Proc West Pharmacol Soc 26:95, 1983.
76. Bayon A, Rossier J, Mauss A, et al: *In vitro* release of [5-methionine]enkephalin and [5-leucine]-enkephalin from the rat globus pallidus. Proc Natl Acad Sci USA 75:3503, 1978.
77. Simantov R: Basal and potassium stimulated, calcium dependent, endorphins release from pituitary cells. Life Sci 23:2503, 1978.
78. Matsumura M, Fukuda N, Saito S, et al: Effect of a test meal, duodenal acidification, and tetragastrin on the plasma concentration of β-endorphin-like immunoreactivity in man. Regul Pept 4:173, 1982.
79. Guillemin R, Vargo T, Rossier J, et al: β-endorphin and adrenocorticotropin are secreted concomitantly by the pituitary gland. Science 197:1367, 1977.
80. Nakao K, Nakai Y, Oki S, et al: Presence of immunoreactive β-endorphin in normal human plasma. A concomitant release of β-endorphin with adrenocorticotropin after metyrapone administration. J Clin Invest 62:1395, 1978.
81. Rossier J, French ED, Rivier C, et al: Foot-shock induced stress increases β-endorphin levels in blood but not brain. Nature 270:618, 1977.
82. Laasberg LH, Johnson EE, Hedley-Whyte J: Effect of morphine and naloxone on leu-enkephalin-like immunoreactivity in dogs. J Pharmacol Exp Ther 212:496, 1980.
83. Smith SS, Awoke S, Wade A, et al: Opiate peptides are released by the perfused rat ileum-jejunum in response to chemical and physical stimuli. Horm Metab Res 15:257, 1983.
84. Schulz R, Wuster M, Herz A: Detection of a long acting endogenous opioid in blood and small intestine. Life Sci 21:105, 1977.
85. Puig MM, Gascon P, Musacchio JM: Electrically induced opiate-like inhibition of the guinea-pig ileum: Cross-tolerance to morphine. J Pharmacol Exp Ther 206:289, 1978.
86. Edin R: The vagal control of the pyloric motor function. A physiological and immunohistochemical study in cat and man. Acta Physiol Scand (Suppl 485):1, 1980.
87. Govoni S, Hanbauer I, Hexum TD, et al: *In vivo* characterization of the mechanisms that secrete enkephalin-like peptides stored in dog adrenal medulla. Neuropharmacology 20:639, 1981.
88. Rees WDW, Sharpe GR, Christofides ND, et al: The effects of an opiate agonist and antagonist on the human upper gastrointestinal tract. Eur J Clin Invest 13:221, 1983.
89. Konturek SJ, Tasler J, Cieszkowski M, et al: Comparison of methionine-enkephalin and morphine in the stimulation of gastric acid secretion in the dog. Gastroenterology 78:294, 1980.
90. Kostritsky-Pereira A, Woussen-Colle MC, de Graef J: Effects of morphine, enkephalins and naloxone on postprandial gastric acid secretion, gastric emptying and gastrin release in dogs. Arch Int Physiol Biochim 92:19, 1984.
91. Materia A, Jaffe BM, Modlin IM, et al: Effect of methionine-enkephalin and naloxone on bombesin-stimulated gastric acid secretion, gastrin, and pancreatic polypeptide release in the dog. Ann Surg 196:48, 1982.
92. Anderson W, Molina E, Rentz J, et al: Analysis of the 2-deoxy-D-glucose-induced vagal stimulation of gastric secretion and gastrin release in dogs using methionine-enkephalin, morphine and naloxone. J Pharmacol Exp Ther 222:617, 1982.
93. Konturek SJ, Kwiecien N, Obtułowicz W, et al: Effect of enkephalin and naloxone on gastric acid and serum gastrin and pancreatic polypeptide concentrations in humans. Gut 24:740, 1983.
94. Chiba T, Taminato T, Kadowaki S, et al: Effects of various gastrointestinal peptides on gastric somatostatin release. Endocrinology 106:145, 1980.
95. McIntosh CHS, Kwok YN, Mordhorst T, et al: Enkephalinergic control of somatostatin secretion from the perfused rat stomach. Can J Physiol Pharmacol 61:657, 1983.
96. Ferri S, Arrigo-Reina R, Candeletti S, et al: Central and peripheral sites of action for the protective effect of opioids of the rat stomach. Pharmacol Res Commun 15:409, 1983.
97. Chey WY, Coy DH, Konturek SJ, et al: Enkephalin inhibits the release and action of secretin on pancreatic secretion in the dog. J Physiol 298:429, 1980.
98. Materia A, Modlin IM, Sank AC, et al: Opiate modulation of pancreatic polypeptide release by a meal in the dog. J Pharmacol Exp Ther 223:355, 1982.
99. Roze C, Dubrasquet M, Chariot J, et al: Central inhibition of basal pancreatic and gastric secretions by β-endorphin in rats. Gastroenterology 79:659, 1980.
100. Ipp E, Dobbs R, Unger RH: Morphine and β-endorphin influence the secretion of the endocrine pancreas. Nature 276:190, 1978.
101. Feldman M, Kiser RS, Unger RH, et al: Beta-endorphin and the endocrine pancreas. Studies in healthy and diabetic human beings. N Engl J Med 308:349, 1983.
102. Green IC, Perrin D, Pedley KC, et al: Effect of enkephalins and morphine on insulin secretion from isolated rat islets. Diabetologia 19:158, 1980.
103. Beubler E, Lembeck F: Inhibition of stimulated fluid secretion in the rat small and large intestine by opiate agonists. Naunyn Schmiedebergs Arch Pharmacol 306:113, 1979.
104. McKay JS, Linaker BD, Higgs NB, et al: Studies of the anti-secretory activity of morphine in rabbit ileum in vitro. Gastroenterology 82:243, 1982.
105. Barbezat GO, Reasbeck PG: Effects of bombesin,

calcitonin, and enkephalin on canine jejunal water and electrolyte transport. Dig Dis Sci 28:273, 1983.
106. Dobbins JW, Dharmsathaphorn K, Racusen L, et al: The effect of somatostatin and enkephalin on ion transport in the intestine. Ann NY Acad Sci 372:594, 1981.
107. Miller RJ, Kachur JF, Field M: Neurohumoral control of ileal electrolyte transport. Ann NY Acad Sci 372:571, 1981.
108. Kachur JF, Miller RJ: Characterization of the opiate receptor in the guinea-pig ileal mucosa. Eur J Pharmacol 81:177, 1982.
109. Paton WDM, Zar MA: The origin of acetylcholine released from guinea-pig intestine and longitudinal muscle strips. J Physiol 194:13, 1968.
110. Waterfield AA, Kosterlitz HW: Stereospecific increase by narcotic antagonists of evoked acetylcholine output in guinea-pig ileum. Life Sci 16:1787, 1975.
111. Kromer W, Schmidt H: Opioids modulate intestinal peristalsis at a site of action additional to that modulating acetylcholine release. J Pharmacol Exp Ther 223:271, 1982.
112. Bartho L, Holzer P, Donnerer J, et al: Evidence for the involvement of substance P in the atropine-resistant peristalsis of the guinea-pig ileum. Neurosci Lett 32:69, 1982.
113. Gintzler AR, Scalisi JA: Effects of opioids on noncholinergic excitatory responses of the guinea-pig isolated ileum: Inhibition of release of enteric substance P. Br J Pharmacol 75:199, 1982.
114. Monier S, Kitabgi P: Effects of β-endorphin, met-enkephalin and somatostatin on the neurotensin-induced neurogenic contraction in the guinea-pig ileum. Regul Pept 2:31, 1981.
115. Yau WM, Lingle PF, Youther ML: Interaction of enkephalin and caerulein on guinea pig small intestine. Am J Physiol 244:G65, 1983.
116. Mitznegg P, Domschke W, Sprugel W, et al: Enkephalins inhibit intestinal motility: Mode of action. Acta Hepato-Gastroenterol 24:119, 1977.
117. Jaques R: Inhibitory effect of enkephalins on contractions of the guinea-pig ileum elicited by PGE_1. Agents Actions 7:317, 1977.
118. Zetler G: Antagonism of the gut-contracting effects of bombesin and neurotensin by opioid peptides, morphine, atropine or tetrodotoxin. Pharmacology 21:348, 1980.
119. Chipkin RE, Stewart JM, Morris DH: Substance P and opioid interaction on stimulated and non-stimulated guinea pig ileum. Eur J Pharmacol 53:21, 1978.
120. Zhu Y-X, Huidobro-Toro JP, Lee NM, et al: Interaction of dynorphin with neurotensin on the guinea pig ileum myenteric plexus. Life Sci 31:1825, 1982.
121. Kromer W, Hollt V, Schmidt H, et al: Release of immunoreactive-dynorphin from the isolated guinea-pig small intestine is reduced during peristaltic activity. Neurosci Lett 25:53, 1981.
122. Hellstrom PM, Rosell S: Effects of neurotensin, substance P and methionine-enkephalin on colonic motility. Acta Physiol Scand 113:147, 1981.
123. Daniel EE, Gonda T, Domoto T, et al: The effects of substance P and met^5-enkephalin in dog ileum. Can J Physiol Pharmacol 60:830, 1982.
124. Gillan MGC, Pollock D: Acute effects of morphine and opioid peptides on the motility and responses of rat colon to electrical stimulation. Br J Pharmacol 68:381, 1980.
125. Huidobro-Toro JP, Way EL: Contractile effect of morphine and related opioid alkaloids, β-endorphin and methionine enkephalin on the isolated colon from Long Evans rats. Br J Pharmacol 74:681, 1981.
126. Bitar KN, Makhlouf GM: Specific opiate receptors on isolated mammalian gastric smooth muscle cells. Nature 297:72, 1982.
127. Davis TP, Culling AJ, Schoemaker H, et al: β-endorphin and its metabolites stimulate motility of the dog small intestine. J Pharmacol Exp Ther 227:499, 1983.
128. Rees WDW, Gibbons LC, Turnberg LA: Influence of opiates on alkali secretion by amphibian gastric and duodenal mucosa in vitro. Gastroenterology 90:323, 1986.
129. Flemstrom G, Jedstedt G, Nylander O: β-endorphin and enkephalins stimulate duodenal mucosal alkaline secretion in the rat in vivo. Gastroenterology 90:368, 1986.
130. Konturek SJ, Tasler J, Cieszkowski M, et al: Opiate peptides and gastrointestinal functions in the dog, in Miyoshi A (ed): *Gut Peptides. Secretion, Function and Clinical Aspects.* Tokyo: Kodansha Ltd; New York Elsevier North-Holland Biomedical Press, 1979, pp 293–302.
131. Cai W, Gu J, Huang W, et al: Peptide immunoreactive nerves and cells of the guinea pig gall bladder and biliary pathways. Gut 24:1186, 1983.
132. Behar J, Biancani P: Effect of naloxone on the cat sphincter of Oddi (SO): Evidence for a physiological role of opioid peptides in the regulation of the sphincter of Oddi, in Wienbeck M (ed): *Motility of the Digestive Tract.* New York, Raven Press, 1982, pp 397–403.
133. Worobetz LJ, Baker RJ, McCallum JA, et al: The effect of naloxone, morphine, and an enkephalin analogue on cholecystokinin octapeptide-stimulated gallbladder emptying. Am J Gastroenterol 77:509, 1982.
134. Crochelt RF, Shaw E, Peikin SR: Enkephalins mediate cholecystokinin induced gallbladder contraction in the guinea pig. Gastroenterology 84:1403, 1983.

Chapter 28

Miscellaneous Peptides

George H. Greeley, Jr., Ph.D.

Several peptides whose locus is not primarily in the gut act to influence gut function. We have grouped here a few such peptides.

THYROTROPIN-RELEASING HORMONE (TRH)

TRH (pGlu-His-Pro-NH_2) was the first hypophysiotropic peptide to be isolated from ovine and porcine hypothalamic extracts. TRH is a tripeptide that causes release and synthesis of an anterior pituitary hormone, thyrotropin (TSH) [1–5]. More recently, mammalian TRH has been shown to result from post-translational processing of a larger precursor protein that contained five copies of TRH [6]. TRH immunoreactivity has also been found in the gut, with the greatest amount in the pancreas of numerous mammals [7–11]. The primary site of TRH in the pancreas appears to be the islets of Langerhans [8,12]. It is not clear whether TRH is localized within the islet or is strictly found in nerves that innervate the islets [8,12]. Serotonin can stimulate TRH release from the pancreas, whereas carbachol inhibits it [13].

Several radioimmunoassays have been developed for TRH [14–17]. According to one report, the plasma half-life of TRH in the normal rat is 3 min, the metabolic clearance rate is 2.02 mL/min, and the renal clearance rate is 2.53 mL/min [18].

TRH appears to affect pancreatic endocrine secretion [19,20] and may act as a fine-tuning regulator for the release of pancreatic glucagon. TRH, in an isolated perfused rat pancreas, did not influence insulin or glucagon release; however, it enhanced arginine-induced glucagon release.

In humans, TRH inhibits both basal and pentagastrin-stimulated gastric acid secretion, and in some cases it inhibits pepsin release in a dose-dependent manner [12,21,22]. TRH is as potent as a standard dose of cimetidine in patients with gastric acid hypersecretion (Zollinger-Ellison syndrome, systemic mastocytosis) [23]. The inhibitory action of TRH on gastric output appears to be independent of gastrin release [23,24]. Konturek et al [24] showed that IV TRH inhibits gastric secretion induced by pentagastrin or by liver extract. In contrast, Tache et al showed that TRH, given intracisternally, actually stimulated gastric acid secretion in a vagally dependent manner [25]. Her group was unable to show any effect of systemic (IV) TRH on gastric secretion in rats [25]. She has recently reported that gastric acid secretion induced by intracisternal TRH is not related to release of gastrin or TSH [26]. TRH apparently activates efferent vagal circuits that stimulate parietal cell secretion [26].

TRH also decreases the pancreatic exocrine response to secretin, caerulein, a meat meal, or duodenal acidification [24]. IV TRH may release somatostatin in the gastric mucosa to act locally to inhibit gastric acid secretion [27]. TRH may cause release of gastric somatostatin, since TRH and somatostatin appear to reciprocally regulate each other's secretion in the hypothalamus [28]. In addition, TRH may inhibit the action of enteric enkephalins, since it has some enkephalin antagonistic properties [29]. Enkephalins can increase gastric secretion in dogs [30].

With regard to gastric motility, TRH can inhibit gastric motor activity and exhibit a relaxing action on the gastric wall [31,32]. In the rat and the dog, TRH can stimulate antral motility [33,34]. In rabbits, intracerebroventricular (ICV) administration of TRH leads to stimulation of colonic and duodenal motility, whereas systemic TRH is ineffective [35]. TRH apparently can inhibit pancreatic enzyme secretion [24]. It can cause a relaxation effect on the isolated rat duodenum in vitro [34], an effect not influenced by tetrodotoxin, phenoxybenzamine, or propranolol.

ICV administration of TRH can result in a dose-dependent elevation of basal gastric acid secretion; activation of the central dopamine receptor appears to inhibit this TRH-induced gastric secretion in rats [36]. In dogs, the central inhibitory effect of TRH or gastric acid secretion appears to be mediated via the vagus nerve [37].

We should note that TRH, given intravenously in humans, is accompanied by ill-defined subjective gastrointestinal symptoms, such as nausea, vomiting, hunger, and others [38]. These effects of IV TRH may reflect a direct action of TRH on smooth muscle [38] as well as a central neural action [35]. Even more important, this is an example in which a brain-gut peptide participates both peripherally and centrally in the regulation of the gut.

GROWTH HORMONE-RELEASING FACTOR (GHRF)

GHRF was recently isolated and characterized as 44-, 40-, and 37-residue peptides from two human pancreatic tumors in patients with acromegaly [39–43]. Their primary structures are identical from their amino terminal. GHRF is structurally similar to the family of peptides embracing secretin-glucagon-vasoactive intestinal peptide (VIP), peptide histidine leucine (PHI), and gastric inhibitory polypeptide (GIP). It has been shown to bind to VIP receptors in human and rat intestinal membranes [44]; however, the high concentration of GHRF needed to stimulate adenylate cyclase through VIP receptors (10^{-8}–10^{-5} M) suggests that GHRF does not act physiologically via VIP receptors. We have recently shown that GHRF (500 pmol/kg-h) augmented both pancreatic bicarbonate and protein output, stimulated by intraduodenal infusions of both HCl and amino acids (44a).

GHRF has been found in pancreatic endocrine tumors, appendiceal carcinoids, and a cecal carcinoid [45]. In addition, a gastrin-producing metastatic islet cell carcinoma removed from an acromegalic patient with Zollinger-Ellison syndrome [46] has been shown to contain GHRF as well as gastrin-releasing peptide and gastrin. One study reports that the greatest concentration of GHRF in humans occurs in the jejunum (2.2 ± 0.64 pmol/g), with smaller amounts in the duodenum and stomach [47]. GHRF was not detected in the ileum or colon. A wide variety of gut and pancreatic tumors also contain GHRF [47].

Structure of GHRF

GHRF-44:

Tyr-Ala-Asp-Ala-Ile-Phe-Asn-Ser-Tyr-Arg-Lys-
Val-Leu-Gly-Gln-Leu-Ser-Ala-Arg-Lys-Leu-Leu-
Gln-Asp-Ile-Met-Ser-Arg-Gln-Gln-Gly-Glu-Ser-
Asn-Gln-Glu-Arg-Gly-Ala-Arg-Ala-Arg-Leu-NH_2

Bosman et al [48] indicate that GHRF is found in the human antrum and in human and rat pancreatic islets. GHRF appears to be colocalized with gastrin in the G cells and with pancreatic polypeptide (PP) in islets.

CORTICOTROPIN-RELEASING FACTOR, SAUVAGINE, AND UROTENSIN I

Corticotropin-releasing factor (CRF) sauvagine, and urotensin are structurally similar peptides (see below). Ovine CRF is a 41 amino acid peptide recently isolated and characterized from the sheep hypothalamus [49–51]. CRF of other species has been isolated and characterized as well [52]. As expected, CRF is a strong stimulant of pituitary ACTH and β-endorphin release [49–51]. Sauvagine is a 40 amino acid peptide isolated and characterized from the skin of the frog [53]. Urotensin I is a neuropeptide isolated from the urophysis of the teleost fish (*Catostomus commersoni*) [54,55].

As expected, CRF has been localized in the CNS [56–60]. In addition, CRF has been found dispersed throughout all the pancreatic islets of primates and cats [61] and in the liver, stomach, duodenum, and pancreas of humans and rats [60,62] as well as in other extragastrointestinal sites. In the rat and mouse, CRF-containing cells are primarily found in the periphery of the islets, mimicking the localization of glucagon, somatostatin, and PP-containing cells [61]. In the chicken and catfish, CRF cells are found centrally within the islets. CRF-containing cells appear to be related to glucagon-containing cells, but their exact identity is unclear. CRF has also been demonstrated in the pancreas of fish, amphibians, reptiles, and birds, and, based on their distribution and morphologic appearance, the CRF-containing cells appear to be similar to the glucagon-containing cells [63]. CRF-containing cells are also seen scattered in the exocrine pancreas of all species studied so far [61]. Since CRF possesses mesenteric vasomotor properties [54,64], pancreatic CRF may have a paracrine role in the regulation of blood flow through the pancreas. CRF cells have also been localized in the gastric antrum and small intestine of human specimens [65].

Similar to CRF and sauvagine, urotensin is a strong stimulant of ACTH release [55]. In mammals, urotensin, CRF, and sauvagine have a specific vasodilatory, hypotensive action on the superior mesenteric vascular bed [54,64,66–69].

Urotensin and sauvagine appear to be 5 to 10 times more potent than CRF [64].

Radioimmunoassays for CRF have been developed [70,71] and CRF levels have been measured in tissue, cerebrospinal fluid, and in plasma [72,73]. The plasma half-life of CRF is apparently longer than that of other small peptides, and its metabolic clearance rate (MCR) is exceptionally low [74]. According to one report, plasma half-lives of CRF are 17.1 ± 2.44 for the short phase and 198 ± 5.3 min for the long phases. The MCR is 0.44 ± 0.06 L/kg/d (pulse injection technique), and the volume of distribution is 213.5 ± 12 mL. The MCR, using the continuous infusion technique, is 2.23 to 5.08 L/kg/d.

Intracerebroventricular (ICV) and subcutaneous (SC) injections of sauvagine (ICV: 0.5, 2.5, and 5 μg/kg; SC: 2.5 and 5 μg/kg) have been shown to decrease gastric emptying in rats [75]. CRF, given intravenously, inhibits gastric emptying in dogs by a mechanism that is independent of opiates [76]. Naloxone alone does not interfere with the inhibitory action of sauvagine on gastric emptying, suggesting that opioid mechanisms do not participate. Tache et al [77] have shown that systemic CRF (IV) inhibits gastric acid secretion in rats and dogs. The inhibitory action of CRF is dose-dependent, persistent, and reversible. Adrenalectomy, hypophysectomy, naloxone pretreatment, or indomethacin pretreatment does not influence CRF action. However, vagotomy partially blocks the action of CRF. Todisco [78] has also shown that the inhibitory action of CRF is not mediated by a direct action on parietal cells or via release of gastric somatostatin or gastrin. Konturek et al [79] have shown that IV CRF (50–200 pmol/kg) inhibited pentagastrin and meal-induced acid from both the vagally denervated and intact stomachs in dogs. CRF also increased gastrin levels. CRF inhibits gastric emptying in dogs [80]. This effect is only one fourth as potent as that of CCK-8, but it does inhibit emptying by 29–52 percent; the mechanism of inhibition is unrelated to opiates. CRF also had mild effects on pancreatic exocrine secretion [79].

ICV administration of CRF results in an elevation in arterial pressure and heart rate [81], which is inhibited by chlorisondamine (ganglionic blocker). Hence, in addition to the action of CRF on ACTH and on β-endorphin release from the pituitary, it acts within the CNS to stimulate sympathetic nervous activity. Tache et al [82] have shown that CRF, given intracisternally, inhibits gastric acid secretion via vagal and adrenal mechanisms in rats. Gunion et al [83] have also shown that administration of CRF into the rat hypothalamus elevates the concentration and output of gastric bicarbonate under normal or achlorhydric conditions.

CRF, given intravenously to normal humans, results in an elevation of PP; however, alterations in the circulating levels of insulin, glucagon, gastrin, somatostatin, motilin, neurotensin, GIP, or CCK were not observed [84]. Peptide histidine isoleucine can potentiate the ACTH-releasing action of CRF in isolated pituitary fragments [85]. Moltz and Fawcett [86] have shown that CRF causes a rapid, dose-dependent inhibition of insulin release, whereas Torres-Aleman [87] reported that CRF resulted in a stimulation of insulin secretion.

Structures of CRF, Sauvagine, and Urotensin I

Homologous residues are underlined (____) and (_ _ _).

CRF:

H-Ser-Gln-Glu-Pro-Pro-Ile-Ser-Leu-Asp-Leu-Thr-Phe-His-Leu-Leu-Arg-Glu-Val-Leu-Glu-Met-Thr-Lys-Ala-Asp-Gln-Leu-Ala-Gln-Gln-Ala-His-Ser-Asn-Arg-Lys-Leu-Leu-Asp-Ile-Ala-NH_2

Sauvagine:

Pyr-Gly-Pro-Pro-Ile-Ser-Ile-Asp-Leu-Ser-Leu-Glu-Leu-Leu-Arg-Lys-Met-Ile-Glu-Ile-Glu-Lys-Gln-Glu-Lys-Glu-Lys-Gln-Gln-Ala-Ala-Asn-Asn-Arg-Leu-Leu-Leu-Asp-Thr-Ile-NH_2

Urotensin I:

H-Asn-Asp-Asp-Pro-Pro-Ile-Ser-Ile-Asp-Leu-Thr-Phe-His-Leu-Leu-Arg-Asn-Met-Ile-Glu-Met-Ala-Arg-Ile-Glu-Asn-Glu-Arg-Glu-Gln-Ala-Gly-Leu-Asn-Arg-Lys-Tyr-Leu-Asp-Glu-Val-NH_2

GALANIN

Galanin is a 29 amino acid peptide that was isolated from porcine upper small bowel by Tatemoto et al [88]. It was named galanin because it had an N-terminal glycine and a C-terminal alanine amide (see structure below). Galanin-containing nerve fibers are seen in the mucosa, smooth muscle, and intramural ganglia and surrounding blood vessels of the gastrointestinal tract [89,90]. Galanin can stimulate contraction of rat stomach, ileum, colon, and urinary bladder muscle strips [89], as well as a potent contractile response in rat jejunal longitudinal muscle preparations [91]. Given intravenously, it can cause a dose-dependent hyperglycemia that appears due to a reversible suppression of release of insulin [92].

Structure of Galanin

Galanin:

Gly-Trp-Thr-Leu-Asn-Ser-Ala-Gly-Tyr-Leu-Leu-Gly-Pro-His-Ala-Ile-Asp-Asn-His-Arg-Ser-Phe-His-Asp-Lys-Tyr-Gly-Leu-Ala-NH_2

REFERENCES

1. Schally AV, Bowers CY, Redding TW, et al: Isolation of thyrotropin releasing factor (TRF) from porcine hypothalamus. Biochem Biophys Res Commun 25:165, 1966.
2. Bøler J, Enzmann F, Folkers K, et al: The identity of chemical and hormonal properties of the thyrotropin releasing hormone and pyroglutamyl-histidyl-proline amide. Biochem Biophys Res Commun 37:705, 1969.
3. Schally AV, Redding TW, Bowers CY, et al: Isolation and properties of porcine thyrotropin-releasing hormone. J Biol Chem 244:4077, 1969.
4. Burgus R, Dunn TF, Desiderio D, et al: Characterization of ovine hypothalamic hypophysiotropic TSH-releasing factor. Nature 226:321, 1970.
5. Nair RMG, Barrett JF, Bowers CY, et al: Structure of porcine thyrotropin releasing hormone. Biochemistry 9:1103, 1970.
6. Lechan RM, Wu P, Jackson IMD, et al: Thyrotropin-releasing hormone precursor: Characterization in rat brain. Science 231:159, 1986.
7. Morley JE, Garvin TJ, Pekary AE, et al: Thyrotropin-releasing hormone in the gastrointestinal tract. Biochem Biophys Res Commun 79:314, 1977.
8. Martino E, Lernmark A, Seo H, et al: High concentration of thyrotropin-releasing hormone in pancreatic islets. Proc Natl Acad Sci 75:4265, 1978.
9. Leppaluoto J, Koivusalo F, Kraama R: Thyrotropin-releasing factor: Distribution in neural and gastrointestinal tissues. Acta Physiol Scand 104:175, 1978.
10. Koivusalo F, Leppaluoto J: High TRF immunoreactivity in purified pancreatic extracts of fetal and newborn rats. Life Sci 24:1655, 1979.
11. Koivusalo F: Evidence of thyrotropin-releasing hormone activity in autopsy pancreata from newborns. J Clin Endocrinol Metab 53:734, 1981.
12. Dolva LØ, Hanssen KF: Thyrotropin-releasing hormone: Distribution and actions in the gastrointestinal tract. Scand J Gastroenterol 17:705, 1982.
13. Lamberton P, Wu P, Jackson IMD: Thyrotropin-releasing hormone release from rat pancreas is stimulated by serotonin but inhibited by carbachol. Endocrinology 117:1834, 1985.
14. Bassiri RM, Utiger RD: The preparation and specificity of antibody to thyrotropin releasing hormone. Endocrinology 90:722, 1972.
15. Koch Y, Baram T: Generation of specific antiserum to thyrotropin releasing-hormone and its use in a radioimmunoassay. FEBS Lett 63:295, 1976.
16. Jackson IMD, Reichlin S: Thyrotropin-releasing hormone (TRH): Distribution in hypothalamic and extrahypothalamic brain tissues of mammalian and submammalian chordates. Endocrinology 95:854, 1974.
17. Kizer JS, Palkovits M, Tappaz M, et al: Distribution of releasing factors, biogenic amines, and related enzymes in the bovine median eminence. Endocrinology 98:685, 1976.
18. Jackson IMD, Papapetrou PD, Reichlin S: Metabolic clearance of thyrotropin-releasing hormone in the rat in hypothyroid and hyperthyroid states: Comparison with serum degradation *in vitro*. Endocrinology 104:1292, 1979.
19. Dolva O, Hanssen KF, Frey HMM: Actions of thyrotropin-releasing-hormone on gastrointestinal function in man. I. Inhibition of glucose and xylose absorption from the gut. Scand J Gastroenterol 13:599, 1978.
20. Morley JE, Levin SR, Pehlevanian M, et al: The effects of thyrotropin-releasing hormone on the endocrine pancreas. Endocrinology 104:137, 1979.
21. Dolva LØ, Hanssen KF, Flaten O, et al: Effect of thyrotropin-releasing hormone on gastric acid secretion in man. Scand J Gastroenterol 17:775, 1982.
22. Dolva LØ, Hanssen KF, Berstad A, et al: Thyrotrophin-releasing hormone inhibits the pentagastrin stimulated gastric secretion in man. A dose response study. Clin Endocrinol 10:281, 1979.
23. Hutton SW, Morley JE, Parent MK, et al: Thyrotropin-releasing hormone suppressed gastric acid output in patients with Zollinger-Ellison syndrome and systemic mastocytosis. Am J Med 71:957, 1981.
24. Konturek SJ, Jaworek J, Cieszkowski M, et al: Effect of thyrotropin-releasing hormone on gastro-intestinal secretions in dogs. Life Sci 29:2289, 1981.
25. Tache Y, Vale W, Brown M: Thyrotropin-releasing hormone—CNS action to stimulate gastric acid secretion. Nature 287:149, 1980.
26. Tache Y, Goto Y, Hamel D, et al: Mechanisms underlying intracisternal TRH-induced stimulation of gastric acid secretion in rats. Regul Pept 13:21, 1985.
27. Khardori R, Khardori N: Mechanism of gastric acid secretion by thyrotropin-releasing hormone. Am J Med 74:988, 1983.
28. Hollander CS, Greene LW, Rosman L, et al: Reciprocal local feedback of somatostatin (SRIF) and thyrotropin releasing hormone (TRH) in dispersed cell culture of rat hypothalamus. Clin Res 28:479A, 1980.
29. Holaday JW, D'Amato RJ, Faden AI: Thyrotropin-releasing hormone improves cardiovascular function in experimental endotoxic and hemorrhagic shock. Science 213:216, 1981.
30. Konturek SJ, Tasler J, Cieszkowski M, et al: Comparison of methionine-enkephalin and morphine in the stimulation of gastric acid secretion in the dog. Gastroenterology 78:294, 1980.
31. Dolva LØ, Stadaas JO: Actions of thyrotropin-releasing hormone on gastrointestinal functions in man. III. Inhibition of gastric motility in response to distension. Scand J Gastroenterol 14:419, 1979.

32. Dolva LØ, Stadaas J, Hanssen KF: Effect of thyrotropin-releasing hormone and atropine on the gastric motility stimulated by insulin-induced hypoglycemia. Scand J Gastroenterol 17:769, 1982.
33. Morley JE, Steinbach JH, Feldman EJ, et al: The effects of thyrotropin releasing hormone (TRH) on the gastrointestinal tract. Life Sci 24:1059, 1979.
34. Tonoue T, Furukawa K, Nomoto T: The direct influence of thyrotropin-releasing hormone (TRH) on the smooth muscle of rat duodenum. Life Sci 25:2011, 1979.
35. Smith JR, La Hann TR, Chesnut RM, et al: Thyrotropin-releasing hormone: Stimulation of colonic activity following intracerebroventricular administration. Science 196:660, 1977.
36. Maeda-Hagiwara M, Watanabe K: Influence of dopamine receptor agonists on gastric acid secretion induced by intraventricular administration of thyrotropin-releasing hormone in the perfused stomach of anaesthetized rats. Br J Pharmacol 79:297, 1983.
37. Soldani G, Del Tacca M, Martino E, et al: The involvement of the vagal pathway in the antisecretory effect of thyrotropin-releasing hormone on gastric secretion in the dog. J Pharm Pharmacol 35:119, 1983.
38. Almqvist S: Clinical side effects of TRH. Front Horm Res 1:38, 1972.
39. Rivier J, Spiess J, Thorner M, et al: Characterization of a growth hormone-releasing factor from a human pancreatic islet tumour. Nature 300:276, 1982.
40. Thorner MO, Perryman RL, Cronin MJ, et al: Somatotroph hyperplasia. Successful treatment of acromegaly by removal of a pancreatic islet tumor secreting a growth hormone-releasing factor. J Clin Invest 70:965, 1982.
41. Esch FS, Bohlen P, Ling NC, et al: Characterization of a 40 residue peptide from a human pancreatic tumor with growth hormone releasing activity. Biochem Biophys Res Commun 109:152, 1982.
42. Guillemin R, Brazeau P, Bohlen P, et al: Growth hormone-releasing factor from a human pancreatic tumor that caused acromegaly. Science 218:585, 1982.
43. Esch FS, Bohlen P, Ling NC, et al: Primary structures of three human pancreas peptides with growth hormone-releasing activity. J Biol Chem 258:1806, 1983.
44. Laburthe M, Amiranoff B, Boige N, et al: Interaction of GRF with VIP receptors and stimulation of adenylate cyclase in rat and human intestinal epithelial membranes. Comparison with PHI and secretin. FEBS Lett 159:89, 1983.
44a. Nealon WH, Beauchamp RD, Greeley GH Jr, et al: Growth hormone releasing factor augments meal-stimulated pancreatic secretion in the dog. Can J Physiol Pharmacol 64 (Suppl July 1986):168, 1986.
45. Bostwick DG, Quan R, Hoffman AR, et al: Growth-hormone-releasing factor immunoreactivity in human endocrine tumors. Am J Pathol 117:167, 1984.
46. Wilson DM, Ceda GP, Bostwick DG, et al: Acromegaly and Zollinger-Ellison syndrome secondary to an islet cell tumor: Characterization and quantification of plasma and tumor human growth hormone-releasing factor. J Clin Endocrinol Metab 59:1002, 1984.
47. Christofides ND, Stephanou A, Suzuki H, et al: Distribution of immunoreactive growth hormone-releasing hormone in the human brain and intestine and its production by tumors. J Clin Endocrinol Metab 59:747, 1984.
48. Bosman FT, van Assche C, Nieuwenhuyzen Kruseman AC, et al: Growth hormone releasing factor (GRF) immunoreactivity in human and rat gastrointestinal tract and pancreas. J Histochem Cytochem 32:1139, 1984.
49. Spiess J, Rivier J, Rivier C, et al: Primary structure of corticotropin-releasing factor from ovine hypothalamus. Proc Natl Acad Sci USA 78:6517, 1981.
50. Vale W, Spiess J, Rivier C, et al: Characterization of a 41-residue ovine hypothalamic peptide that stimulates secretion of corticotropin and β-endorphin. Science 213:1394, 1981.
51. Rivier C, Brownstein M, Spiess J, et al: *In vivo* corticotropin-releasing factor-induced secretion of adrenocorticotropin, β-endorphin, and corticosterone. Endocrinology 110:272, 1982.
52. Ling N, Esch F, Bohlen P, et al: Isolation and characterization of caprine corticotropin-releasing factor. Biochem Biophys Res Commun 122:1218, 1984.
53. Montecucchi PC, Henschen A, Erspamer V: Structure of sauvagine, a vasoactive peptide from the skin of a frog. Hoppe Seylers Z Physiol Chem 36:1178, 1979.
54. MacCannell KL, Lederis K: Mammalian pharmacology of the fish neuropeptide urotensin I. Fed Proc 42:91, 1983.
55. Lederis K, Letter A, McMaster D, et al: Complete amino acid sequence of urotensin I, a hypotensive and corticotropin-releasing neuropeptide from *Catostomus*. Science 218:162, 1982.
56. Merchenthaler I, Vigh S, Petrusz P, et al: Immunocytochemical localization of corticotropin-releasing factor (CRF) in the rat brain. Am J Anat 165:385, 1982.
57. Burlet A, Tonon M-C, Tankosic P, et al: Comparative immunocytochemical localization of corticotropin releasing factor (CRF-41) and neurohypophysial peptides in the brain of Brattleboro and Long-Evans rats. Neuroendocrinology 37:64, 1983.
58. Antoni FA, Palkovits M, Makara GB, et al: Immunoreactive corticotropin-releasing hormone in the hypothalamoinfundibular tract. Neuroendocrinology 36:415, 1983.
59. Cummings S, Elde R, Ells J, et al: Corticotropin-releasing factor immunoreactivity is widely distributed within the central nervous system of the rat: An immunohistochemical study. J Neurosci 3:1355, 1983.
60. Suda T, Tomori N, Tozawa F, et al: Distribution and characterization of immunoreactive corticotropin-

releasing factor in human tissues. J Clin Endocrinol Metab 55:861, 1984.

61. Petrusz P, Merchenthaler I, Maderdrut JL, et al: Corticotropin-releasing factor (CRF)-like immunoreactivity in the vertebrate endocrine pancreas. Proc Natl Acad Sci USA 80:1721, 1983.
62. Wolter HJ: Corticotropin-releasing factor is contained within perikarya and nerve fibres of rat duodenum. Biochem Biophys Res Commun 122:381, 1984.
63. Petrusz P, Merchenthaler I, Ordronneau P, et al: Corticotropin-releasing factor (CRF)-like immunoreactivity in the gastro-entero-pancreatic endocrine system. Peptides 5(Suppl 1):71, 1984.
64. MacCannell KL, Lederis K, Hamilton PL, et al: Amunine (ovine CRF), urotensin I and sauvagine, three structurally-related peptides, produce selective dilation of the mesenteric circulation. Pharmacology 25:116, 1982.
65. Nieuwenhuijzen Kruseman AC, Linton EA, Rees LH, et al: Corticotropin-releasing factor immunoreactivity in human gastrointestinal tract. Lancet 2:1245, 1982.
66. Melchiorri P, Negri L: Action of sauvagine on the mesenteric vascular bed of the dog. Regul Pept 2:1, 1981.
67. Brown MR, Fisher LA, Spiess J, et al: Comparison of the biologic actions of corticotropin-releasing factor and sauvagine. Regul Pept 4:107, 1982.
68. MacCannell K, Giraud G, Lederis K, et al: Use of a specific mesenteric vasodilator peptide, urotensin I, to reduce afterload in the dog. Can J Physiol Pharmacol 58:1412, 1980.
69. MacCannell K, Lederis K: Dilatation of the mesenteric vascular bed of the dog produced by a peptide, urotensin I. J Pharmacol Exp Ther 203:38, 1977.
70. Suda T, Tomori N, Tozawa F, et al: Effects of bilateral adrenalectomy on immunoreactive corticotropin-releasing factor in the rat median eminence and intermediate-posterior pituitary. Endocrinology 113:1182, 1983.
71. Vale W, Vaughan J, Yamamoto G, et al: Assay of corticotropin releasing factor. Methods Enzymol 103:565, 1983.
72. Nemeroff CB, Widerlov E, Bissette G, et al: Elevated concentrations of CSF corticotropin-releasing factor-like immunoreactivity in depressed patients. Science 226:1342, 1984.
73. Suda T, Tomori N, Yajima F, et al: Immunoreactive corticotropin-releasing factor in human plasma. J Clin Invest 76:2026, 1985.
74. Schulte HM, Chrousos GP, Gold PW, et al: Metabolic clearance rate and plasma half-life of radioiodinated corticotropin releasing factor in a primate. J Clin Endocrinol Metab 55:1023, 1982.
75. Broccardo M, Improta G, Melchiorri P: Effect of sauvagine on gastric emptying in conscious rats. Eur J Pharmacol 85:111, 1982.
76. Pappas T, Debas H, Tache Y: Corticotropin-releasing factor inhibits gastric emptying in dogs. Regul Pept 11:193, 1985.
77. Tache T, Goto Y, Gunion M, et al: Inhibition of gastric acid secretion in rats and in dogs by corticotropin-releasing factor. Gastroenterology 86:281, 1984.
78. Todisco A: Inhibition of gastric acid secretion by corticotropin releasing factor (CRF) is not mediated by direct action on parietal cells or by regulation of gastric somatostatin and gastrin. Gastroenterology 88:1719, 1985.
79. Konturek SJ, Pawlik W, Thor PJ, et al: Effects of corticotropin releasing factor (CRF) on gastrointestinal secretion, motility and circulation in dogs. Gastroenterology 88:1453, 1985.
80. Pappas T, Debas H, Tache Y: Corticotropin-releasing factor inhibits gastric emptying in dogs. Regul Pept 11:193, 1985.
81. Fisher LA, Rivier J, Rivier C, et al: Corticotropin-releasing factor (CRF): Central effects on mean arterial pressure and heart rate in rats. Endocrinology 110:2222, 1982.
82. Tache Y, Goto Y, Gunion MW, et al: Inhibition of gastric acid secretion in rats by intracerebral injection of corticotropin-releasing factor. Science 222:935, 1983.
83. Gunion MW, Tache Y, Kauffman GL: Intrahypothalamic corticotropin-releasing factor (CRF) increases gastric bicarbonate content. Gastroenterology 88:1407, 1985.
84. Lytras N, Grossman A, Rees LH, et al: Corticotrophin releasing factor: Effects on circulating gut and pancreatic peptides in man. Clin Endocrinol 20:725, 1984.
85. Tilders F, Tatemoto K, Berkenbosch F: The intestinal peptide PHI-27 potentiates the action of corticotropin-releasing factor on ACTH release from rat pituitary fragments in vitro. Endocrinology 115:1633, 1984.
86. Moltz JH, Fawcett CP: Corticotropin-releasing factor inhibits insulin release from perfused rat pancreas. Am J Physiol 248:E741, 1985.
87. Torres-Aleman I, Mason-Garcia M, Schally AV: Stimulation of insulin secretion by corticotropin-releasing factor (CRF) in anesthetized rats. Peptides 5:541, 1984.
88. Tatemoto K, Rokaeus A, Jornvall H, et al: Galanin—a novel biologically active peptide from porcine intestine. FEBS Lett 164:124, 1983.
89. Rokaeus A, Melander T, Hokfelt T, et al: A galanin-like peptide in the central nervous system and intestine of the rat. Neurosci Lett 47:161, 1984.
90. Ekblad E, Rokaeus A, Håkanson R, et al: Galanin nerve fibers in the rat gut: Distribution, origin and projections. Neuroscience 16:355, 1985.
91. Ekblad E, Håkanson R, Sundler F, et al: Galanin: Neuromodulatory and direct contractile effects on smooth muscle preparations. Br J Pharmacol 86:241, 1985.
92. McDonald TJ, Dupre J, Tatemoto K, et al: Galanin inhibits insulin secretion and induces hyperglycemia in dogs. Diabetes 34:192, 1985.

Section Seven

Nonpeptide Agents

We have placed in this section nonpeptide compounds that influence gut function by endocrine and paracrine actions. Included are two vasoactive amines (histamine and serotonin) and the prostaglandin family of 20-carbon-atom fats.

Chapter 29

Histamine

Laszlo Mate, M.D., Donald G. MacLellan, M.D., and James C. Thompson, M.D.

HISTORY

In 1910, Dale and Laidlaw [1] examined the effect of a new chemical substance, imidazolylethylamine (histamine), on various pharmacologic models. They drew attention to the finding that the pharmacologic action of histamine was similar to the symptom complex seen in an animal that had received injections of protein to which it had been sensitized. They thus anticipated the discovery of the important role of histamine in allergic reactions and anaphylaxis. Popielski [2], in 1920, reported that histamine was a powerful stimulant of gastric acid secretion.

There are two types of histamine receptors. Those effects that can be abolished by the traditional antihistamine agents (for example, the classic symptoms associated with allergic reactions) are mediated through H_1 receptors [3]. A second type of histamine receptor, the H_2 receptor, was described in 1972 by Black et al [4] in studies that used the selective H_2 antagonist, burimamide. H_2 receptors can be found in gastric mucosa, in the rat uterus, and in the guinea pig atrium. Smooth muscle tissues in the ileum and bronchi are unaffected by H_2 antagonists, indicating that they have H_1 receptors [4]. In the cardiovascular system, the effects of histamine appear to be mediated by both types of receptors [5]. Several specific types of H_1 and H_2 receptor antagonists are now commercially available (for example, diphenhydramine and pyrilamine selectively block H_1 receptors, and cimetidine, ranitidine, and famotidine selectively block H_2 receptors [6]).

DISTRIBUTION

Histamine is stored and synthesized mainly in tissue mast cells and in circulating basophils. In the gastrointestinal tract of the rat, histamine is stored in enterochromaffin-like cells [7]. In rabbits and pigs uniquely, blood platelets have the capacity to synthesize, store, and take up histamine from the circulation [8,9]. Gastric histamine is found in mast cells [10], which may differ from nongastric mast cells in that they appear not to release histamine after administration of compound 48/80 [11]. Histamine has been found to be present throughout the length of the gut, with the greatest concentration in the acid-secreting gastric mucosa [12–14].

ASSAY

The first assay for histamine was developed using atropinized guinea pig ileum. Although this bioassay is still in use on occasion, newer methods are now available that are more accurate and that avoid the pitfalls of bioassays, for example, fluorometry [15,16] and enzymatic isotope assay [17,18], thin layer chromatography [19], gas-liquid chromatography [20], and cation [21] and ion exchange chromatography [22]. The enzymatic isotope assay is widely used because of its relative simplicity and its accuracy. Histamine can also be measured by high speed liquid chromatography [23] and by gas chromatography-mass spectrometry [24].

CATABOLISM

Histamine is catabolized either by diamine oxidase or by histamine methyltransferase. The main catabolites are *N*-methylimidazole acetic acid and *N*-methylhistamine, which are excreted in the urine [25].

RELEASE

Histamine is released from the stomach after a meal, especially after the ingestion of meat [26]. Gastrin has been shown to release histamine from the rat stomach [27], and vagotomy blocks histamine release.

ACTIONS

The major physiologic role for histamine in the gastrointestinal tract is its participation in the regulation of gastric secretion. This effect is mostly mediated by H_2 receptors, although there may also be an H_1 component [28].

In 1920, the gastric secretagogue effect of histamine was established by Popielski [2], who suggested that histamine was the final common mediator of gastric acid secretion, through which all other secretagogues acted. Ekblad [29] still supports this hypothesis. On the other hand, Soll [30] has provided evidence that parietal cells have separate receptors for acetylcholine, gastrin, and histamine. Soll has also shown potentiation between gastrin and histamine and acetylcholine and histamine, but little between gastrin and acetylcholine (Fig 29-1) [30,31]. The synergism between gastrin and histamine has been confirmed in vivo [32]. Whether the responses of the isolated cells actually reflect the responses of their counterparts in intact mucosa remains a major consideration. Nevertheless, the primacy of histamine as an important initiator and component of the acid secretory system is well accepted.

Gastric secretion may be stimulated by the newly described although chemically not identified antral histamine [33]. Stimulation by antral histamine is expressed more in the denervated than in the innervated stomach, in contrast to gastrin stimulation, in which vagal innervation enhances the stimulatory action [33]. Vatier et al [34] proposed that antral histamine enhances gastric acid secretion by suppressing the inhibitory action of somatostatin. Somatostatin has an inhibitory effect on histamine-stimulated activity in the enriched parietal cell preparation, while gastrin stimulation is not affected [35].

Although some studies have shown pentagastrin infusion to cause release of histamine into the gastric lumen, the output of acid and levels of histamine release in these studies did not correlate, so that histamine appears to be an unlikely candidate

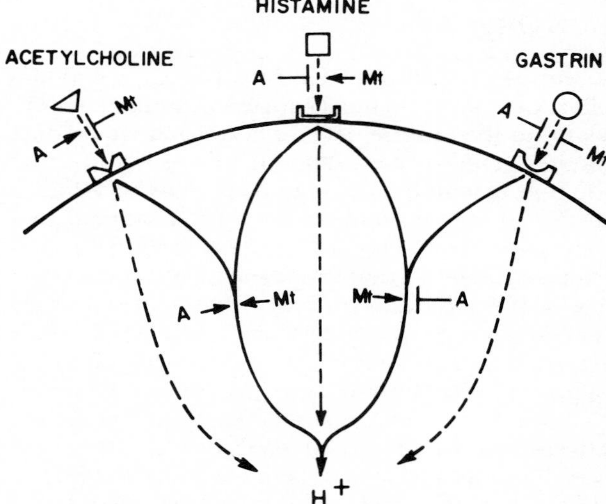

Figure 29-1. A working model for the actions and interactions of secretagogues on the isolated parietal cell. The dashed lines represent independent actions of secretagogues, and the solid lines represent interactions. Sites at which atropine (A) and metiamide (Mt) are respectively inhibitory (arrows) and at which these agents are not inhibitory (——) are indicated. (From Soll [31], by permission of the Rockefeller University Press.)

for the final mediator in gastrin-induced gastric secretion [36]. More recent studies failed to demonstrate histamine release by pentagastrin, either in vivo or in vitro [37]. Furthermore, histamine administration causes a reduction in gastrin release after bombesin stimulation [38].

Histamine, in the gastric mucosa, seems to act in a true paracrine manner. It is stored in close proximity to its target, the parietal cells. Parietal cells have high enzyme activity for the catabolism of histamine, which apparently prevents elevation of systemic histamine levels after stimulation of gastric secretion. In addition to stimulating acid secretion, histamine also increases output of pepsin in humans [39] and in dogs [40].

Histamine alone is capable of causing peptic ulceration in various animals [41]. Recently, a reproducible model of duodenal ulceration in rats was described using histamine and indomethacin [42]. In experimental stress ulcers, the histamine and serotonin content of the gastric mucosa decreases, which may suggest increased release [43].

Histamine increases gastric mucosal blood flow in dogs, while cimetidine decreases it [44]. On the other hand, the vasodilatation caused by histamine in the small intestine appears to be mediated by H_1 receptors, although the experimental results are species-dependent to a great extent [45].

Unlike acetylcholine, which stimulates both acid and alkaline secretion in the frog stomach (the latter secretion is mediated by cGMP), histamine has no effect on alkaline secretion. The intracellular mediator of histamine-induced gastric acid secretion is cAMP [46], which then activates type 1 cAMP-dependent protein kinase [47]. Whether this is the sole pathway for histamine-stimulated acid secretion is still controversial [48].

Both H_1 and H_2 receptors are present in the biliary tract. The dominant effect on the gallbladder, following histamine administration, is contraction, both in vivo and in vitro. This contraction can be inhibited by H_1 receptor antagonists, while H_2 antagonists enhance the histamine-induced contraction, indicating an inhibitory H_2 mechanism [49]. These results can be reproduced using selective H_1 and H_2 agonists [50]. Histamine decreases the activity of the sphincter of Oddi via H_1 receptors [51,52].

Histamine exerts a mainly stimulatory action on gastrointestinal motility, which is predominantly H_1-mediated [53]. Ileal motility is noncholinergic but can be prevented by tetrodotoxin and morphine, suggesting a neural pathway [54]. Histamine increases enzyme and bicarbonate output in the isolated pancreas from dogs [55] and rabbits [56].

REFERENCES

1. Dale HH, Laidlaw PP: The physiological action of β-imidazolyl-ethylamine. J Physiol (Lond) 41:318, 1910.
2. Popielski L: β-Imidazolylethylamin und die organextrakte. Pflugers Arch 178:214, 1920.
3. Ash ASF, Schild HO: Receptors mediating some actions of histamine. Br J Pharmacol 27:427, 1966.
4. Black JW, Duncan WAM, Durant CJ, et al: Definition and antagonism of histamine H_2-receptors. Nature 236:385, 1972.
5. Summers RJ, Kaliner M: Current concepts of histamine actions through H_1 and H_2 receptors. Compr Ther 8:6, 1982.
6. Douglas WW: Histamine and 5-hydroxytryptamine (serotonin) and their antagonists, in Gilman AG, Goodman LS, and Gilman A (eds): *The Pharmacological Basis of Therapeutics.* 6th Ed. New York, MacMillan Publishing Co, Inc, 1980, pp 609–646.
7. Aures D, Håkanson R: Amine formation in polypeptide-producing endocrine cells of the digestive tract. Eur J Pharmacol 3:316, 1968.
8. Almeida AP, Flye W, Deveraux D, et al: Distribution of histamine and histaminase (diamine oxidase) in blood of various species. Comp Biochem Physiol 67C:187, 1980.
9. Goth A: Histamine release. 1. On the general problem of the release of histamine. Handbook Exp Pharmacol 18:57, 1978.
10. Beaven MA, Soll AH, Lewin KJ: Histamine synthesis by intact mast cells from canine fundic mucosa and liver. Gastroenterology 82:254, 1982.
11. Soll AH, Lewin KJ, Beaven MA: Isolation of histamine-containing cells from rat gastric mucosa: Biochemical and morphologic differences from mast cells. Gastroenterology 80:717, 1981.
12. Douglas WW, Feldberg W, Paton WDM, et al: Distribution of histamine and substance P in the wall of the dog's digestive tract. J Physiol 115:163, 1951.
13. Feldberg W, Harris GW: Distribution of histamine in the mucosa of the gastro-intestinal tract of the dog. J Physiol 120:352, 1953.
14. Smith AN: The distribution and release of histamine in human gastric tissues. Clin Sci 18:533, 1959.
15. Shore PA, Burkhalter A, Cohn VH Jr: A method for the fluorometric assay of histamine in tissues. J Pharmacol Exp Ther 127:182, 1959.
16. Endo Y: Simple method for the simultaneous determination of histamine, polyamines and histone H1. J Chromatogr 205:155, 1981.
17. Snyder SH, Baldessarini RJ, Axelrod J: A sensitive and specific enzymatic isotopic assay for tissue histamine. J Pharmacol Exp Ther 153:544, 1966.
18. Beaven MA, Jacobsen S, Horakova Z: Modification of the enzymatic isotopic assay of histamine and its application to measurement of histamine in tissues, serum and urine. Clin Chim Acta 37:91, 1972.
19. Schwartzman RM: Quantitative thin-layer chromatography of histamine and its metabolites. J Chromatogr 86:263, 1973.
20. Navert H: New approach to the separation and iden-

tification of some methylated histamine derivatives by gas chromatography. J Chromatogr 106:218, 1975.
21. Mett CL, Sturgeon RJ: Cation-exchange chromatography of histamine in the presence of ethylammonium chloride. J Chromatogr 235:536, 1982.
22. Deelder RS, van den Berg JHM: Study on the retention of amines in reversed-phase ion-pair chromatography on bonded phases. J Chromatogr 218:327, 1981.
23. Tsuruta Y, Kohashi K, Ohkura Y: Determination of histamine in plasma by high-speed liquid chromatography. J Chromatogr 146:490, 1978.
24. Mita H, Yasueda H, Shida T: Simultaneous determination of histamine and N^T-methylhistamine in human plasma and urine by gas chromatography—mass spectrometry. J Chromatogr 221:1, 1980.
25. Schayer RW, Cooper JAD: Metabolism of C^{14} histamine in man. J Appl Physiol 9:481, 1956.
26. Irvine WT, Code CF: Gastric secretion and free histamine in urine. Am J Physiol 195:202, 1958.
27. Haverback BJ, Tecimer LB, Dyce BJ, et al: The effect of gastrin on stomach histamine in the rat. Life Sci 3:637, 1964.
28. Vinik AI, Heldsinger A, Skoglund ML: Evidence for both H_2 and H_1 histamine activation of oxyntic cells. Gastroenterology 80:1309, 1981.
29. Ekblad EBM: Histamine: The sole mediator of pentagastrin-stimulated acid secretion. Acta Physiol Scand 125:135, 1985.
30. Soll AH: The actions of secretagogues on oxygen uptake by isolated mammalian parietal cells. J Clin Invest 61:370, 1978.
31. Soll AH: The interaction of histamine with gastrin and carbamylcholine on oxygen uptake by isolated mammalian parietal cells. J Clin Invest 61:381, 1978.
32. Vatier J, Bonfils S: Role de l'histamine antrale et de la gastrine dans la secretion acide gastrique: Realites experimentales et hypotheses. Gastroenterol Clin Biol 7:474, 1983.
33. Vatier J, Poitevin CH, Robert JC, et al: Histamine is able to suppress the inhibitory effect of somatostatin on exogenous gastrin: Comparison between extractive antral histamine and synthetic histamine. Agents Actions 13:1, 1983.
34. Vatier J, Poitevin C, Accary JP, et al: Antramine (antral histamine) antagonizes somatostatin inhibition on endogenous gastrin-induced gastric secretion. A new hypothesis for the role of histamine in gastric secretion regulation. Scand J Gastroenterol 20:671, 1985.
35. Chew CS: Inhibitory action of somatostatin on isolated gastric glands and parietal cells. Am J Physiol 245:G221, 1983.
36. Peden NR, Boyd EJS, Callachan H, et al: The effects of impromidine and pentagastrin on gastric output of histamine, acid and pepsin in man. Hepatogastroenterology 29:30, 1982.
37. Redfern JS, Thirlby R, Feldman M, et al: Effect of pentagastrin on gastric mucosal histamine in dogs. Am J Physiol 248:G369, 1985.
38. Kleibeuker JH, Kauffman GL: Intravenous histamine reduces bombesin-stimulated gastrin release in dog. Gastroenterology 84:1209, 1983.
39. Hirschowitz BI: Pepsinogen: Its origin, secretion and excretion. Physiol Rev 37:475, 1957.
40. Thompson JC, Davidson WD, Patton JJ, et al: Histamine stimulation of gastric pepsin secretion in the dog. Arch Surg 97:805, 1968.
41. Schwartz JC: Gastric histamine in the pathogenesis of experimental ulcers, in Pfeiffer CJ (ed): *Peptic Ulcer*. Philadelphia, J. B. Lippincott Co, 1971, pp 190–198.
42. Takeuchi K, Furukawa O, Tanaka H, et al: A new model of duodenal ulcers induced in rats by indomethacin plus histamine. Gastroenterology 90:836, 1986.
43. Hirvonen J, Elfving R: Histamine and serotonin in the gastric erosions of rats dead from exposure to cold: A histochemical and quantitative study. Z Rechtsmed 74:273, 1974.
44. Cheung LY, Sonnenschein L: Effects of histamine and cimetidine on gastric blood flow and intramural pH in dogs. Gastroenterology 80:1123, 1981.
45. Mortillaro NA, Granger DN, Kvietys PR, et al: Effects of histamine and histamine antagonists on intestinal capillary permeability. Am J Physiol 240:G381, 1981.
46. Ekblad EBM: Histamine and cAMP as possible mediators of acetylcholine-induced acid secretion. Am J Physiol 239:G255, 1980.
47. Chew CS: Parietal cell protein kinases. Selective activation of type I cAMP-dependent protein kinase by histamine. J Biol Chem 260:7540, 1985.
48. Sewing K-F, Beil W, Hannemann H, et al: The adenylate cyclase-cyclic AMP-protein kinase system in different cell populations of the guinea pig gastric mucosa. Life Sci 12:1097, 1985.
49. Waldman DB, Zfass AM, Makhlouf GM: Stimulatory (H_1) and inhibitory (H_2) histamine receptors in gallbladder muscle. Gastroenterology 72:932, 1977.
50. Schoetz DJ Jr, Wise WE Jr, La Morte WW, et al: Histamine receptors in primate gallbladder. Dig Dis Sci 28:353, 1983.
51. Toouli J, Dodds WJ, Honda R, et al: Effect of histamine on motor function of opossum sphincter of Oddi. Am J Physiol 241:G122, 1981.
52. LaMorte WW, Gaca JM, Wise WE, et al: Choledochal sphincter relaxation in response to histamine in the primate. J Surg Res 28:373, 1980.
53. Hirschowitz BI: An update on histamine receptors and the gastrointestinal tract. Dig Dis Sci 30:998, 1985.
54. Sakai K: A pharmacological analysis of the contractile action of histamine upon the ileal region of the isolated, blood-perfused small intestine of the rat. Br J Pharmacol 67:587, 1979.
55. Iwatsuki K, Ikeda K, Chiba S: Effect of histamine on pancreatic exocrine secretion in the dog. Acta Int Pharmacodyn 251:166, 1981.
56. Liebow C, Franklin JE Jr: Histamine stimulation of digestive enzyme secretion by *in vitro* rabbit pancreas. Dig Dis Sci 27:234, 1982.

Chapter 30

Serotonin

Laszlo Mate, M.D., Graeme J. Poston, F.R.C.S., and James C. Thompson, M.D.

HISTORY

A long-known but incompletely characterized vasoconstrictor agent, the vasoactive amine serotonin, was ultimately identified and chemically characterized in 1949 as 5-hydroxytryptamine (5-HT) by Rapport [1] and subsequently synthesized in 1951 by Hamlin and Fischer [2]. Serotonin is not a gastrointestinal peptide, but it has actions that overlap those of many gastrointestinal hormones and it influences gut function, so it is included in this survey.

DISTRIBUTION

About 90 percent of the total serotonin content of mammals is located in the gastrointestinal tract, mostly in enterochromaffin cells distributed throughout the gut [3] and, to a lesser extent, in the myenteric plexus. Mast cells of the rat and mouse contain serotonin, whereas mast cells of other species do not. Serotonin is also located in the central nervous system and is found in platelets [4]. Several plants (banana, plum, avocado, tomato) are rich in serotonin [5], although dietary consumption of serotonin is not known to have any physiologic significance. Serotonin plays an important role in the immune response and in the central nervous system, but in this chapter only its gastrointestinal activities will be considered.

ASSAY

The first techniques for measurement of serotonin were bioassays [6], which were later superceded by chemical procedures such as spectrophotometry and spectrofluorometry [7–9]. A sensitive radioimmunoassay has been available since 1973 [10].

PHARMACOKINETICS AND CATABOLISM

Serotonin is synthesized from tryptophan by tryptophan-5-hydrolase and 5-hydroxytryptophan decarboxylase. The main catabolic pathways are through monoamine oxidase to 5-hydroxyindole acetaldehyde, and then either oxidation to 5-hydroxyindole acetic acid (5-HIAA), which is the main catabolite, or reduction to 5-hydroxytryptophol, which is significantly increased after consumption of alcohol [11]. Both metabolites are excreted primarily in the urine [12], but several ancillary paths have been demonstrated [13].

Serotonin is synthesized chiefly within the enterochromaffin cells of the gut, which are considered by some to be part of the so-called amine precursor uptake and decarboxylation (APUD) system [14]. These cells are capable of synthesizing several humoral agents (polypeptides, vasoactive amines), and serotonin is certainly stored together with other agents and may be released with them [15,16]. Platelets also contain the enzymes necessary for serotonin synthesis; serotonin may be released from platelets on stimulation [17].

After release from the gastrointestinal tract, the bulk of serotonin is eliminated from the circulation in a single passage through the liver or lungs. Serotonin is also partially eliminated by platelet uptake [18,19], so its circulating levels remain low [20]. Significant amounts do escape immediate inactivation, which enables it to function as a circulating hormone [21].

At least two different subtypes of serotonin receptors (5-HT_1 and 5-HT_2) exist in the central nervous system, and similar receptor populations exist in the gut [22–25]. Recent work has suggested the existence of a third as yet unclassified serotonin receptor in the guinea pig ileum [26].

RELEASE

Release of serotonin can be stimulated via both adrenergic and cholinergic pathways [16], but the latter are significantly more effective [27]. Vagal stimulation depletes intestinal mucosal serotonin content, with a subsequent rise of serotonin concentrations in both portal venous blood and the intestinal lumen [28,29]. Furthermore, direct cholinergic stimulation with carbamylcholine of the rabbit duodenum stimulates release of serotonin, and this effect can be antagonized by atropine [30]. Adrenergic-stimulated release of serotonin occurs via both alpha and beta receptors in the cat, being potentiated by isoproterenol and antagonized by propranolol [31,32]. Adrenalectomy resulted in a decrease in the release of serotonin (while, interestingly, causing a corresponding increase in release of substance P) (Fig 30-1). Recently, the existence of a mucosal inhibitory mechanism that is neither cholinergic nor adrenergic was demonstrated in vitro in the rabbit duodenum [33].

Vagal stimulation [28] and increased intraluminal pressure in the gut [34] both produce an increase in the intraluminal content of serotonin.

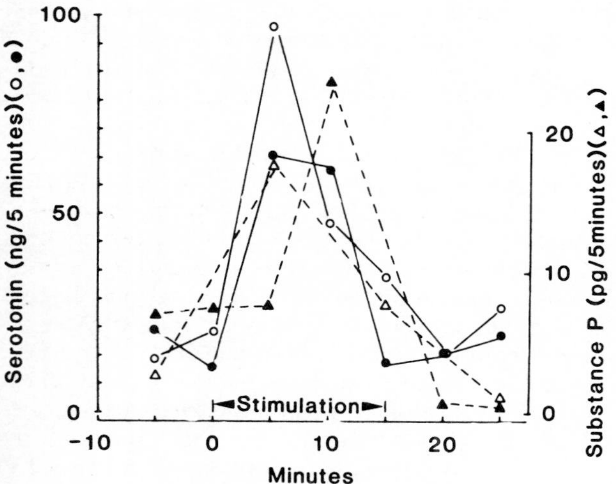

Figure 30-1. Synchronous changes in immunoreactive serotonin (○ — ○) and substance P (△ — △) in intestinal perfusates in one cat during vagal nerve stimulation before (open symbols) and after (closed symbols) bilateral adrenalectomy. (From Ahlman H et al [28], by permission of the American Association for the Advancement of Science.)

Direct acid stimulation of duodenal mucosa causes serotonin release in both rabbits [35] and dogs, and a similar effect is seen when fat is administered intraduodenally to dogs [21,36]. In vitro release of serotonin is calcium-dependent, and this release can be suppressed by somatostatin [37].

ACTIONS

The effect of serotonin on gastric secretion is still not clearly understood. In rats 1–10 mg/kg serotonin was reported to suppress basal, urecholine-, gastrin-, and histamine-induced gastric secretion (volume, acid, and pepsin output) [38–40]. Serotonin abolishes insulin-stimulated gastric secretion.

The relationship between serotonin and gastric secretion has been studied extensively in dogs. In the innervated canine stomach, serotonin decreases gastric secretion [41], but this inhibition is reduced after vagotomy and is not seen in a Heidenhain pouch [21,42]. Jaffe et al [21] have suggested that serotonin may play an important role in the duodenal mechanisms for feedback inhibition of gastric acid secretion (Fig 30-2).

Although both secretin and serotonin are released during duodenal acidification, they each have an independent inhibitory effect on gastric secretion [43]. Serotonin is likely to exert a background restraining effect on basal gastric secretion, since the administration of the specific serotonin antagonist, methysergide, increases gastric acid secretion in several species (rats, dogs, and even humans) [44,45]. Serotonin increases the secretion of mucin from the pyloric mucosa. This effect is not dependent on increased motility, since it is present in the everted pouch and is not abolished by hexamethonium, which decreases motility [46].

Introduction of acid or fat into the duodenum inhibits gastric acid, stimulates pepsin secretion, and increases blood levels of serotonin. Serotonin antagonists cause this inhibitory effect to disappear, which suggests mediation by serotonin [37,47]. Serotonin releases gastrin and decreases release of somatostatin from isolated stomachs of rats [48].

Serotonin stimulates intestinal secretion and may be responsible, at least in part, for the diarrhea observed in some diseases (for example, amebiasis [49], cholera [50], and celiac disease [51]), but no serotonergic receptors have been found in the

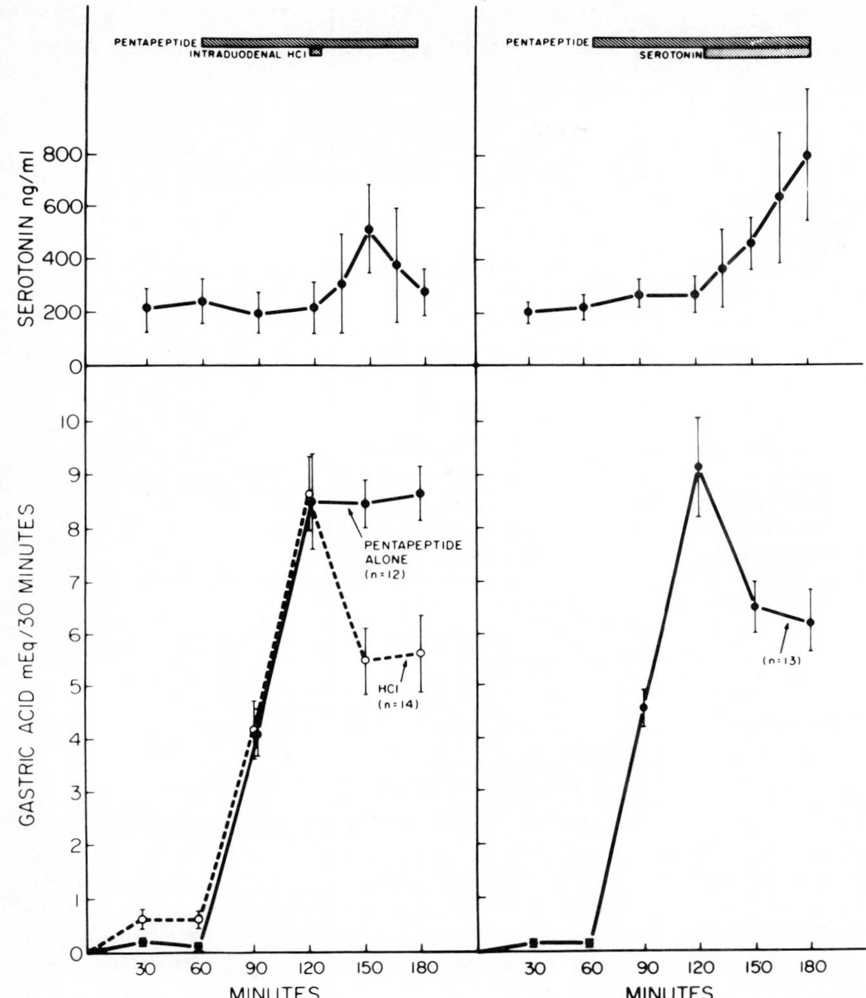

Figure 30-2. The effect of duodenal acidification and serotonin infusion on peripheral venous serotonin levels (upper panels), and gastric fistula output (lower panels). (From Jaffe BM et al [21], by permission of The CV Mosby Co.)

intestinal epithelial cells of rats, suggesting an indirect effect [52]. Besides stimulation of intestinal secretion, serotonin inhibits absorption of sodium chloride [53].

The mechanisms of interaction between serotonin and prostaglandins in the gastrointestinal tract and central nervous system are not clear. In isolated rat stomachs, indomethacin blocked the inhibitory effect of serotonin on gastric secretion [54], but in in vivo studies on rat stomachs, serotonin appeared to mediate the inhibitory effect of prostaglandin E_1 on gastric secretion [55]. Nonsteroidal anti-inflammatory drugs eliminate the contractile effect of serotonin on isolated guinea pig ileum [56].

Serotonin causes the redistribution of systemic blood flow. In anesthetized dogs, it increases perfusion of the stomach, brain, heart, and skeletal muscle, while decreasing perfusion of the kidney, spleen, and liver [57]. In the rat stomach, serotonin inhibits epinephrine-induced vasoconstriction [58] and increases gastric mucosal blood flow [59].

Serotonin-containing cells are widely distributed in the pancreas [60]. Serotonin decreases pancreatic output of water and bicarbonate, while secretion of protein remains unchanged [61,62]. Serotonin decreases blood flow in the isolated, perfused pancreas [63] and causes mesenteric vasoconstriction [28]; in the cat, however, dilatation of the small vessels overshadowed this effect [29].

The effects of serotonin on gut motility are variable. Serotonin was first measured by bioassay, measuring contraction of strips of rat fundus [64]. In the guinea pig and mouse stomach, serotonin

Table 30-1. Characteristics of carcinoid syndrome produced by tumors arising from different sites

	Midgut	*Foregut*		*Hindgut*
	Ileal	*Bronchial*	*Gastric*	*(Rectal)*
Flush	Brief, multiple	Prolonged, severe, with facial edema, lacrimation, fever	Bright red, face and neck	Carcinoid syndrome is *very rare*
Metastases	Usually in abdomen	Osteoblastic and skin, as well as abdomen	Usually in abdomen	Abdomen, but osteoblastic and skin common
Histology	Usually typical argentaffin	Tendency to trabecular pattern; may be very atypical		Tendency to argentaffin
Metabolic features	Indole secretion largely serotonin	May secrete other polypeptide hormones; symptoms respond to corticosteroids	Frequently secrete 5-hydroxy-tryptophan and histamine; increased incidence of peptic ulcer	Serotonin secretion *very* rare

(Data from Brown [74].)

causes both contraction and relaxation [65]. In the guinea pig colon, serotonin first causes relaxation, followed by contraction [66], while in the cat colon, it causes contraction but relaxes the rectum [67]. In the rat small intestine, serotonin stimulates motility [68], but in the dog small intestine, it stimulates activity only in the muscularis mucosa [69]. These effects can be abolished by several agents blocking neural pathways [67,70].

Serotonin slightly decreases the flow of bile [71], but it has no effect on the gallbladder in humans [72] or isolated muscle strips of rabbit gallbladder (unpublished studies from our laboratory).

CARCINOID SYNDROME

In 1953, serotonin was identified in a carcinoid tumor [73]; later studies in patients with the carcinoid syndrome showed that serotonin was elevated in the serum and its metabolite, 5-HIAA, was elevated in the urine. Serotonin was considered for years to be the agent responsible for this syndrome, but more recent studies [74] suggest that the symptoms are the result of secretion of several agents, with the variable manifestations of the disease reflecting the predominant agent.

Next to thyroid tumors, carcinoid tumors are the most common endocrine tumors. Only about one of 10 tumors of endocrine tissue is functional, and the ratio is far lower in carcinoids. Carcinoid tumors occur in the entire gut; the appendix is the most common site (45 percent of carcinoids are in the appendix, 10 percent in the ileum, and 15 percent in the rectum). The carcinoid syndrome usually occurs with widespread metastatic tumors, especially those arising from the mid gut. Primary tumors from the bronchus and ovary may rarely give rise to the syndrome. The syndrome is characterized by flushing (confined to the upper half of the body) that is precipitated by certain foods, alcohol, exertion, and IV administration of epinephrine, and it is abolished by administration of somatostatin. Somatostatin is effective in alleviating all symptoms. The long-acting somatostatin analog (SMS-201-995, "Sandostatin") has been particularly effective in long-term symptomatic therapy in a selected group of patients [74a]. The compound is immensely promising in these patients and in others with secretory diarrhea. Gastric carcinoid, which is rare in humans, causes a localized bright red rash of the face and neck, probably produced by the large amounts of histamine that carcinoids characteristically produce (Table 30-1) [74].

The carcinoid syndrome is further associated with diarrhea, abdominal pain, myocardial fibrosis (pulmonary stenosis, bicuspid regurgitation, and constrictive pericarditis), generalized sclerosis with a scleroderma-like syndrome, and pellagra (nicotinic acid deficiency). Carcinoid disturbs tryptophan metabolism, and, since the essential amino acid tryptophan is a precursor of both serotonin and the vitamin nicotinic acid, the diversion of tryptophan from nicotinic acid production results in pellagra.

Tryptophan is initially hydroxylated to 5-hydroxytryptophan, the principal metabolite of foregut carcinoid, but midgut carcinoids can further decarboxylate this to 5-hydroxytryptamine, which explains the biochemical differences between the two types (Table 30-1). Gastrointestinal symptoms of the carcinoid syndrome can be reduced by both 5-HT_1 antagonists (methysergide) [75] and 5-HT_2 antagonists (ketanserin) [76].

REFERENCES

1. Rapport MM: Serum vasoconstrictor (serotonin). V. The presence of creatinine in the complex. A proposed structure of the vasoconstrictor principle. J Biol Chem 180:961, 1949.
2. Hamlin KE, Fischer FE: The synthesis of 5-hydroxytryptamine. J Am Chem Soc 73:5007, 1951.
3. Sjolund K, Sanden G, Håkanson R, et al: Endocrine cells in human intestine: An immunocytochemical study. Gastroenterology 85:1120, 1983.
4. Essman WB: Serotonin distribution in tissues and fluids, in Essman WB (ed): *Serotonin in Health and Disease. Volume I: Availability, Localization and Disposition.* New York, SP Medical & Scientific Books, 1978, pp 15–180.
5. Udenfriend S, Lovenberg W, Sjoerdsma A: Physiologically active amines in common fruits and vegetables. Arch Biochem Biophys 85:487, 1959.
6. Erspamer V: Pharmakologische Studien uber Enteramin. I. Mitteilung: Uber die Wirkung von Acetonextrakten der Kaninchenmagenschleimhaut auf den Blutdruck und auf isolierte uberlebende Organe. Naunyn Schmiedebergs Arch Pharmacol 196:343, 1940.
7. Dalgliesh CE, Toh CC, Work TS: Fractionation of the smooth muscle stimulants present in extracts of gastro-intestinal tract. Identification of 5-hydroxytryptamine and its distinction from substance P. J Physiol 120:298, 1953.
8. Wise CD: An improved and simplified method for the fluorometric determination of brain serotonin. Anal Biochem 18:94, 1967.
9. Udenfriend S, Weissbach H, Clark CT: The estimation of 5-hydroxytryptamine (serotonin) in biological tissues. J Biol Chem 215:337, 1955.
10. Peskar B, Spector S: Serotonin: Radioimmunoassay. Science 179:1340, 1973.
11. Davis VE, Brown H, Huff JA, et al: The alteration of serotonin metabolism to 5-hydroxytryptophol by ethanol ingestion in man. J Lab Clin Med 69:132, 1967.
12. Keglevic D, Supek Z, Kveder S, et al: The metabolism of exogenous ^{14}C-labelled 5-hydroxytryptamine in rats. Biochem J 73:53, 1959.
13. Bosin TR: Serotonin metabolism, in Essman WB (ed): *Serotonin in Health and Disease. Volume I: Availability, Localization and Disposition.* New York, SP Medical & Scientific Books, 1978, pp 181–300.
14. Pearse AGE: The diffuse neuroendocrine system and the APUD concept: Related "endocrine" peptides in brain, intestine, pituitary, placenta, and anuran cutaneous glands. Med Biol 55:115, 1977.
15. Polak JM, De Mey J, Bloom SR: 5-Hydroxytryptamine in mucosal endocrine cells of the gut and lung, in De Clerck F, Vanhoutte PM (eds): *5-Hydroxytryptamine in Peripheral Reactions.* New York, Raven Press, 1982, pp 23–35.
16. Zinner MJ, DeMagistris L, Ahlman J, et al: Simultaneous release of 5-HT substance P, and motilin into the lumen of the isolated cat jejunum. Gastroenterology 82:1218, 1982.
17. Marmaras VJ, Mimikos N: Enzymic formation of serotonin in mammalian blood platelets and red cells. Experientia 27:196, 1971.
18. Thomas DP, Vane JR: 5-Hydroxytryptamine in the circulation of the dog. Nature 216:335, 1967.
19. Udenfriend S, Weissbach H: Turnover of 5-hydroxytryptamine (serotonin) in tissues. Proc Soc Exp Biol Med 97:748, 1958.
20. Genefke IK, Mandel P: Variations diurnes de la serotonine libre chez des sujets normaux. Clin Chim Acta 19:131, 1968.
21. Jaffe BM, Kopen DF, Lazan DW: Endogenous serotonin in the control of gastric acid secretion. Surgery 82:156, 1977.
22. Middlemiss DN, Fozard JR: 8-Hydroxy-2-(DI-n-propylamino)-tetralin discriminates between subtypes of the 5-HT_1 recognition site. Eur J Pharmacol 90:151, 1983.
23. Peroutka SJ, Snyder SH: Multiple serotonin receptors: Differential binding of [^{3}H]5-hydroxytryptamine,[^{3}H]lysergic acid diethylamide and [^{3}H]spiroperidol. Molec Pharmacol 16:687, 1979.
24. Engel G, Hoyer D, Kalkman H, et al: Identification of 5HT_2 receptors on longitudinal muscle of the guinea pig ileum. J Recept Res 4:113, 1984.
25. Saxena PR, Lawang A: A comparison of cardiovascular and smooth muscle effects of 5-hydroxytryptamine and 5-carboxamido-tryptamine, a selective agonist of 5-HT_1 receptors. Arch Int Pharmacodyn Ther 277:235, 1985.
26. Cohen ML, Schenck KW, Colbert W, et al: Role of 5-HT_2 receptors in serotonin-induced contractions of nonvascular smooth muscle. J Pharmacol Exp Ther 232:770, 1985.
27. Gross KB, Sturkie PD: Concentration of serotonin in intestine and factors affecting its release. Proc Soc Exp Biol Med 148:1261, 1975.
28. Ahlman H, DeMagistris L, Zinner M, et al: Release of immunoreactive serotonin into the lumen of the feline gut in response to vagal nerve stimulation. Science 213:1254, 1981.

29. Ahlman H, Dahlstrom A: Storage and release of 5-hydroxytryptamine in enterochromaffin cells of the small intestine, in De Clerck F, Vanhoutte PM (eds): *5-Hydroxytryptamine in Peripheral Reactions.* New York, Raven Press, 1982, pp 1–21.
30. Kellum J, McCabe M, Schneier J, et al: Neural control of acid-induced serotonin release from rabbit duodenum. Am J Physiol 245:G824, 1983.
31. Kellum JM, Donowitz M, Cerel A, et al: Acid and isoproterenol cause serotonin release by acting on opposite surfaces of duodenal mucosa. J Surg Res 36:172, 1984.
32. Larsson I, Dahlstrom A, Pettersson G, et al: The effects of adrenergic antagonists on the serotonin levels of feline enterochromaffin cells after splanchnic nerve stimulation. J Neural Transm 47:89, 1980.
33. Kellum JM, Wu J, Donowitz M: Enteric neural pathways inhibitory to rabbit duodenal serotonin release. Surgery 96:139, 1984.
34. Bulbring E, Lin RCY: The effect of intraluminal application of 5-hydroxytryptamine and 5-hydroxytryptophan on peristalsis; the local production of 5-HT and its release in relation to intraluminal pressure and propulsive activity. J Physiol 140:381, 1958.
35. Kellum JM, McCabe M, Schneier J, et al: Neural mediation of acid-stimulated serotonin release from rabbit duodenum. Gastroenterology 82:1098, 1982.
36. Wise L, Burkholder J, Zagaloff A, et al: Studies on the role of serotonin in the inhibition of gastric acid secretion by the duodenum. Ann Surg 168:824, 1968.
37. Forsberg EJ, Miller RJ: Regulation of serotonin release from rabbit intestinal enterochromaffin cells. J Pharmacol Exp Ther 227:755, 1983.
38. Thompson JH: Serotonin (5-hydroxytryptamine) and the alimentary system, in Essman WB (ed): *Serotonin in Health and Disease. Volume IV: Clinical Correlates.* New York, Spectrum Publications, Inc, 1977, pp 201–222.
39. Shay H, Sun DCH, Gruenstein M: Effect of serotonin and reserpine on interdigestive gastric secretion in the rat. Fed Proc 16:118, 1957.
40. Haverback BJ, Wirtschafter SK: The gastrointestinal tract and naturally occurring pharmacologically active amines. Adv Pharmacol 1:309, 1962.
41. Black JW, Fisher EW, Smith AN: The effects of 5-hydroxytryptamine on gastric secretion in anaesthetized dogs. J Physiol 141:27, 1958.
42. Sosin H, Nicoloff DM, Peter ET, et al: Effect of serotonin on histamine stimulated secretion in canine Heidenhain pouches. Fed Proc 21:264, 1962.
43. Mate LM, Sakamoto T, Greeley GH Jr, et al: Regulation of gastric acid secretion by secretin and serotonin. Am J Surg 149:40, 1985.
44. Debnath PK, Goel RK, Sanyal AK: Effect of 5-hydroxytryptamine antagonist on gastric secretion in albino rats. Indian J Med Res 63:1688, 1975.
45. Caldara R, Ferrari C, Barbieri C, et al: Effect of two anti-serotoninergic drugs, methysergide and metergoline, on gastric acid secretion and gastrin release in healthy man. Eur J Clin Pharmacol 17:13, 1980.
46. White TT, Magee DF: The influence of serotonin on gastric mucin production. Gastroenterology 35:289, 1958.
47. Wazna MF, Stein T, Wise L: The effect of serotonin on pepsin inhibition by duodenal fat. Ann Surg 186:130, 1977.
48. Koop H, Arnold R: Control of rat gastric somatostatin and gastrin release by serotonin. Gastroenterology 84:1214, 1983.
49. McGowan K, Kane A, Asarkof N, et al: *Entamoeba histolytica* causes intestinal secretion: Role of serotonin. Science 221:762, 1983.
50. Nilsson O, Cassuto J, Larsson P-A, et al: 5-Hydroxytryptamine and cholera secretion: A histochemical and physiological study in cats. Gut 24:542, 1983.
51. Enerback L, Hallert C, Norrby K: Raised 5-hydroxytryptamine concentrations in enterochromaffin cells in adult coeliac disease. J Clin Pathol 36:499, 1983.
52. Gaginella TS, Rimele TJ, Wietecha M: Studies on rat intestinal epithelial cell receptors for serotonin and opiates. J Physiol 335:101, 1983.
53. Zimmerman TW, Binder HJ: Serotonin-induced alteration of colonic electrolyte transport in the rat. Gastroenterology 86:310, 1984.
54. Canfield SP, Spencer JE: The inhibitory effects of 5-hydroxytryptamine on gastric acid secretion by the rat isolated stomach. Br J Pharmacol 78:123, 1983.
55. Goel RK, Debnath PK, Sanyal AK: Role of serotonin in gastric acid secretion inhibition by prostaglandin E_1. Indian J Med Res 78:142, 1983.
56. Famaey JP, Fontaine J, Seaman I, et al: A possible role of prostaglandins in guinea-pig isolated ileum contractions to serotonin. Prostaglandins 14:119, 1977.
57. Zinner MJ, Kasher F, Jaffe BM: The hemodynamic effects of intravenous infusions of serotonin in conscious dogs. J Surg Res 34:171, 1983.
58. Guth PH, Smith E: Vasoactive agents and the gastric microcirculation. Microvasc Res 8:125, 1974.
59. Yano S, Hoshino E, Harada M: Effect of vasoactive drugs on gastric blood flow measured by a cross thermocouple method in rats. Jpn J Pharmacol 31:117, 1981.
60. Puppi A, Tigyi A, Lissak K: 5-Hydroxytryptamine and frog pancreas, I. Acta Physiol Hung 33:285, 1968.
61. Hudock JJ, Khentigan A, Vanamee P, et al: The effect of serotonin and serotonin antagonists on external pancreatic secretion in dogs. J Surg Res 3:307, 1963.
62. Nakano S: Some physiological observations on the exocrine pancreas. The effects of some agents on pancreatic secretion. Nagoya J Med Sci 31:79, 1968.
63. Takeuchi O, Satoh S, Hashimoto K: Secretory and vascular response to various biogenic and foreign substances of the perfused canine pancreas. Jpn J Pharmacol 24:57, 1974.
64. Vane JR: A sensitive method for the assay of 5-hydroxytryptamine. Br J Pharmacol 12:344, 1957.
65. Bulbring E, Gershon MD: 5-hydroxytryptamine participation in the vagal inhibitory innervation of the stomach. J Physiol 192:823, 1967.

66. Furness JB, Costa M: The nervous release and the action of substances which affect intestinal muscle through neither adrenoreceptors nor cholinoreceptors. Philos Trans R Soc Lond [Biol] 265:123, 1973.
67. Fasth S, Hedlund H, Hulten L, et al: The effects of 5-hydroxytryptamine on large intestinal motility and blood flow in the cat. Acta Physiol Scand 118:329, 1983.
68. Sakai K, Akima M, Shiraki Y: Comparative studies with 5-hydroxytryptamine and its derivatives in isolated, blood-perfused small intestine and ileum strip of the rat. Jpn J Pharmacol 29:223, 1979.
69. Tansy MF, Martin JS, Landin WE, et al: Discrete motor effects of neurohumoral and hormonal stimuli on the canine small intestine. Surg Gynecol Obstet 150:827, 1980.
70. Chahl LA: Substance P mediates atropine-sensitive response of guinea-pig ileum to serotonin. Eur J Pharmacol 87:485, 1983.
71. Kortz WJ, Schirmer BD, Feldman JR, et al: Serotonin suppresses bile salt independent bile formation. Gastroenterology 82:1105, 1982.
72. Mack AJ, Todd JK: A study of human gall bladder muscle *in vitro*. Gut 9:546, 1968.
73. Lembeck F: 5-Hydroxytryptamine in a carcinoid tumour. Nature 172:910, 1953.
74. Brown H: Serotonin-producing tumors, in Essman WB (ed): *Serotonin in Health and Disease. Volume IV: Clinical Correlates.* New York, Spectrum Publications, Inc, 1977, pp 393–423.
74a. Creutzfeldt W, Stockmann F: The carcinoid syndrome. Presented at Symposium on Gastrointestinal Endocrine Tumors, Vancouver, Canada, 4–6 July, 1986.
75. Mengel CE: Therapy of the malignant carcinoid syndrome. Ann Int Med 62:587, 1965.
76. Ahlman H, Dahlstrom A, Gronstad K, et al: The pentagastrin test in the diagnosis of the carcinoid syndrome. Blockade of gastrointestinal symptoms by ketanserin. Ann Surg 201:81, 1985.

Chapter 31

Prostaglandins

Laszlo Mate, M.D., R. Daniel Beauchamp, M.D., and James C. Thompson, M.D.

HISTORY

Prostaglandins, a family of unsaturated, oxygenated fatty acids, can be synthesized in all mammalian tissue, in tissues from other vertebrate and invertebrate species, and in plants [1]. The basic structure contains 20 carbon atoms, and the position and type of side ligands and the number of double bonds between the carbon atoms determine the naming of the compound (e.g., PGE_1, PGD_2, PGH_2). The number of prostaglandins so far identified in mammalian tissues is about 20, in major categories named A, B, C, D, E, F, G, H, and I, depending on the functional group of the cyclopentane ring (Fig 31-1). The mammalian designation 1, 2, or 3 (i.e., PGE_1, PGE_2) indicates the position of the desaturated double bonds. The biologically active endoperoxide intermediates of prostaglandin biosynthesis are the thromboxanes.

DISTRIBUTION

In the gastrointestinal tract, PGD, PGE, PGF, PGI_2, and thromboxane A_2 (TxA_2) have been identified, as have the enzymes responsible for their metabolism. The gastric mucosa has the greatest amount of PGE_2, while the muscular layers contain mainly PGI_2 [2].

ASSAY

Prostaglandins can be measured by gas-liquid chromatography, ultraviolet spectroscopy, and radioimmunoassay [3] in addition to traditional bioassays (platelet aggregation and muscle strips, inter alia) [4].

PHARMACOKINETICS AND CATABOLISM

Prostaglandins are formed by the enzyme prostaglandin synthase (a dioxygenase), from arachidonic acid through the unstable metabolites PGG_2 and PGH_2 (Fig 31-2). They are rapidly metabolized to substances of reduced biologic activity in tissue. The chief catabolic pathways convert PGE_2 and $PGF_{2\alpha}$ into dicarbocyclic acid urinary metabolites. Other prostaglandins are metabolized by the same reactions.

RELEASE

Prostaglandins exert most of their activities at or near the site of their synthesis; they are not stored in cells but are synthesized and released locally upon stimulation [5].

ACTIONS

Since prostaglandins do not usually exert their effects at a distant site, they function chiefly as paracrine agents.

Gastric Secretion

Prostaglandins of the A, E, and I types inhibit gastric secretion of water, acid, and pepsin. This effect has been observed in various species using various stimulants (for example, pentagastrin, histamine, vagal stimulation, food) [6].

The natural PGE_1 and PGE_2 are active either parenterally or orally, but in the latter case, only in extremely high doses [5,7]; their synthetic methyl analogues are more potent orally and their effects

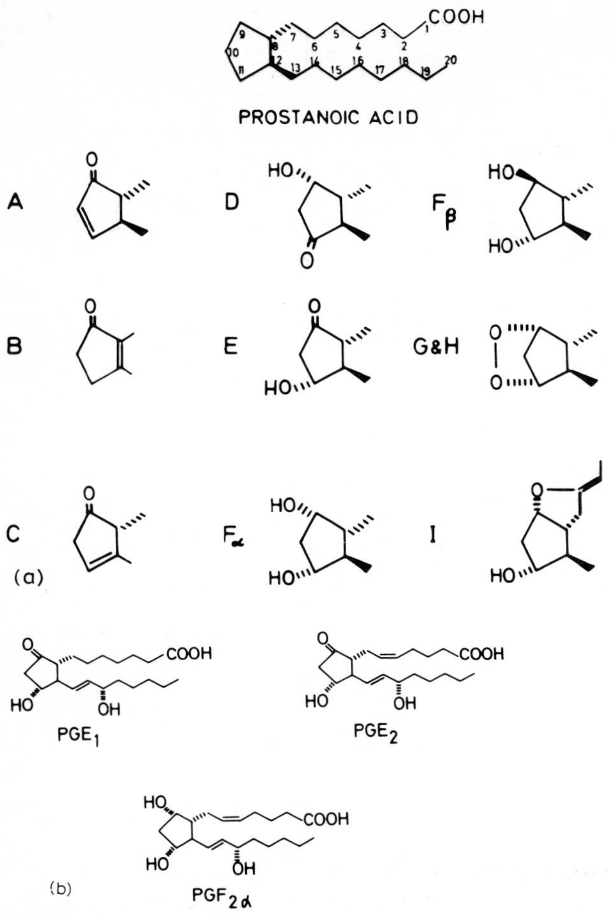

Figure 31-1. **A.** The structure of prostanoic acid, the carbon skeleton of the prostaglandins, and the structure and functional groups of the cyclopentane ring in prostaglandins A to I. **B.** Structures of prostaglandins E_1, E_2, and $F_{2\alpha}$, the first prostaglandins to be identified. (From Oliw E, et al, in Pace-Asciak C, Granstrom E (eds): *Prostaglandins and Related Substances.* New York, Elsevier, 1983.)

longer lasting [8]. Recently, much attention has been given to prostacyclin (PGI_2); among the naturally occurring prostaglandins, it has the most potent antisecretory effect on the stomach [9], and it is an important metabolite of arachidonic acid in the stomach [10].

The mechanism of the antisecretory effect is not fully understood. In 1973 Becker et al [11] from our laboratory showed that an infusion of PGE_1 greatly suppressed food-stimulated acid secretion in dogs and greatly augmented the postprandial release of gastrin. *Unlike all other* known inhibitors of gastric secretion, prostaglandins do not decrease gastric secretion by decreasing gastric mucosal blood flow [12,13]; in fact, the ratio of blood flow to gastric secretion either remains the same or even increases. The target of the prostaglandins is the parietal cell, and the eventual decrease in mucosal blood flow is secondary to the antisecretory action [12]. PGI_2 has strong vasodilator properties and may even increase mucosal blood flow [14–16]. According to in vitro studies, prostaglandins specifically block the histamine-stimulated production of cAMP by the parietal cells, thus decreasing acid output [17,18].

In human studies, prostaglandins were effective in promoting the healing of peptic ulcers, but because of their side effects, the most important of which is diarrhea, they are not in routine clinical use [12–22]. PGE_2 stimulates gastric bicarbonate secretion in a cholinergic manner [23].

Pancreatic Secretion

Naturally existing prostaglandin E [24] and I_2 [25], and a synthetic prostaglandin analogue, 16-16-dimethyl prostaglandin E_2 [24], can inhibit secretin-stimulated pancreatic volume and bicarbonate in conscious dogs. PGI_1 and PGE_2 inhibit secretin-stimulated pancreatic secretion in the anesthetized cat [25]. PGI_2 inhibits caerulein- and secretin-stimulated pancreatic protein secretion [26]. Given alone, these agents seem to be mild stimulants of pancreatic secretion in the conscious dog [24,25,27]. Watson et al [28] from our laboratory reported that an infusion of PGE_1 inhibited pancreatic volume and bicarbonate secretion in response to duodenal acidification in dogs and caused a significant decrease in acid-stimulated release of secretin.

Vascular effects of PGE_1 [24] and PGE_2 [29] result in decreased systemic arterial blood pressure in the anesthetized dog. PGE_1 and PGE_2 cause a decrease in systemic arterial pressure and reduction in pancreatic blood flow and concomitant decreases in secretin-stimulated pancreatic secretion in the anesthetized cat [25]. Conversely, in the saline-perfused isolated cat pancreas model, in which perfusion pressure is kept constant, prostaglandins E_1, E_2, $F_{1\alpha}$, and $F_{2\alpha}$ stimulate pancreatic volume and electrolyte secretion, given individually or in combination with secretin [25]. In the blood-perfused dog pancreas, however, PGE_2 inhibits secretin-stimulated pancreatic secretion [29].

Perfused in vitro preparations of whole pancreas from the rat and mouse are stimulated to

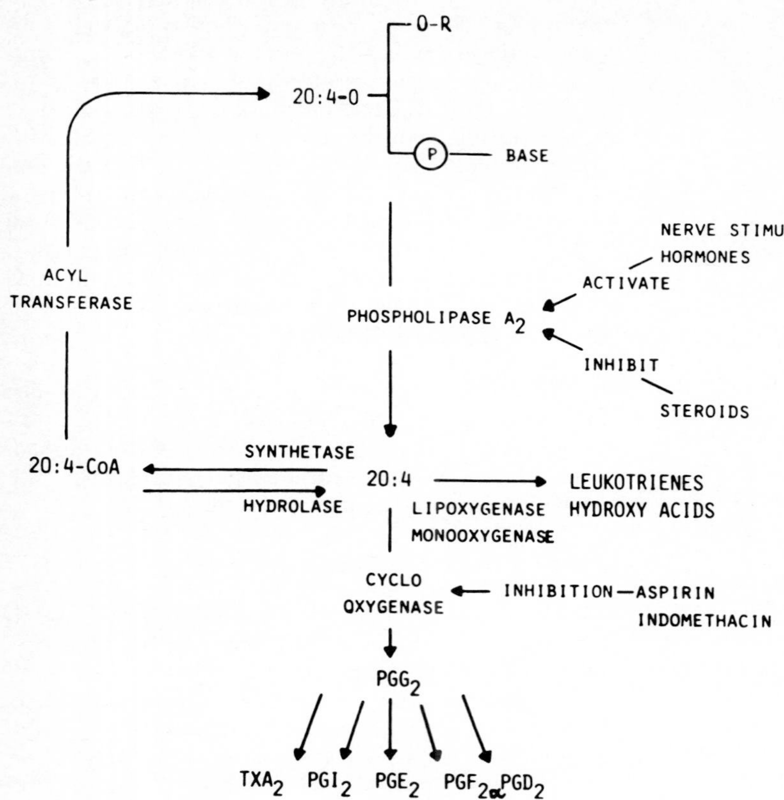

Figure 31-2. Mechanism of release of arachidonic acid from glycerophospholipids for subsequent conversion to oxygenated products or for re-esterification into glycerophospholipids in the 2-acyl position. (From Oliw E, et al, in Pace-Asciak C, Granstrom E (eds): *Prostaglandins and Related Substances.* New York, Elsevier, 1983.)

secrete amylase when treated with PGE_2 [30], an effect that is augmented in an additive fashion with carbamylcholine stimulation. Indomethacin inhibits carbamylcholine-stimulated amylase secretion in the same model [30]. The prostaglandin effects seen in this model require an intact pancreas and do not work in glands that are disrupted [31–34].

Intestinal Secretion

Most prostaglandins induce rapid accumulation of fluid in the small intestine. This effect is called "enteropooling." It is rather similar to the effect of cholera toxin, which may be mediated by prostaglandins [35]. In the gut, prostaglandins act through the stimulation of cAMP synthesis, and cAMP has been proved to cause enteropooling [36–38]. Prostaglandin antagonists can relieve diarrhea associated with food intolerance [39]. Among the known prostaglandins, only PGD_2 and PGI_2 lack this enteropooling effect [40]. PGI_2 has an inhibitory effect on stimulated pancreatic secretion [26], while PGE_2 facilitates it [30]. Prostaglandins can stimulate the release of both insulin and glucagon, depending upon the glucose levels [41,42].

Gastrointestinal Motility

PGF increases lower esophageal sphincter tone, while PGE_2 and PGI_2 relax it [43,44]. In humans, oral administration of indomethacin causes an increase in the lower esophageal sphincter tone [45], and intravenous PGE_2 relieved sphincter spasm in patients with achalasia [46].

Isolated strips of longitudinal smooth muscle from the gut are contracted by all prostaglandins, while circular muscles are relaxed by PGE [47]. The stimulatory action of prostaglandins is generally the result of a direct action, but in some cases it may be cholinergically mediated, at least in part [48]. Several prostaglandins stimulate small intestinal motility, which may allow them to be of therapeutic benefit in patients with ileus [49].

Biliary Motility

On biliary smooth muscles, prostaglandins have an effect similar to that of cholecystokinin (that is, direct contraction of the gallbladder and relaxation of the sphincter of Oddi in vitro) [50], but the effectiveness of the several types of prostaglandins is variable. Their effects on circular and longitudinal muscle are different [51], and the sensitivity depends upon the species studied [52]. Unlike prostaglandin E, which decreases the activity of the sphincter of Oddi, $PGF_{2\alpha}$ caused an increase in its contractility [53].

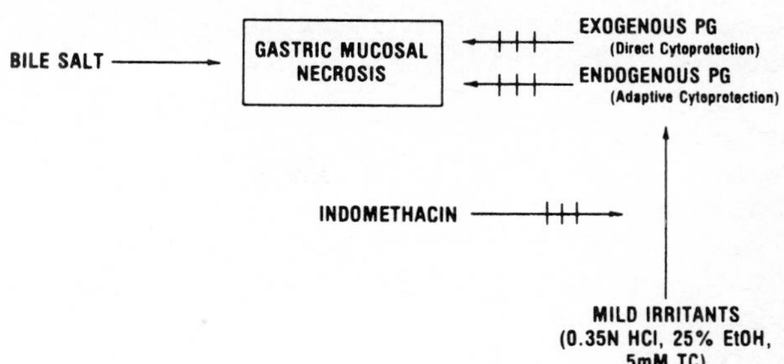

Figure 31-3. Diagram summarizing the two forms of cytoprotection by prostaglandins, namely, that due to exogenous administration of prostaglandins (direct cytoprotection) and that due to endogenous formation of prostaglandins (adaptive cytoprotection). (From Chaudhury TK, Robert A, Dig Dis Sci 25:830, 1980.)

Cytoprotection

A special property of all prostaglandins is cytoprotection. This effect was first noticed when some prostaglandins were found to prevent experimental gastric ulceration [54]. Although ulcer prevention was first ascribed to antisecretory actions, prostaglandins later proved to be cytoprotective, even in doses too low to affect gastric secretion [55], and PGF, which has no effect on gastric secretion, shared this effect as well [56]. Prostaglandins protect the gastric mucosa against all kinds of necrotizing agents (e.g., boiling water, absolute ethanol) [57]. The mechanism for these somewhat puzzling effects is poorly understood. Pretreatment with prostaglandins prevents damage of the mucosa, but only in the presence of glucocorticoids [58]. In addition, it has been shown that nonsteroidal anti-inflammatory compounds (e.g., aspirin, indomethacin), which have well-known ulcerogenic side effects, cause gastric mucosal damage by blocking the synthesis of prostaglandins at the cyclo-oxygenase level [59–61]. A new phenomenon has been recently described, called adaptive cytoprotection, which refers to the cytoprotective effect achieved by pretreatment with mild irritants before the damaging agent is administered. The administration of a subthreshold dose of ulcerogens is shown to increase gastric prostaglandin levels in a dose-dependent manner. Mild irritants prevent mucosal damage, but administration of indomethacin eliminated this effect, giving further support to the concept that the adaptive cytoprotection is mediated by prostaglandins [62] (Fig 31-3).

Several theories have been established to explain cytoprotection. Besides their eventual effect on gastric secretion, prostaglandins may defend mucosal integrity by stimulating gastric and duodenal secretion of bicarbonate [63,64]. They also enhance mucus production [65–68] and mucosal blood flow [16], and they have trophic effects on gastric mucosa [69] and to a lesser extent on the mucosa of the whole gastrointestinal tract [70], so they very likely activate all known defense mechanisms. Recent data suggest that insufficient production of prostaglandins in response to the gastric acid load may have a role in the genesis of duodenal ulcer [71]. Prostaglandin-related cytoprotection was recently shown to be a general phenomenon, protecting parenchymal cells too, probably by stabilization of membranes [72]. Evaluation of the role of cytoprotection in clinical trials with prostaglandins in the treatment of peptic ulcer is complicated by the antisecretory effects of the agents. If an ulcer heals, is it because of cytoprotection or acid reduction? The physiologic significance of cytoprotection is difficult to evaluate and some have expressed skepticism.

Modulators of Peptide Hormone Responses

Prostaglandins may play an important role in modifying or mediating the effects of some peptide hormones in the gastrointestinal tract. Indomethacin (a cyclo-oxygenase inhibitor) abolishes the inhibitory effect of somatostatin in the isolated rat stomach [73]. Furthermore, indomethacin has been shown to decrease basal somatostatin release from the pancreas and stomach, and it abolishes the acetylcholine-stimulated increase in somatostatin from both stomach and pancreas, which suggests that release of somatostatin is dependent upon prostaglandins [74].

Rioux et al [75] found that contraction of the isolated portal vein stimulated by neurotensin was inhibited by indomethacin. Prostaglandins also appear to modify other neurotensin effects. Bardon and Ruckebusch [76] recently reported that pretreatment with prostaglandin synthetase inhibitors reduced the magnitude of both the neurotensin- and meal-stimulated colonic hypermotility responses. We have recently found that indomethacin treatment abolishes the inhibitory action of neurotensin on pentagastrin-stimulated gastric acid secretion, and indomethacin inhibits neurotensin- and secretin-stimulated pancreatic exocrine secretion and neurotensin-stimulated pancreatic polypeptide release in the dog (unpublished results).

The products of metabolism of arachidonate, prostaglandins, and leukotrienes appear to play an important role in the stimulation-secretion coupling of insulin and glucagon from pancreatic islet cells [77].

Leukotrienes

In 1940, Kellaway and Trethewie [78] first described a substance released from the guinea pig lung after antigen stimulation, characterized by a slow onset of the response. Hence, it was named slow-reacting substance of anaphylaxis (SRS-A), but its chemical structure was unknown until 1979 [79], when the term leukotriene (LT) was introduced, referring to its origin from neutrophil leukocytes. Leukotrienes originate from the same arachidonic acid as prostanoids, synthesized by lipoxygenase, but the structures and reactions involved in the metabolism of leukotrienes are completely different from the prostanoid metabolic pathways. Unlike prostanoids, formation of leukotrienes is not blocked by cyclo-oxygenase inhibitors but only by steroids that block arachidonic acid formation, thus preventing both prostaglandin and leukotriene synthesis [80].

The different categories of leukotrienes are named according to the different side ligands (LTA, LTB . . . LTE), and the number of double bonds in the basic 20 carbon atom structure determines the attached number (e.g., LTC_3, LTC_4, LTC_5), in a fashion similar to the naming of the prostaglandins. Leukotrienes have already been identified in leukocytes, macrophages, mastocytes, and lung tissue of different species [81–84]. They are released upon antigenic stimulation from various tissues [78,85]. Extensive studies have shown that the inflammatory-anaphylactic properties of leukotrienes are 30 to 40 times more potent than histamine in edema formation and airway obstruction in the guinea pig, monkey, and in humans; the airways of rats and rabbits were not found to be sensitive to LTC_4 and LTD_4 [86–89].

Although SRS-A was first identified using guinea pig ileal muscle strips, few studies have been published until now on the gastrointestinal effects of leukotrienes. In the ileal smooth muscle, species differences, similar to those mentioned previously in connection with airway musculature, have been shown (that is, guinea pig ileum is very sensitive to leukotrienes, but the same preparation from rats does not respond), whereas rat stomach and colonic muscle contracted in a dose-dependent manner after administration of LTC_4 and LTD_4 [90,91]. Using rabbit parietal cells, LTC_4 and LTD_4 stimulated the ^{14}C aminopyrine uptake of rabbit parietal cells, and this effect was slightly less than that of histamine or carbachol on a molar basis [92].

REFERENCES

1. Christ EJ, van Dorp DA: Comparative aspects of prostaglandin biosynthesis in animal tissues. Biochim Biophys Acta 270:537, 1972.
2. LeDuc LE, Needleman P: Regional localization of prostacyclin and thromboxane synthesis in dog stomach and intestinal tract. J Pharmacol Exp Ther 211:181, 1979.
3. Hensby C: Physical methods in prostaglandin research, in Crabbe P (ed): *Prostaglandin Research*. New York, Academic Press, 1977, p 104.
4. Ferreira SH: Prostaglandin bioassay, in Berti F, Samuelsson B, Velo GP (ed): *Prostaglandins and Thromboxanes*. New York, Plenum Press, 1977, pp 27–40.
5. Johansson C, Bergstrom S: Prostaglandins and protection of the gastroduodenal mucosa. Scand J Gastroenterol (Suppl 77):21, 1982.
6. Robert A: Effects of prostaglandins on the stomach and the intestine. Prostaglandins 6:523, 1974.
7. Robert A, Schultz JR, Nezamis JE, et al: Gastric antisecretory and antiulcer properties of PGE_2, 15-methyl PGE_2, and 16,16-dimethyl PGE_2. Intravenous, oral and intrajejunal administration. Gastroenterology 70:359, 1976.
8. Robert A, Magerlein BJ: 15-methyl PGE_2 and 16,16-dimethyl PGE_2: Potent inhibitors of gastric secretion. Adv Biosci 9:247, 1973.
9. Konturek SJ, Hanchar AJ, Nezamis JE, et al: Comparison of prostacyclin (PGI_2) and prostaglandin E_2 (PGE_2) on gastric secretory and serum gastrin responses to a meal, pentagastrin and histamine. Gastroenterology 76:1173, 1979.
10. Moncada S, Salmon JA, Vane JR, et al: Formation of prostacyclin and its product 6-oxo-$PGF_{1\alpha}$ by the gastric mucosa of several species. J Physiol (Lond) 275:4P, 1977.
11. Becker HD, Reeder DD, Thompson JC: Effect of prostaglandin E_1 on the release of gastrin and gastric secretion in dogs. Endocrinology 93:1148, 1973.
12. Jacobson ED: Comparison of prostaglandin E_1 and norepinephrine on the gastric mucosal circulation. Proc Soc Exp Biol Med 133:516, 1970.
13. Miller TA, Henagan JM, Robert A: Effect of 16,16-dimethyl PGE_2 on resting and histamine-stimulated gastric mucosal blood flow. Dig Dis Sci 25:561, 1980.

14. Whittle BJR: Mechanisms underlying gastric mucosal damage induced by indomethacin and bile-salts, and the actions of prostaglandins. Br J Pharmacol 60:455, 1977.
15. Walus KM, Gustaw P, Konturek SJ: Differential effects of prostaglandins and arachidonic acid on gastric circulation and oxygen consumption. Prostaglandins 20:1089, 1980.
16. Konturek SJ, Robert A, Hanchar AJ, et al: Comparison of prostacyclin and prostaglandin E_2 on gastric secretion, gastrin release, and mucosal blood flow in dogs. Dig Dis Sci 25:673, 1980.
17. Soll AH: Pharmacology of inhibitors of parietal cell function. J Clin Gastroenterol 3(Suppl 2):85, 1981.
18. Major JS, Scholes P: The localization of a histamine H_2-receptor adenylate cyclase system in canine parietal cells and its inhibition by prostaglandins. Agents Actions 8:324, 1978.
19. Vantrappen G, Janssens J, Popiela T, et al: Effect of 15(R)-15-methyl prostaglandin E_2 (Arbaprostil) on the healing of duodenal ulcer. A double-blind multicenter study. Gastroenterology 83:357, 1982.
20. Rybicka J, Gibinski K: Methyl-prostaglandin E_2 analogues for healing of gastroduodenal ulcers. Scand J Gastroenterol 13:155, 1978.
21. Ippoliti AF, Isenberg JI, Maxwell V, et al: The effect of 16,16 dimethyl prostaglandin E_2 on meal-stimulated gastric acid secretion and serum gastrin in duodenal ulcer patients. Gastroenterology 70:488, 1976.
22. Karim SMM, Carter DC, Bhana D, et al: Effect of orally and intravenously administered prostaglandin (15(R)15-methyl E_2) on gastric secretion in man. Adv Biosci 9:255, 1973.
23. Miller TA, Henagan JM, Watkins LA, et al: Prostaglandin-induced bicarbonate secretion in the canine stomach: Characteristics and evidence for a cholinergic mechanism. J Surg Res 35:105, 1983.
24. Rudick J, Gonda M, Dreiling DA, et al: Effects of prostaglandin E_1 on pancreatic exocrine function. Gastroenterology 60:272, 1971.
25. Case RM, Scratcherd T: Prostaglandin action on pancreatic blood flow and on electrolyte and enzyme secretion by exocrine pancreas *in vivo* and *in vitro*. J Physiol 226:393, 1972.
26. Konturek SJ, Tasler J, Jaworek J, et al: Prostacyclin inhibits pancreatic secretion. Am J Physiol 238:G531, 1980.
27. Rosenberg V, Biezunski D, Gonda M, et al: Influence of a synthetic prostaglandin analog on pancreatic secretion. Surgery 79:509, 1976.
28. Watson LC, Miller TA, Rayford PL, et al: Effect of prostaglandin E_1 on plasma secretin and pancreatic exocrine function in dogs. Surg Forum 27:426, 1976.
29. Iwatsuki K, Chiba S: Effects of prostacyclin and prostaglandin E_2 on the secretion of pancreatic juice in the dog. Clin Exp Pharmacol Physiol 9:495, 1982.
30. Marshall PJ, Dixon JF, Hokin LE: Prostaglandin E_2 derived from phosphatidylinositol breakdown in the exocrine pancreas facilitates secretion by an action on the ducts. J Pharmacol Exp Ther 221:645, 1982.
31. Heisler S: Effect of various prostaglandins and serotonin on protein secretion from rat exocrine pancreas. Experientia 29:1234, 1973.
32. Chauvelot L, Heisler S, Huot J, et al: Prostaglandins and enzyme secretion from dispersed rat pancreatic acinar cells. Life Sci 25:913, 1979.
33. Bauduin H, Galand N, Boeynaems JM: In vitro stimulation of prostaglandin synthesis in the rat pancreas by carbamylcholine, caerulein and secretin. Prostaglandins 22:35, 1981.
34. Marshall PJ, Dixon JF, Hokin LE: Evidence for a role in stimulus-secretion coupling of prostaglandins derived from release of arachidonoyl residues as a result of phosphatidyl-inositol breakdown. Proc Natl Acad Sci USA 77:3292, 1980.
35. Bennett A: The relationship of prostaglandins to cholera. Prostaglandins 11:425, 1976.
36. Field M: Ion transport in rabbit ileal mucosa. II. Effects of cyclic 3′,5′-AMP. Am J Physiol 221:992, 1971.
37. Kimberg DV, Field M, Gershon E, et al: Effects of prostaglandins and cholera enterotoxin on intestinal mucosal cyclic AMP accumulation. J Clin Invest 53:941, 1974.
38. Simon B, Kather H: Human gastric mucosal adenylate cyclase activity: Effects of various cytoprotective prostaglandins. Eur J Clin Invest 10:481, 1980.
39. Lessof MH, Anderson JA, Youlten LJF: Prostaglandins in the pathogenesis of food intolerance. Ann Allergy 51:249, 1983.
40. Robert A, Hanchar AJ, Lancaster C, et al: Prostacyclin (PGI_2) and PGD_2 prevent enteropooling and diarrhea caused by prostaglandins and cholera toxin. Fed Proc 38:1239, 1979.
41. Pek S, Tai T-Y, Elster A: Stimulatory effects of prostaglandins E-1, E-2, and F-2-alpha on glucagon and insulin release in vitro. Diabetes 27:801, 1978.
42. Horie H, Matsuyama T, Namba M, et al: Modulation by prostaglandin D_2 of glucagon and insulin secretion in the perfused rat pancreas. Prostaglandins Leukotrienes Med 12:315, 1983.
43. Daniel EE, Crankshaw J, Sarna S: Prostaglandins and myogenic control of tension in lower esophageal sphincter *in vitro*. Prostaglandins 17:629, 1979.
44. Goyal RK, Rattan S, Hersh T: Comparison of the effects of prostaglandins E_1, E_2, and A_2, and of hypovolumic hypotension on the lower esophageal sphincter. Gastroenterology 65:608, 1973.
45. Kruidinier J, Tao P, Wilson DE: The role of prostaglandins in lower esophageal sphincter pressure in man. Clin Res 26:663A, 1978.
46. Goyal RK, Mukhopadhyay A, Rattan S: Effect of prostaglandin E_2 on the lower esophageal sphincter in normal subjects and patients with achalasia. Clin Res 22:358A, 1974.
47. Bennett A, Eley KG, Scholes GB: Effect of prostaglandins E_1 and E_2 on intestinal motility in the guinea-pig and rat. Br J Pharmacol 34:639, 1968.
48. Bennett A, Eley KG, Scholes GB: Effects of prosta-

glandins E_1 and E_2 on human, guinea-pig and rat isolated small intestine. Br J Pharmacol 34:630, 1968.
49. Ruwart MJ, Klepper MS, Rush BD: The beneficial effects of prostaglandins in post-operative ileus. Gastroenterology 74:1088, 1978.
50. Andersson K-E, Andersson R, Hedner P, et al: Parallelism between mechanical and metabolic responses to cholecystokinin and prostaglandin E_2 in extrahepatic biliary tract. Acta Physiol Scand 89:571, 1973.
51. Wood JR, Saverymuttu SH, Ashbrooke AB, et al: Effects of various prostanoids on gallbladder muscle, in Samuelsson B, Ramwell PW, Paoletti R (eds): *Advances in Prostaglandin and Thromboxane Research.* New York, Raven Press, 1980, pp 1569–1571.
52. Mroczka J, Baer HP, Scott GW: Effects of prostaglandins on isolated dog gallbladder and cystic duct, in Wienbeck M (ed): *Motility of the Digestive Tract.* New York, Raven Press, 1982, pp 421–426.
53. Martinez E, Sarles JC: Effect of prostaglandins E_1, E_2 and $F_{2\alpha}$ on the electric activity of the sphincter of Oddi in living rabbit. Eur Surg Res 15:322, 1983.
54. Jacobson ED, Chaudhury TK, Thompson WJ: Mechanism of gastric mucosal cytoprotection by prostaglandins. Gastroenterology 70:897, 1976.
55. Odonkor P, Mowat C, Himal HS: Prevention of sepsis-induced gastric lesions in dogs by cimetidine via inhibition of gastric secretion and by prostaglandin via cytoprotection. Gastroenterology 80:375, 1981.
56. Robert A, Nezamis JE, Lancaster C, et al: Cytoprotection by prostaglandins in rats. Prevention of gastric necrosis produced by alcohol, HCl, NaOH, hypertonic NaCl, and thermal injury. Gastroenterology 77:433, 1979.
57. Robert A: Cytoprotection by prostaglandins. Scand J Gastroenterol 16(Suppl 67):223, 1981.
58. Szabo S, Gallagher GT, Horner HC, et al: Role of the adrenal cortex in gastric mucosal protection by prostaglandins, sulfhydryls, and cimetidine in the rat. Gastroenterology 85:1384, 1983.
59. Vane JR: Inhibition of prostaglandin synthesis as a mechanism of action for aspirin-like drugs. Nature New Biol 231:232, 1971.
60. Whittle BJR: Relationship between the prevention of rat gastric erosions and the inhibition of acid secretion by prostaglandins. Eur J Pharmacol 40:233, 1976.
61. Guth PH, Aures D, Paulsen G: Topical aspirin plus HCl gastric lesions in the rat. Cytoprotective effect of prostaglandin, cimetidine, and probanthine. Gastroenterology 76:88, 1979.
62. Robert A, Nezamis JE, Lancaster C, et al: Mild irritants prevent gastric necrosis through "adaptive cytoprotection" mediated by prostaglandins. Am J Physiol 245:G113, 1983.
63. Kauffman GL Jr, Reeve JJ Jr, Grossman MI: Gastric bicarbonate secretion: Effect of topical and intravenous 16,16-dimethyl prostaglandin E_2. Am J Physiol 239:G44, 1980.
64. Rees WDW, Warhurst G, Turnberg LA: Demonstration of HCO_3^- secretion by the human stomach in vivo. Gut 22:A882, 1981.
65. Bolton JP, Palmer D, Cohen MM: Effect of the E_2 prostaglandins on gastric mucus production in rats. Surg Forum 27:402, 1976.
66. Bolton JP, Cohen MM: Stimulation of non-parietal cell secretion in canine Heidenhain pouches by 16,16-dimethyl prostaglandin E_2. Digestion 17:291, 1978.
67. Johansson C, Kollberg B: Stimulation by intragastrically administered E_2 prostaglandins of human gastric mucus output. Eur J Clin Invest 9:229, 1979.
68. Ruppin H, Person B, Robert A, et al: Gastric cytoprotection in man by prostaglandin E_2. Scand J Gastroenterol 16:647, 1981.
69. Konturek SJ, Brzozowski T, Piastucki I, et al: Role of mucosal prostaglandins and DNA synthesis in gastric cytoprotection by luminal epidermal growth factor. Gut 22:927, 1981.
70. Reinhart WH, Muller O, Halter F: Influence of long-term 16,16-dimethyl prostaglandin E_2 treatment on the rat gastrointestinal mucosa. Gastroenterology 85:1003, 1983.
71. Ahlquist DA, Dozois RR, Zinsmeister AR, et al: Duodenal prostaglandin synthesis and acid load in health and in duodenal ulcer disease. Gastroenterology 85:522, 1983.
72. Muller P, Dammann HG, Simon B: Wirken prostaglandine auch auberhalb des magen-darm-epithels zytoprotektiv? Leber Magen Darm 12:154, 1982.
73. Ligumski M, Goto Y, Debas H, et al: Prostaglandins mediate inhibition of gastric acid secretion by somatostatin in the rat. Science 219:301, 1983.
74. Schusdziarra V, Stapelfeldt W, Klier M, et al: Effect of acetylcholine on the release of pancreatic and gastric somatostatin-like immunoreactivity in normal, chemically sympathectomized and indomethacin-treated dogs. Hepatogastroenterology 29:153, 1982.
75. Rioux F, Quirion R, Leblanc MA, et al: Possible interactions between neurotensin and prostaglandins in the isolated rat portal vein. Life Sci 27:259, 1980.
76. Bardon T, Ruckebusch Y: Neurotensin-induced colonic motor responses in dogs: A mediation by prostaglandins. Regul Pept 10:107, 1985.
77. Pek SB, Walsh MF: Eicosanoids as regulators of pancreatic islet hormone secretion. Adv Prostaglandin, Thromboxane Leukotriene Res 13:221, 1985.
78. Kellaway CH, Trethewie ER: The liberation of a slow-reacting smooth muscle-stimulating substance in anaphylaxis. Quart J Exp Physiol 30:121, 1940.
79. Morris HR, Taylor GW, Piper PJ, et al: Structure of slow-reacting substance of anaphylaxis from guinea-pig lung. Nature 285:104, 1980.
80. Blackwell GJ, Carnuccio R, Di Rosa M, et al: Macrocortin: A polypeptide causing the anti-phospholipase effect of glucocorticoids. Nature 287:147, 1980.
81. Morris HR, Taylor GW, Piper PJ, et al: Slow reacting substances (SRSs): The structure identification of SRSs from rat basophil leukaemia (RBL-1) cells. Prostaglandins 19:185, 1980.

82. Lewis RA, Austen KF, Drazen JM, et al: Slow reacting substances of anaphylaxis: Identification of leukotrienes C-1 and D from human and rat sources. Proc Natl Acad Sci USA 77:3710, 1980.
83. Orning L, Hammarstrom S, Samuelsson B: Leukotriene D: A slow reacting substance from rat basophilic leukemia cells. Proc Natl Acad Sci USA 77:2014, 1980.
84. Borgeat P, Samuelsson B: Arachidonic acid metabolism in polymorphonuclear leukocytes: Effects of ionophore A23187. Proc Natl Acad Sci USA 76:2148, 1979.
85. Wolbling RH, Aehringhaus U, Peskar BA, et al: Release of slow-reacting substance of anaphylaxis and leukotriene C_4-like immunoreactivity from guinea pig colonic tissue. Prostaglandins 25:809, 1983.
86. Smedegård G, Hedqvist P, Dahlen S-E, et al: Leukotriene C_4 affects pulmonary and cardiovascular dynamics in monkey. Nature 295:327, 1982.
87. Dahlen S-E, Hedqvist P, Hammarstrom S, et al: Leukotrienes are potent constrictors of human bronchi. Nature 288:484, 1980.
88. Jones TR, Davis C, Daniel EE: Pharmacological study of the contractile activity of leukotriene C_4 and D_4 on isolated human airway smooth muscle. Can J Physiol Pharmacol 60:638, 1982.
89. Hedqvist P, Dahlen S-E, Gustafsson L, et al: Biological profile of leukotrienes C_4 and D_4. Acta Physiol Scand 110:331, 1980.
90. Goldenberg MM, Subers EM: The reactivity of rat isolated gastrointestinal tissues to leukotrienes. Eur J Pharmacol 78:463, 1982.
91. Holme G, Brunet G, Piechuta H, et al: The activity of synthetic leukotriene C-1 on guinea pig trachea and ileum. Prostaglandins 20:717, 1980.
92. Magous R, Bali J-P, Rossi J-C, et al: Leukotrienes stimulate acid secretion from isolated gastric parietal cells. Biochem Biophys Res Commun 114:897, 1983.

Section Eight

Regulatory Interrelationships

Every metabolic function in an organism is related to all other functions. The regulation of gut function is influenced by some specific interactions, those, for example that exist between the brain and the gut, the gut and the endocrine pancreas, those among gastrin, calcium, and calcium regulatory hormones; and even some between the gut and the reproductive system. Those interrelationships are discussed in this section.

Chapter 32

Gastrin-Calcium-Calcitonin Axis

Marilyn Marx, M.D., Cary W. Cooper, Ph.D., and James C. Thompson, M.D.

HISTORICAL BACKGROUND

Reeder et al [1] showed in 1970 that intravenous infusion of calcium stimulated the release of gastrin in humans. Shortly thereafter, they demonstrated that calcium given by mouth also directly stimulated release of gastrin from antral mucosa, and that calcium given intravenously, orally, or intragastrically, would enhance gastrin release and gastric acid secretion [2,3]. Further, Cooper et al [4] have shown that infusion of low doses of parathyroid hormone stimulated gastrin release, even in the absence of hypercalcemia. This finding, together with the fact that gastrin can stimulate release of calcitonin [5,6], suggests a physiologic interrelationship, that is, a feedback loop, among calcium, calcium-regulating hormones, and gastrin (Fig 32-1). In addition, Inoue et al [7], in our laboratory, have recently systematically studied the effects of divalent cations other than calcium on the release of gastrointestinal hormones. They showed that the divalent cations, calcium, magnesium, and zinc, when given either intraduodenally or intravenously, stimulated release of cholecystokinin (CCK), pancreatic polypeptide, and gastrin in a qualitatively similar way.

More than a decade ago, Care et al [5] and Cooper et al [6,8] independently provided evidence suggesting that certain gastrointestinal hormones could serve as calcitonin secretagogues. Both groups clearly showed that the gastrointestinal hormones, CCK and gastrin, were potent calcitonin-releasing agents in the pig. Studies revealed that the amino acid residues responsible for causing calcitonin release were C-terminal residues common to both CCK and gastrin, which also are found in active natural or synthetic analogues such as caerulein and pentagastrin (Table 32-1) [9].

FACTORS INFLUENCING CALCITONIN RELEASE

Calcitonin release is tied to feeding and gastrointestinal activity. Gastrointestinal hormones, including gastrin and CCK, may play a role in promoting calcitonin release during feeding and intestinal absorption of nutrients and calcium. In

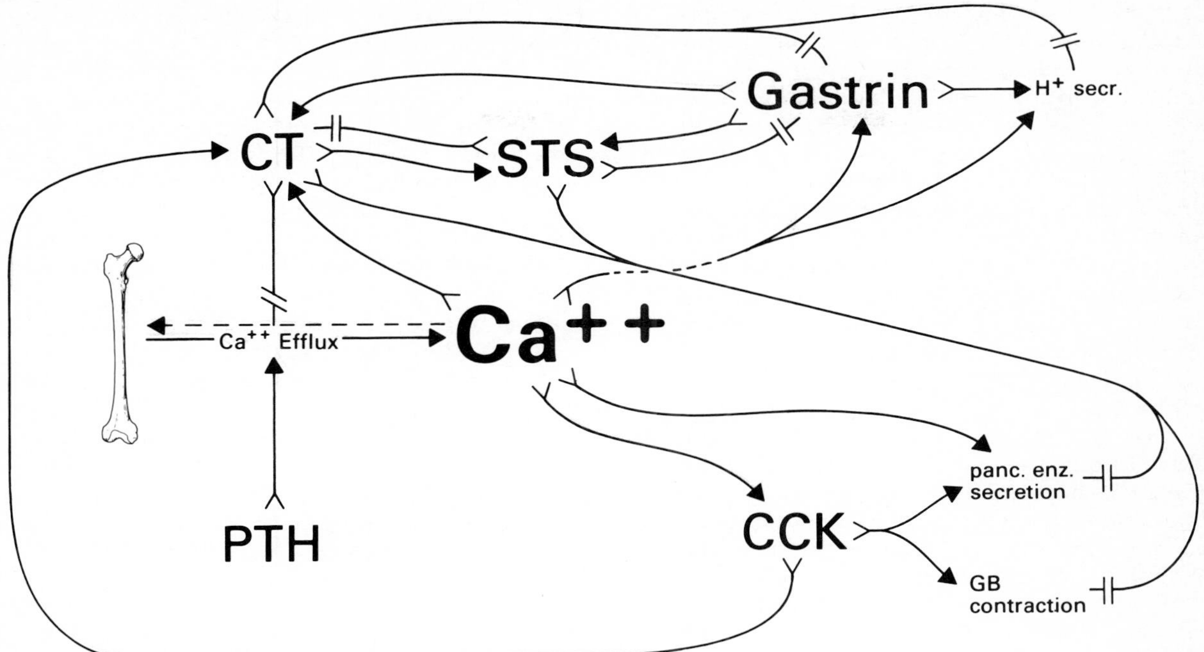

Figure 32-1. Diagrammatic representation of the interrelationship between calcium, calcium-regulating hormones, and gastrointestinal hormones. (CT = calcitonin; PTH = parathyroid hormone; CCK = cholecystokinin; STS = somatostatin.) Calcium stimulates gastrin release and acid secretion, while CT inhibits both. Gastrin stimulates the release of CT, a function that is utilized in the pentagastrin infusion test for medullary carcinoma of the thyroid. Calcium also releases CT. CT restricts efflux of calcium from bone and PTH stimulates calcium efflux and resorption of calcium from bone. In addition, calcium stimulates release of CCK and is a requisite for pancreatic enzyme secretion. CCK, like gastrin, can promote secretion of CT. Both CT and somatostatin inhibit gallbladder function and pancreatic enzyme secretion. CT effects on gastric and pancreatic functions may be direct or via enhanced release of somatostatin. Somatostatin actually inhibits release of all the agents shown. (By permission of Thompson JC and Marx M: Gastrointestinal hormones, in MM Ravitch et al (eds): *Current Problems in Surgery.* Chicago, Year Book Medical Publishers Inc, 1984.)

some species such as the pig, there is strong evidence that gastrin is a physiologically effective calcitonin secretagogue because 1) provoking endogenous gastrin release from the porcine gastric antrum causes calcitonin secretion [5,6], and 2) increases in blood gastrin no larger than those found

Table 32-1. **Relationships between C-terminal structure of analogs of gut peptides and their activity as calcitonin secretagogues**

Peptide	*Structure*	*Calcitonin-Releasing Activity*
Caerulein	pGlu-Glu-Asp-Tyr-Thr-Gly-Trp-Met-Asp-Phe-NH_2 HSO_3	+
CCK-8	-Asp-Tyr-Met-Gly-Trp-Met-Asp-Phe-NH_2 HSO_3	+
Pentagastrin	t-boc-βAla-Trp-Met-Asp-Phe-NH_2	+
Tetragastrin	-Trp-Met-Asp-Phe-NH_2	+
Trigastrin	-Met-Asp-Phe-NH_2	−
Modified tetragastrin	-Trp-Met-Asn-Phe-NH_2	−

Data from Talmage et al [9]. Peptides were tested by infusion into the pig thyroid artery; calcitonin was measured in thyroid venous effluent blood before and after infusion of test agents.

after a meal are sufficient to evoke an increase in calcitonin release [10]. In addition, Cooper et al [10] showed that concentrations of gastrin and calcitonin in pig thyroid venous blood show a strong positive correlation under a variety of experimental circumstances, and studies of temporal relationships have revealed that increased secretion of gastrin precedes the increased release of calcitonin (Cooper, unpublished data). Therefore, at least in the pig, gastrin is a physiologic regulator of postprandial calcitonin release. Because gastrin acts directly when infused into the thyroid artery [6,8], it seems clear that its action is directly on the thyroid C cells and not via some extrathyroidal intermediate.

Once gastrin was established as a potent, rapid-acting secretagogue for calcitonin, clinical interest was aroused. Hennessy et al [11] showed, for the first time, that pentagastrin could induce a rapid and abnormally large increase in plasma calcitonin in patients with medullary carcinoma of the thyroid. Currently, the preferred test uses a combined administration of pentagastrin and calcium [12].

Although it is clear that gastrin and CCK can elicit secretion of calcitonin in the pig, and that, in the pig, physiologic amounts of gastrin are sufficient to stimulate calcitonin release, the evidence that these gut hormones play a physiologic role in other species is unclear. In humans, there is evidence both for and against such findings, but the majority of studies emphasize the lack of clinical and physiologic relationships between gastrin and calcitonin. The findings of Heynen et al [13] suggest that the stimulation of calcitonin secretion by gastrin and its synthetic analogue, pentagastrin, is a pharmacologic rather than a physiologic phenomenon. More clinical studies will be needed in order to resolve this issue.

The postprandial gastrointestinal signals for C cell secretion of calcitonin may not be entirely humoral. In the rat, neurogenic stimuli may also be involved. Rats conditioned to eat at a specific time each day show a rise in calcitonin at the usual postprandial time, even when they are not given food and when they do not release gastrin [14]. In addition, studies in the pig [15] and in humans [16] suggest that adrenergic stimuli can elicit calcitonin release.

CALCITONIN ON GASTROINTESTINAL FUNCTION

The consequences of postprandial secretion of calcitonin are teleologically beneficial, both for the skeleton and for extraskeletal tissues. Calcitonin restricts efflux of calcium from the skeleton into the bloodstream; this is its best-established biologic effect. Not as widely accepted is its ability, at least in large amounts, to reduce both gastrin and gastric acid secretion [17,18] and to restrict pancreatic enzyme secretion and gallbladder contraction [19]. Jansen and Lamers [20] showed that calcitonin could inhibit bombesin-stimulated serum gastrin and gastric acid secretion in humans. Chiba et al [21] demonstrated that in the isolated perfused rat stomach, calcitonin caused a simultaneous dose-dependent increase in gastric somatostatin release and a decrease in gastrin secretion, with a significant inverse correlation evident between the two. They suggest the possibility that somatostatin mediates the suppression of gastrin secretion produced by calcitonin [21]. Thus, calcitonin inhibits a variety of gastrointestinal functions. The reason these actions are not widely appreciated may be because most of these studies have used high, nonphysiologic doses of calcitonin. Therefore, until more extensive studies are conducted using physiologic amounts of calcitonin, these gastrointestinal effects remain interesting pharmacologic phenomena.

Calcitonin Gene-Related Peptide (CGRP)

In the early 1980s, molecular biologic studies by Rosenfeld et al [22] revealed that primary transcripts of the calcitonin gene could code for an additional peptide, which they named CGRP. This 37-residue peptide was somewhat homologous to salmon calcitonin and bore some structural features (N-terminal S-S and C-terminal amide) essential for biologic activity of authentic calcitonin. According to Rosenfeld et al, brain and other nervous tissue processed the primary gene transcript in a tissue-specific fashion, so that mature mRNA in nerves coded for a prohormonal sequence, CGRP, and a C-terminal flanking peptide, while thyroid C cells processed the transcript so that mature mRNA coded for the same prohormonal sequence, calcitonin, and a flanking peptide. Posttranslational enzymatic processing in the brain then led to production of CGRP, while C-cell processing produced calcitonin. The existence of CGRP predicted by Rosenfeld et al from rat nucleotide sequences was confirmed by extraction and sequencing of human CGRP [23]. Rat and human CGRPs differ by 4 residues out of 37.

CGRP exists in nervous tissue in the peripheral as well as in the central nervous system (CNS). Many workers now believe that CGRP is the endogenous calcitonin-like ligand detected in earlier experimental studies, which indicated calcitonin immunoreactivity in the CNS and which showed marked effects when calcitonin was administered into the CNS of animals. This belief is supported by recent studies indicating that CGRP, given centrally, can mimic inhibition of both feeding [24] and of gastric acid secretion [25,26] and that CGRP and calcitonin can interact with the same binding site (receptor) in some tissues [27].

Numerous studies within the last few years suggest that CGRP may be produced in nervous tissue throughout the body, that it may be found in endocrine cells [28,29] and vasculature [30], and that it is likely to be not only ubiquitous but also an important regulator of various physiologic processes. In nerves, CGRP may function as a neuromodulator. In endocrine cells of the pancreas, CGRP has been colocalized with somatostatin [31] and has been found to inhibit release of insulin by β cells [32] and to stimulate acinar production of amylase [33]. In vivo studies have shown an inhibitory effect on gastric [25] and pancreatic [33a] secretion. CGRP has been shown to be a potent vasodilator [34]. These exciting new studies leave open the possibility that CGRP, produced in nerves, blood vessels, or endocrine cells of the gut, may prove to be an important local regulator of numerous gastrointestinal functions.

HYPOCALCEMIA AND ACUTE PANCREATITIS

Hypocalcemia frequently is observed in severe attacks of acute pancreatitis [35–37], although the etiology remains obscure. Almost 40 years ago, Edmondson and Berne [36] suggested that fatty acids, liberated by the action of pancreatic lipase, bound calcium as a soap. More recently, the acute fall in plasma calcium in acute pancreatitis at various times has been attributed to hyperglucagonemia [38], hypoalbuminemia [39], hypomagnesemia [40], parathyroid hormone deficiency [37], or hypercalcitoninemia [41]. However, the evidence for each explanation has remained controversial and unconvincing. Obviously, the factors involved in the homeostatic response of blood calcium during acute pancreatitis need further clarification.

The antisecretory actions of calcitonin on both gastric and pancreatic secretion prompted a prospective, randomized clinical evaluation of calcitonin in acute pancreatitis by Goebell et al [42]. Calcitonin did not influence mortality rate, but some favorable effects were observed, which included a more rapid decline of urinary and serum amylase activity, faster normalization of the leukocyte count and temperature, a more rapid disappearance of abdominal pain, a decreased frequency of pleural effusion, and a shorter hospital stay. No adverse effects of calcitonin treatment were observed. The authors concluded that calcitonin may be added as an adjuvant to the usual medical management of acute pancreatitis. Despite this report, there seems to be little enthusiasm for calcitonin therapy, and numerous anecdotal reports give no grounds for optimism.

GASTRIN-CALCITONIN INTERRELATIONSHIPS

Calcitonin may have a regulatory function in the release of gastrin. Becker et al [18] studied the effect of intravenous infusion of large doses of calcitonin on gastric secretion and serum gastrin levels in patients with duodenal ulcer disease, primary hyperparathyroidism, or the Zollinger-Ellison syndrome. Gastric secretion was greatly inhibited in all three groups of patients, and serum gastrin levels were depressed in all patients with elevated basal gastrin levels. In normal subjects, calcitonin strongly inhibited the serum gastrin response to food.

REFERENCES

1. Reeder DD, Jackson BM, Ban J, et al: Influence of hypercalcemia on gastric secretion and serum gastrin concentrations in man. Ann Surg 172:540, 1970.
2. Reeder D, Conlee JL, Thompson JC: Changes in gastric secretion and serum gastrin concentration in duodenal ulcer patients after oral calcium antacid, in Demling L (ed): *Gastrointestinal Hormones.* Stuttgart, Georg Thieme Verlag, 1972, pp 19–22.
3. Reeder DD, Conlee JL, Thompson JC: Calcium carbonate antacid and serum gastrin concentration in duodenal ulcer. Surg Forum 22:308, 1971.
4. Cooper CW, Bolman RM III, Lineham WM, et al: Interrelationships between calcium, calcemic hormones and gastrointestinal hormones. Recent Prog Horm Res 34:259, 1978.
5. Care AD, Bates RFL, Swaminathan R, et al: The role of gastrin as a calcitonin secretagogue. J Endocrinol 51:735, 1971.
6. Cooper CW, Schwesinger WH, Mahgoub AM, et al: Thyrocalcitonin: Stimulation of secretion by pentagastrin. Science 172:1238, 1971.
7. Inoue K, Fried GM, Wiener I, et al: Effect of divalent cations on gastrointestinal hormone release and exocrine pancreatic secretion in dogs. Am J Physiol 248:G28, 1985.
8. Cooper CW, Schwesinger WH, Ontjes DA, et al: Stimulation of secretion of pig thyrocalcitonin by gastrin and related hormonal peptides. Endocrinology 91:1079, 1972.
9. Talmage RV, Cooper CW, Toverud SU: The physiological significance of calcitonin, in Peck WA (ed): *Bone and Mineral Research. Annual 1. A Yearly Sur-*

vey of Developments in the Field of Bone and Mineral Metabolism. Amsterdam, Excerpta Medica, 1983, pp 74–143.

10. Cooper CW, McGuigan JE, Schwesinger WH, et al: Correlation between levels of gastrin and thyrocalcitonin in pig thyroid venous blood. Endocrinology 95:302, 1974.
11. Hennessy JF, Wells SA Jr, Ontjes DA, et al: A comparison of pentagastrin injection and calcium infusion as provocative agents for the detection of medullary carcinoma of the thyroid. J Clin Endocrinol Metab 39:487, 1974.
12. Wells SA Jr, Baylin SB, Linehan WM, et al: Provocative agents and the diagnosis of medullary carcinoma of the thyroid gland. Ann Surg 188:139, 1978.
13. Heynen G, Brassine A, Daubresse JC, et al: Lack of clinical and physiological relationship between gastrin and calcitonin in man. Eur J Clin Invest 11:331, 1981.
14. Talmage RV, Hirsch PF, VanderWiel CJ: Calcitonin, feeding and calcium conservation, in Pecile A (ed): *Calcitonin.* International Congress Series 540, Amsterdam, Excerpta Medica, 1980, pp 96–109.
15. Care AD, Bates RFL, Gitelman HJ: A possible role for the adenyl cyclase system in calcitonin release. J Endocrinol 48:1, 1970.
16. Vora NM, Williams GA, Hargis GK, et al: Comparative effect of calcium and of the adrenergic system on calcitonin secretion in man. J Clin Endocrinol Metab 46:567, 1978.
17. Hesch RD, Hufner M, Hasenhager B, et al: Inhibition of gastric secretion by calcitonin in man. Horm Metab Res 3:140, 1971.
18. Becker HD, Reeder DD, Scurry MT, et al: Inhibition of gastrin release and gastric secretion by calcitonin in patients with peptic ulcer. Am J Surg 127:71, 1974.
19. Hufner M, Hesch RD, Schmidt H, et al: The gastrointestinal effects of calcitonin. Acta Endocrinol (Copenh) Suppl 159:65, 1972.
20. Jansen JBMJ, Lamers CBHW: Calcitonin and secretin inhibit bombesin-stimulated serum gastrin and gastric acid secretion in man. Regul Pept 1:415, 1981.
21. Chiba T, Taminato T, Kadowaki S, et al: Effects of [$Asu^{1,7}$]-eel calcitonin on gastric somatostatin and gastrin release. Gut 21:94, 1980.
22. Rosenfeld MG, Mermod J-J, Amara SG, et al: Production of a novel neuropeptide encoded by the calcitonin gene via tissue-specific RNA processing. Nature 304:129, 1983.
23. Morris HR, Panico M, Etienne T, et al: Isolation and characterization of human calcitonin gene-related peptide. Nature 308:746, 1984.
24. Krahn DD, Gosnell BA, Levine AS, et al: Effects of calcitonin gene-related peptide on food intake. Peptides 5:861, 1984.
25. Lenz HJ, Mortrud MT, Rivier J, et al: Calcitonin gene-related peptide (CGRP) inhibits gastric acid secretion (GAS). Clin Res 32:26A, 1984.
26. Tache Y, Gunion M, Lauffenburger M, et al: Inhibition of gastric acid secretion by intracerebral injection of calcitonin gene related peptide (CGRP) in rats. Gastroenterology 86:1272, 1984.
27. Goltzman D, Mitchell J: Interactions of calcitonin and calcitonin gene-related peptide at receptor sites in target tissues. Science 227:1343, 1985.
28. Cooper CW, Borosky SA, Peng T-C: Presence of calcitonin gene-related peptide in the rat thyroid and its secretion from baby rat thyroids in vitro. Abstract Booklet, 7th Annual Meeting of the American Society of Bone and Mineral Research, A377, 1985.
29. Sabate MI, Stolarsky LS, Polak JM, et al: Regulation of neuroendocrine gene expression by alternative RNA processing. Colocalization of calcitonin and calcitonin gene-related peptide in thyroid C-cells. J Biol Chem 260:2589, 1985.
30. Mulderry PK, Ghatei MA, Rodrigo J, et al: Calcitonin gene-related peptide in cardiovascular tissues of the rat. Neuroscience 14:947, 1985.
31. Fujimura M, Hancock MB, Cooper CW, et al: Immunocytochemical localization of calcitonin gene-related peptide in pancreatic islet cells of the rat. Gastroenterology 88:1390, 1985.
32. Greeley GH Jr, Alwmark A, Cooper CW, et al: Calcitonin and calcitonin-gene related peptide inhibition of insulin secretion in vitro. Fed Proc 44:1391, 1985.
33. Seifert H, Sawchenko P, Chesnut J, et al: Receptor for calcitonin gene-related peptide: Binding to exocrine pancreas mediates biological actions. Am J Physiol 249:G147, 1985.

33a. Nealon WH, Beauchamp RD, Townsend CM Jr., et al: Comparative potencies of calcitonin gene-related peptide and calcitonin in the regulation of canine pancreatic exocrine function. Surg Forum 36:142, 1985.

34. Brain SD, Williams TJ, Tippins JR, et al: Calcitonin gene-related peptide is a potent vasodilator. Nature 313:54, 1985.
35. Edmondson HA, Fields IA: Relation of calcium and lipids to acute pancreatic necrosis. Report of fifteen cases, in one of which fat embolism occurred. Arch Int Med 69:177, 1942.
36. Edmondson HA, Berne CJ: Calcium changes in acute pancreatic necrosis. Surg Gynecol Obstet 79:240, 1944.
37. Condon JR, Ives D, Knight MJ, et al: The aetiology of hypocalcaemia in acute pancreatitis. Br J Surg 62:115, 1975.
38. Cortes EP: Pancreatitis and calcium metabolism. Ann Int Med 74:1014, 1971.
39. Imrie CW, Allam BF, Ferguson JC: Hypocalcaemia of acute pancreatitis: The effect of hypoalbuminaemia. Curr Med Res Opin 4:101, 1976.
40. Edmondson HA, Berne CJ, Homann RE Jr, et al: Calcium, potassium, magnesium and amylase disturbances in acute pancreatitis. Am J Med 12:34, 1952.
41. deBoer AC, Mulder H, Fischer HRA, et al: Characteristic changes in the concentrations of some peptide hormones, in particular those regulating serum calcium, in acute pancreatitis and myocardial infarction. Acta Med Scand 209:193, 1981.
42. Goebell H, Ammann R, Herfarth C, et al: A double-blind trial of synthetic salmon calcitonin in the treatment of acute pancreatitis. Scand J Gastroenterol 14:881, 1979.

Chapter 33

Brain-Gut Axis

Marilyn Marx, M.D., and George H. Greeley, Jr., Ph.D.

HISTORY

Although most if not all peripheral organ systems are influenced, to some degree, by the central nervous system (CNS), there seems to be a special connection between the CNS and the gut in mammals as well as in lower nonmammalian vertebrates and in nonvertebrates. This special relationship stems from the finding that many of the small peptides discovered initially in the CNS are also present in the gut; conversely, many of the peptides first isolated from the gut have also been localized in the CNS. The study of this aspect of gut physiology has received dramatic attention during the last decade, due in part to technical advances in immunocytochemistry, radioimmunoassay, neurophysiology, and molecular biology [1–11].

In most animals, the intake of foodstuffs brings about changes in gastric motility and secretion. The arrival of partially digested food into the small bowel is accompanied by a stimulation of pancreatic exocrine secretion, mucosal blood flow, and bowel motor activity [12]. Gastric and pancreatic phases of the response of the gut that accompany food ingestion are controlled partially by humoral mechanisms that involve, inter alia, gastrin, cholecystokinin (CCK), secretin, gastric inhibitory polypeptide (GIP), insulin, and glucagon, as well as the intrinsic or enteric nervous systems. The importance of the CNS seems limited to the cephalic phase, at least in terms of our current understanding. The gut is innervated by an immense local, somewhat autonomous nervous system, which is called the enteric nervous system (ENS) [13,14]. The activity of the enteric nervous system is probably regulated, in part, by the CNS [12].

Brown [15] states that the CNS may regulate visceral functions by one of three efferent control systems. These three systems are 1) the brain-hypothalamic-pituitary hormone circuit (for example, TRH-TSH-T_4); 2) the autonomic nervous system; and 3) the putative direct action of brain factors that exert their influence upon their peripheral targets via the bloodstream. It seems intriguing that peptides that are common to the CNS and gut probably play intermediary roles as neurotransmitters or neuromodulators in the regulation of gut function by the CNS and ENS [9,11,14]. For instance, in humans, gastric acid secretion often increases during or following stressful episodes (trauma, injuries, or emotional stress) [16]. The CNS also participates in the production of nausea and vomiting and other maladies of gastroduodenal motility. Although both humoral and neural pathways interface with the CNS and gut, whether these brain-gut peptides are the substrate in the response of the CNS and ENS is not clear.

From an historical perspective, the initial contribution to the development of the brain-gut axis occurred in 1931 when von Euler and Gaddum [17] discovered that both brain and intestinal extracts of the horse stimulated contractions of rabbit intestine that were not blocked by atropine and were, therefore, not due to acetylcholine. The material, which they called substance P (for preparation), was the first example of a biologically active peptide found in both brain and gut. The dual distribution of substance P and many other peptides is an example of biologic conservation whereby a substance is used by two or more anatomically distant systems.

Cholecystokinin is an excellent example of a peptide that may play a role as a gastrointestinal endocrine effector and as a neurotransmitter in the CNS [18]. CCK appeared early in phylogenetic evolution, within the neuronal elements of invertebrates. Immunocytochemical studies have localized CCK-like immunoreactivity in nerve cells of the hydra, a coelenterate, which has the most primitive nervous system in the animal kingdom [19]. The distribution of CCK in the CNS is different from that of all other known peptides, except for vasoactive intestinal peptide, in that both CCK and vasoactive intestinal peptide (VIP) are predominantly cerebral cortical peptides, although both have a wide extracortical distribution [20,21]. Outside of the cerebral cortex, the highest concentration is in the caudate nucleus [22]. Substantial amounts of CCK-like immunoreactivity are also present in the posterior lobe of the pituitary gland [22], and the majority of the CCK found in the posterior lobe has been shown to originate in the periventricular nuclei of the hypothalamus. Simon-Assmann et al [23] from our laboratory have studied the distribution and molecular heterogeneity of CCK in different regions of the CNS in rats and cows. They found CCK-8 and CCK-33 to be widely distributed throughout the CNS of both species; the CCK was biologically active in all regions of the brain. The distribution of the two molecular forms was similar, and they were present in similar concentrations.

Specific high-affinity cholecystokinin binding sites are present in rat and guinea pig brains [24,25]. In addition to the presence of CCK receptors in the brain and pancreas, CCK receptors have been identified in the rat vagus nerve [26]. More importantly, CCK has been reported to produce a variety of behavioral and physiologic effects after administration into the CNS. These CNS effects are appetite regulation [27,28]; hyperglycemia [29]; hypothermia [30]; analgesia [31]; CNS depression [31,32]; ptosis [31]; rotational syndrome [33]; and changes in anterior pituitary hormone release [34]. Lu et al [35] from our laboratory found that intracerebroventricular (ICV) administration of CCK-8 results in a dose-related release of pancreatic polypeptide (PP) from the pancreas in conscious dogs. There is abundant evidence, therefore, to suggest that CCK plays a role as a neurotransmitter or neuromodulator in the CNS.

Any concept that a gut peptide exerts a single biologic effect is certainly an oversimplification. Gut peptides in the brain may have central neural functions that are related to their gastrointestinal action in controlling digestion. For example, CCK-8 or bombesin, when given intracerebroventricularly, result in an inhibition of feeding in sheep and rats [36]. Since there are substantial quantities of CCK and bombesin in the CNS, it is not unlikely that in some species, or under specific circumstances, CCK and other peptides act as central satiety signals [18,28,36]. Peptides in the nervous system may also have trophic actions on their postsynaptic targets.

EFFECTS OF BRAIN-GUT PEPTIDES

In the following paragraphs, we will describe some of the CNS effects of the brain-gut peptides on gut function.

Numerous studies have addressed the effects of ICV administration of various peptides on gastric secretion [37,38]. The effects of neurotensin [39], thyrotropin-releasing hormone (TRH) [40,41], calcitonin [42], gastrin [43], somatostatin [44], bombesin [45,46], gastrin-releasing peptide (GRP) [47], and calcitonin-gene-related peptide (CGRP) [48] have been reported. Neurotensin may act via central catecholaminergic systems, since reserpine or 6-hydroxydopamine pretreatment abolishes the inhibitory effect of neurotensin [39]. Neurotensin can increase turnover of dopamine, noradrenaline, and serotonin in the CNS [49]. Noradrenaline, given in the lateral hypothalamic area, also inhibits gastric acid secretion in rats [50]. Morley et al [40] report that TRH, given intracerebroventricularly, causes a dose-dependent stimulation of gastric secretion that is blocked by opiates and is insensitive to bombesin. Tache et al [41] report that intracisternal TRH promotes gastric secretion in rats and that the stimulatory action of TRH is vagally dependent. ICV TRH also stimulates colonic motility in rats [51]. ICV calcitonin also inhibits gastric acid secretion and is 1,000 times more potent than when administered peripherally [42,52]. Gastrin or pentagastrin, injected into the hypothalamus, causes gastric acid secretion in rats [43], and somatostatin, surprisingly, when placed in the lateral hypothalamus, also stimulates a vagally dependent gastric acid secretion in rats [44]. Tache et al have shown that bombesin [45] and GRP [47] can inhibit gastric acid secretion when given intracisternally in rats. Pappas et al [53] have shown that ICV bombesin also inhibits gastric acid secretion in dogs.

Tache et al [37,46] have indicated that the central effects of bombesin and GRP are independent of interaction with CNS catecholaminergic, serotoninergic, dopaminergic, gabaergic, and cholinergic circuits in rats. The finding that regulation of gastric acid secretion in rats by these peptides is independent of other brain circuits is a mystery, since one would imagine an interaction between peptide and brain aminergic neurotransmitter pathways. Other data indicate that central noradrenergic [50,54] and gabaergic [55,56] pathways participate. The gastrin-releasing action of bombesin requires the intact pathways crossing the posterior, lateral, and medial borders of the lateral hypothalamus and is independent of changes in gastric pH. The lateral hypothalamus itself is not obligatory for the action of bombesin or gastric acid secretion [57].

Substance P [58], CGRP [59–61], and corticotropin-releasing factor (CRF) [62] also inhibit gastric acid secretion. It is not known whether these inhibitors of gastric secretion affect enteric release of serotonin, secretin, or gastric inhibitory polypeptide, which are all inhibitors of gastric acid secretion.

Brain lesion studies [63–65], stimulation of specific brain nuclei [65–69], and pharmacologic manipulation studies [70–72] also indicate that signals originating within the CNS participate in the regulation of gastric secretion.

ICV calcitonin can block ICV calcium-induced feeding in satiated rats and sheep [73,74], suggesting that calcitonin exerts its central influence by regulating calcium fluxes across neuronal membranes. In sheep, calcium-induced feeding was blocked by intrahypothalamic atropine and was reduced by phentolamine [74]. Calcium may alter excitability of CNS centers which regulate feeding.

Scant information is available with regards to central neural regulation of pancreatic exocrine secretion. Substances that activate the central vagal system (insulin, 2-DG) cause pancreatic release of water, bicarbonate, and enzymes in rats [75]. The central action of insulin and 2-DG on the vagal pathway is blocked by methadone at the central level. It appears that methadone exerts its effects on some aminergic or cholinergic circuit located between the lateral hypothalamus and the dorsal motor nucleus of the vagus. β-Endorphin and morphine also inhibit basal pancreatic exocrine secretion in dogs [76]. This effect is reversible by naloxone and α-endorphin, and met- and leu-enkephalin are ineffective. The central action of β-endorphin and morphine agrees with the data regarding the central action of small doses of β-endorphins and morphine on gastrointestinal motility and transit [77].

Intraventricular morphine also causes spike potentials and affects intestinal transit in the small intestine of the cat [78], which is naloxone- and naltrexone-sensitive. Bombesin, given centrally, also inhibits vagally stimulated contractions of the antrum [79]. Other studies in the rat indicate that ICV bombesin (0.1-1.0 μg) can slow gastric emptying, delay small bowel transit (0.01-3.0 μg), and increase the time of large bowel transit (1.0 μg) [80]. Calcitonin, given intracerebroventricularly, alters the intestinal motility pattern from a fasting to a fed pattern [81–83]. ICV CCK-8 promotes gastric emptying in dogs [84]. The exact mechanism of the central actions of morphine on gastrointestinal motility and pancreatic and gastric secretion is unclear. It may be that the CNS effects are mediated via neural (vagal), hormonal, or a combination of pathways.

The regulation of patterns of gut motility has been thought to be under the primary influence of neural and hormonal factors. A few studies now indicate that the CNS may affect motility patterns via its action on the ENS. Classically, the messages regulating gastric and small bowel motility were considered to travel via the vagus nerve, with acetylcholine as the only transmitter [85]. Recently, however, Schirmer et al [85] showed that stimulation of the periventricular hypothalamus affected gastric myoelectric and motor activity even in the face of atropine. CCK-8 has been shown to modulate the neurons in the dorsal vagal nucleus in response to gastric distention [86]. In sheep, ICV tetra- and pentagastrin and G-17 caused a premature short period of rumination, which suggests that G-17 and its C-terminal fragments may have a physiologic role in the central control of rumination [87]. In rats, somatostatin, given as a constant infusion, can increase the frequency of the myoelectric migrating complex (MMC) of the small bowel, whereas CCK-8 decreased the frequency of the MMC [88]. This finding is interesting, since the systemic actions of CCK-8 and somatostatin on intestinal motility can be reproduced by central administration. Bueno et al [89] have shown that 1) met-enkephalin appears to reorganize the MMC in fed dogs; 2) leu-enkephalin stimulates colonic motility, whereas met-enkephalin affects it by a peripheral action. In rats, ICV neurotensin and calcitonin restore the fasting pattern of MMC, and substance P shortens the postprandial pattern [90]. The central actions of neurotensin and calcitonin are abolished by vagotomy. In dogs, neurotensin can act centrally to regulate the pattern of antral and jejunal motility [91]. Bueno et al [92] also reported that neurotensin and calcitonin influenced the motility pattern of the small bowel by stimulating release of prostaglandin in the brain.

Certainly many questions need to be answered regarding proposed physiologic roles of brain-gut peptides. Whether peptides that are released from the gastrointestinal tract during a meal actually alter gut motility by a CNS action is not known. Do these peptides exert their effects on neural circuits between the CNS and ENS? It may be useful also to determine which pharmacologic manipulations modify motility by acting on the CNS, the ENS, or their connections.

Several studies have considered the possible presence and sites of actions of gut hormones on the pituitary and hypothalamus. A physiologic role for VIP in neuroendocrine events has been suggested by its ability to stimulate prolactin release in vitro [93–95] and in vivo [96,97], in addition to its ability to stimulate growth hormone [86] and luteinizing hormone (LH) secretion [97–99]. Samson et al [100] have shown that secretin, a close structural homologue of VIP, may also play a role in neuroendocrine physiology. The ability of secretin to stimulate adenylate cyclase activity in preparations of pituitary membranes [101] and to displace labeled VIP binding in rat brain membranes [102] suggests the presence and a site of action of secretin within the hypothalamo-pituitary axis. Samson et al [100] extended these observations by demonstrating the ability of secretin to stimulate the release of prolactin in a dose-related fashion from cultured, dispersed, rat pituitary cells. They conclude, however, that the possibility that secretin of gastrointestinal origin plays a physiologic role in the control of prolactin secretion is unlikely, since circulating levels were well below the doses required for the in vitro effect, and raising the circulating exogenous levels had little effect on prolactin release.

Morley et al [34] studied the effects of five peptides originally isolated from the gastrointestinal tract on the secretion of hormones from incubated rat anterior pituitary. They showed that CCK-8, as well as tetragastrin, stimulated release of growth hormone from cultured pituitary quarters, but neither bombesin, secretin, nor PP altered growth hormone secretion. At high concentrations, bombesin, secretin, CCK-8, and PP increased release of gonadotropin (LH, FSH). Gastrin-17 and CCK-39 were found to be potent stimulants of growth hormone release, whereas gut caerulein, a peptide related to CCK-8, failed to do so. CCK-8 released growth hormone from monolayer cultures of GH3 pituitary tumor cells [34]. Morley et al [34] showed that the inhibitory effect of somatostatin at 10^{-5} M was reversed by the addition of CCK-8 at 10^{-7} M and by the GH3 tumor system in vitro.

A large number of peptides have been shown to release growth hormone in vivo, but only TRH and arginine vasopressin have been demonstrated to have a direct effect on the pituitary in vitro [103,104]. Morley et al [34] suggested that CCK-8 may play a role as an endogenous growth hormone-releasing factor. The ability of CCK-8 at 10^{-7} M to neutralize the inhibitory effect of somatostatin at 10^{-5} M indicates that CCK-8 may have a physiologic role in the modulation of growth hormone secretion [34].

REFERENCES

1. Dockray GJ: Brain-gut peptides. Viewpoints Dig Dis 13:5, 1981.
2. Dockray GJ, Gregory RA: Relations between neuropeptides and gut hormones. Proc R Soc Lond [Biol] 210:151, 1980.
3. Pearse AGE: Peptides in brain and intestine. Nature 262:92, 1976.
4. Bloom SR: Gut and brain—Endocrine connections. The Goulstonian lecture 1979. J R Coll Physicians Lond 14:51, 1980.
5. Schwyzer R: Peptides and the new endocrinology. Naturwissenschaften 69:15, 1982.
6. Yanaihara N, Sato H, Inoue A, et al: Comparative study on distribution of bombesin-, neurotensin- and α-endorphin-like immunoreactivities in canine tissues. Adv Exp Med Biol 120:29, 1979.
7. Brown M, Allen R, Villarreal J, et al: Bombesin-like activity: Radioimmunologic assessment in biological tissues. Life Sci 23:2721, 1978.
8. Pearse AGE, Takor TT: Embryology of the diffuse neuroendocrine system and its relationship to the common peptides. Fed Proc 38:2288, 1979.
9. Snyder SH: Brain peptides as neurotransmitters. Science 209:976, 1980.
10. Track NS: Regulatory peptides of the gut and brain. Can J Surg 26:211, 1983.
11. Krieger DT: Brain peptides: What, where, and why? Science 222:975, 1983.
12. Ewart WR, Wingate DL: Central representation of arrival of nutrient in the duodenum. Am J Physiol 246:G750, 1984.
13. Goyal RK: Neurology of the gut, in Sleisenger M, Fordtran J (eds): *Gastrointestinal Disease.* 3rd Ed. Philadelphia, WB Saunders, 1983, pp 97–115.
14. Gershon MD, Erde SM: The nervous system of the gut. Gastroenterology 80:1571, 1981.
15. Brown M: Neuropeptides: Central nervous system effects on nutrient metabolism. Diabetologia 20:299, 1981.
16. Oektedalen O, Opstad PK, Schaffalitzky de Muckadell OB, et al: Basal hyperchlorhydria and its relation to the plasma concentrations of secretin, vasoactive intestinal polypeptide (VIP) and gastrin during prolonged strain. Regul Pept 5:235, 1983.
17. von Euler US, Gaddum JH: An unidentified depressor substance in certain tissue extracts. J Physiol 72:74, 1931.
18. Morley JE: Minireview. The ascent of cholecystokinin (CCK)—from gut to brain. Life Sci 30:479, 1982.

19. Grimmelikhujzen CJP, Sundler F, Rehfeld JF: Gastrin/CCK-like immuno-reactivity in the nervous system of coelenterates. Histochemistry 69:61, 1980.
20. Beinfeld MC, Meyer DK, Brownstein MJ: Cholecystokinin in the central nervous system. Peptides 2(Suppl 2):77, 1981.
21. Besson J, Rotsztejn W, Leburthe M, et al: Vasoactive intestinal peptide (VIP): Brain distribution, subcellular localization and effect of deafferentation of the hypothalamus in male rats. Brain Res 165:79, 1979.
22. Beinfeld MC, Meyer DK, Eskay RL, et al: The distribution of cholecystokinin immunoreactivity in the central nervous system of the rat as determined by radioimmunoassay. Brain Res 212:51, 1981.
23. Simon-Assmann PM, Yazigi R, Greeley GH Jr, et al: Biologic and radioimmunologic activity of cholecystokinin in regions of mammalian brains. J Neurosci Res 10:165, 1983.
24. Saito A, Sankaran H, Goldfine ID, et al: Cholecystokinin receptors in the brain: Characterization and distribution. Science 208:1155, 1980.
25. Innis RB, Snyder SH: Cholecystokinin receptor binding in brain and pancreas: Regulation of pancreatic binding by cyclic and acyclic guanine nucleotides. Eur J Pharmacol 65:123, 1980.
26. Zarbin MA, Wamsley JK, Innis RB, et al: Cholecystokinin receptors: Presence and axonal flow in the rat vagus nerve. Life Sci 29:697, 1981.
27. Mueller K, Hsiao S: Current status of cholecystokinin as a short-term satiety hormone. Neurosci Biobehav Rev 2:79, 1978.
28. Morley JE: Minireview. The neuroendocrine control of appetite: The role of the endogenous opiates, cholecystokinin, TRH, gamma-amino-butyric-acid and the diazepam receptor. Life Sci 27:355, 1980.
29. Morley JE, Levine AS: Intraventricular cholecystokinin-octapeptide produces hyperglycemia in rats. Life Sci 28:2187, 1981.
30. Katsuura G, Hirota R, Itoh S: Cholecystokinin-induced hypothermia in the rat. Experientia 37:60, 1981.
31. Zetler G: Analgesia and ptosis caused by caerulein and cholecystokinin octapeptide (CCK-8). Neuropharmacology 19:415, 1980.
32. Zetler G: Anticonvulsant effects of caerulein and cholecystokinin octapeptide, compared with those of diazepam. Eur J Pharmacol 65:297, 1980.
33. Mann JFE, Boucher R, Schiller PW: Rotational syndrome after central injection of C-terminal 7-peptide of cholecystokinin. Pharmacol Biochem Behav 13:125, 1980.
34. Morley JE, Melmed S, Briggs J, et al: Cholecystokinin octapeptide releases growth hormone from the pituitary *in vitro*. Life Sci 25:1201, 1979.
35. Lu Q-H, Greeley GH Jr, Zhu X-G, et al: Intracerebroventricular administration of cholecystokinin-8 elevates plasma pancreatic polypeptide levels in awake dogs. Endocrinology 114:2415, 1984.
36. Della-Fera MA, Baile CA: CCK-octapeptide injected in CSF and changes in feed intake and rumen motility. Physiol Behav 24:943, 1980.
37. Tache Y, Vale W, Rivier J, et al: Brain regulation of gastric acid secretion in rats by neurogastrointestinal peptides. Peptides 2(Suppl 2):51, 1981.
38. Morley JE, Levine AS, Silvis SE: Central regulation of gastric acid secretion: The role of neuropeptides. Life Sci 31:399, 1982.
39. Osumi Y, Nagasaka Y, Wang LH, et al: Inhibition of gastric acid secretion and mucosal blood flow induced by intraventricularly applied neurotensin in rats. Life Sci 23:2275, 1978.
40. Morley JE, Levine AS, Silvis SE: Endogenous opiates inhibit gastric acid secretion induced by central administration of thyrotropin-releasing hormone (TRH). Life Sci 29:293, 1981.
41. Tache Y, Vale W, Brown M: Thyrotropin-releasing hormone—CNS action to stimulate gastric acid secretion. Nature 287:149, 1980.
42. Morley JE, Levine AS, Silvis SE: Intraventricular calcitonin inhibits gastric acid secretion. Science 214:671, 1981.
43. Tepperman BL, Evered MD: Gastrin injected into the lateral hypothalamus stimulates secretion of gastric acid in rats. Science 209:1142, 1980.
44. Tache Y, Rivier J, Vale W, et al: Is somatostatin or a somatostatin-like peptide involved in central nervous system control of gastric secretion? Regul Pept 1:307, 1981.
45. Tache Y, Vale W, Rivier J, et al: Brain regulation of gastric secretion: Influence of neuropeptides. Proc Natl Acad Sci USA 77:5515, 1980.
46. Tache Y, Collu R: CNS mediated inhibition of gastric secretion by bombesin: Independence from interaction with brain catecholaminergic and serotoninergic pathways and pituitary hormones. Regul Pept 3:51, 1982.
47. Tache Y, Marki W, Rivier J, et al: Central nervous system inhibition of gastric secretion in the rat by gastrin-releasing peptide, a mammalian bombesin. Gastroenterology 81:298, 1981.
48. Lenz HJ, Mortrud MT, Rivier JE, et al: Central nervous system actions of calcitonin gene-related peptide on gastric acid secretion in the rat. Gastroenterology 88:539, 1985.
49. Garcia-Sevilla JA, Magnusson T, Carlsson A, et al: Neurotensin and its amide analogue [Gln^4]-neurotensin: Effects on brain monoamine turnover. Naunyn-Schmiedebergs Arch Pharmacol 305:213, 1978.
50. Osumi Y, Aibara S, Sakae K, et al: Central noradrenergic inhibition of gastric mucosal blood flow and acid secretion in rats. Life Sci 20:1407, 1977.
51. Smith JR, La Hann TR, Chesnut RM, et al: Thyrotropin-releasing hormone: Stimulation of colonic activity following intracerebroventricular administration. Science 196:660, 1977.
52. Hesch RD, Hufner M, Hasenhager B, et al: Inhibition

of gastric secretion by calcitonin in man. Horm Metab Res 3:140, 1971.
53. Pappas T, Hamel D, Debas H, et al: Cerebroventricular bombesin inhibits gastric acid secretion in dogs. Gastroenterology 89:43, 1985.
54. Yamaguchi I, Hiroi J, Kumada S: Central and peripheral adrenergic mechanisms regulating gastric secretion in the rat. J Pharmacol Exp Ther 203:125, 1977.
55. Levine AS, Morley JE, Kneip J, et al: Muscimol induces gastric acid secretion after central administration. Brain Res 229:270, 1981.
56. Kimura H, Kuriyama K: Distribution of gamma-aminobutyric acid (GABA) in the rat hypothalamus: Functional correlates of GABA with activities of appetite controlling mechanisms. J Neurochem 24:903, 1975.
57. Tache Y, Grijalva CV, Gunion MW, et al: Lateral hypothalamic mediation of hypergastrinemia induced by intracisternal bombesin. Neuroendocrinology 39:114, 1984.
58. Goto Y, Garcia R, Debas HT: Specificity of substance P (SP) inhibition to neural mechanisms of gastric acid secretion. Gastroenterology 86:1094, 1984.
59. Tache Y, Gunion M, Lauffenburger M, et al: Inhibition of gastric acid secretion by intracerebral injection of calcitonin gene related peptide (CGRP) in rats. Gastroenterology 86:1272, 1984.
60. Lenz HJ, Vale WW, Rivier JE, et al: Calcitonin gene-related peptide (CGRP), a novel neuropeptide, acts within the brain to inhibit gastric acid secretion (GAS). Gastroenterology 86:1158, 1984.
61. Lenz HJ, Webb VJ, Hester SE, et al: Calcitonin gene-related peptide: Inhibition of gastric acid secretion in the dog. Gastroenterology 86:1158, 1984.
62. Tache Y, Goto Y, Gunion MW, et al: Inhibition of gastric acid secretion in rats by intracerebral injection of corticotropin-releasing factor. Science 222:935, 1983.
63. Ridley PT, Brooks FP: Alterations in gastric secretion following hypothalamic lesions producing hyperphagia. Am J Physiol 209:319, 1965.
64. Davis RA, Brooks FP, Steckel DC: Gastric secretory changes after anterior hypothalamic lesions. Am J Physiol 215:600, 1968.
65. Grijalva CV, Lindholm E, Novin D: Physiological and morphological changes in the gastrointestinal tract induced by hypothalamic intervention: An overview. Brain Res Bull 5(Suppl 1):19, 1980.
66. Feldman S, Conforti N, Birnbaum D: Gastric secretion and acid output in the rat following hippocampal, septal and mid-brain stimulation. Isr J Med Sci 7:1276, 1971.
67. Stephens DN, Morrissey SM: Hypothalamic stimulation induces acid secretion, hypoglycemia, and hyperinsulinemia. Am J Physiol 228:1206, 1975.
68. Misher A, Brooks FP: Electrical stimulation of hypothalamus and gastric secretion in the albino rat. Am J Physiol 211:403, 1966.
69. Carmona A, Slangen J: Effects of chemical stimulation of the hypothalamus upon gastric secretion. Physiol Behav 10:657, 1973.
70. del Tacca M, Soldani G, Bernardini C, et al: Pharmacological studies on the mechanisms underlying the inhibitory and excitatory effects of clonidine on gastric acid secretion. Eur J Pharmacol 81:255, 1982.
71. Nakadate T, Nakaki T, Muraki T, et al: Inhibitory α_2-adrenergic mechanism regulating gastric secretion in pylorus-ligated rats. Naunyn-Schmiedebergs Arch Pharmacol 320:170, 1982.
72. Thompson JH, George R: Chronic effects of nicotine on gastric secretion in rats with hypothalamic lesions. Am J Dig Dis 17:513, 1972.
73. Myers RD, Bender SA, Krstic MK, et al: Feeding produced in the satiated rat by elevating the concentration of calcium in the brain. Science 176:1124, 1972.
74. Seoane JR, McLaughlin CL, Baile CA: Feeding following intrahypothalamic injections of calcium and magnesium ions in sheep. J Dairy Sci 58:349, 1975.
75. Roze C, Chariot J, de la Tour J, et al: Methadone blockade of 2-deoxyglucose-induced pancreatic secretion in the rat. Evidence for a central site of action. Gastroenterology 74:215, 1978.
76. Roze C, Dubrasquet M, Chariot J, et al: Central inhibition of basal pancreatic and gastric secretions by β-endorphin in rats. Gastroenterology 79:659, 1980.
77. Burks TF: Central sites of action of gastrointestinal drugs. Gastroenterology 74:322, 1978.
78. Stewart JJ, Weisbrodt NW, Burks TF: Centrally mediated intestinal stimulation by morphine. J Pharmacol Exp Ther 202:174, 1977.
79. Aronchick C, Feng H-S, Brooks FP, et al: Bombesin in the 4th ventricle of cats inhibits vagally stimulated antral contractions and acid secretion. Gastroenterology 84:1093, 1983.
80. Porreca F, Burks TF: Centrally administered bombesin affects gastric emptying and small and large bowel transit in the rat. Gastroenterology 85:313, 1983.
81. Demol P, Hotz J, Goebell H: Calcitonin induces activity fronts in the upper intestine and inhibits the interdigestive acid and pancreatic secretion in man. Gastroenterology 86:1060, 1984.
82. Bueno L, Fioramonti J, Ferre JP: Calcitonin—C.N.S. action to control the pattern of intestinal motility in rats. Peptides 4:63, 1983.
83. Bernier JJ, Rambaud JC, Cattan D, et al: Diarrhoea associated with medullary carcinoma of the thyroid. Gut 10:980, 1969.
84. Pappas TN, Melendez R, Debas HT: Cerebroventricular administration of CCK-8 accelerates gastric emptying. Gastroenterology 86:1206, 1984.
85. Schirmer BD, Iacono RP, Nashold BS, et al: Neural control of gastrointestinal motility: Evidence for noncholinergic regulatory influences. Surgery 94:191, 1983.
86. Ewart WR, Wingate DL: Cholecystokinin octapep-

tide and gastric mechanoreceptor activity in rat brain. Am J Physiol 244:G613, 1983.
87. Honde C, Bueno L: Evidence for central neuropeptidergic control of rumination in sheep. Peptides 5:81, 1984.
88. Bueno L, Ferre J-P: Central regulation of intestinal motility by somatostatin and cholecystokinin octapeptide. Science 216:1427, 1982.
89. Bueno L, Fioramonti J, Honde C, et al: Central and peripheral control of gastrointestinal and colonic motility by endogenous opiates in conscious dogs. Gastroenterology 88:549, 1985.
90. Bueno L, Ferre JP, Fioramonti J, et al: Effects of intracerebroventricular administration of neurotensin, substance P and calcitonin on gastrointestinal motility in normal and vagotomized rats. Regul Pept 6:197, 1983.
91. Bueno L, Fioramonti J, Fargeas MJ, et al: Neurotensin: A central neuromodulator of gastrointestinal motility in the dog. Am J Physiol 248:G15, 1985.
92. Bueno L, Fargeas MJ, Fioramonti J, et al: Central control of intestinal motility by prostaglandins: A mediator of the actions of several peptides in rats and dogs. Gastroenterology 88:1888, 1985.
93. Ruberg M, Rotsztejn WH, Arancibia S, et al: Stimulation of prolactin release by vasoactive intestinal peptide (VIP). Eur J Pharmacol 51:319, 1978.
94. Schaar CJ, Clemens JA, Dininger NB: Effect of vasoactive intestinal polypeptide on prolactin release in vitro. Life Sci 25:2071, 1979.
95. Samson WK, Said SI, Snyder G, et al: *In vitro* stimulation of prolactin release by vasoactive intestinal peptide. Peptides 1:325, 1980.
96. Kato Y, Iwasaki Y, Iwasaki J, et al: Prolactin release by vasoactive intestinal polypeptide in rats. Endocrinology 103:554, 1978.
97. Vijayan E, Samson WK, Said SI, et al: Vasoactive intestinal peptide: Evidence for a hypothalamic site of action to release growth hormone, luteinizing hormone, and prolactin in conscious ovariectomized rats. Endocrinology 104:53, 1979.
98. Epelbaum J, Tapia-Arancibia L, Besson J, et al: Vasoactive intestinal peptide inhibits release of somatostatin from hypothalamus in vitro. Eur J Pharmacol 58:493, 1979.
99. Samson WK, Burton KP, Reeves JP, et al: Vasoactive intestinal peptide stimulates luteinizing hormone–releasing hormone release from median eminence synaptosomes. Regul Pept 2:253, 1981.
100. Samson WK, Lumpkin MD, McCann SM: Presence and possible site of action of secretin in the rat pituitary and hypothalamus. Life Sci 34:155, 1984.
101. Deschodt-Lanckman M, Robberecht P, Christophe J: Characterization of VIP-sensitive adenylate cyclase in guinea pig brain. FEBS Lett 83:76, 1977.
102. Taylor DP, Pert CB: Vasoactive intestinal polypeptide: Specific binding to rat brain membranes. Proc Natl Acad Sci USA 76:660, 1979.
103. Carlson HE, Mariz IK, Daughaday WH: Thyrotropin-releasing hormone stimulation and somatostatin inhibition of growth hormone secretion from perfused rat adenohypophyses. Endocrinology 94:1709, 1974.
104. Martin JB, Brazeau P, Tannenbaum GS, et al: Neuroendocrine organization of growth hormone regulation, in Reichlin S, Baldessarini RJ, Martin JB (eds): *The Hypothalamus*. New York, Raven Press, 1978, pp 329–357.

Chapter 34

Entero-Insulinar Axis: Incretin Candidates

George H. Greeley, Jr., Ph.D.

Eating a meal causes secretion of insulin by the pancreatic beta cell, not only as a direct result of the hyperglycemia but also as a direct effect of gastrointestinal and pancreatic peptides that are released in response to the meal [1–3]. In fact, the classic observation of Scow and Cornfield [4] was that oral glucose stimulates the pancreatic beta cell more profoundly than intravenous (IV) glucose, despite identical blood glucose levels. Gastrointestinal peptides are believed to control at least 50 percent of the pancreatic insulin secreted after oral glucose [4–8]. These findings form the basis, in part, of the concept that gastrointestinal peptides play an important role in the overall insulin response after ingestion of a meal. The secretion of such gut factors, as well as their insulin-releasing action, is probably triggered by the ingestion (and preferably, the absorption) of certain nutrients, especially glucose. In fact, the insulinotropic action of a gut peptide should be dependent upon the circulating glucose level, since insulin release in the face of normoglycemia may result in hypoglycemia.

The entero-insulinar axis hypothesis proposes that gastrointestinal peptides play a significant role in insulin secretion and glucoregulation. Actually, the entero-insulinar axis is composed of several physiologic stimuli (endocrine, nutrients, and neural signals) that pass from the gut to the pancreatic islets. The pancreatic islet target sites are α, β, delta, PP, and possibly other cell types.

The insulinogenic factor (or factors) of the gut were called "incretin" by La Barre [9,10], and the term incretin can be applied to any insulin-releasing humoral factor derived from the intestinal mucosa. If a particular peptide brings about insulin release via peptidergic nerve fibers, the substance cannot be considered an incretin. As originally defined, incretin candidates refer only to those substances that act as endocrine effectors of insulin release. According to Creutzfeldt [1], some of the criteria for an incretin candidate are 1) the enteric substance is released by the absorption of nutrients, especially carbohydrates, and 2) the substance stimulates insulin release in the presence of glucose in amounts that mimic circulating levels seen after a meal. Although a gut peptide, gastric inhibitory polypeptide (GIP, also called glucose-dependent insulinotropic polypeptide) is a potent glucose-dependent releaser of insulin [11–13]; other gastrointestinal peptides are also potent stimulants of insulin secretion. In fact, Szecowka et al [14] have reported that cholecystokinin (CCK-33) is as potent as GIP in releasing insulin, and Ebert and Creutzfeldt [15] suggested that GIP is not the major incretin. Hence, it is important to recognize that more than one gut peptide exerts an incretin effect. Whether many of these incretin candidates exert an insulinotropic action at physiologic dosages is debatable. Physiologic doses of many of the gut and pancreatic peptides are not yet determined, and the significance of reported postprandial concentrations of some gut peptides is still controversial.

McIntyre et al [5,16] suggested that a humoral substance was released from the jejunal wall, which enhanced glucose-induced insulin secretion. Dupre et al [17] suggested that this substance was located in the upper small bowel, and Moody et al [18] postulated that a factor from the ileum-jejunum enhanced glucose-induced insulin release; they further stated that this insulinotropic substance was not secretin or CCK.

Breuer et al [19,20] reported that patients who had gastrectomy with pyloroplasty exhibited hyperinsulinemia and glucose intolerance, suggesting that an intestinal factor released during glucose absorption facilitated glucose deposition.

They also found unusually high glicentin levels in these particular postoperative patients and showed that exogenous secretin lowered glicentin levels. However, Marco et al [21] found no evidence that glicentin is an insulinotropic substance.

INSULINOTROPIC ENTERIC PEPTIDES

GIP

GIP has been shown to be a potent insulinotropic factor in humans and in a variety of laboratory animals when the elevation in blood glucose is 20 percent above resting levels [11,22]. The insulinotropic action of GIP is glucose-dependent, and the magnitude of the insulin response to GIP is related to the circulating glucose levels [11]. Hence, a threshold concentration of glucose appears necessary for GIP-induced insulin release [12]. The insulinotropic action of GIP is absent when GIP is given as a single bolus in the normoglycemic condition [3]. In contrast to other gastrointestinal peptides, GIP can cause insulin release during the second prolonged phase. Both oral glucose and triglycerides promote GIP release [11], whereas IV glucose does not elevate plasma GIP levels [11,23]. In the fed rat (glucose, 6.6 ± 1 mmol/L), infusion of GIP (100 pmol/kg/min) alone caused insulin secretion, whereas infusion of GIP (in doses of 10 and 100 pmol/kg/min) potentiated glucose-induced insulin secretion [14]. Pederson and Brown [12] showed that GIP can elevate insulin release in a dose-dependent manner in the presence of glucose. Dupre et al [13] showed that GIP potentiated glucose-induced insulin secretion and enhanced glucose tolerance in humans. In adult goats (which are ruminants), GIP lacks an incretin effect, whereas in young goats (which are not), GIP participates in glucose-stimulated insulin release [24]. Apparently, adult goats and perhaps all ruminants lack an incretin system.

Secretin

Numerous studies have indicated that secretin can be insulinotropic in humans and in laboratory animals. In humans, secretin can cause insulin secretion in both the fed and fasting state [25]. Secretin can also enhance glucose-induced insulin secretion [25, 26]. Secretin can cause a rapid, short-lived release of insulin in humans [27,28]. Interestingly, insulin responses to a pulse or infusion of secretin resemble each other [27,28]. Dupre et al [29] showed that secretin administration to patients caused insulin but not glucagon release. Raptis et al [30] showed that the insulin responses to IV CCK or secretin were completely absent in patients with pancreatic insufficiency, suggesting that some factor originating in the exocrine pancreas facilitates CCK- or secretin-induced insulin release. In awake dogs, secretin has a minimal insulinotropic action [31], and in rats, secretin alone, or in combination with glucose, did not affect insulin secretion, in vivo or in vitro [14,32]. Secretin can stimulate glucagon release, however [32].

Doses of secretin that are effective exocrine stimulants fail to cause insulin release [32,33]. Secretin infusion (10 CU/min) for 20 minutes can suppress basal and hyperglycemic levels of glucagon [34]; however, these doses of secretin are pharmacologic. Endogenously released secretin, brought about by intraduodenal infusion of hydrochloric acid in anesthetized dogs, elevates portal but not peripheral plasma insulin levels [35].

Gastrin

Gastrin-induced insulin secretion is monophasic, transient, and independent of circulating glucose levels [36]. Chronic hypergastrinemia can lead to inhibition of insulin secretion in response to glucose-induced hyperglycemia in a patient with a gastrojejunostomy and a gastrinoma [36]. Infusion of supraphysiologic doses of gastrin into normal humans raised insulin levels and potentiated glucose-induced insulin secretion [37]. Tetragastrin also causes a rapid and short-lived elevation in plasma insulin in dogs and humans [38,39].

CCK

Infusion of caerulein (an analog of CCK, in doses of 10 and 100 ng/kg/min) into anesthetized rats provokes secretion of pancreatic glucagon and insulin [40]. These doses of caerulein are supraphysiologic, at least in terms of exocrine pancreas secretion. Infusion of equimolar doses of CCK-33 or CCK-8 can increase insulin secretion in dogs [31]. Although CCK can enhance glucose-induced insulin secretion in the rat [14], CCK is insulinotropic at fasting levels of glucose [31] in contrast to GIP. In fact, CCK-33 seems more potent, on a molar basis, than GIP [14]. IV glucose also potentiates CCK-8-induced insulin release [31], whereas equimolar doses of GIP did not enhance IV glucose-induced insulin release.

In awake dogs, impure CCK (i.e., CCK-PZ [0.5 U/kg]) is a stronger stimulant of insulin release than 0.5 g/kg glucose [41]. CCK-PZ also potentiates glucose-induced insulin secretion, and a constant infusion of CCK-PZ is no more effective than a single injection. Caerulein, at doses supramaximal for exocrine pancreatic secretion, stimulates pancreatic insulin release [42]. Glucose does not augment caerulein-induced insulin secretion; however, caerulein exposure augments glucose-induced insulin release. CCK-33 causes insulin and glucagon release at doses that were supramaximal for pancreatic exocrine secretion. The glucagon and insulin responses were immediate and transient despite constant infusion of CCK. In fed rats, CCK-33 (1 pmol/kg/min) augments glucose or arginine-induced insulin secretion [14]. Higher doses of CCK-33 (10 to 100 pmol/kg/min) are more effective. In fact, GIP, at a dose of 1 pmol/kg/min, does not cause insulin release. CCK-33 also causes glucagon release.

Okabayashi et al [43] have shown that the primary structure of CCK that is required for CCK-induced exocrine pancreatic secretion is also required for endocrine effects. Preservation of amino acid residues, in positions 5 to 8, and the amidated residue of the C terminal are necessary. CCK-4 is 100,000 times less potent than CCK-8 [43]. Lindkaer Jensen et al [44], using an isolated perfused pig pancreas, showed that CCK-39 stimulates insulin release in the presence of glucose; however, CCK-33 and CCK-8 were ineffective. CCK-33 (99 percent pure) was 43 percent as potent as GIP, on a molar basis, in bringing about insulin release [45]. Interestingly, the insulin responses to GIP and CCK-33 were biphasic and sustained as well as glucose-dependent. More recently, Hermansen [46] has reported that CCK-8 sulfate and CCK-8 desulfated (0.1, 1.0, 10 nm), in the presence of 5.5 mM glucose, can cause dose-dependent elevations in somatostatin, glucagon, and insulin secretion from the isolated perfused pancreas of the dog.

MISCELLANEOUS

Somatostatin, Substance P, Pancreatic Polypeptide (PP), Neurotensin

Somatostatin, substance P, and PP (4.25 and 42.5 mmol/kg) inhibit glucose-induced insulin release [47]. In this particular study, neurotensin was ineffective. Somatostatin inhibits carbachol-induced insulin release, whereas substance P and PP are without effect. Neurotensin potentiates the response to carbachol. Brown and Vale [48] indicate that substance P and neurotensin can evoke hypoinsulinemia, hypergluconemia, and hyperglycemia in the rat. High doses of neurotensin result in an elevation of plasma glucose and glucagon levels and reduce circulating insulin levels in rats [49,50]. In dogs, IV neurotensin increases glucagon levels but reduces insulin levels [49]. In isolated rat islets, neurotensin can inhibit insulin release and stimulate glucagon release.

Peptide Histidine Isoleucine (PHI)

PHI (3 ng/mL) can induce insulin release in the presence of glucose and can also enhance arginine-induced glucagon release [51,52]. PHI, in the absence of glucose, stimulates glucagon release; however, in the presence of glucose, PHI causes release of insulin and somatostatin. PHI can also potentiate arginine-induced somatostatin, insulin, and glucagon release [52].

Bombesin and GRP-like Peptides

The insulinotropic action of these peptides is discussed in Chapter 25.

Relative Incretin Potencies of Different Peptides in Vitro

Alwmark et al [53] in our laboratory tested the relative insulin-releasing potencies of 11 different peptides in suspensions of isolated rat islets (Table 34-1). Gastrin-releasing peptide was the most potent. Contrary to findings from the isolated perfused rat pancreas [43], CCK-4 was more potent than CCK-8.

Table 34-1. **Relative incretin potencies of various gut peptides tested with isolated rat islets**

Gut peptide	*Lowest concentration that causes insulin release*
GRP	10^{-11} M
CCK-4	10^{-11} M
CCK-8	10^{-10} M
VIP	10^{-10} M
Bombesin	10^{-9} M
PHI	10^{-9} M
GIP	10^{-8} M
Secretin	10^{-8} M
Gastrin	10^{-7} M
Neurotensin	10^{-6} M
Somatostatin	Does not cause release

REFERENCES

1. Creutzfeldt W: The incretin concept today. Diabetologia 16:75, 1979.
2. Makhlouf GM: The neuroendocrine design of the gut. The play of chemicals in a chemical playground. Gastroenterology 67:159, 1974.
3. Andersen DK, Elahi D, Brown JC, et al: Oral glucose augmentation of insulin secretion. Interactions of gastric inhibitory polypeptide with ambient glucose and insulin levels. J Clin Invest 62:152, 1978.
4. Scow RO, Cornfield J: Quantitative relations between the oral and intravenous glucose tolerance curves. Am J Physiol 179:435, 1954.
5. McIntyre N, Holdsworth CD, Turner DS: New interpretation of oral glucose tolerance. Lancet 2:20, 1964.
6. Elrick H, Stimmler L, Hlad CJ Jr, et al: Plasma insulin response to oral and intravenous glucose administration. J Clin Endocrinol 24:1076, 1964.
7. Perley MJ, Kipnis DM: Plasma insulin responses to oral and intravenous glucose: Studies in normal and diabetic subjects. J Clin Invest 46:1954, 1967.
8. Lickley HLA, Chisholm DJ, Robinovitch A, et al: Effects of portacaval anastomosis on glucose tolerance in the dog: Evidence of an interaction between the gut and the liver in oral glucose disposal. Metabolism 24:1157, 1975.
9. La Barre J, Ledrut J: A propos de l'action hypoglycemiante des extraits duodenaux. Comptes Rendus des Scans de la Societe de Biologie 115:750, 1934.
10. La Barre J, Still EU: Studies on the physiology of secretin. III. Further studies on the effects of secretin on the blood sugar. Am J Physiol 91:649, 1930.
11. Pederson RA, Schubert HE, Brown JC: Gastric inhibitory polypeptide. Its physiologic release and insulinotropic action in the dog. Diabetes 24:105, 1975.
12. Pederson RA, Brown JC: The insulinotropic action of gastric inhibitory polypeptide in the perfused isolated rat pancreas. Endocrinology 99:780, 1976.
13. Dupre J, Ross SA, Watson D, et al: Stimulation of insulin secretion by gastric inhibitory polypeptide in man. J Clin Endocrinol Metab 37:826, 1973.
14. Szecowka J, Lins PE, Efendic S: Effects of cholecystokinin, gastric inhibitory polypeptide, and secretin on insulin and glucagon secretion in rats. Endocrinology 110:1268, 1982.
15. Ebert R, Creutzfeldt W: Influence of gastric inhibitory polypeptide antiserum on glucose-induced insulin secretion in rats. Endocrinology 111:1601, 1982.
16. McIntyre N, Holdsworth CD, Turner DS: Intestinal factors in the control of insulin secretion. J Clin Endocrinol 25:1317, 1965.
17. Dupre J: An intestinal hormone affecting glucose disposal in man. Lancet 2:672, 1964.
18. Moody AJ, Markussen J, Schaich Fries A, et al: The insulin releasing activities of extracts of pork intestine. Diabetologia 6:135, 1970.
19. Breuer RI, Moses H III, Hagen TC, et al: Gastric operations and glucose homeostasis. Gastroenterology 62:1109, 1972.
20. Breuer RI, Zuckerman L, Hauch TW, et al: Gastric operations and glucose homeostasis. II. Glucagon and secretin. Gastroenterology 69:598, 1975.
21. Marco J, Baroja IM, Diaz-Fierros M, et al: Relationship between insulin and gut glucagon-like immunoreactivity (GLI) secretion in normal and gastrectomized subjects. J Clin Endocrinol 34:188, 1972.
22. Flaten O, Tronier B: Dose-dependent increase in concentrations of gastric inhibitory polypeptide and pancreatic polypeptide after small amounts of glucose intraduodenally in man. Scand J Gastroenterol 17:677, 1982.
23. Cataland S, Crockett SE, Brown JC, et al: Gastric inhibitory polypeptide (GIP) stimulation by oral glucose in man. J Clin Endocrinol Metab 39:223, 1974.
24. Nilssen KJ, Hove K, Jorde R: Insulin and gastric inhibitory polypeptide secretion in young milk-fed and adult goats. Am J Physiol 244:E209, 1983.
25. Dupre J, Curtis JD, Unger RH, et al: Effects of secretin, pancreozymin, or gastrin on the response of the endocrine pancreas to administration of glucose or arginine in man. J Clin Invest 48:745, 1969.
26. Shima K, Tarui S: The effect of secretin on glucose-stimulated insulin secretion in man. Endocrinol Jpn 21:13, 1974.
27. Lerner RL, Porte D Jr: Uniphasic insulin responses to secretin stimulation in man. J Clin Invest 49:2276, 1970.
28. Lerner RL, Porte D Jr: Studies of secretin-stimulated insulin responses in man. J Clin Invest 51:2205, 1972.
29. Dupre J, Rojas L, White JJ, et al: Effects of secretin on insulin and glucagon in portal and peripheral blood in man. Lancet 2:26, 1966.
30. Raptis S, Rau RM, Schroder KE, et al: The role of the exocrine pancreas in the stimulation of insulin secretion by intestinal hormones. III. Insulin responses to secretin and pancreozymin, and to oral and intravenous glucose, in patients suffering from chronic insufficiency of the exocrine pancreas. Diabetologia 7:160, 1971.
31. Williams RH, Champagne J: Effects of cholecystokinin, secretin, and pancreatic polypeptide on secretion of gastric inhibitory polypeptide, insulin, and glucagon. Life Sci 25:947, 1979.
32. Otsuki M, Sakamoto C, Ohki A, et al: Effects of porcine secretin on exocrine and endocrine function in the isolated perfused rat pancreas. Am J Physiol 241:G43, 1981.
33. Buchanan KD, Vance JE, Morgan A, et al: Effect of pancreozymin on insulin and glucagon levels in blood and bile. Am J Physiol 215:1293, 1968.
34. Santeusanio F, Faloona GR, Unger RH: Suppressive effect of secretin upon pancreatic alpha cell function. J Clin Invest 51:1743, 1972.
35. Boden G, Essa N, Owen OE, et al: Effects of intraduodenal administration of HCl and glucose on circulat-

ing immunoreactive secretin and insulin concentrations. J Clin Invest 53:1185, 1974.

36. Massaro RP: Hormonal responses to intravenous and oral glucose tolerance testing in a patient with a gastrinoma and a gastrojejunostomy. Gastroenterology 66:1058, 1974.
37. Rehfeld JF, Stadil F: The effect of gastrin on basal- and glucose-stimulated insulin secretion in man. J Clin Invest 52:1415, 1973.
38. Kaneto A, Tasaka Y, Kosaka K, et al: Stimulation of insulin secretion by the C-terminal tetrapeptide amide of gastrin. Endocrinology 84:1098, 1969.
39. Rehfeld JF: Effect of gastrin and its C-terminal tetrapeptide on insulin secretion in man. Acta Endocrinol 66:169, 1971.
40. Otsuki M, Sakamoto C, Maeda M, et al: Effect of caerulein on exocrine and endocrine pancreas in the rat. Endocrinology 105:1396, 1979.
41. Meade RC, Kneubuhler HA, Schulte WJ, et al: Stimulation of insulin secretion by pancreozymin. Diabetes 16:141, 1967.
42. Otsuki M, Sakamoto C, Yuu H, et al: Discrepancies between the doses of cholecystokinin or caerulein-stimulating exocrine and endocrine responses in perfused isolated rat pancreas. J Clin Invest 63:478, 1979.
43. Okabayashi Y, Otsuki M, Ohki A, et al: Effects of C-terminal fragments of cholecystokinin on exocrine and endocrine secretion from isolated perfused rat pancreas. Endocrinology 113:2210, 1983.
44. Jensen S, Rehfeld JF, Holst JJ, et al: Secretory effects of cholecystokinins on the isolated perfused porcine pancreas. Acta Physiol Scand 111:225, 1981.
45. Pederson RA, Brown JC: Effect of cholecystokinin, secretin, and gastric inhibitory polypeptide on insulin release from the isolated perfused rat pancreas. Can J Physiol Pharmacol 57:1233, 1979.
46. Hermansen K: Effects of cholecystokinin (CCK)-4, nonsulfated CCK-8, and sulfated CCK-8 on pancreatic somatostatin, insulin, and glucagon secretion in the dog: Studies *in vitro*. Endocrinology 114:1770, 1984.
47. Lundquist I, Sundler F, Ahren B, et al: Somatostatin, pancreatic polypeptide, substance P, and neurotensin: Cellular distribution and effects on stimulated insulin secretion in the mouse. Endocrinology 104:832, 1979.
48. Brown M, Vale W: Effects of neurotensin and substance P on plasma insulin, glucagon and glucose levels. Endocrinology 98:819, 1976.
49. Fernstrom MH, Carraway RE, Leeman SE: Neurotensin, in Martini L, Ganong WF (eds): *Frontiers in Neuroendocrinology*. New York, Raven Press, 1980, pp 103–127.
50. Nagai K, Frohman LA: Hyperglycemia and hyperglucagonemia following neurotensin administration. Life Sci 19:273, 1976.
51. Szecowka J, Tatemoto K, Mutt V, et al: Interaction of a newly isolated intestinal polypeptide (PHI) with glucose and arginine to effect the secretion of insulin and glucagon. Life Sci 26:435, 1980.
52. Szecowka J, Tendler D, Efendic S: Effects of PHI on hormonal secretion from perfused rat pancreas. Am J Physiol 245:E313, 1983.
53. Alwmark A, Khalil T, Mate L, et al: Gut hormones as incretin candidates. Surg Forum 35:209, 1984.

Chapter 35

Gonad-Gut Axis

Pomila Singh, Ph.D., and James C. Thompson, M.D.

Regulatory systems for one organ system appear to interrelate with other regulatory systems. The sharing of regulatory peptides by the central nervous system and the gut has been studied and codified into the brain-gut axis. Similar interactions may occur between the gut and the reproductive system. We will review the information that supports the concept of a gonad-gut axis.

Decrease in plasma glucose levels related to hyperinsulinemia and increased insulin secretions in response to glucose in late pregnancy have been reported both in women [1,2] and laboratory animals [3,4]. Distinct changes in the endocrine pancreas during pregnancy have been reported, which include progressive rise in the ratio of endocrine to exocrine tissue, β cell hypertrophy, β cell hyperplasia, increased secretory activity of β cells, swollen mitochondria, increased amount of light (pale) β granules, and increased incidence of rough endoplasmic reticulum [5–7]. In vitro pancreatic islets from pregnant rats have been shown to respond to glucose or amino acids with significantly higher release of insulin when compared with islets from nonpregnant animals (Fig 35-1) [8–10]. Islets from pregnant rats compared to those of nonpregnant rats were found to be much more metabolically active, as indicated by significantly higher concentrations of adenylate cyclase and of basal and cyclic AMP-dependent protein kinase, which correlates with increased insulin response to glucose. Phosphodiesterase and phosphatase activity, on the other hand, was not significantly different [11]. Pregnancy-associated changes in the α cell function of glucagon release have also been reported [8,12].

The mechanism of the observed changes in pancreatic function during pregnancy appears to involve gonadal, adrenal, and placental hormones, while hypophyseal hormones do not appear to play an important role, as ascertained from experiments in hypophysectomized pregnant rats [3]. In a study of cultured islets, only placental lactogen of the placental hormones was shown to cause hyperplasia and hypertrophy of β cells directly, while progesterone was without effect [13]. Overwhelming evidence, however, indicates a definite role for sex steroids and glucocorticoids in glucose homeostasis, both in pregnant and nonpregnant animals. The functional role of each hormone individually is, however, as yet undecided, and the mechanism of action at the cellular level is unknown.

ROLE OF SEX STEROIDS

Long-term in vivo treatment of spayed animal models with various combinations of sex steroids has provided the most convincing evidence for a role of sex steroids in endocrine pancreatic functions. In ovariectomized rats [14] and mice [15], a decrease in the plasma insulin levels and a decreased insulin response (to glucose or amino acids) from isolated islets have been shown, indicating a role of gonadal hormones in normal glucose homeostasis. Administration of estradiol or progesterone to the ovariectomized rats restores most of the deleterious effects of ovariectomy on pancreatic functions [14–17]. Along the same lines, in vitro administration of estradiol or progesterone has been shown to cause hyperinsulinism, hypertrophy, and hyperplasia of the pancreas [10,15,18–20]. Treatment of rats with estradiol and progesterone has also been shown to be associated with ultrastructural changes in the pancreatic islets resembling those seen during pregnancy. These changes are apparently predominantly due to an estradiol effect, and progesterone may have

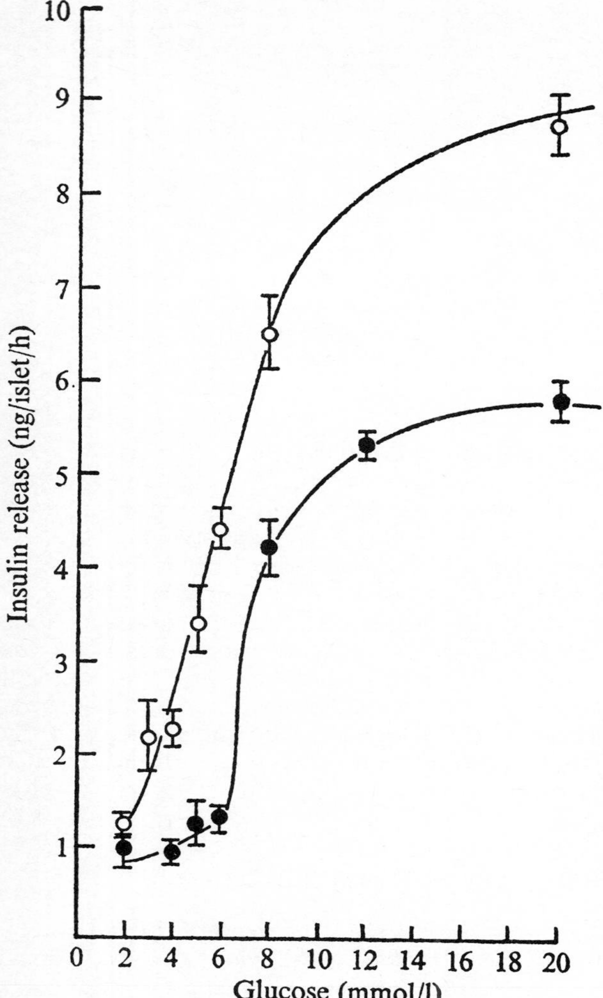

Figure 35-1. Effect of varying glucose concentrations on insulin release from normal rats (closed circle) and pregnant female rats (open circle). Each point represents a mean of at least 12 observations, with ±SEM shown as vertical bars. (From Green and Taylor [9], by permission of the Journal of Endocrinology.)

only a synergistic effect [21]. A predominant role of estradiol is also indicated from findings that insulin levels and the insulin response to glucose are highest during proestrus and estrus and are significantly lower during diestrus in four-day-cycling rats [16]. In one study, the in vivo role of progesterone in augmenting the effect of estradiol on insulin release was not observed [14]. The hyperinsulinism induced by estrogens, however, is believed to result from the direct trophic action of estrogens on the endocrine pancreas [4]. A direct effect of estrogens on insulin secretion is not observed in the absence of adrenals [22], which supports the view that the increase in insulin that follows estrogen treatment of ovariectomized rats is secondary to trophic effects on the pancreatic cells. Similarly, the severe hypoglycemic effects of streptozotocin in intact and ovariectomized mice and the cytotoxic effects of the drug on the β cells have been shown to be countered effectively by administration of estradiol-17β [23].

As opposed to the described insulinotropic effects of estradiol in ovariectomized animals, progesterone alone appears to be required in the intact animals in order to allow for enhanced insulin release in response to glucose, increased plasma insulin levels, and higher cyclic AMP (cAMP) content of the pancreas [4,24–27]. In one study, estradiol was reported to oppose the insulinotropic effects of progesterone in intact rats [25]. Thus, in intact animals, estradiol may have a priming effect on the positive insulinotropic effect of progesterone, since in ovariectomized animals, progesterone has not been reported to significantly increase insulin response to glucose without estradiol. Neither of the sex steroid hormones given to ovariectomized rats was observed to significantly increase the insulin response to glucose; this may be related to the very high doses of steroids used [28]. In another recent study, ovariectomy in rats was found to result in increased calcium uptake, high insulin content, enhanced glucose oxidation, enhanced glucose-induced secretion of insulin, and ultrastructural changes in β cells, all of which changes were restored to normal with estradiol and progesterone treatment [29]. These observations, however, appear to contradict the findings of most other workers.

Direct effects of sex steroid hormones in organ or tissue culture have also been studied recently. Most reports have not confirmed an acute insulin release from the islets during short-term (<2 hr) incubation of the islets with steroids [4,19]. However, at longer incubation periods (20 hr) with progesterone and estradiol, insulin release was enhanced without concomitant changes in the adenylate cyclase activity [19]. On long-term (15 days) tissue culture of mouse islets, an increase in insulin release has been reported in the presence of progesterone but not in the presence of estradiol or testosterone [30].

The role of androgens in pancreatic function is not clear. Exogenous testosterone has been shown to have a deleterious effect on glucose tolerance both in male and female spayed rats [16]. In tissue culture studies of islets, testosterone has not been found to have any effect on insulin release [30]. Thus, an effect, if any, of androgens on the endocrine pancreatic function in normal male rats remains to be shown.

The *importance of glucocorticoids* in the observed hyperinsulinemic response of ovariectomized rats to estradiol has been demonstrated in one study in which adrenalectomy caused estradiol to have the opposite effect [17]. Corticoids have, in fact, been shown to cause hyperinsulinemia [31–33], β cell hyperplasia [34], a decrease in glucagon levels [33], and ultrastructural changes in the pancreas similar to those seen with gonadal hormones [35]. Adrenalectomy has been shown to cause a decrease in glucose oxidation, calcium uptake, insulin response to glucose, and cAMP concentrations, which were all reversed by dexamethasone [36]. The in vivo, long-term effects of gonadal hormone, may, in fact, be mediated by a number of hormones, including glucocorticoids, since estradiol is known to cause an increase in the concentration of cortisol [35] and growth hormone [37] and a decrease in glucagon [17], all of which result in an increase in insulin levels; progesterone reduces growth hormone secretions [38]. Since a protective effect of estradiol in experimentally diabetic animals has been observed even in adrenalectomized and hypophysectomized animals [39], an important role of estradiol in the insulinotropic effects cannot be ignored.

Corticosterone and cortisone have been found to have a negative effect on the secretion of insulin in response to glucose or amino acids in vitro [40,41], which is contrary to the observed hyperinsulinemic effects of glucocorticoids in vivo [31–33]. The in vivo effect may be caused by peripheral resistance to the action of insulin that is induced by corticoids to insulin [34]. ACTH and dexamethasone are known to cause a 50 to 60 percent decrease in insulin binding to receptors on hepatocytes by changing the affinity of the binding sites [42], thus inducing a peripheral resistance effect. The direct negative effect on insulin release observed in vitro appears to be produced by an impairment of calcium influx into the islet cells [41].

STEROID BINDING PROTEINS

Strong evidence for a direct role of gonadal steroids in the endocrine functions of pancreas is provided by the finding of specific binding proteins for steroids in the islets. Estrogen receptors with a relatively high binding affinity ($K_d = 20$ nM), high binding capacity (170 fmol/mg protein), and a 4S molecular form have been described in the pancreatic islets of rats [43,44]. The number of unoccupied binding sites was found to decrease significantly during premajority of the sites by high circulating levels of endogenous estradiol. In streptozotocin-induced diabetes in rats, estrogen receptors were greatly reduced in a similar fashion, which strongly suggested a primary location of estrogen receptors in β cells, since β cells are eliminated on streptozotocin treatment [45].

In male and female baboons, the possible presence of estrogen but not androgen receptors has been demonstrated by autoradiographic localization of specifically bound estradiol in the nuclei of islet cells [46]. Extracellular calcium-dependent uptake of ^{3}H-progesterone by rat islets that specifically translocates to the nucleus has also been demonstrated [47]. The binding to the cytosol protein appears to be saturable, indicating the presence of high-affinity progesterone receptors in the islets of Langerhans from female rats [47]. An extremely high concentration and uptake of ^{3}H-testosterone by castrated male and female rat pancreas, even higher than that by the classic androgen target organs such as prostate, has been reported [48]; this indicates the presence of androgen-binding proteins in the pancreas. This has been confirmed by the finding (both in the cytosol and nuclei of rat pancreas) of high-affinity ($K_d = 2$ nM) and low-capacity (4.7 fmol/mg protein) androgen receptors that bind testosterone and 5α-dihydrotestosterone (DHT) with equal affinity, have a 3–5S sedimentation value, and have been described similarly [49]. Though both aromatase and 5α-reductase activities have been described in normal pancreas to a small extent [50], 5α-reductase does not appear to be very active in the pancreas, since 70–90 percent of ^{3}H-testosterone that was localized in the pancreatic nuclei was unmetabolized and only traces of 5α-DHT were observed [49]. In another study, however, significant uptake of androgens in the pancreatic tissue was not observed, while significant uptake and retention of estradiol by the pancreas, especially the exocrine pancreas, was seen in dogs and baboons [51].

STEROIDS AND EXOCRINE PANCREATIC FUNCTIONS

A possible role for steroids in exocrine pancreatic function has only recently become apparent. The presence of zymogen granules in the pancreatic acini has been shown to be dependent on glucocorticoids or estrogenic steroids [52,53]. Adrenalectomy in male rats and ovariectomy in female rats caused a marked depletion of the zymogen granules, and within 9 hours of treatment with triamcinolone or estradiol, complete restoration of granules was observed; restoration was unaffected by actinomycin D [53]. Uptake of amino acid was also found to be significantly affected by the steroid hormone status of the animals, which indicates a role for steroid hormones in the synthesis and secretion of proteins by the exocrine pancreas.

The action of glucocorticoids has been examined extensively [52,53]. In adrenalectomized animals, protein synthesis and secretion from the pancreas were greatly enhanced, resulting in loss of zymogen granules. Administration of triamcinolone restored these effects. Thus, it appears that under normal conditions, endogenous steroids exert a negative modulatory effect on protein synthesis. The ability of acinar cells to secrete in the apparent absence of secretory vesicles (zymogen granules) and under conditions of steroid depletion may signify that secretion of proteins does not always require the presence of secretory vesicles [54,55]. In a study of cultured mouse acini, a similar dramatic reduction in rates of amylase release and ^{3}H-leucine incorporation after corticosterone has been shown [56]. Epidermal growth factor significantly increases androgen release, especially in the presence of insulin and carbachol, while glucagon, growth hormone, T_3, and secretin were without effect [56]. Similarly, administration of estrogens to dogs reportedly results in decreased protein, zinc, and bicarbonate and increased amylase and lipase levels in the pancreas, while amylase release is inhibited [57].

Pancreatitis, an acinar disease, has been shown to be associated on occasion with estrogen administration given for contraceptive purposes, for treatment of postmenopausal syndrome, or for treatment of prostatic carcinoma [58,59]. The mechanism of action of estrogen, however, may be peripherally related to the associated hypertriglyceridemia, caused by a number of hormonal changes induced by estradiol, such as increase in insulin and growth hormone levels and decrease in glucagon levels [59].

Steroid Binding in the Exocrine Pancreas

Demonstration of specific uptake and retention of estriol (E_3) and estrone (E_1) and of diethylstilbestrol (DES) (but not testosterone and 5α-dihydrotestosterone) in pancreatic tissues [51] resulted in a search for specific estradiol-binding proteins in the pancreas. In 1973, a cytosol-receptor protein for E_3 and estradiol (E_2) was described in the pancreas of dogs, baboons, and humans. The receptor has a sedimentation coefficient of 3.7 to 4.2S, and is apparently translocated to the nucleus, since a 4.6S binding protein could be extracted from the nucleus [60]. The exact number of the receptor sites or the cellular location was not described, but an acinar localization appeared likely. Later, the same group described the presence of a 4S binding protein in the cytosol and in microsomal and nuclear extracts. Both a high-affinity ($K_d = 10^{-7}$ to 10^{-9} M), low-capacity E_2-binder and a very large capacity, nonsaturable, E_2-binder with a low affinity were described [61]. Thus, for the first time, it became clear that pancreatic tissue has more than one type of E_2-binder, but its cellular localization was not clear [61]. Later studies localized the high-capacity E_2-binder to the cytosol and microsomal fractions, with a capacity of approximately 1,000 fmol/mg cytosol protein [57,62]. The microsomal E_2-binder was studied in some detail and found to be specific to its localization in the pancreas and to be immunologically distinct from microsomal proteins from other glands [57,62].

High-capacity, low-affinity E_2-binders have been similarly described in the liver [63], while low-affinity, high-capacity androgen binding proteins have been described in male reproductive tract tissues [64]. These binding sites may play a role in the secretory function of the tissues, since estrogens and androgens have been shown to affect the attachment of ribosomes to liver endoplasmic reticulum [65]; or the role may be in the movement of electrolytes, since in the kidney, estrogenic influence on the electrolyte movement has been shown [66].

Nuclear estrogen receptors in the acinar cells either have not been observed [67] or low levels (18–38 fmol) have been described [57]. Boctor et al [67] have not observed the presence of high-affinity E_2-binders in either the cytosol or nuclei of pancreatic acini but have described the presence of soluble, high-capacity, low-affinity E_2-binders that do not translocate to the nucleus and require the presence of an endogenous factor for binding to estradiol, as demonstrated by their elegant experiments (Fig 35-2) [68].

The number of binding sites appeared to increase in the presence of increasing concentrations of an accessory cofactor, the activity of which could be mimicked by a serum protease substrate such as the oligopeptide *N*-benzoyl-L-phenylail-

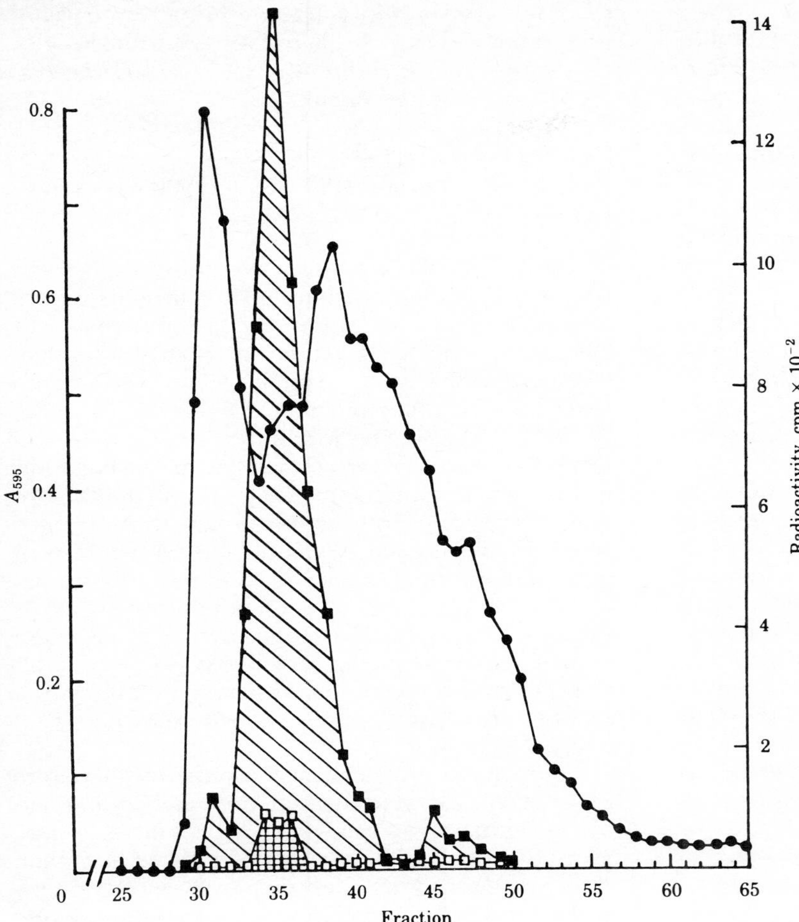

Figure 35-2. Elution pattern of [^{3}H]estradiol-binding protein chromatography on Sephacryl S-200. One milliliter of the 100,000 × *G* supernatant from rat pancreas, initially homogenized in buffer *b*, was charged onto a Sephacryl S-200 (Pharmacia) column (1.6 × 82 cm) equilibrated at 8°C with 10 mM Tris, pH 7.4/0.05 percent NaN_3. Elution was with buffer A at a flow rate of 8 mL/hr (approximately 1.8 mL per fraction). To 100-μL aliquots of each fraction was added 50 μL of buffer (open square) or 50 μL of accessory factor (closed square); 50 μL of [^{3}H]estradiol (final concentration, 10 nM), and, after 1 hr at room temperature, 300 μL of charcoal suspension. The suspension was chilled for 30 minutes at 0°C and centrifuged, and 100-μL aliquots of the supernatant were assayed. Protein was determined in 100 μL aliquots treated with 2.5 mL of Bio-Rad protein reagent (A_{595}) (closed circle) or 100 μL of [^{3}H]estradiol [68]. Recovery of protein was >90 percent. (From Boctor et al [68], by permission of The National Academy of Sciences.)

anyl-L-valyl-L-arginyl *P*-nitroanilide [69]. In the absence of the cofactor, ^{3}H-E_2 binding was negligible; it was increased significantly in the presence of the cofactor. Binding was found to range from 0.6 pmol (K_d of 7 nM) to almost 12 pmol/mg protein (K_d of 200 nM) in relation to cofactor concentration [69]. The significance of the high-capacity E_2-binders, however, remains questionable, since the serum concentration of estradiol in male and female rats between 30 and 90 days of age is only 1 to 2 × 10^{-10} M [70]; at such concentration only 1 percent of the total binding sites would be occupied under physiologic conditions.

In the human pancreas obtained from cadavers 24 to 28 hours after death, a high-capacity (4 percent of the total cytosol protein) and low-affinity estrogen binding protein has been described [71]. This binding protein has a sedimentation coefficient of 3S and a Stokes radius of 52 Å and was not found to bind to either DNA cellulose or phosphocellulose [71].

STEROIDS AND PANCREATIC CARCINOMA

High-affinity estrogen binding proteins with a high capacity of 157 to 2,769 fmol/mg protein have been observed in malignant and fetal pancreatic cytosols, and no 5α-dihydrotestosterone binding has been observed [72,73]. Similarly, Molteni et al [74] reported the presence of 4S and 8S estrogen-binding proteins with high-binding capacities (approximately 1,000 fmol/g tissue) in both the normal pancreas and in transplantable acinar carcinoma of rats. In 1980, Stedman et al reported 4S and 8S estrogen receptors (220 to 1,000 fmol/g tissue) in two specimens of human pancreatic cancer [75], while Satake et al [76] observed estrogen receptors with low capacity (4 fmol) and high affinity (0.04 nM) in only one out of seven human pancreatic ductal cancers. In another study, however, no estrogen receptors were detected in two human pancreatic cancers [77].

In about 43 percent of rat pancreatic carcinomas induced by DMBA (9,10-dimethyl-1,2-benzanthracene) and determined to be of ductal origin, high-affinity (K_d = 0.1–0.5 nM) estrogen receptors, with binding sites ranging from 8 to 34 fmol have been described [76]. Molteni et al [78], on the other hand, did not find estrogen binding in ductal pancreatic carcinoma but did report a high degree of E_2-positive binding in rat pancreatic acinar carcinoma.

A recent study suggests a further possible role for testosterone in pancreatic carcinoma [79]: in both men and women with pancreatic carcinoma, a significantly lower level of serum testosterone was present compared to that in healthy controls or patients with other malignancies. Serum estradiol concentrations were, on the other hand, within normal range in both men and women with pancreatic and other malignant cancers. Since a high content of 5α-reductase and aromatase levels has also been reported in pancreatic carcinoma tissue of patients [50], the low testosterone levels observed could be a result of high uptake by the pancreatic cancer tissues. In breast carcinoma also, abnormalities have been found in the estrogen receptor levels, aromatase and 5α-reductase levels [80–85], and androgen levels [86]. These studies suggest a possible role of steroids and steroid receptors in the development or treatment of pancreatic cancer.

PEPTIDES AND STEROID INTERACTIONS IN PANCREATIC FUNCTION

We know of only one study on the important aspect of possible interactions of steroids and peptides in the control of pancreatic function. Somatostatin, in the high concentrations of 2–25 μM, has been reported to enhance specific binding of ^{3}H-E_2 to cytosolic protein, while at higher concentrations it inhibits the binding [87]. These effects may be caused by degradation products of somatostatin. Since somatostatin has been shown to be internalized into mucosal cells [88] in a manner similar to the entrance of insulin into the hepatocytes [89], and since somatostatin has been shown to activate phosphatase activity at 0.1 nM concentration [88], the internalized somatostatin may possibly interact with estradiol-binding protein and inhibit exocytosis by anchoring to the membrane structures [87]. In another system, E_2 has been shown to inhibit the binding and mitogenic effects of epidermal growth factor (a peptide hormone) on primary cultures of *Xenopus* hepatocytes [90], which indicates once again that steroid hormones may indeed interact directly with the binding systems of gut peptide hormones.

ROLE OF STEROIDS IN NORMAL AND CANCEROUS GUT TISSUES

Little information exists regarding the role of steroids, if any, in normal gut function. Estrogen, however, has been shown to cause movement of calcium in another system, i.e., diethylstilbestrol (DES) was observed to inhibit calcium influx into and cause the efflux of calcium from uterine mitochondria [91,92]. The inhibitory effect of DES on histamine release from rat peritoneal mast cells, in proportion to its negative effect on atropine content, has been recently reported [93]; this indicates a direct effect of estrogens on the metabolism of cells, which results in an inhibition of degranulation. The effect of estrogen on gut mast cells, however, is unknown, but since estrogen has been shown to alter membrane transport [94], a generalized effect of estrogen on secretory functions in a number of tissues, including pancreas, could be envisaged.

Men have an increased incidence of peptic ulcer as compared to women, especially women in the child-bearing years [95]. This difference may be due to an action of testosterone or estradiol. Through ages 15–60, men secrete more acid in response to a test meal than women [96]. Pregnancy has a protective effect against peptic ulcers [97]. These observations suggest a possible role of estrogenic and androgenic hormones in peptic ulcer and in the secretion of gastric acid as well. This possibility is enhanced by our recent finding of specific estradiol-binding proteins in the stomach of both male and female rats [98], which appear to be directly under the control of the sex steroid hormones [99].

Progesterone has been shown to inhibit motility of human gastric and colonic smooth muscle in vitro, while estradiol and corticoids were found to be without effect [100]. In another study, estrogens have been shown to stimulate intestinal motility, as does cholecystokinin (CCK) [101].

Significant effects of steroids on the ion transport and absorptive capacity of the proximal and distal colon have also been demonstrated [102–104]. Mineralo- and glucocorticoids affect absorption of sodium by the proximal and distal colon of rabbits [102]. Corticosteroids have also been shown to significantly affect the enzymatic and morphologic maturation as well as the osmoregulatory function of mammalian and nonmammalian intestine [103]. The reported presence of type I (high-affinity) mineralocorticoid receptors and of type II (low-affinity) glucocorticoid receptors in the cytosol of jejunum and colon of the domestic duck [103] and of type I glucocorticoid receptors in isolated intestinal epithelial cells of rats [104] further corroborates an important and direct role of steroid hormones in the absorptive function of the intestine.

In cancer tissues, only an 8S estrogen binding protein has been reported in colonic neoplasms ranging from 16 to 69 fmol/g tissue; the protein was present in 24 percent of tumors [105]. Colon cancer is reportedly more common in women, while pancreatic and rectal cancers are more common in men [106]. Either a 4S, or an 8S, or both 4S and 8S estrogen-binding proteins have been reported in 50 percent of colon and rectal carcinomas, ranging from 78 to 1,394 fmol/g tissue [78].

In a study by Alford et al [107], 33 primary human colon cancers were examined for the presence of estradiol, progesterone, and dihydrotestosterone receptors. Seventy percent were positive for one or the other steroid receptors, 30 percent were positive for high-affinity estradiol receptors, 26 percent contained all three receptors, and 23 percent were positive for glucocorticoid receptors [107]. Thus some large bowel cancers may be endocrine-dependent [107]. In a follow-up study, six of eight patients whose tumors showed steroid-binding activity for at least one steroid were free of disease 1 to 3 years postoperatively, but only two of 12 patients who were negative for steroid-binding proteins were free of disease [108]. In another recent study, an increase in the percentage of samples containing estradiol and progesterone receptors was reported in both normal and malignant tissues from patients with adenocarcinoma of the colon compared to samples from normal tissues from patients without colon disease [109]. The authors suggest that the presence of estrogen and progesterone receptors may be indicative of a precancerous condition, contrary to the conclusions of Geelhoed et al [108].

These results suggest a possible therapeutic significance of steroid-binding proteins in colon cancers, in a manner analogous to the role of steroid receptors in breast cancer. In preliminary studies, however, we have found a high percentage of fundic and colon carcinomas to be positive for specific progesterone binding sites rather than estradiol binding sites [110]. Steroid receptors have, in fact, been described in a number of soft tissue sarcomas and meningiomas [111,112]. The significance of the steroid receptors in the various cancer tissue is, as yet, not understood. They may be related either to dedifferentiation as a result of oncogenesis [105] or to a hormonal dependence of the cancer, as seen in breast, endometrial, and prostatic cancers [113–115].

Estrogens and androgens have been implicated in the etiology of colon cancer. Davidson et al [116] support the concept that estrogens have a promoting effect on cancer of the right side of the colon. They suggest that another explanation for the sex and site distribution of colorectal cancer may be the androgenic stimulation of the left side of the colon relative to that of the right. Based on their findings, Stebbings et al [117], on the other hand, concluded that androgens may actually promote the formation of colorectal adenomas, which may partly explain the predominance of colorectal adenomas in male patients aged 65 years and over.

STEROIDS AND GALLBLADDER FUNCTIONS

Gallbladder disease is more prevalent in women than in men [118,119]. Gallbladder emptying is impaired during pregnancy (Fig 35-3) [101,120,121], and the lithogenicity of bile decreases in the second and third trimesters of pregnancy [121]. The increase in lithogenicity could be an estrogen effect, since estradiol administration results in decreased bile acid synthesis and secretion [121,122]. Decreased bile acid secretion could

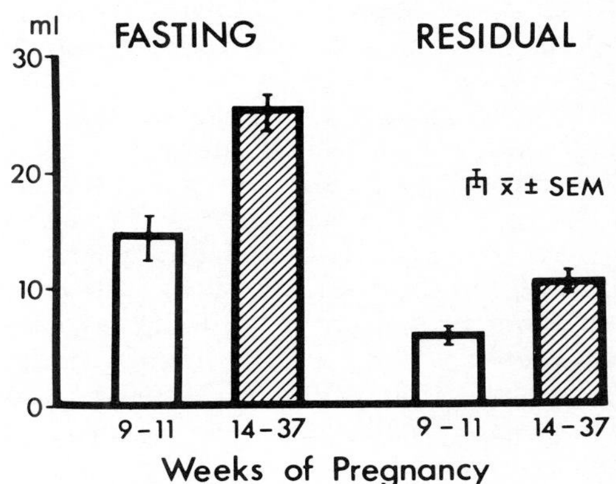

Figure 35-3. Fasting and residual gallbladder volumes during pregnancy. Both volumes are much larger in the last two thirds of pregnancy than in early pregnancy ($p < 0.0005$ for both). (From Braverman et al [101], by permission of the Massachusetts Medical Society.)

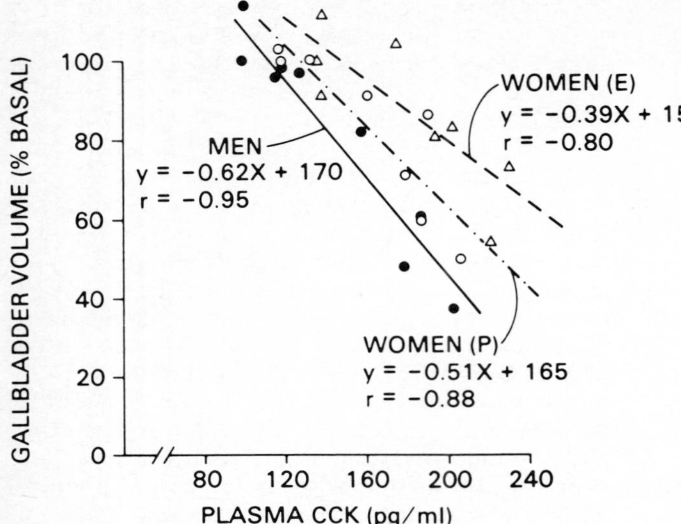

Figure 35-4. Linear regression analysis of gallbladder volume (expressed as % basal volume) versus plasma concentration of CCK. Slope for men (black circle) is significantly different from that for women (E) (triangle) but not from that for women (P) (open circle). (From Fried et al [127], by permission of the The CV Mosby Co.)

then lead to lithogenic bile because of relatively greater cholesterol secretion [121], or it could be due to higher cholesterol synthesis and turnover rate. Both of these functions are E_2-dependent and have been shown to occur [120,123,124]. Estrogens have been shown to significantly increase the prostaglandin activity of rabbit gallbladder; the biosynthesis of prostaglandins was found to be 20-fold higher in female rabbits compared to male rabbits [125]. This indicates that the sex-dependent differences in the observed activity of the gallbladder could be attributable to the prostaglandin effect of estrogens.

Gallbladder motility was reportedly impaired during the ovulatory cycle [126], while in a study from our laboratory, impaired gallbladder emptying in response to CCK was observed at the progesterone peak of the menstrual cycle in women (Fig 35-4). Men had a larger fasting gallbladder volume than women and showed greater gallbladder contractility in response to endogenous release of CCK [127]. In vitro studies with gallbladder strips have reported that gallbladders from pregnant rabbits show diminished sensitivity to CCK, and estrogen, but not progesterone, diminished gallbladder contractility [128]. Another in vitro study, however, reported that gallbladder strips from progesterone-treated male guinea pigs contracted less in response to CCK and acetylcholine than strips from untreated males [129].

Preliminary studies in our laboratory indicate an increased presence of progesterone receptors in diseased gallbladder muscle, while estrogen receptors and CCK receptor levels are unaffected, further indicating the role of female gonadal steroids in the gallbladder function. A negative effect of progesterone on fluid transport rates in vitro, in the gallbladder, has been reported in guinea pigs [130].

REFERENCES

1. Spellacy WN, Goetz FC: Plasma insulin in normal late pregnancy. N Eng J Med 268:988, 1963.
2. Kalkhoff R, Schalch DS, Walker JL, et al: Diabetogenic factors associated with pregnancy. Trans Assoc Am Physicians 77:271, 1964.
3. Malaisse WJ, Malaisse-Lagae F, Picard C, et al: Effects of pregnancy and chorionic growth hormone upon insulin secretion. Endocrinology 84:41, 1969.
4. Costrini NV, Kalkhoff RK: Relative effects of pregnancy, estradiol and progesterone in plasma insulin and pancreatic islet insulin secretion. J Clin Invest 50:992, 1971.
5. Aerts L, Van Assche FA: Ultrastructural changes of the endocrine pancreas in pregnant rats. Diabetologia 11:285, 1975.
6. Van Assche FA, Aerts L, Gepts W: Morphological changes in the endocrine pancreas in pregnant rats with experimental diabetes. J Endocrinol 80:175, 1979.
7. Marynissen G, Aerts L, Van Assche FA: The endocrine pancreas during pregnancy and lactation in the rat. J Dev Physiol 5:373, 1983.
8. Kalkhoff RK, Kim H-J: Effects of pregnancy on insulin and glucagon secretion by perfused rat pancreatic islets. Endocrinology 102:623, 1978.
9. Green IC, Taylor KW: Effects of pregnancy in the rat on the size and insulin secretory response to the islets of Langerhans. J Endocrinol 54:317, 1972.
10. Sutter-Dub M-T: Effects of pregnancy and progesterone and/or oestradiol on the insulin secretion

and pancreatic insulin content in the perfused rat pancreas. Diabete Metab 5:47, 1979.
11. Lipson LG, Sharp GWG: Insulin release in pregnancy: Studies on adenylate cyclase, phosphodiesterase, protein kinase, and phosphoprotein phosphatase in isolated rat islets of Langerhans. Endocrinology 103:1272, 1978.
12. Mandour T, Kissebah AH, Wynn V: Mechanism of oestrogen and progesterone effects on lipid and carbohydrate metabolism: Alteration in the insulin: glucagon molar ratio and hepatic enzyme activity. Eur J Clin Invest 7:181, 1977.
13. Nielsen JH: Effects of growth hormone, prolactin and placental lactogen on insulin content and release, and deoxyribonucleic acid synthesis in cultured pancreatic islets. Endocrinology 110:600, 1982.
14. Basabe JC, Chieri RA, Foglia VG: Action of sex hormones on the insulinemia of castrated female rats. Proc Soc Exp Biol Med 130:1159, 1969.
15. Bailey CJ, Ahmed-Sorour H: Role of ovarian hormones in the long-term control of glucose homeostasis. Effects on insulin secretion. Diabetologia 19:475, 1980.
16. Bailey CJ, Matty AJ: Glucose tolerance and plasma insulin of the rat in relation to the oestrous cycle and sex hormones. Horm Metab Res 4:266, 1972.
17. Faure A, Sutter-Dub M-T, Sutter BCJ, et al: Ovarian-adrenal interactions in regulation of endocrine pancreatic function in the rat. Diabetologia 24:122, 1983.
18. Green IC, El Seifi S, Perrin D, et al: Cell replication in the islets of Langerhans of adult rats: Effects of pregnancy, ovariectomy, and treatment with steroid hormones. J Endocrinol 88:219, 1981.
19. Howell SL, Tyhurst M, Green IC: Direct effects of progesterone on rat islets of Langerhans in vivo and in tissue culture. Diabetologia 13:579, 1977.
20. Sutter-Dub M-T, Faure A, Aerts L, et al: Effects of progesterone and 17-β-oestradiol treatments on the pancreatic B cell in castrated female rats. Biochemical variations. J Physiol (Paris) 74:725, 1978.
21. Aerts L, Van Assche FA, Faure A, et al: Effects of treatment with progesterone and oestradiol-17β on the endocrine pancreas in ovariectomized rats: Ultrastructural variations in the B cells. J Endocrinol 84:317, 1980.
22. Faure A, Haouari M, Sutter BCJ: Insulin secretion and biosynthesis after oestradiol treatment. Horm Metab Res 17:378, 1985.
23. Puah JA, Bailey CJ: Insulinotropic effect of ovarian steroid hormones in streptozotocin diabetic female mice. Horm Metab Res 17:216, 1985.
24. Ashby JP, Shirling D, Baird JD: Effect of progesterone on insulin secretion in the rat. J Endocrinol 76:479, 1978.
25. Hager D, Georg RH, Leitner JW, et al: Insulin secretion and content in isolated rat pancreatic islets following treatment with gestational hormones. Endocrinology 91:977, 1972.
26. Hamburger AD, Kuipers ACJ, van der View J: The effect of progesterone on plasma insulin in the rabbit. Experientia 31:602, 1975.
27. Beck P: Progestin enhancement of the plasma insulin response to glucose in rhesus monkeys. Diabetes 18:146, 1969.
28. Lenzen S: Effects of ovariectomy and treatment with progesterone or oestradiol-17β on the secretion of insulin by the perfused rat pancreas. J Endocrinol 78:153, 1978.
29. Garcia ME, Borelli MI, Dumm CLG, et al: Functional and ultrastructural changes induced by short term ovariectomy on pancreatic islets. Horm Metab Res 15:76, 1983.
30. Nielsen JH: Direct effect of gonadal and contraceptive steroids on insulin release from mouse pancreatic islets in organ culture. Acta Endocrinologica 105:245, 1984.
31. Malaisse WJ, Malaisse-Lagae F, McCraw EF, et al: Insulin secretion in vitro by pancreatic tissue from normal, adrenalectomized, and cortisol-treated rats. Proc Soc Exp Biol Med 124:924, 1967.
32. Sutter BCJ: Surrenale et insulinemie chez le rat. II. Corticosurrenale et insuline serique. Diabetologia 4:295, 1968.
33. Lenzen S: The effect of hydrocortisone treatment and adrenalectomy on insulin and glucagon secretion from the perfused rat pancreas. Endokrinologie 68:189, 1976.
34. Tomita T, Visser P, Friesen S, et al: Cortisone-induced islet cell hyperplasia in hamsters. Virchows Arch [Cell Pathol] 45:85, 1984.
35. Bencosme SA, Martinez-Palomo A: Formation of secretory granules in pancreatic islet B cells of cortisone-treated rabbits. Lab Invest 18:746, 1968.
36. Borelli MI, Garcia ME, Dumm CLG, et al: Glucocorticoid-induced changes in insulin secretion related to the metabolism and ultrastructure of pancreatic islets. Horm Metab Res 14:287, 1982.
37. Frantz AG, Rabkin MT: Effects of estrogen and sex difference on secretion on human growth hormone. J Clin Endocrinol 25:1470, 1965.
38. Bhatia SK, Moore D, Kalkhoff RK: Progesterone suppression of the plasma growth hormone response. J Clin Endocrinol Metab 35:364, 1972.
39. Rodriguez RR: Influence of oestrogens and androgens on the production and prevention of diabetes, in Leibel BS, Wrenshall GA (eds): *On the Nature and Treatment of Diabetes*. Amsterdam, Excerpta Medica, 1965, pp 288–307.
40. Barseghian G, Levine R, Epps P: Direct effect of cortisol and cortisone on insulin and glucagon secretion. Endocrinology 111:1648, 1982.
41. Billaudel B, Mathias PCF, Sutter BCJ, et al: Inhibition by corticosterone of calcium inflow and insulin release in rat pancreatic islets. J Endocrinol 100:227, 1984.
42. Kahn CR: Role of insulin receptors in insulin-resistant states. Metabolism 29:455, 1980.
43. Tesone M, Chazenbalk GD, Ballejos G, et al: Estro-

gen receptor in rat pancreatic islets. J Steroid Biochem 11:1309, 1979.
44. El Seifi S, Green IC, Perrin D: Insulin release and steroid-hormone binding in isolated islets of Langerhans in the rat: effects of ovariectomy. J Endocrinol 90:59, 1981.
45. Agarwal MK (ed): *Streptozotocin. Fundamentals and Therapy*. New York, Elsevier/North-Holland, 1981.
46. Winborn WB, Sheridan PJ, McGill HC: Estrogen receptors in the islets of Langerhans of baboons. Cell Tissue Res 230:219, 1983.
47. Green IC, Howell SL, El Seifi S, et al: Binding of ^{3}H-progesterone by isolated rat islets of Langerhans. Diabetologia 15:349, 1978.
48. Gustafsson J-A, Pousette A: Demonstration and partial characterization of cytosol receptors for testosterone. Biochemistry 14:3094, 1975.
49. Pousette A: Demonstration of an androgen receptor in rat pancreas. Biochem J 157:229, 1976.
50. Iqbal MJ, Greenway B, Wilkinson ML, et al: Sex-steroid enzymes, aromatase and 5α-reductase in the pancreas: A comparison of normal adult, foetal and malignant tissue. Clin Sci 65:71, 1983.
51. Kirdani RY, Varkarakis MJ, Murphy GP, et al: Distribution of simultaneously injected androgens and estrogens in animal tissues. Endocrinology 90:1245, 1972.
52. Grossman A, Boctor AM, Lane B: Dependence of pancreatic integrity on adrenal and ovarian secretions. Endocrinology 85:956, 1969.
53. Grossman A, Boctor AM, Band P, et al: Role of steroids in secretion-modulating effect of triamcinolone and estradiol on protein synthesis and secretion from the rat exocrine pancreas. J Steroid Biochem 19:1069, 1983.
54. Rothman SS: Protein transport by the pancreas. The current paradigm is analyzed and an alternative hypothesis is proposed. Science 190:747, 1975.
55. Rothman SS: Passage of proteins through membranes—old assumptions and new perspectives. Am J Physiol 238:G391, 1980.
56. Logsdon CD, Williams JA: Pancreatic acini in short-term culture: Regulation by EGF, carbachol, insulin, and corticosterone. Am J Physiol 244:G675, 1983.
57. Sandberg AA, Rosenthal HE: Steroid receptors in exocrine glands: The pancreas and prostate. J Steroid Biochem 11:293, 1979.
58. Mallory A, Kern F: Drug-induced pancreatitis: A critical review. Gastroenterology 78:813, 1980.
59. Parker WA: Estrogen-induced pancreatitis. Clin Pharmacol 2:75, 1983.
60. Sandberg AA, Kirdani RY, Varkarakis MJ, et al: Estrogen receptor protein of pancreas. Steroids 22:259, 1973.
61. Sandberg AA, Rosenthal HE: Estrogen receptors in the pancreas. J Steroid Biochem 5:969, 1974.
62. Rosenthal HE, Sandberg AA: Estrogen binding proteins in rat pancreas. J Steroid Biochem 9:1133, 1978.
63. Gschwendt M: A cytoplasmic oestrogen-binding component in chicken liver. Hoppe Seylers Z Physiol Chem 356:157, 1975.
64. Ritzen EM, Hagenas L: Androgen binding and transport in testis and epididymis. Vitam Horm 33:283, 1975.
65. Blyth CA, Freedman RB, Rabin BR: Sex specific binding of steroid hormones to microsomal membranes of rat liver. Nature New Biol 230:137, 1971.
66. DeVries JR, Ludens JH, Fanestil DD: Estradiol renal receptor molecules and estradiol-dependent antinatriuresis. Kidney Int 2:95, 1972.
67. Boctor AM, Band P, Grossman A: Specific binding of ^{3}H-estradiol to the cytosol of rat pancreas and uterus: Bound sites in pancreatic extracts do not translocate ^{3}H-estradiol to nuclei suggesting a basic difference in mode of action. J Recep Res 2:453, 1981–82.
68. Boctor AM, Band P, Grossman A: Requirement for an accessory factor for binding of ^{3}H-estradiol to protein in the cytosol fraction of rat pancreas. Proc Natl Acad Sci USA 78:5648, 1981.
69. Boctor AM, Band P, Grossman A: Specific binding of [^{3}H]-estradiol to the cytosol of rat pancreas: Alteration of the apparent number of binding sites by an endogenous factor and oligopeptide derivatives. J Steroid Biochem 18:245, 1983.
70. Dohler KD, Wuttke W: Changes with age in levels of serum gonadotropins, prolactin, and gonadal steroids in prepubertal male and female rats. Endocrinology 97:898, 1975.
71. Pousette A, Carlstrom K, Skoldefors H, et al: Purification and partial characterization of a 17β-estradiol-binding macromolecule in the human pancreas. Cancer Res 42:633, 1982.
72. Greenway BA, Iqbal MJ, Johnson PJ, et al: Pancreatic carcinoma—A sex-steroid responsive tumour? Proc ASCO 1:6, 1982.
73. Greenway B, Iqbal MJ, Johnson PJ, et al: Oestrogen receptor proteins in malignant and fetal pancreas. Br Med J 283:751, 1981.
74. Molteni A, Rao MS, Reddy JK, et al: Estradiol receptors in the transplantable pancreatic carcinoma of the rat. Fed Proc 37:897, 1978.
75. Stedman KE, Moore GE, Morgan RT: Estrogen receptor proteins in diverse human tumors. Arch Surg 115:244, 1980.
76. Satake K, Yoshimoto T, Mukai R, et al: Estrogen receptors in 7,12-dimethylbenz (a) anthracene (DMBA) induced pancreatic carcinoma in rats and in human pancreatic carcinoma. Clin Oncol 8:49, 1982.
77. Kiang DT, Kennedy BJ: Estrogen receptor assay in the differential diagnosis of adenocarcinomas. JAMA 238:32, 1977.
78. Molteni A, Bahu RM, Battifora HA, et al: Estradiol receptor assays in normal and neoplastic tissues. A possible diagnostic aid for tumor differentiation. Ann Clin Lab Sci 9:103, 1979.
79. Greenway B, Iqbal MJ, Johnson PJ, et al: Low

serum testosterone concentrations in patients with carcinoma of the pancreas. Br Med J 286:93, 1983.
80. Singh P, Chattopadhyay T, Kapur MM, et al: Cytosol and nuclear estradiol receptors in normal and cancerous breast tissue of women. Ind J Med Res 68:97, 1978.
81. Singh P: Interaction of androgens with the normal and cancerous tissues of women. Ph.D. Thesis. All India Institute of Medical Sciences, India, 1978.
82. Singh P, Laumas KR, Muldoon TG: Metabolic pathway of androgens in non-cancerous and cancerous human mammary gland tissues. Endocrinology 114(Suppl):1522, 1984.
83. McGuire WL: An update on estrogen and progesterone receptors in prognosis for primary and advanced breast cancer, in Iacobelli S, King RJB, Lippman ME (eds): *Hormones and Cancer.* New York, Raven Press, 1980.
84. Wittliff JL, Savlov ED: Estrogen-binding capacity of cytoplasmic forms of the estrogen receptors in human breast cancer, in McGuire WL, Carbone PP, Vollmer EP (eds): *Estrogen Receptors in Human Breast Cancer.* New York, Raven Press, 1975.
85. Miller WR, Hawkins RA, Forrest APM: Steroid metabolism and oestrogen receptors in human breast carcinomas. Eur J Cancer Clin Oncol 17:913, 1981.
86. Bulbrook RD, Hayward JL, Spicer CC: Relation between urinary androgen and corticoid excretion and subsequent breast cancer. Lancet 2:395, 1971.
87. Band P, Richardson SB, Boctor AM, et al: Somatostatin enhances binding of [^{3}H]estradiol to a cytosolic protein in rat pancreas. J Biol Chem 258:7284, 1983.
88. Reyl JF, Lewin MJM: Intracellular receptor for somatostatin in gastric mucosal cells: Decomposition and reconstitution of somatostatin-stimulated phosphoprotein phosphatase. Proc Natl Acad Sci USA 79:978, 1982.
89. Schlessinger J, Shechter Y, Willingham MC, et al: Direct visualization of binding, aggregation, and internalization of insulin and epidermal growth factor on living fibroblastic cells. Proc Natl Acad Sci USA 75:2659, 1978.
90. Wolffe AP, Bersimbaev RI, Tata JR: Inhibition by estradiol of binding and mitogenic effect of epidermal growth factor in primary cultures of *Xenopus* hepatocytes. Mol Cell Endocrinol 40:167, 1985.
91. Batra S, Bengtsson LP: Inhibition by diethylstilbestrol of calcium uptake by human myometrial mitochondria. Eur J Pharmacol 18:281, 1972.
92. Batra SC: Effect of some estrogens and progesterone on calcium uptake and calcium release by myometrial mitochondria. Biochem Pharmacol 22:803, 1973.
93. Suzuki T, Uchida MK: Inhibitory effect of diethylstilbestrol on histamine release by rat mast cells and its relation to the cellular ATP content. Biochim Biophys Acta 803:323, 1984.
94. Pietras RJ, Szego CM: Steroid hormone-responsive, isolated endometrial cells. Endocrinology 96:946, 1975.
95. Ivy AC, Martin CG: Sex as a constitutional factor for susceptibility to peptic ulcer. Gastroenterology 13:215, 1949.
96. Vanzant FR, Alvarez WC, Eusterman GB, et al: The normal range of gastric acidity from youth to old age. Arch Int Med 49:345, 1932.
97. Sandweiss DJ, Saltzstein HC, Farbman AA: The relation of sex hormones to peptic ulcer. Am J Dig Dis 6:6, 1939.
98. Singh P, Afinni B, Thompson JC: Estradiol binding proteins in the GI tract of rats. Gastroenterology 88:1589, 1985.
99. Singh P, Afinni B, Thompson JC: Effect of steroids on estradiol (E_2) and progesterone (Pg) binding sites in the fundus and pancreas of castrated male and female rats. Gastroenterology 88:1589, 1985.
100. Kumar D: In vitro inhibitory effect of progesterone on extrauterine human smooth muscle. Am J Obstet Gynecol 84:1300, 1962.
101. Braverman DZ, Johnson ML, Kern F Jr: Effects of pregnancy and contraceptive steroids on gallbladder function. N Engl J Med 302:362, 1980.
102. Sellin JH, DeSoignie RC: Steroids alter ion transport and absorptive capacity in proximal and distal colon. Am J Physiol 249:G113, 1985.
103. DiBattista JA, Mehdi AZ, Sandor T: A profile of the intestinal mucosal corticosteroid receptors in the domestic duck. Gen Comp Endocrinol 59:31, 1985.
104. Lentze MJ, Colony P, Trier JS: Glucocorticoid receptors in isolated intestinal epithelial cells in rats. Am J Physiol 249:G58, 1985.
105. McClendon JE, Appleby D, Claudon DB, et al: Colonic neoplasms. Tissue estrogen receptor and carcinoembryonic antigen. Arch Surg 112:240, 1977.
106. Morson BC, Dawson IMP (eds): *Gastrointestinal Pathology.* London, Blackwell Scientific Publications, 1972.
107. Alford TC, Do H-M, Geelhoed GW, et al: Steroid hormone receptors in human colon cancers. Cancer 43:980, 1979.
108. Geelhoed GW, Alford C, Lippman ME: Biologic implications of steroid hormone receptors in cancers of the colon. South Med J 78:252, 1985.
109. Marugo M, Molinari F, Fazzuoli L, et al: Estradiol and progesterone receptors in normal and pathologic colonic mucosa in humans. J Endocrinol Invest 8:117, 1985.
110. Singh P, Rae-Venter B, Townsend CM Jr, et al: Estrogen and progesterone binding in human GI cancers. Gastroenterology 88:1589, 1985.
111. Chaudhuri PK, Walker MJ, Beattie CW, et al: Distribution of steroid hormone receptors in human soft tissue sarcomas. Surgery 90:149, 1981.
112. Donnell MS, Meyer GA, Donegan WL: Estrogen-receptor protein in intracranial meningiomas. J Neurosurg 50:499, 1979.
113. Ekman P, Dahlberg E, Gustafsson J-A, et al: Present and future clinical value of steroid receptor assays in human prostatic carcinoma, in Iacobelle S, King RJB, Lindner HR, Lippman ME (eds): *Hormones and Cancer.* New York, Raven Press, 1980, pp 361–370.

114. Siiteri PK, Nisker JA, Hammond GL: Hormonal basis of risk factors for breast and endometrial cancer, in Iacobelle S, King RJB, Lindner HR, Lippman ME (eds): *Hormones and Cancer.* New York, Raven Press, 1980, pp 499–505.
115. James VHT, Reed MJ: Steroid hormones and human cancer, in Iacobelle S, King RJB, Lindner HR, Lippman ME (eds): *Hormones and Cancer.* New York, Raven Press, 1980, pp 471–487.
116. Davidson M, Yoshizawa CN, Kolonel LN: Do sex hormones affect colorectal cancer? Br Med J 290:1868, 1985.
117. Stebbings WSL, Farthing MJG, Vinson GP, et al: Do sex hormones affect colorectal cancer? Br Med J 291:138, 1985.
118. Bennion LJ, Grundy SM: Risk factors for the development of cholelithiasis in man. N Engl J Med 299:1161; 1221, 1978.
119. Friedman GD, Kannel WB, Dawber TR: The epidemiology of gallbladder disease: Observations in the Framingham study. J Chron Dis 19:273, 1966.
120. Gerdes MM, Boyden EA: The rate of emptying of the human gallbladder in pregnancy. Surg Gynecol Obstet 66:145, 1938.
121. Kern F Jr, Everson GT, DeMark B, et al: Biliary lipids, bile acids, and gallbladder function in the human female. J Clin Invest 68:1229, 1981.
122. Lynn J, Williams L, O'Brien J, et al: Effects of estrogen upon bile: Implications with respect to gallstone formation. Ann Surg 178:514, 1973.
123. Nilsson S, Stattin S: Gallbladder emptying during the normal menstrual cycle. A cholecystographic study. Acta Chir Scand 133:648, 1967.
124. Kritchevsky D, Staple E, Rabinowitz JL, et al: Differences in cholesterol oxidation and biosynthesis in liver of male and female rats. Am J Physiol 200:519, 1961.
125. Myers SI: Effect of estrogen on rabbit gallbladder prostaglandin biosynthesis. J Surg Res 38:630, 1985.
126. Everson GT, McKinley C, Lawson M, et al: Gallbladder function in the human female: Effect of the ovulatory cycle, pregnancy, and contraceptive steroids. Gastroenterology 82:711, 1982.
127. Fried GM, Ogden WD, Fagan CJ, et al: Comparison of cholecystokinin release and gallbladder emptying in men and in women at estrogen and progesterone phases of the menstrual cycle. Surgery 95:284, 1984.
128. Zhu XG, Fried GM, Greeley G, et al: Effect of estrogen and progesterone on cholecystokinin-stimulated gallbladder contraction in vitro. Gastroenterology 82:1218, 1982.
129. Ryan JP, Pellecchia D: Effect of progesterone pretreatment on guinea pig gallbladder motility in vitro. Gastroenterology 83:81, 1982.
130. Mat CRBC, France VM: Effect of 17β-oestradiol priming on progesterone induced inhibition of fluid transport by male guinea-pig gall-bladder *in vitro.* J. Physiol 278:30P, 1978.

Section Nine

Clinical Issues

Chapter 36

Clinical Significance of Gastrointestinal Hormones

Marilyn Marx, M.D., Jan B. Newman, M.D., Karen S. Guice, M.D., William H. Nealon, M.D., Courtney M. Townsend, Jr., M.D., and James C. Thompson, M.D.

Gastrointestinal hormones may be involved in many diseases of the gut. So far, however, we can identify significant roles only in peptic ulcer disease, syndromes caused by gastrointestinal hormone-producing tumors, chronic pancreatitis, and sprue.

PEPTIC ULCER DISEASE

Radioimmunoassay (RIA), which allows for quantitative determination of peptide hormones, has expanded our knowledge regarding the pathogenesis of ulcer disease. Yet, instead of a clearer definition of ulcer disease, the new discoveries raise new questions in regard to mechanisms and previously unknown hormonal relationships. Peptic ulcer disease affects 10 million people in the United States, but the exact etiology remains a mystery.

We know that peptic ulcer disease results from an abnormal relationship between parietal cell acid production and mucosal resistance to acid injury [1,2]. In simplistic terms, we may say that peptic ulcers occur when acid-peptic forces attacking the mucosa overcome mucosal defense mechanisms (Table 36-1).

Normal Acid Secretion

Gastric acid is normally produced by the parietal cells in the fundic mucosa. Parietal cells are receptive to three types of control: neuroendocrine, endocrine, and paracrine (Fig 36-1). These signals may function independently or together to regulate acid production.

Parietal cells concentrate hydrogen ions more than one million times. Grossman [3] has suggested that the parietal cell is probably stimulated by five chemical agents: acetylcholine released from cho-

Table 36-1. **Factors involved in the pathogenesis of peptic ulceration**
Enzymatic digestion of mucous membrane

Attack	*Defense*
Acid peptic digestion (pH < 4)	Dilution (nonparietal secretion)
Drugs (salicylates, steroids)	Emptying
Direct trauma	Neutralization (HCO_3^- from bile and pancreas)
Ischemia	Mucosal barrier (probably most important)
	Rich blood supply

No acid—no ulcer

linergic nerve endings; gastrin from G cells in the antrum and duodenum; so-called intestinal phase hormones [4,5]; ingested protein, which apparently may stimulate the parietal cell directly; and histamine, which binds to specific histamine type 2 (H_2) receptors on the parietal cell. Grossman and Konturek [6] suggested that parietal cells do not secrete with maximal efficiency unless all receptors are occupied. It is thought that for maximal acid secretion to occur, all receptors must be occupied by their respective secretagogues; however, in the face of blockade of one receptor, some acid secretion may still occur. This theory, though unproven, is helpful in explaining why vagotomy and H_2-receptor antagonists (cimetidine, ranitidine, and famolidine) work. Vagotomy removes vagal acetylcholine, and the receptor antagonists block histamine from its receptor. The histamine receptor is clearly the most important, because when it is blocked, acid output is nearly abolished (see Fig 9-3).

Neurocrine stimulation through vagal nerve fibers, mediated by acetylcholine, occurs during the cephalic and gastric phases of gastric secretion. Vagal excitation of the parietal cells is both direct via acetylcholine and indirect via release of gastrin [7]. Atropine blocks the parietal cell response both to direct vagal excitation and to gastrin [8,9]. Vagal denervation, which lowers acid secretion, also inhibits the parietal cell response to gastrin. Recent immunohistochemical studies have located substance P, vasoactive intestinal peptide (VIP), somatostatin, and enkephalin in nerves of the gastric myenteric plexus [10,11], but the function of these neuropeptides in this location remains uncertain.

Endocrine control of acid production is primarily due to the release and actions of gastrin, which is produced in G cells of the antrum and released by mechanical, neural, or chemical stimuli. Stimulation of gastrin release is mediated by gastric and intestinal intraluminal peptides and amino acids [12], gastric distention, vagal cholinergic effects, blood-borne calcium [13], and epinephrine [14]. Inhibition of gastrin release may be accomplished by intraluminal acid, acting directly upon G cells, or by release of secretin [15]. Other blood-borne mediators, gastric inhibitory polypeptide (GIP), VIP, glucagon, or calcitonin [16], also inhibit gastrin release. Acid inhibition is the only mechanism yet shown to have important physiologic action as feedback.

The major physiologic action of gastrin is to stimulate gastric acid production. Additionally, it causes pepsin release and increases gastric mucosal blood flow. Gastrin is rapidly catabolized by a widespread, nonspecific mechanism acting in the circulation.

One paracrine effect on the parietal cell is illustrated by the mast cell, which has a long axonlike projection that appears to touch the parietal cell in histologic sections. It is believed that this "connection" is part of a histamine-mediated regulatory feedback mechanism for control of parietal cell function.

Negative regulation of acid output by control feedback is typified by somatostatin [17]. Somatostatin is produced by the "D" cells of the gastric mucosa, which are distributed in the antrum in a

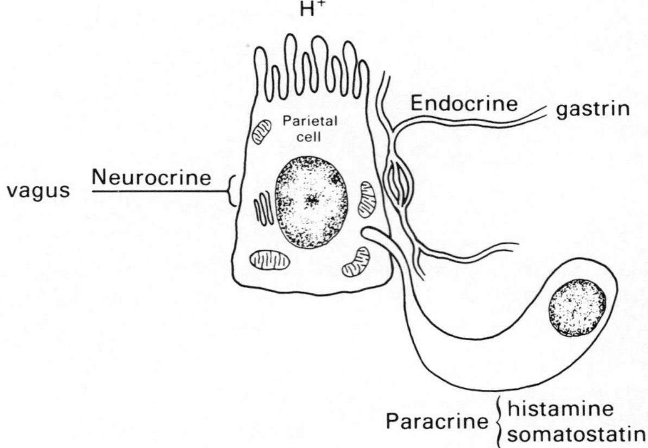

Figure 36-1. Acid secretion from the parietal cell is controlled by neurocrine, endocrine, and paracrine factors.

pattern similar to that of the G cells. These D cells also exhibit paracrine control [11,18,19]. Somatostatin, in addition to its direct paracrine effects, appears to function locally via intramural portal venous connections [20] to inhibit gastric acid secretion. This results from both a direct effect on the parietal cell and indirectly via suppression of gastrin release. Somatostatin may be the long-sought antral chalone [4]. Somatostatin is released by vagal stimulation, secretin, pentagastrin, bombesin, calcitonin, and apomorphine [17]. It is also released by duodenal acidification [10,21].

Abnormal Acid Secretion

In 1910, Schwarz [22] gave us the dictum: "no acid-no ulcer." Even though we know that peptic ulceration occurs only in the presence of acid, quantitative studies of acid, of acid-control mechanisms, and of the role of gastrointestinal hormones in acid regulation have failed to delineate completely the pathophysiology of peptic ulcer disease.

Duodenal ulcers generally occur in the presence of excess gastric acid, but they may also occur with normal acid output. Only one third of patients with clinical duodenal ulcer disease secrete excessive amounts of acid [23]. Despite hypersecretion of acid caused by gastrin released by gastrinoma, 5 to 10 percent of patients with the Zollinger-Ellison (ZE) syndrome do not have peptic ulcers [24]. This implies that there is not a simple linear relationship between peptic ulcer disease and acid production. Several additional mechanisms are involved in producing the clinical picture of peptic ulcer disease. For purposes of simplification, we will examine several of the relationships between the control mechanisms and the gastrointestinal hormones that allow production of excess acid.

First, there may be excess acid synthesis for one of several reasons: increased parietal cell mass, greater sensitivity of the parietal cells to acid-releasing stimuli, or an increased capacity of the parietal cell to release acid with normal stimuli [25]. Second, there may be an increase in release or an increased sensitivity of the mechanisms to release acid stimuli. Finally, a defect in negative feedback may exist, resulting in a relative increase in the release of acid.

Duodenal ulcer patients, as a population, have an increased capacity to secrete gastric acid [1], but only one third of individuals with duodenal ulcers actually hypersecrete [23]. The fasting gastric acid secretion of some duodenal ulcer patients is greater than controls [26]; a greater parietal cell mass appears to be at least a partial explanation [25,27]. Increased parietal cell mass may explain why duodenal ulcer patients have an increased basal acid output and a greater maximal capacity for acid production. The increased parietal cell mass in patients with gastrinoma has been attributed to the known tropic effects of gastrin on gastric and duodenal mucosa [28].

Gastric acid secretion is probably, in part, genetically determined. Full-blooded Pima Indians do not develop peptic ulcer disease but may develop chronic gastritis and gastric cancer. Basal and betazole-stimulated gastric acid outputs are significantly lower in these Indians than those found in age- and weight-matched Caucasian controls (basal and meal-stimulated plasma gastrin levels were higher in Pima Indians) [29]. This would imply that this particular genetically homogeneous group has either a smaller parietal cell mass or a decrease in parietal cell sensitivity to gastrin that may convey protection from peptic ulcer disease.

The relationship of gastrin to common acid-peptic disease is only partially defined. While it is clear that elevated serum gastrin levels are associated with increased acid production and release, hypergastrinemia is a term that requires definition. Because there are many different molecular forms of gastrin (G-17 and G-34, for example) and many radioimmunoassays in use, it is important to realize that some gastrins have more physiologic significance than others. The full significance of this molecular heterogeneity has yet to be described [30–32]. Clearance studies of synthetic human gastrin, G-17, demonstrated that the half-life was the same for duodenal ulcer patients and normal controls [33], while other studies have shown an increase in both the antral and serum concentrations of the N-terminal fragment of G-17 in duodenal ulcer patients [34]. Several studies have suggested that gastrin may be processed in an abnormal fashion by duodenal ulcer patients. Most of the studies are based on small samples. Since duodenal ulcer is a disease noted for its heterogeneity, we must await studies on large numbers of patients before we can accept these implications of gastrin's involvement.

Immediate postprandial release of gastrin is not increased in duodenal ulcer disease, but acid secretion is increased during the second to fourth hour after ingestion of a meal [1]. There appears to be no correlation between basal or postprandial serum gastrin concentration and maximal acid output in ordinary duodenal ulcer disease [28].

However, if the sensitivity of the parietal cell is increased in duodenal ulcer disease, then normal gastrin concentrations could cause a greater acid response. In a study comparing serum gastrin levels after insulin-induced hypoglycemia in patients with duodenal disease and normal controls, when complete neutralization of intragastric acid was done, serum gastrin levels rose higher in the duodenal ulcer patients than in the controls, but there was no difference before neutralization. This suggests that there is a greater gastrin response to vagal stimulation but that the excess acid effectively provides rapid negative feedback [35].

Duodenal ulcer patients are more sensitive than normal subjects to both exogenous and endogenous gastrins. This may be because of increased vagal tone, increased affinity of parietal cell gastrin receptors, or high levels of second messengers, such as calcium. Increases in acid secretion in these patients also appear to be more sensitive to antral distention when their duodenal ulcer disease is active [36].

The classic illustration of hypergastrinemia and ulcer disease is the ZE syndrome, seen with a gastrin-secreting, non-β cell tumor. Hypergastrinemia is also seen in patients with antral G cell hyperplasia, retained antrum after antrectomy and vagotomy, massive small bowel resection, or renal failure.

The clinical manifestations of the ZE syndrome are variable. Causes of hypergastrinemia are shown in Table 36-2. Peptic ulcers may be found in the duodenum or stomach as well as in atypical locations, such as the jejunum. Other patients (about 7 percent) have diarrhea as the only complaint. The diagnosis of ZE syndrome requires reproducible fasting hypergastrinemia, elevated basal acid output, and elevated stimulated maximal acid output [24,37]. The diagnosis is confirmed by secretin-stimulated increases in serum gastrin. About 25 percent of patients with ZE syndrome have the multiple endocrine neoplasia I syndrome (MEN I), the most common manifestation of which is parathyroid adenoma [38].

Table 36-2. Causes of hypergastrinemia

Increased stimulation of gastrin release
- ZE syndrome (gastrinoma)
- Antral G cell hyperplasia ± pheochromocytoma
- Pyloric obstruction

Decreased inhibition of gastrin release
- Hypo- or achlorhydria (atrophic gastritis, pernicious anemia, gastric carcinoma, vitiligo)
- Antral exclusion operation
- Vagotomy

Possible decreased catabolism
- Chronic renal failure

Unknown
- Rheumatoid arthritis
- Small bowel resection (temp.)

Antral G cell hyperplasia is a rare condition but should be considered if other causes of hypergastrinemia are absent [37,39]. Secondary G cell hyperplasia occurs in patients with pernicious anemia due to the loss of acid feedback inhibition of gastrin [15,37].

If a portion of antrum is left in continuity with the duodenum and both are excluded from the remaining stomach, as may occur with a Billroth II reconstruction, hypergastrinemia will result, again due to loss of acid feedback inhibition [37]. This situation can usually be avoided by obtaining histologic confirmation of duodenal mucosa at the distal resection margin at the time of antrectomy.

Massive small bowel resection also leads to hypergastrinemia. Occasionally, peptic ulcer results, but the pathogenesis is not entirely clear. This hypergastrinemic effect is usually transient and can be successfully treated by H_2-receptor blockage.

Because the kidneys are responsible for the clearance of gastrin, nephrectomy [40] or renal failure [37] may lead to hypergastrinemia.

The concept of vagal hyperfunction, initially proposed by Dragstedt [41], although not proved, is still quite attractive. During a sham feeding-pentagastrin study, duodenal ulcer patients not only showed higher basal acid outputs but also a greater response to vagal stimulation than controls [30]. Duodenal ulcer patients given small doses of atropine demonstrate a significant rise in serum gastrin concentrations compared to normals. Basal secretion of acid and pepsin in normal controls is diminished with small amounts of atropine, whereas patients with duodenal ulcer disease require five times the amount of atropine to achieve a comparable 50 percent inhibition of basal acid and pepsin output [9].

Additional information regarding the importance of vagal innervation comes from studies of ulcer patients before and after vagotomy. Postvagotomy basal acid and pepsin outputs were reduced by 78 and 62 percent, respectively. These levels were returned almost to preoperative values when secretion was measured after urecholine treatment simulating vagal stimulation [42]. Vagotomy in some form is the key to surgical management of peptic ulcer disease. Clinical evidence and probable pathophysiology of vagal influence in peptic ulcer disease favor the most specific approach, a highly selective vagal denervation of the parietal cell mass.

Impairment of feedback has yet to be demonstrated clinically. Somatostatin inhibits gastrin release as well as acid secretion and is thought to act through both hormone and paracrine pathways. Serum somatostatin levels, both basal and food-stimulated, are the same in patients with duodenal ulcers and normal controls, despite the high basal, food-stimulated and peak pentagastrin-stimulated gastric acid secretion rates observed in the patient with ulcer disease [43]. Exogenous somatostatin given to the same group of patients inhibits blood-stimulated gastric acid secretion and gastrin release to the same extent in ulcer patients and normal controls [43].

Other hormonal feedback mechanisms include secretin, which is normally released by acidification of the duodenum. In one study [44], secretin release was found to be less in patients with duodenal ulcer disease than in normals. However, when the technique of intragastric titration was used, there was no evidence for defective feedback inhibition of gastric secretion on gastrin release. Furthermore, secretin release was the same in duodenal ulcer patients and normal controls [45].

Gastric emptying is more rapid in duodenal ulcer patients [46]. Postprandial secretion-emptying kinetic studies have determined the rate at which acid is delivered to the duodenum. Duodenal ulcer patients have an abnormally prolonged gastric secretory response to food; acid secretion returns to fasting levels more slowly than in controls [1].

The role of mucosal resistance is less well understood than that of acid secretion. The protective mucus coating of the gastric epithelium, the vascular supply of the stomach, and the rate of epithelial regeneration are probably all protective mechanisms. The relative contribution of each to protection from ulcer disease has not, however, been firmly established. Most investigators in the area of mucosal resistance have examined gastric ulcers. Primary gastric ulcers are characterized by a low acid output, both basal [47] and maximal [48], so that these models may not explain the pathogenesis of duodenal ulcer disease.

Reflux of duodenal contents into the stomach is thought to be one mechanism by which gastric mucosa is damaged and made susceptible to ulceration [49]. Bile acids and lysolecithin have been implicated as specific agents in duodenal contents that destroy the normal protective barrier [50,51].

In rabbits subjected to hemorrhagic shock, diminished mucosal blood flow has been shown to be an important factor in acute stress ulceration [52]. Conversely, selective vasodilation of gastric blood vessels with isoproterenol protected the gastric mucosa in a similar hemorrhagic shock model in rabbits [53].

Both ischemic and bile-induced gastric ulcers, however, require the addition of acid. Ulcers produced by constant intragastric infusion of 0.1 M hydrochloric acid are prevented in dogs by the simultaneous administration of intravenous sodium bicarbonate [54].

There is not a simple explanation for the pathogenesis of peptic ulcer disease. Acid is important, but it is only one mechanism by which ulcers are produced. Hypergastrinemia, likewise, accounts for only a small proportion of ulcers. Peptic ulcer disease is produced by a complex set of interactions between neural and hormonal regulatory mechanisms, many of which are not currently understood.

POSSIBLE ROLES OF GUT PEPTIDES IN DUODENAL ULCER DISEASE

There has been recent interest in the influence of various newly discovered peptides in the pathogenesis of duodenal ulcer disease [28,55]. Basal acid hypersecretion in duodenal ulcer disease is unrelated to elevated gastrin levels. Alternate explanations for this phenomenon have included the intestinal phase hormone entero-oxyntin, the proposed acid secretagogue released from the small intestine [56,57]. Controversy has surrounded the existence of this peptide, particularly in view of the fact that IV amino acids may mimic at least some of that peptide's putative actions [58]. Another candidate for this nongastrin stimulation of basal acid output is endogenous endorphins, based upon the observation that naloxone inhibits basal acid secretion [59].

The finding of increased postprandial acid secretion has also correlated poorly with serum gastrin determinations and may be explained by numerous hypothetical mechanisms (see above). Earlier in this chapter, we discussed the possibility of an increased sensitivity of the parietal cell to gastrin. Another possible mechanism is a disproportionate release of a more potent form of gastrin. Three molecular forms of gastrin predominate in the circulation of higher mammals, G-34, G-17, and G-14, with the number referring to the number of amino acids in each molecular form. Each fragment has preserved the intact carboxyl-terminal amino acids and all are biologically active. The two larger forms, G-17 and G-34, predominate in humans, with G-17 largely in the antral G cells and G-34 in the duodenal G cells; the site of origin gains biologic significance only after a Billroth I antrectomy reconstruction. Using two antisera to gastrin, one specific for G-17 and one that measures both G-17 and G-34, Taylor et al [60] were able to demonstrate a significantly elevated response of the combined G-17/G-34 to a meal in duodenal ulcer patients compared to normal controls, with no difference in the G-17 fraction. This suggests a postprandial hypersecretion of G-34. Recent studies suggest that these two fragments have a comparable molar potency [61]; this is in contrast to the traditional belief that G-34 was a minimally effective acid secretagogue. This finding has sparked renewed interest in this hypothesis.

The list of gastrointestinal peptides that have been shown to exert an inhibitory action on the gastric parietal cell has grown. Postprandial hypersecretion of gastric acid may result from a diminished postprandial release of an inhibitory peptide. Kihl et al [62] made the observation that intraduodenal oleate inhibited gastric acid secretion less effectively in duodenal ulcer patients than in controls, and they found close correlation between the degree of inhibition and postprandial release of neurotensin, a known inhibitor of acid output. More recently discovered peptides, such as peptide YY and calcitonin gene-related peptide (CGRP), are also known to act as inhibitors of gastric secretion. Peptide YY is present in the distal gut and is released by fat. Postprandial release of CGRP has not been clearly demonstrated, and neither peptide has been studied in duodenal ulcer patients. The increased rate of gastric emptying observed in duodenal ulcer patients may be explained by a loss of inhibitors of motility; the majority of peptides that inhibit secretion have a similar effect on gastric emptying.

The concept of mucosal integrity is a factor in the pathogenesis of duodenal ulcer disease. The gastrointestinal mucosa has the capacity for extremely rapid cell turnover, and peptides that enhance the regenerative process may be expected to preserve the mucosal barrier. Epidermal growth factor is trophic to rat gastric mucosa [63] and is a potent antagonist of acid secretion. The potential role for such an agent in the treatment of duodenal ulcer disease and the possible consequences of a deficiency of this substance in the pathophysiology of duodenal ulcer disease are intriguing, but as yet unexplored.

GASTROINTESTINAL HORMONE-PRODUCING TUMORS

Endocrine tumors may arise from any portion of the gastrointestinal tract or pancreas. The great majority of gastrointestinal hormone-producing tumors are found in the pancreas (Table 36-3). The cells that give rise to these neoplasms are members of a diffuse neuroendocrine system with similar biochemical and histologic characteristics [64,65]. Specifically, they have the capacity for amine precursor uptake and decarboxylation (APUD). "APUD cell" is a collective term for components of this diffuse neuroendocrine system. Another common feature of all APUD cells is the presence of neuron-specific enolase, a glycolytic enzyme first recognized in brain tissue [66]. Many objections have been raised to the APUD concept, and there now appear to be as many arguments against it as in its favor.

Most gastrointestinal hormone-producing tumors secrete a single peptide that is responsible for the clinical and biochemical features that characterize each syndrome. These cells also have polyhormonal potential [67], and multiple hormones may often be extracted from a tumor of a patient in whom one hormone alone is responsible for the clinical features of the syndrome.

The islets of Langerhans of the adult human pancreas contain four different types of endocrine cells that secrete specific types of hormones: α cells (glucagon), β cells (insulin), Δ_1 cells (somatostatin), and Δ_2 cells (VIP). G cells, which secrete gastrin, are found in the fetal but not the adult human pancreas [68]; G cells in the adult are concentrated in the mucosa of the antrum of the stomach. Tumors that arise from these specific endocrine cells and secrete biologically active peptides are named for the peptides secreted. These tumors

Table 36-3. Pancreatic islet cell tumors

α cell:	Glucagon	Glucagonoma
β cell:	Insulin	Insulinoma
Δ cell:	Somatostatin	Somatostatinoma
Δ_2 cells:	VIP	WDHA
G cell:	Gastrin	ZE syndrome

are insulinomas, gastrinomas, VIPomas, and somatostatinomas.

There are as yet only five clear-cut, well-recognized clinical syndromes that involve tumors of the gastrointestinal tract and pancreas. The hormones involved and the diseases are 1) insulin in patients with insulinoma; 2) gastrin in patients with the ZE syndrome; 3) VIP in the watery diarrhea (WDHA or Verner-Morrison) syndrome caused by VIP-producing tumor (VIPoma), which may be in the pancreas or which may be a ganglioneuroblastoma; 4) glucagon in the glucagonoma syndrome (diabetes, dermatitis, glossitis, and anemia); and 5) somatostatin in the somatostatinoma syndrome (mild diabetes, dyspepsia, and gallstones). Tumors from cells producing PP, calcitonin, GRF, and neurotensin have also been reported. Clinical features of noninsulin-producing islet cell tumors are summarized in Table 36-4. After briefly discussing the five well-recognized endocrinopathies, we will also describe abnormalities of gastrointestinal hormones seen in sprue-like syndromes and in chronic pancreatitis.

Neoplasms arising from endocrine cells may be benign or malignant, and different endocrine tumors tend to exhibit one biologic behavior or the other (for example, 90 percent of insulinomas are benign, whereas at least 60 percent of gastrinomas are malignant). The majority of these peptide-producing tumors occur in the pancreas, but primary tumors have been found in the wall of the duodenum, in the stomach, in solitary lymph nodes, in the liver, in the ovary, and in other ectopic sites as well.

The biologic behavior of gastrointestinal hormone-producing tumors is now relatively well defined [24,55]. In the period of initial recognition of each syndrome, almost all the early cases manifested full-blown, almost over-ripe, expressions of hormone excess. A high percentage of tumors were malignant. With more experience, we recognize earlier and less flagrant examples that are often atypical. In pure form, the separate patterns of behavior of the different syndromes are easily recognized. Surgical management is directed primarily at tumor removal in order to effect cure of the syndromes as well as to prevent complications of persistent tumor growth and, subsequently, metastasis [69]. For patients with unresectable tumors, systemically active therapy has been developed that is directed at the product of the tumor (for example, H_2-receptor antagonists for ZE syndrome patients and diazoxide for patients with hyperinsulinism), and that is cytotoxic for the tumor itself. The long-acting analog of somatostatin ("Sandostatin," SMS 201-995) is effective in treating many symptoms (especially secretory diarrhea) of nonresectable functioning endocrine tumors.

Insulinoma

The syndrome of insulinoma is caused by an overproduction of insulin, usually by a solitary, benign β cell neoplasm of the islets of Langerhans. The clinical symptoms are largely neurologic, are caused by acute and chronic episodes of hypoglycemia, and may be present for years [70–72]. These symptoms, which occur in the majority of patients, are nonfocal and transient (apathy, dizziness, cloudy sensorium, behavioral disorders, coma, or seizures). On the other hand, temporary, focal symptoms, such as paralysis, sensory loss, or diplopia, may also occur. Many patients with insulinoma have been found in mental hospitals, where they were placed because of bizarre behavior disorders or decreased mental ability due to prolonged periods of hypoglycemia that resulted in permanent neurologic deficits. Patients may also show symptoms of catecholamine excess, including episodic palpitations, pallor, chest pain, nausea, vomiting, and diarrhea.

Symptoms of hypoglycemia caused by excess circulating insulin are often precipitated by prolonged fasting or by exercise. Observations of patients with insulinomas led Whipple and Frantz [73] in 1935 to propose a diagnostic triad bearing Whipple's name: a) symptoms of hypoglycemia brought about by fasting or exercise, b) the presence of a low blood glucose (less than 45 mg/dL), and c) symptoms that are relieved by administration of glucose. Symptoms are precipitated by a 12-hr fast in 37 percent of patients, in 73 percent by a 24-hr fast, and in 95 percent by a fast of 72 hr [70,74]. The ability to measure insulin by specific RIA has improved the specificity of diagnosis of insulinoma. Hypoglycemia brought about by prolonged fasting is, however, the most reliable diagnostic test for the presence of an insulinoma. By simultaneous measurement of blood glucose and insulin levels, an inappropriately high insulin level for the existing glucose level can be detected. The insulin-glucose ratio thus derived is a highly specific diagnostic test for insulinoma. The normal insulin-glucose ratio is equal to or less than 0.4, and patients with insulinoma often exhibit ratios higher than 1.0.

Studies of the biosynthesis and secretion of insulin in normal and abnormal states have led to further accuracy in the differential diagnosis of

Table 36-4. Characteristics of islet cell tumors

Tumor	*Clinical Features*	*Diagnostic Features*	*Ectopic*	*Malignant, %*	*Multiple, %*	*Localization*	*Resectable, %*
Insulinoma	Symptoms of hypoglycemia (catecholamine release) plus mental confusion and obtundation (late)	Absolute (unusual) or relative (common) hyperinsulinism, appropriate levels of C-reactive protein	rare (<5%)	10	10	Percutaneous transhepatic venous sampling, angiography	>90
Gastrinoma	Severe peptic ulcer disease, secretory diarrhea	Serum gastrin rise after IV secretin, high basal and peak acid secretion, secretory diarrhea stops on H_2 receptor antagonists	10% are paraduodenal, stomach, omental	70	70	Difficult	Pancreatic < 20; duodenal—all; ectopic 80
Glucagonoma	Necrolytic migratory erythema, mild diabetes, psychiatric disturbances, diarrhea, venous thrombosis	Excessive glucagon release after IV tolbutamide	Rare	Nearly all	Rare	Easy, large tumors	25
VIPoma	Large volume secretory diarrhea, hypokalemia, metabolic acidosis, hypochlorhydria	Stool electrolytes [(Na + K) × 2] account for osmolality of stool water without gap, fecal pH <8 on fasting (colonic HCO_3^- secretion), concomitant plasma PHM elevation	10% retroperitoneal, lung	40	Rare	Angiography	70
Somatostatinoma	Dyspepsia, diabetes, gallstones, steatorrhea, hypochlorhydria	Hyperglycemia without hyperketonemia, stool weight usually 400–800 g/day, stool fat 10–30 g/day	15% duodenal	Nearly all	0	—	60
PPoma	None recognized (secretory diarrhea in one case)	None known for pure PPoma	—	—	—	—	—
Calcitoninoma	Diarrhea	Secretory diarrhea while fasting, additional osmotic component while eating (decreased small bowel transit time)	—	—	—	—	—
Neurotensinoma	Esophageal reflux (in one case)	None known for pure neurotensinoma	—	—	—	—	—
GRFoma	Acromegaly	Normal sella, normal head in CT scan, no GH release by exogenous GRF (pituitary tumors respond)	—	—	—	—	—

hypoglycemia. Proinsulin is formed within the rough endoplasmic reticulum of β cells. Proteolytic enzymes convert proinsulin molecules into insulin and a connecting peptide, C-peptide. C-peptide is a major part of the connection between the α and β chains of the insulin molecule. After proteolytic cleavage, C-peptide is stored in specific granules within the β cells and is normally released in equimolar concentrations with insulin. Proinsulin, insulin, and C-peptide can be measured in blood by specific RIA. Almost all insulinoma patients have elevated proinsulin levels, and the proinsulin proportion of total circulating insulin is increased in most cases.

Measurement of concentrations of C-peptide in blood has further aided in the diagnosis, since changes reflect β cell activity and can be used in the differential diagnosis of hypoglycemia in the following manner: in the C-peptide suppression test, commercial insulin is infused into a patient to produce hypoglycemia, and when blood glucose levels reach 40 mg/dL or lower, normal individuals reduce secretion of endogenous insulin and C-peptide by 50 to 70 percent. Insulinoma patients, however, do not suppress secretion of C-peptide. In patients who are injecting themselves with insulin to produce factitial hypoglycemia, determination of C-peptide levels is also valuable. In these patients, hypoglycemia is associated with high insulin levels, and a distinction between exogenous or endogenous insulin cannot be made. However, if low C-peptide values are found, the diagnosis of exogenous administration of insulin is firm.

Although other provocative tests, such as administration of tolbutamide, glucagon, calcium, or L-leucine, have variously been touted as superior diagnostic tests, the most reliable test remains a prolonged fast [75]. During fasting, which may require up to 72 hours, periodic determinations of blood glucose and blood insulin levels are made. In order to judge the effectiveness of the fast, blood glucose must reach a level of less than 50 mg/dL in men and less than 40 mg/dL in women. At the same time, inappropriately high insulin levels for the measured glucose levels (insulin-glucose ratio equal to or greater than 1.0) confirm the diagnosis of insulinoma.

Once the biochemical diagnosis of insulinoma appears likely, attempts to localize the tumor by visceral angiography are usually carried out. These attempts are especially important because of the small size of the tumors (the majority are less than 2 cm). With insulinoma, successful localization can be achieved in about 90 percent of patients in whom a clinical and biochemical diagnosis is firm [76]. Preoperative localization is important not only because of the small size of the tumor but also because of the relatively uniform distribution of insulinomas throughout the gland. Stefanini et al [70] reported that in 951 patients reviewed, about one third of the tumors were found in the head, a third in the body, and a third in the tail of the pancreas. The tumors are usually reddish-brown in color and encapsulated; 90 percent are single, and only 10 percent are malignant.

Cure can be effected by enucleation of the tumor or by partial pancreatectomy. If a tumor is not found at operation, an empiric ("blind") distal pancreatectomy with excision of the body and tail of the pancreas should be carried out. The pancreas is divided at the level of the superior mesenteric vessels, leaving the head of the gland in situ. The pancreatic specimen should then be sliced in bread-loaf fashion in order to identify the tumor, which may be buried deep within the gland. Blind resections of the head of the gland (a so-called Whipple procedure or radical pancreaticoduodenectomy) should not be performed because of the high risk of death or of serious complications that are associated with this operation.

All patients with insulinomas should receive high concentrations of glucose preoperatively and intraoperatively until the tumor is found. This is especially important the night before the operation. Periodic determinations of blood glucose and insulin levels throughout the operative procedure (and after excision of the tumor) confirm, usually within 2 hours [77], that the tumor has been removed. Rapid techniques for insulin RIA are available. Permanent cure rates approach 90 percent [71].

Gastrinoma

In 1955, Zollinger and Ellison [78] operated on two patients with fulminant peptic ulcer diatheses who had islet cell tumors of the pancreas. Severe peptic ulcer disease caused by a non-β cell tumor of the pancreas became known as the Zollinger-Ellison syndrome. Gregory and Tracy [79] isolated gastrin from a pancreatic tumor of a patient with ZE syndrome and established this peptide as the ulcerogenic substance in these patients. Shortly afterwards, RIAs were developed for the measurement of gastrin in serum as well as in tissue extracts. Subsequently, specific RIAs have been developed for most gastrointestinal hormone-producing peptides.

Only about one patient out of 1,000 with peptic ulcer disease will have ZE syndrome. The diagnostic triad proposed by Zollinger and Ellison [78] has proved useful: 1) massive gastric hypersecretion, 2) multiple peptic ulcer, and 3) non-β cell tumors of the pancreas, often associated with diarrhea. The biologic basis and the natural history of the ZE syndrome and a summary of our clinical management of ZE patients have been recently reported [24,80,81]. Two questions naturally arise early in the care of patients with peptic ulcer disease who may have ZE syndrome: 1) which patients should have measurements of plasma gastrin?, and 2) which patients should have provocative testing with secretin? Rayford and Thompson [82] advocate that gastrin determinations should be performed in patients with

1) recurrent peptic ulcers or recurrent ulcer symptoms after an acid-reducing operation;
2) duodenal ulcer and hypersecretion of acid (especially those with basal acid secretion that is greater than 15 meq/hr);
3) duodenal ulcer and diarrhea;
4) duodenal ulcer and hypercalcemia;
5) relatives who have ZE syndrome or the multiple endocrine neoplasia (MEN) I syndrome;
6) duodenal ulcers who are under 20 years old and postoperative patients in whom antral exclusion is suspected.

We currently add to this list patients with

7) acid hypersecretion and diarrhea;
8) acid hypersecretion and any of the stigmata of the MEN syndromes;
9) duodenal ulcer of sufficient severity to require operation.

Elevated gastrin levels may be present in patients with achlorhydria, hypochlorhydria (with or without pernicious anemia) [83], chronic atrophic gastritis [30], gastric carcinoma [84], vitiligo [85], antral G cell hyperplasia [86], pyloric obstruction [87], chronic renal failure [88], pheochromocytoma [89], small intestinal resection [90], rheumatoid arthritis [91], and postvagotomy [92]. This problem is compounded by some patients with ZE syndrome who have normal gastrin determinations [93,94]. Acid studies can also be misleading [94]. In our laboratory, the upper limit of normal for fasting serum gastrin is 150 pg/mL. With repeated testing, most ZE patients show elevated fasting levels of serum gastrin, usually ranging from 200 pg/mL to over 1,000 pg/mL. As with gastric secretory activity, basal serum gastrin levels may be highly variable [80], and at times, several of our patients have had normal levels. Therefore, repeated (three fasting serum gastrin levels) demonstration of fasting hypergastrinemia in patients with acid hypersecretion provides the best laboratory confirmation of the presence of a gastrinoma.

Even in the presence of hypergastrinemia and high gastric acid output, antral G cell hyperplasia and (in previously operated on patients) antral exclusion [95] cannot be ruled out. For these reasons, provocative testing is required in patients in whom ZE syndrome is strongly suspected, regardless of the gastrin levels. Secretin is preferable to calcium because of lack of side effects and brevity of action. A bolus injection of pure GIH secretin (1 CU/kg) with a rise of serum gastrin of 100 pg/mL was our previous standard [81]. We now prefer an infusion of 2 CU secretin per kilogram for one hour. Patients with G cell hyperplasia and retained antrum and duodenal ulcer patients should not have positive secretin tests. A test meal that may cause gastrin release in patients with antral G cell hyperplasia and duodenal ulcer does not cause significant elevations of gastrin in patients with gastrinoma, since the amount of gastrin released from the antrum is such a small fraction of total serum gastrin in patients with tumors that elaborate gastrin.

Percutaneous transhepatic venous sampling of gastrin has been advocated by Glowniak [96] and Burcharth [97] and their colleagues. The value of this procedure remains questionable [81,98]. Perhaps the addition of a secretin infusion during sampling to cause release of gastrin from the tumor, as suggested by Thompson et al [81], will increase the yield.

We have recently reviewed the oncologic aspects of gastrinoma [24]. Unlike insulinomas, at least 60 percent of gastrinomas are malignant, and half of the patients have metastases at the time of initial diagnosis [24,38,99,100]. As for all tumors that produce gastrointestinal hormones, the malignant potential of gastrinomas cannot be determined by histologic examination. If tumors metastasize, they are malignant. We decide if a patient is "cured" after tumor resection by following serial gastrin measurements. If a patient has normal levels for a year after operation, we consider him cured. Only four of 30 patients we have operated on have had normal postoperative serum gastrin levels, and all had isolated extrapancreatic gastrinomas. One had an omental nodule, one a hepatic tumor that we excised, one a cystic tumor arising from the lesser curvature of the stomach, and one a paraduodenal nodule. Three of the tumors were considered metastatic at operation [81].

We believe that all patients who have ZE syndrome should undergo operation for two reasons: 1) to identify and resect all tumor, since persistent tumor growth or subsequent metastases often lead ultimately to death; and 2) in patients in whom no tumor is found or in whom all tumor cannot be resected, the most reliable relief of hypersecretory symptoms for the life of the patient can be achieved by total gastrectomy. Of the 30 ZE patients we have followed, 26 have had total gastrectomy (with Roux-en-Y esophagojejunostomy), with no operative deaths [81]. Review of the reports of operations on ZE patients published since 1978 reveals an operative mortality for total gastrectomy of 5 percent out of 257 patients reported, and if the patients who had emergency total gastrectomy are excluded, the operative mortality in these collected patients is only 2.5 percent. We do not advocate gastrectomy in patients whose secretory symptoms are easily managed by H_2-receptor antagonists, but we have operated on eight patients who developed life-threatening complications after having been placed on cimetidine. We found that the patient either had not been given an adequate dose or had failed to comply with the regimen prescribed. We have previously discussed therapeutic alternatives [81].

The long-term nutritional results in our ZE patients after total gastrectomy have been surprisingly good (Fig 36-2). The mean postoperative weight loss has been 14 percent [81].

We have summarized arguments supporting total gastrectomy for the hypersecretory aspects of the ZE syndrome [81]. It is clear that most patients will be treated by H_2-receptor antagonists (cimetidine, ranitidine, or famotidine) or by the proton-pump blocker omeprazole. All of these drugs are effective. Should the hypersecretory aspects of the disease be managed pharmacologically, it is vital that the *tumor* be managed surgically. Every attempt should be made to excise the tumors. All other endocrine tumors of the pancreas are managed by operation, and there is no evidence that gastrinoma should be treated differently. Gastrinomas, in fact, have the highest incidence of malignancy and deserve, therefore, the greatest efforts at removal.

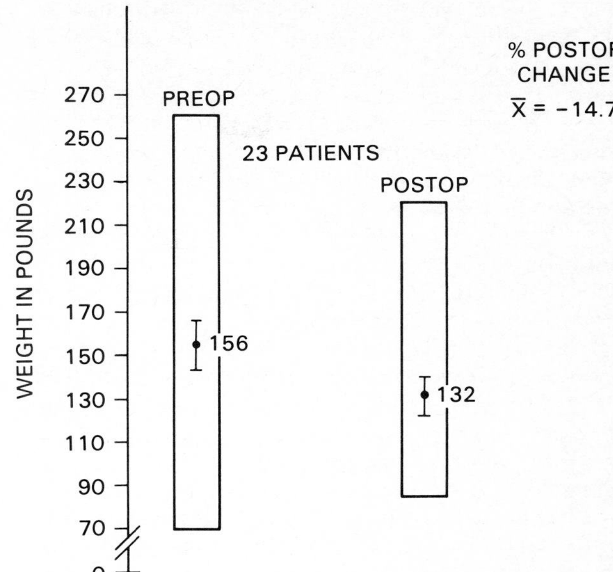

Figure 36-2. Mean weight loss in 23 patients who underwent total gastrectomy for the Zollinger-Ellison syndrome. The mean preoperative weight was 156 pounds, range 70–258 pounds, and the mean postoperative weight was 132 pounds, range 88–220 pounds. This represents a mean postoperative weight loss of 14.7 percent.

VIPoma

In 1958, Verner and Morrison [101] reported two patients who died of watery diarrhea and hypokalemia. They were found at autopsy to have benign islet cell tumors of the pancreas. In 1966 Matsumoto et al [102] suggested that the name pancreatic cholera would appropriately describe the Verner-Morrison syndrome. The acronym, WDHA (watery diarrhea, hypokalemia achlorhydria), was suggested by Marks et al [103] in 1967. Most patients are actually hypo-, not achlorhydric (Table 36-4).

In 1973, VIP was first proposed as the diarrheagenic agent by Bloom et al [104], who measured high levels of VIP in plasma and tumor extracts of six patients with WDHA; they suggested the name VIPoma for the responsible tumor. Kane et al [105] have recently shown that infusion of doses of VIP, which produce blood levels in normal humans equal to those of patients with VIPomas, reproduces the symptoms of WDHA syndrome.

The diagnosis of the Verner-Morrison syndrome is made by demonstrating elevated levels of VIP in plasma, levels usually above 150 pg/mL in a patient with watery diarrhea. Not all tumors that produce VIP and the syndrome of WDHA are located in the pancreas; ganglioneuroblastomas may also produce this syndrome, particularly in children [106]. In all, only about 100 patients with the Verner-Morrison syndrome have been described.

Glucagonoma

Glucagon-producing α cell tumors are often slow-growing, but over 50 percent are malignant [107,108]. In 1942, Becker et al [109] reported, in a dermatology journal, the case of a 45-year-old woman with chronic erythematous papulovesicular dermatitis, anemia, glucose intolerance, cheilitis, and glossitis (Table 36-4). At autopsy, she was found to have an islet cell carcinoma of the body and tail of the pancreas. Sweet [110], in 1974, observed the resolution of these skin lesions after surgical extirpation of a pancreatic α cell tumor, and Mallinson et al [111] coined the term, glucagonoma, in the same year. Seven years later, 55 patients with the glucagonoma syndrome had been reported. The clinical syndrome is characterized by diabetes, dermatitis (termed necrolytic migratory erythema), weight loss, anemia, diarrhea, an increased tendency to thrombosis [112], and elevated blood glucagon levels. Secretin has been reported to produce a rise in circulating glucagon levels in patients with glucagonoma [113]. As with all gastrointestinal hormone-producing tumors of the pancreas, localization of the tumor may be achieved by CT scanning (Fig 36-3) and by selective angiography (Fig 36-4). Surgical excision can completely reverse all clinical manifestations of the syndrome when all tumor can be removed.

Somatostatinoma

Fewer than 30 patients with somatostatinoma syndrome have been reported. The first report was in 1977 [114]. The term somatostatinoma was coined by Ganda et al [115] in the same year. Only two years later, Krejs et al [116] reviewed six cases of somatostatinoma. Diagnosis is difficult because the clinical features are nonspecific: they are dyspepsia, mild diabetes, cholelithiasis, diarrhea, weight loss, and hypo- or achlorhydria [114–118] (Table 36-4). In all patients studied, elevated blood levels of somatostatin have been found. Elevated plasma somatostatin levels have also been found in patients with other tumors: medullary carcinoma of the thyroid [119,120], pheochromocytoma [119], small cell carcinoma of the lung [120,121], bronchial tumor [121], and thymic tumor [121]. Somatostatin-like immunoreactivity has been found by immunocytochemistry or extraction techniques in mixed pancreatic tumors [122] and in midgut [123], rectal carcinoid tumors [124], and mucinous ovarian tumors [125]. These patients did not exhibit the so-called somatostatinoma syndrome. Since all neuroendocrine tumors may be polyhormonal, somatostatin production may occur in virtually any tumor of neuroendocrine origin. The somatostatin produced may cause no symptoms or be masked by other hormone products. The clinical and pathologic features of somatostatinoma are summarized in Table 36-5.

Pancreatic Polypeptide as a Tumor Marker

Elevated plasma levels of pancreatic polypeptide (PP) have been found in patients with islet cell

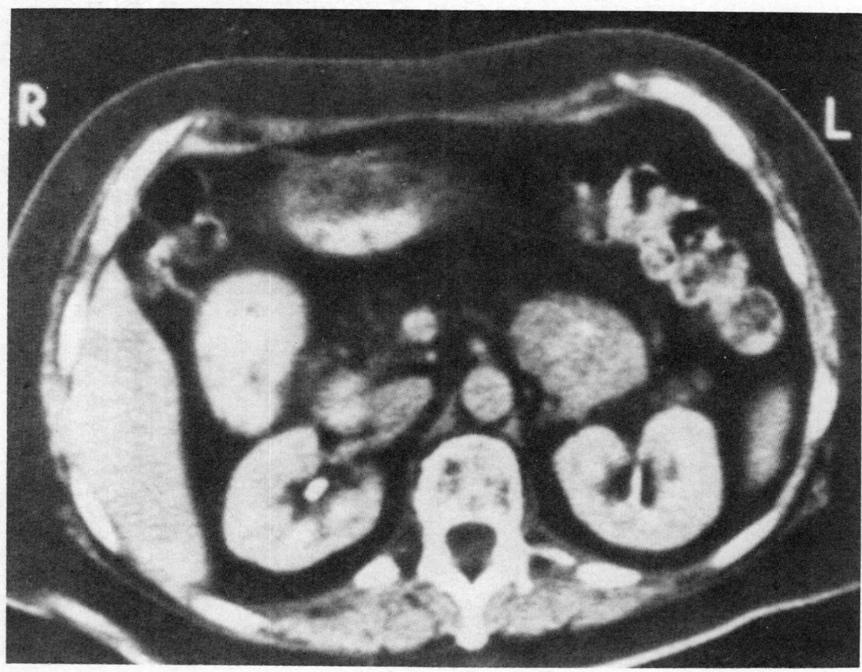

Figure 36-3. Computed axial tomogram of the abdomen demonstrating a mass in the tail of the pancreas. A nidus of calcium is present within the mass. (By permission of CM Parker et al, J Dermatol Surg Oncol 10:884, 1984.)

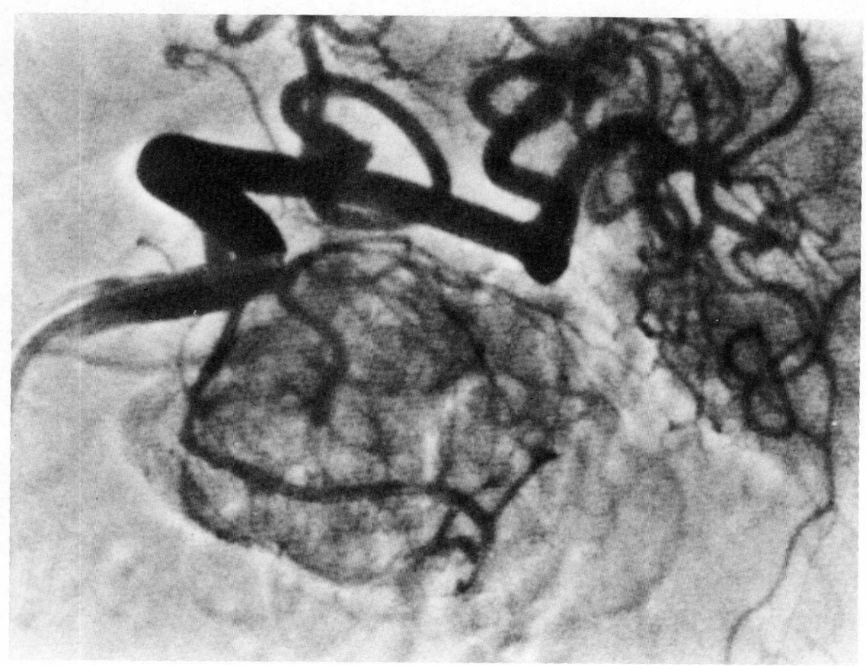

Figure 36-4. Summation film of a selective splenic-pancreatic arteriogram showing a homogeneous vascular tumor fed by a splenic vessel. Tumor mass is seen above the large vessel in the center of the photograph. (By permission of CM Parker et al, J Dermatol Surg Oncol 10:884, 1984.)

tumors of the pancreas and carcinoids [126,127]. There have been no clinical syndromes attributed to excess production of PP; in fact, the physiologic significance of PP has yet to be determined in humans. Elevated levels of PP have been suggested as a marker for endocrine pancreatic tumors, but only about half of all patients with pancreatic endocrine tumors have abnormally high levels of PP. Another problem is that elevated levels of plasma PP have also been found in aging patients [128] and in patients with diabetes mellitus [129], renal failure [130], carcinoid tumors [131], and inflammatory disease (subacute lupus erythematosus and rheumatoid arthritis) [132], and in laxative abusers [131] and patients with peptic ulcer disease [127]. Atropine suppression of PP has been suggested to determine whether elevated PP levels truly point to a tumor [126], but this suppression may not be specific. Measurement of PP is not useful for screening for pancreatic endocrine tumors.

CHRONIC PANCREATITIS

Chronic pancreatitis can result in decreased pancreatic enzyme secretion and malabsorption caused by loss of pancreatic tissue. Collection of pancreatic secretions after stimulation with secretin and/or CCK has been disappointing as a diagnostic aid in chronic pancreatitis [133,134]. The possible roles of gastrointestinal hormones in the etiology and pathogenesis of chronic pancreatitis have been studied; the results have been conflicting and confusing, due in part to the variable extent of disease, different classification systems for disease, and problems with assays. Fasting PP levels have almost universally been reported to be normal. Adrian et al [135] reported diminished meal-stimulated PP responses in patients with chronic pancreatitis who had steatorrhea, but normal responses in patients without steatorrhea. CCK-8-stimulated release of PP is apparently diminished in patients regardless of the presence or absence of steatorrhea [136]. Thus, the so-called PP stimulation test appears to have limited clinical applicability.

GIP has been reported to be increased in patients with chronic pancreatitis [137]. Patients have been classified into two groups, those with mild steatorrhea (who have elevated GIP release) and those with severe steatorrhea (who have low release) [138]. In patients with chronic pancreatitis, improvement of pancreatogenic insufficiency reverses the impaired GIP response [139]. Enteroglucagon may be normal or elevated in chronic pancreatitis [140], and motilin is elevated in some patients with chronic pancreatitis [141].

Nealon et al [141a] from our group have demonstrated depressed release of neurotensin in patients with advanced injury to the gland, as well as

Table 36-5. Some clinical and pathologic features of somatostatinoma in cases*

Ref	Pt. age, years	Sex	Primary pancreas	Metastasis in: Liver	Bone	Other	Gallbladder disease	Diabetes	Anemia	Hypertension	Diarrhea or steatorrhea	Other hormone excess	Survival
(15)	55	F	+	+	−	—	+	+	−	NS	+	—	Few hours post-op
(16)	46	F	+	−	−	—	+	+	+	−	−	—	4 yr (SA)
(17)	54	M	+	+	−	—	NS	+	NS	+	−	ACTH	6 days postop
(18)	63	F	+	+	−	—	+	+	+	NS	+	—	30 wk (SA)
(19)	52	M	+	+	−	—	+	+	+	−	+	Calcitonin	10 mo (SA)
(20)	33	F	+	+	−	Nodes	−	°	NS	NS	NS	Insulin	NS
(20)	36	M	+	−	−	—	−	+	NS	NS	NS	ACTH	2 yr (SA)
(21)	70		+	+	−	Duodenum	+	+	−	−	+	Calcitonin	4 wk postop
(22)	NS	NS	+	−	−	—	NS	+	NS	NS	+	—	—
(23)	68	F	+	+	−	Nodes	NS	+	+	−	+	Endorphin, calcitonin, ACTH, gastrin	20 mo
(14)	54	F	+	+	+	Kidney, adrenal, thyroid, skin, ovary	+	+	+	−	+	—	15 mo
(118)	51	F	?	+	+	—	−	+	+	+	+	Calcitonin, PRL±	5 mo (SA)

Key: +, yes; −, no; NS, not stated; SA, still alive at time of report; ACTH, adrenocorticotropic hormone; PRL, prolactin; °, patient had hypoglycemia.
* (From Reynolds et al [118])

an enhanced release of PP in patients with moderate pancreatic insufficiency.

CELIAC DISEASE AND NONTROPICAL SPRUE

In addition to the clear-cut endocrinopathies described above, gut hormones may be involved in other disease states. Celiac disease and nontropical sprue are diseases of malabsorption in children and adults caused by sensitivity to gluten. Diagnosis requires evidence of malabsorption, small bowel mucosal atrophy (flattening and blunting of small bowel villi are seen in biopsy specimens), and clinical improvement on a gluten-free diet. Although the diseases have been reported to be due to either toxic or immunologic reactions, the etiology is unknown. These patients have decreased pancreatic enzyme secretion as well as decreased gallbladder motility; however, the response to exogenous CCK is normal [141,142]. Tropical sprue is clinically similar to nontropical sprue. It is thought to be caused by an infection, but the etiology is unknown. It is usually less severe than nontropical sprue, occurs only in patients who have been to endemic areas, and responds to long-term antibiotic and folate treatment.

Because of the diffuse gastrointestinal effects of these three diseases and changes in proximal small bowel histology, the patterns of gastrointestinal hormone release have been explored. Besterman et al [142] studied the "gut hormone profile" in patients with celiac disease and found normal PP and gastrin levels, but levels of secretin, insulin, and GIP were decreased. Enteroglucagon was significantly increased and neurotensin was variably increased. After adequate treatment, only GIP remained decreased. Lauritsen et al [143] found decreased GIP but normal insulin levels and a normal incretin index, which he attributed to actions of other gastrointestinal hormones. Meal-stimulated and duodenal mucosal CCK concentrations were diminished in celiac sprue [141,142].

THERAPEUTIC USES

The gastrointestinal hormones that are of current therapeutic use are CCK-8, caerulein, glucagon, and somatostatin. Intranasal CCK-8 (one drop [1 mg/mL]), three times daily, improved pancreatic function in 22 of 30 patients with chronic pancreatitis (as measured by the Lundh test) [144]. Over 50 percent of 13 patients retested 3 months after treatment continued to have better function than they had before treatment. CCK promotes satiety [145–148]. Despite one early negative study in humans [149], more recent studies in which CCK was given intravenously have shown it to decrease food intake in normal individuals [150] and in obese patients [148]. Although the effects appear promising, we believe that CCK is unlikely to be of reliable long-term therapeutic use.

The effects of gastrointestinal hormones on gut motility have been put to diagnostic and therapeutic use. Glucagon suppresses bowel motility and is used by radiologists and endoscopists to paralyze the bowel for hypotonic studies of the duodenum and colon [151]. CCK-8 and its analogue, caerulein, have been used to stimulate peristalsis in patients with postoperative or drug-induced ileus [152,153].

Somatostatin is generally a suppressive agent and it decreases release of gastrin, glucagon, and other peptides in patients with pancreatic endocrine tumors [154]; it also relieves flushing in carcinoid syndrome [155]. A new long-acting somatostatin analogue (SMS 201-995) has been successfully used to decrease diarrhea in VIPoma patients for preoperative preparation [156]. Somatostatin and its analogues may be used to terminate carcinoid crisis or prevent bronchoconstriction and hypotension, which may occur with surgical procedures in patients with carcinoid tumors [155], and for symptomatic treatment in patients with metastatic VIPoma or carcinoid [157].

Somatostatin has been used to control hypoglycemia caused by insulin-producing tumors [158,159] and by nesidioblastosis [160]. It suppresses growth hormone release in patients with acromegaly [161].

Somatostatin treatment rapidly improves skin lesions associated with glucagonoma [162] and the so-called pseudoglucagonoma syndrome (patients with normal levels of glucagon but who have skin lesions usually associated with glucagonoma) [163]. The results have persisted for long periods after cessation of infusions (7 weeks in a glucagonoma patient and over 5 months in a pseudoglucagonoma patient). Somatostatin has also been effective in the treatment of psoriasis, which is thought by some investigators to be due to excess of growth hormone [164] or to epidermal growth factor [165].

Somatostatin has also been successfully utilized in the treatment of gastrointestinal disorders. Di Costanzo et al [166] reported closure of gastrointestinal fistulas in five out of six patients (who had been on total parenteral nutrition) within 24 hours of the onset of somatostatin therapy. Somatostatin may slow diarrhea in patients with Crohn's disease who have had multiple small bowel resections [167].

In a randomized controlled trial, somatostatin was compared with cimetidine in the treatment of severe persistent gastrointestinal hemorrhage in patients who were not candidates for surgery. Somatostatin stopped bleeding in eight out of ten patients, whereas cimetidine was effective in only one out of ten patients [168]. Other later studies have failed to provide clear evidence for a role for somatostatin in patients with upper gastrointestinal bleeding.

Somatostatin has been used in the treatment of severe acute pancreatitis, with promising results. It has produced clinical improvement and decreased levels of amylase and lipase [169]. A multicenter double-blind trial of somatostatin treatment for acute pancreatitis demonstrated good results [170]. Somatostatin has been shown to decrease insulin requirements in juvenile onset diabetics [171]. When somatostatin is combined with insulin, it decreases the duration of ketosis and hyperglycemia associated with diabetic ketoacidosis [172,173].

Clinical use of somatostatin in humans has been without side effects. The use has been limited by the necessity of intravenous injection, lack of specificity, and short half-life. The long-acting analogue provided by Sandoz, SMS 201-995, answers these objections. Currently, somatostatin is being used only experimentally, but SMS 201-995 should be available soon. In the future, somatostatin and its longer-acting analogues may be used to terminate carcinoid crisis or prevent bronchoconstriction and hypotension that may occur with surgical procedures in carcinoid patients, for preoperative preparation in VIPoma patients, and for symptomatic treatment in patients with metastatic VIPoma or carcinoids. A long-acting, orally effective analogue, which has specific growth hormone suppressive action without insulin suppression, has been developed [174]; this compound may be of value in the treatment of acromegaly and diabetes.

In summary, the clinical roles for gastrointestinal hormones are few, but we are learning more and more about them. Yalow and Berson [175] reported the technique for RIA of insulin in 1960. The roles of gastrin, VIP, glucagon, and somatostatin in clinical disease states are established. CCK analogues may be of help with ileus and possibly in chronic pancreatitis and obesity. Somatostatin therapy in pancreatitis, diarrhea, gastrointestinal hemorrhage, carcinoid, MEN syndromes, diabetes, and other conditions appears promising.

REFERENCES

1. Malagelada J-R: Pathophysiology of duodenal ulcer. Scand J Gastroenterol 14(Suppl 55):39, 1979.
2. Thompson JC: Stomach and duodenum, in Sabiston DC Jr (ed): Davis-Christopher's *Textbook of Surgery*. 13th Ed. Philadelphia, WB Saunders Co, 1985, pp 810–874.
3. Grossman MI: The chemicals that activate the "on" switches of the oxyntic cell. Mayo Clin Proc 50:515, 1975.
4. Grossman MI and others: Candidate hormones of the gut. Gastroenterology 67:730, 1974.
5. Rayford PL, Miller TA, Thompson JC: Secretin, cholecystokinin and newer gastrointestinal hormones. N Engl J Med 295:1093; 1157, 1976.
6. Grossman MI, Konturek SJ: Inhibition of acid secretion in dog by metiamide, a histamine antagonist acting on H_2 receptors. Gastroenterology 66:517, 1974.
7. Emås S: Vagal influences on gastric acid secretion. Scand J Gastroenterol 8:1, 1973.
8. Håkanson R, Liedberg G: Mechanism of activation of rat stomach histidine decarboxylase after vagal denervation. Eur J Pharmacol 16:78, 1971.
9. Hirschowitz BI, Molina E, Tim LO, et al: Effects of very low doses of atropine on basal acid and pepsin secretion, gastrin, and heart rate in normals and DU. Dig Dis Sci 29:790, 1984.
10. Larsson L-I: Peptide secretory pathways in GI tract: Cytochemical contributions to regulatory physiology of the gut. Am J Physiol 239:G237, 1980.
11. Håkanson R, Alumets J, Ekelund M, et al: Stimulation of gastric acid secretion. Scand J Gastroenterol 14(Suppl 55):21, 1979.
12. Konturek SJ, Kaess H, Kwiecien N, et al: Characteristics of intestinal phase of gastric secretion. Am J Physiol 230:335, 1976.
13. Christiansen J, Kirkegaard P, Olsen PS, et al: Interaction of calcium and gastrin on gastric acid secretion in duodenal ulcer patients. Gut 25:174, 1984.
14. Brandsborg O: Control of gastrin secretion by catecholamines with special reference to duodenal ulcer. Dan Med Bull 26:333, 1979.
15. Straus E: Gastrointestinal hormones, in Brodoff BN, Bleicher SJ (eds): *Diabetes Mellitus and Obesity*. Baltimore, Williams & Wilkins, 1982, pp 79–88.
16. Austin LA, Heath H III: Calcitonin. Physiology and pathophysiology. N Engl J Med 304:269, 1981.
17. Guslandi M: Inhibition of gastric acid secretion by somatostatin: A puzzle? Int J Clin Pharmacol Ther Toxicol 20:339, 1982.
18. Larsson L-I, Goltermann N, de Magistris L, et al: Somatostatin cell processes as pathways for paracrine secretion. Science 205:1393, 1979.
19. Alumets J, Ekelund M, El Munshid HA, et al: Topography of somatostatin cells in the stomach of the rat: Possible functional significance. Cell Tissue Res 202:177, 1979.
20. Schusdziarra V, Harris V, Conlon JM, et al: Pancreatic and gastric somatostatin release in response to intragastric and intraduodenal nutrients and HCl in the dog. J Clin Invest 62:509, 1978.
21. Schusdziarra V, Rouiller D, Harris V, et al: Release of gastric somatostatin-like immunoreactivity during acidification of the duodenal bulb. Gastroenterology 76:950, 1979.
22. Schwarz K: Über penetrierende Magen- und Jejunalgeschwure. Beitr Klin Chir 67:96, 1910.
23. Grossman MI: Peptic ulcer: The pathophysiological background. Scand J Gastroenterol Suppl 58:7, 1980.
24. Townsend CM Jr, Lewis BG, Gourley WK, Thompson JC: Gastrinoma. Curr Probl Cancer 7:1, 1982.
25. Schmidt-Wilcke HA, Haake U, Riecken EO: Investigations on the relationship between maximal acid output and parietal cells in gastric mucosal biopsies with special reference to duodenal ulcer. Acta Hepato-Gastroenterol 21:297, 1974.
26. Baron JH: An assessment of the augmented histamine test in the diagnosis of peptic ulcer. Correlations between gastric secretion, age and sex of patients, and site and nature of the ulcer. Gut 4:243, 1963.
27. Card WI, Marks IN: The relationship between the acid output of the stomach following "maximal" histamine stimulation and the parietal cell mass. Clin Sci 19:147, 1960.
28. Taylor IL: Gastrointestinal hormones in the pathogenesis of peptic ulcer disease. Clin Gastroenterol 13:355, 1984.
29. Sasaki H, Nagulesparan M, Samloff IM, et al: Low acid output in Pima Indians. A possible cause for the rarity of duodenal ulcer in this population. Dig Dis Sci 29:785, 1984.
30. Walsh JH, Grossman MI: Gastrin. N Engl J Med 292:1324; 1377, 1975.
31. Walsh JH, Grossman MI: Circulating gastrin in peptic ulcer disease. Mt Sinai J Med 40:374, 1973.
32. Rehfeld JF: What is gastrin? A progress report on the heterogeneity of gastrin in serum and tissue. Digestion 11:397, 1974.
33. Walsh JH, Isenberg JI, Ansfield J, et al: Clearance and acid-stimulating action of human big and little gastrins in duodenal ulcer subjects. J Clin Invest 57:1125, 1976.
34. Petersen B, Andersen BN: Abnormal processing of antral gastrin in active duodenal ulcer disease. Eur J Clin Invest 14:214, 1984.
35. Hansky J, Korman MG, Cowley DJ, et al: Serum gastrin in duodenal ulcer. Gut 12:959, 1971.
36. Bergegardh S, Olbe L: Gastric acid response to antrum distension in man. Scand J Gastroenterol 10:171, 1975.
37. Debas HT: Clinical implications of the gastrointestinal hormones. Can J Surg 22:10, 1979.

38. Wilson SD: Ulcerogenic tumors of the pancreas: The Zollinger-Ellison syndrome, in Carey LC (ed): *The Pancreas.* St. Louis, CV Mosby Co, 1973, pp 295–318.
39. Walsh JH, Nair PK, Kleibeuker J, et al: Pathological acid secretion not due to gastrinoma. Scand J Gastroenterol 18(Suppl 82):45, 1982.
40. El Munshid HA, Liedberg G, Rehfeld JF, et al: Effect of bilateral nephrectomy on serum gastrin concentration, gastric histamine content, histidine decarboxylase activity, and acid secretion in the rat. Scand J Gastroenterol 11:87, 1976.
41. Dragstedt LR: Peptic ulcer. An abnormality in gastric secretion. Am J Surg 117:143, 1969.
42. Hirschowitz BI, Helman CA: Effects of fundic vagotomy and cholinergic replacement on pentagastrin dose responsive gastric acid and pepsin secretion in man. Gut 23:675, 1982.
43. Colturi TJ, Unger RH, Feldman M: Role of circulating somatostatin in regulation of gastric acid secretion, gastrin release, and islet cell function. Studies in healthy subjects and duodenal ulcer patients. J Clin Invest 74:417, 1984.
44. Bloom SR, Ward AS: Failure of secretin release in patients with duodenal ulcer. Br Med J 1:126, 1975.
45. Thompson JC, Swierczek JS: Acid and endocrine responses to meals varying in pH in normal and duodenal ulcer subjects. Ann Surg 186:541, 1977.
46. Kurokawa M, Saito R, Shinomura Y, et al: Effect of intraduodenal load of endogenous acid on secretin release in patients with peptic ulcer. Am J Gastroenterol 77:471, 1982.
47. Johnson HD: Gastric ulcer: Classification, blood group characteristics, secretion patterns and pathogenesis. Ann Surg 162:996, 1965.
48. Wormsley KG, Grossman MI: Maximal histalog test in control subjects and patients with peptic ulcer. Gut 6:427, 1965.
49. Du Plessis DJ: Pathogenesis of gastric ulceration. Lancet 1:974, 1965.
50. Davenport HW: Back diffusion of acid through the gastric mucosa and its physiological consequences, in Jerzy Glass GB (ed): *Progress in Gastroenterology.* New York, Grune & Stratton, 1970, pp 42–56.
51. Kivihaakso E, Silen W: Pathogenesis of experimental gastric-mucosal injury. N Engl J Med 301:364, 1979.
52. Harjola P-T, Sivula A: Gastric ulceration following experimentally induced hypoxia and hemorrhagic shock: *In vivo* study of pathogenesis in rabbits. Ann Surg 163:21, 1966.
53. Ritchie WP Jr, Shearburn EW III: Influence of isoproterenol and cholestyramine on acute gastric mucosal ulcerogenesis. Gastroenterology 73:62, 1977.
54. Cummins GM, Grossman MI, Ivy AC: An experimental study of the acid factor in ulceration of the gastrointestinal tract in dogs. Gastroenterology 10:714, 1948.
55. Thompson JC, Marx M: Gastrointestinal hormones. Curr Probl Surg 21:1, 1984.
56. Debas HT, Slaff GF, Grossman MI: Intestinal phase of gastric acid secretion: Augmentation of maximal response of Heidenhain pouch to gastrin and histamine. Gastroenterology 68:691, 1975.
57. Orloff MJ, Hyde PVB, Kosta LD, et al: The intestinal phase hormone. World J Surg 3:523, 1979.
58. Mariano EC, Beloni A, Lander JH: Some properties shared by amino acids and entero-oxyntin. Ann Surg 188:181, 1978.
59. Feldman M, Walsh JH, Taylor IL: Effect of naloxone and morphine on serum gastrin and pancreatic polypeptide concentrations in humans. Gastroenterology 79:294, 1980.
60. Taylor IL, Dockray GJ, Calam J, et al: Big and little gastrin response to food in normal and ulcer subjects. Gut 20:957, 1979.
61. Eysselein VE, Maxwell V, Reedy T, et al: Similar acid stimulatory potencies of synthetic big and little gastrins in humans. Gastroenterology 84:1147, 1983.
62. Kihl B, Rokaeus A, Rosell S, et al: Fat inhibition of gastric acid secretion in man and plasma concentrations of neurotensin-like immunoreactivity. Scand J Gastroenterol 16:513, 1981.
63. Johnson LR, Guthrie PD: Stimulation of rat oxyntic gland mucosal growth by epidermal growth factor. Am J Physiol 238:G45, 1980.
64. Pearse AGE: Common cytochemical and ultrastructural characteristics of cells producing polypeptide hormones (the *APUD* series) and their relevance to thyroid and ultimobranchial C cells and calcitonin. Proc Roy Soc Lond [Biol] 170:71, 1968.
65. Polak JM, Bloom SR: Pathology of peptide-producing neuroendocrine tumours. Br J Hosp Med 33:78, 1985.
66. Tapia FJ, Polak JM, Barbosa AJA, et al: Neuron-specific enolase is produced by neuroendocrine tumours. Lancet 1:808, 1981.
67. Larsson L-I, Grimelius L, Håkanson R, et al: Mixed endocrine pancreatic tumors producing several peptide hormones. Am J Pathol 79:271, 1975.
68. Creutzfeldt W, Arnold R, Creutzfeldt C, et al: Pathomorphologic, biochemical, and diagnostic aspects of gastrinomas (Zollinger-Ellison syndrome). Human Pathol 6:47, 1975.
69. Townsend CM Jr, Thompson JC: Surgical management of tumors that produce gastrointestinal hormones. Annu Rev Med 36:111, 1985.
70. Stefanini P, Carboni M, Patrassi N, et al: Beta-islet cell tumors of the pancreas: Results of a study on 1,067 cases. Surgery 75:597, 1974.
71. Edis AJ, McIlrath DC, van Heerden JA, et al: Insulinoma—Current diagnosis and surgical management. Curr Probl Surg 13:1, 1976.
72. Chong PN, Cheah JS, Ng SC, et al: Problems in the management of insulinoma. Singapore Med J 26:312, 1985.
73. Whipple AO, Frantz VK: Adenoma of islet cells with hyperinsulinism. A review. Ann Surg 101:1299, 1935.
74. ReMine WH, Scholz DA, Priestley JT: Hyperinsulin-

ism. Clinical and surgical aspects. Am J Surg 99:413, 1960.

75. Kaplan EL, Fredland A: The diagnosis and treatment of insulinomas, in Thompson NW, Vinik AI (eds): *Endocrine Surgery Update.* New York, Grune & Stratton, 1983, pp 245–268.
76. Vinik AI, Stroedel WE, Cho KJ, et al: Localization of hormonally active gastrointestinal tumors, in Thompson NW, Vinik AI (eds): *Endocrine Surgery Update.* New York, Grune & Stratton, 1983, pp 195–218.
77. Tutt GO Jr, Edis AJ, Service FJ, et al: Plasma glucose monitoring during operations for insulinoma: A critical reappraisal. Surgery 88:351, 1980.
78. Zollinger RM, Ellison EH: Primary peptic ulcerations of the jejunum associated with islet cell tumors of the pancreas. Ann Surg 142:709, 1955.
79. Gregory RA, Tracy HJ: The constitution and properties of two gastrins extracted from hog antral mucosa: Part I. The isolation of two gastrins from hog antral mucosa. Part II. The properties of two gastrins isolated from hog antral mucosa. Gut 5:103; 107, 1964.
80. Thompson JC, Reeder DD, Villar HV, et al: Natural history and experience with diagnosis and treatment of the Zollinger-Ellison syndrome. Surg Gynecol Obstet 140:721, 1975.
81. Thompson JC, Lewis BG, Wiener I, et al: The role of surgery in the Zollinger-Ellison syndrome. Ann Surg 197:594, 1983.
82. Rayford PL, Thompson JC: Gastrin. Surg Gynecol Obstet 145:257, 1977.
83. McGuigan JE, Trudeau WL: Serum gastrin concentrations in pernicious anemia. N Engl J Med 282:358, 1970.
84. McGuigan JE, Trudeau WL: Serum and tissue gastrin concentrations in patients with carcinoma of the stomach. Gastroenterology 64:22, 1973.
85. Howitz J, Rehfeld JF: Serum-gastrin in vitiligo. Lancet 1:831, 1974.
86. Ganguli PC, Pearse AGE, Polak JM, et al: Antral-gastrin-cell hyperplasia in peptic-ulcer disease. Lancet 1:583, 1974.
87. Feurle G, Ketterer H, Becker HD, et al: Circadian serum gastrin concentrations in control persons and in patients with ulcer disease. Scand J Gastroenterol 7:177, 1972.
88. Korman MG, Laver MC, Hansky J: Hypergastrinaemia in chronic renal failure. Br Med J 1:209, 1972.
89. Hayes JR, Kennedy TL, Ardill J, et al: Stimulation of gastrin release by catecholamines. Lancet 1:819, 1972.
90. Straus E, Gerson CD, Yalow RS: Hypersecretion of gastrin associated with the short bowel syndrome. Gastroenterology 66:175, 1974.
91. Rooney PJ, Kennedy AC, Hayes JR, et al: Hypergastrinaemia in rheumatoid arthritis. Scott Med J 18:132, 1973.
92. Stern DH, Walsh JH: Gastrin release in postoperative ulcer patients: Evidence for release of duodenal gastrin. Gastroenterology 64:363, 1973.
93. Modlin IM, Jaffe BM, Sank A, et al: The early diagnosis of gastrinoma. Ann Surg 196:512, 1982.
94. McGuigan JE, Wolfe MM: Secretin injection test in the diagnosis of gastrinoma. Gastroenterology 79:1324, 1980.
95. Korman MG, Scott DF, Hansky J, et al: Hypergastrinaemia due to an excluded gastric antrum: A proposed method for differentiation from the Zollinger-Ellison syndrome. Aust NZ J Med 3:266, 1972.
96. Glowniak JV, Shapiro B, Vinik AI, et al: Percutaneous transhepatic venous sampling of gastrin. N Engl J Med 307:293, 1982.
97. Burcharth F, Stage JG, Stadil F, et al: Localization of gastrinomas by transhepatic portal catheterization and gastrin assay. Gastroenterology 77:444, 1979.
98. Silen W: Percutaneous transhepatic venous sampling of gastrin. N Engl J Med 307:1586, 1982 (Letter).
99. Ellison EH, Wilson SD: The Zollinger-Ellison syndrome: Re-appraisal and evaluation of 260 registered cases. Ann Surg 160:512, 1964.
100. Fox PS, Hofmann JW, Wilson SD, et al: Surgical management of the Zollinger-Ellison syndrome. Surg Clin North Am 54:395, 1974.
101. Verner JV, Morrison AB: Islet cell tumor and a syndrome of refractory watery diarrhea and hypokalemia. Am J Med 25:374, 1958.
102. Matsumoto KK, Peter JB, Schultze RG, et al: Watery diarrhea and hypokalemia associated with pancreatic islet cell adenoma. Gastroenterology 50:231, 1966.
103. Marks IN, Bank S, Louw JH: Islet cell tumor of the pancreas with reversible watery diarrhea and achlorhydria. Gastroenterology 52:695, 1967.
104. Bloom SR, Polak JM, Pearse AGE: Vasoactive intestinal peptide and watery-diarrhoea syndrome. Lancet 2:14, 1973.
105. Kane MG, O'Dorisio TM, Krejs GJ: Production of secretory diarrhea by intravenous infusion of vasoactive intestinal polypeptide. New Engl J Med 309:1482, 1983.
106. Long RG, Bryant MG, Mitchell SJ, et al: Clinicopathological study of pancreatic and ganglioneuroblastoma tumours secreting vasoactive intestinal polypeptide (VIPomas). Br Med J 282:1767, 1981.
107. Parker CM, Hanke CW, Madura JA, et al: Glucagonoma syndrome: Case report and literature review. J Dermatol Surg Oncol 10:884, 1984.
108. Vandersteen PR, Scheithauer BW: Glucagonoma syndrome. A clinicopathologic, immunocytochemical, and ultrastructural study. J Am Acad Dermatol 12:1032, 1985.
109. Becker SW, Kahn D, Rothman S: Cutaneous manifestations of internal malignant tumors. Arch Dermatol Syph 45:1069, 1942.
110. Sweet RD: A dermatosis specifically associated with a tumour of pancreatic alpha cells. Br J Dermatol 90:301, 1974.
111. Mallinson CN, Bloom SR, Warin AP, et al: A glucagonoma syndrome. Lancet 2:1, 1974.
112. Prinz RA, Dorsch TR, Lawrence AM: Clinical

aspects of glucagon-producing islet cell tumors. Am J Gastroenterol 76:125, 1981.

113. Stacpoole PW, Jaspan J, Kasselberg AG, et al: A familial glucagonoma syndrome. Genetic, clinical and biochemical features. Am J Med 70:1017, 1981.

114. Kovacs K, Horvath E, Ezrin C, et al: Immunoreactive somatostatin in pancreatic islet-cell carcinoma accompanied by ecotopic A.C.T.H. syndrome. Lancet 1:1365, 1977.

115. Ganda OP, Weir GC, Soeldner JS, et al: "Somatostatinoma": A somatostatin-containing tumour of the endocrine pancreas. N Engl J Med 296:963, 1977.

116. Krejs GJ, Orci L, Conlon JM, et al: Somatostatinoma syndrome. Biochemical, morphologic and clinical features. N Engl J Med 301:285, 1979.

117. Editorial: Somatostatin: Hormonal and therapeutic roles. Lancet 2:77, 1985.

118. Reynolds C, Pratt R, Chan-Yan C, et al: Somatostatinoma—The most recently described pancreatic islet cell tumor. West J Med 142:393, 1985.

119. Saito H, Saito S: Plasma somatostatin in normal subjects and in various diseases: Increased levels in somatostatin-producing tumors. Horm Metabol Res 14:71, 1982.

120. Roos BA, Lindall AW, Ells J, et al: Increased plasma and tumor somatostatin-like immunoreactivity in medullary thyroid carcinoma and small cell lung cancer. J Clin Endocrinol Metab 52:187, 1981.

121. Penman E, Wass JAH, Besser GM, et al: Somatostatin secretion by lung and thymic tumours. Clin Endocrinol 13:613, 1980.

122. Yano T, Yamamoto N, Fujimori K, et al: Glucagon-secreting pancreatic islet cell carcinoma, containing insulin and somatostatin, with hypoglycemic attack. Am J Gastroenterol 77:387, 1982.

123. Lundqvist M, Wilander E: Somatostatin-like immunoreactivity in mid-gut carcinoids. Acta Pathol Microbiol Immunol Scand [A] 89:335, 1981.

124. O'Briain DS, Dayal Y, DeLellis RA, et al: Rectal carcinoids as tumors of the hindgut endocrine cells. A morphological and immunohistochemical analysis. Am J Surg Pathol 6:131, 1982.

125. Takeda A, Matsuyama M, Chihara T, et al: Ultrastructure and immunohistochemistry of gastro-entero-pancreatic (GEP) endocrine cells in mucinous tumors of the ovary. Acta Pathol Jpn 32:1003, 1982.

126. Floyd JC Jr: Pancreatic polypeptide. Clinics Gastroenterol 9:657, 1980.

127. Lonovics J, Devitt P, Watson LC, et al: Pancreatic polypeptide. A review. Arch Surg 116:1256, 1981.

128. Berger D, Crowther R, Floyd JC Jr, et al: Effects of age on fasting levels of pancreatic hormones in healthy subjects. Diabetes 26:381, 1977.

129. Floyd JC, Fajans SS, Pek S, et al: A newly recognized pancreatic polypeptide; Plasma levels in health and disease. Rec Prog Horm Res 33:519, 1977.

130. Hallgren R, Lundqvist G, Chance RE: Serum levels of human pancreatic polypeptide in renal disease. Scand J Gastroenterol 12:923, 1977.

131. Oberg K, Grimelius L, Lundqvist G, et al: Update on pancreatic polypeptide as a specific marker for endocrine tumours of the pancreas and gut. Acta Med Scand 210:145, 1981.

132. Hallgren R, Lundqvist G: Elevated levels of circulating pancreatic polypeptide in inflammatory and infectious disorders. Regul Pept 1:159, 1980.

133. Denyer ME, Cotton PB: Pure pancreatic juice studies in normal subjects and patients with chronic pancreatitis. Gut 20:89, 1979.

134. Mee AS, Klaff LJ, Girdwood AH, et al: Comparative study of pancreatic polypeptide (PP) secretion, endocrine and exocrine function, and structural damage in chronic alcohol induced pancreatitis (CAIP). Gut 24:642, 1983.

135. Adrian TE, Besterman HS, Mallinson CN, et al: Impaired pancreatic polypeptide release in chronic pancreatitis with steatorrhoea. Gut 20:98, 1979.

136. Owyang C, Scarpello JH, Vinik AI: Correlation between pancreatic enzyme secretion and plasma concentration of human pancreatic polypeptide in health and in chronic pancreatitis. Gastroenterology 83:55, 1982.

137. Botha JL, Vinik AI, Brown JC: Gastric inhibitory polypeptide (GIP) in chronic pancreatitis. J Clin Endocrinol Metab 42:791, 1976.

138. Ebert R, Creutzfeldt W, Brown JC, et al: Response of gastric inhibitory polypeptide (GIP) to test meal in chronic pancreatitis—Relationship to endocrine and exocrine insufficiency. Diabetologia 12:609, 1976.

139. Ebert R, Creutzfeldt W: Reversal of impaired GIP and insulin secretion in patients with pancreatogenic steatorrhea following enzyme substitution. Diabetologia 19:198, 1980.

140. Besterman HS, Adrian TE, Bloom SR, et al: Pancreatic and gastrointestinal hormones in chronic pancreatitis. Digestion 24:195, 1982.

141. Calam J, Ellis A, Dockray GJ: Identification and measurement of molecular variants of cholecystokinin in duodenal mucosa and plasma. J Clin Invest 69:218, 1982.

141a. Nealon WH, Beauchamp RD, Townsend CM Jr, et al: Diagnostic role of gastrointestinal hormones in patients with chronic pancreatitis. Ann Surg 204:90, 1986.

142. Besterman HS, Bloom SR, Sarson DL, et al: Gut-hormone profile in coeliac disease. Lancet 1:785, 1978.

143. Lauritsen KB, Lauritzen JB, Christensen KC: Gastric inhibitory polypeptide and insulin release in response to oral and intravenous glucose in coeliac disease. Scand J Gastroenterol 17:241, 1982.

144. Pap A, Berger Z, Varro V: Trophic effect of cholecystokinin-octapeptide in man—A new way in the treatment of chronic pancreatitis? Digestion 21:163, 1981.

145. Gibbs J, Young RC, Smith GP: Cholecystokinin decreases food intake in rats. J Comp Physiol Psychol 84:488, 1973.

146. Gibbs J, Falasco JD, McHugh PR: Cholecystokinin-decreased food intake in rhesus monkeys. Am J Physiol 230:15, 1976.

147. Smith GP, Gibbs J, Jerome C, et al: The satiety effect of cholecystokinin: A progress report. Peptides 2(Suppl 2):57, 1981.
148. Pi-Sunyer X, Kissileff HR, Thornton J, et al: C-terminal octapeptide of cholecystokinin decreases food intake in obese men. Physiol Behav 29:627, 1982.
149. Goetz H, Sturdevant R: Effect of cholecystokinin on food intake in man. Clin Res 23:98A, 1975.
150. Stacher G, Steinringer H, Schmierer G, et al: Cholecystokinin octapeptide decreases intake of solid food in man. Peptides 3:133, 1982.
151. Modlin IM, Jaffe BM: Clinical usefulness of glucagon. Surgery 87:470, 1980.
152. Henrichs I, Teller WM: Pathophysiology of gastrointestinal hormones. Implications for paediatrics. Eur J Pediatr 135:3, 1980.
153. Jackson DV Jr, Wu WC, Spurr CL: Treatment of vincristine-induced ileus with sincalide, a cholecystokinin analog. Cancer Chemother Pharmacol 8:83, 1982.
154. Fallucca F, Delle Fave G, Giangrande L, et al: Effect of somatostatin on gastrin, insulin and glucagon secretion in two patients with Zollinger-Ellison syndrome. J Endocrinol Invest 4:451, 1981.
155. Long RG, Peters JR, Bloom SR, et al: Somatostatin, gastrointestinal peptides, and the carcinoid syndrome. Gut 22:549, 1981.
156. Bloom SR, Polak JM: VIPomas, in Said SI (ed): *Vasoactive Intestinal Peptide.* New York, Raven Press, 1982, pp 457–468.
157. Bloom SR, Adrian TE, Barnes AJ, et al: New specific long-acting somatostatin analogues in the treatment of pancreatic endocrine tumours. Gut 19:446, 1978.
158. Scuro LA, Lo Cascio V, Adami S, et al: Somatostatin inhibition of insulin secretion in insulin-producing tumors. Metabolism 25:603, 1976.
159. Kitson HF, McCrossin RB, Jimenez M, et al: Somatostatin treatment of insulin excess due to β-cell adenoma in a neonate. J Pediatr 96:145, 1980.
160. Roti E, Ghinelli C, Bandini P, et al: Effects of somatostatin in a case of severe hypoglycemia due to nesidioblastosis. J Endocrinol Invest 4:209, 1981.
161. Gaspar L, Laszlo FA: Long-term bromocriptine treatment and somatostatin in acromegaly. Endokrinologie 76:152, 1980.
162. Sohier J, Jeanmougin M, Lombrail P, et al: Rapid improvement of skin lesions in glucagonomas with intravenous somatostatin infusion. Lancet 1:40, 1980.
163. Lubetzki J, Guillausseau PJ, Binet O, et al: Pseudoglucagonoma responsive to somatostatin. Lancet 2:316, 1981.
164. Weber G, Klughardt G, Neidhardt M: Psoriasis and human growth hormone: Aetiology and therapy. Arch Dermatol Res 270:361, 1981.
165. Ghirlanda G, Uccioli L, Perri F, et al: Epidermal growth factor, somatostatin, and psoriasis. Lancet 1:65, 1983.
166. di Costanzo J, Cano N, Martin J: Somatostatin in persistent gastrointestinal fistula treated by total parenteral nutrition. Lancet 2:338, 1982.
167. Dharmsathaphorn K, Gorelick FS, Sherwin RS, et al: Somatostatin decreases diarrhea in patients with the short-bowel syndrome. J Clin Gastroenterol 4:521, 1982.
168. Kayasseh L, Keller U, Gyr K, et al: Somatostatin and cimetidine in peptic-ulcer haemorrhage. A randomised controlled trial. Lancet 1:844, 1980.
169. Limberg B, Kommerell B: Treatment of acute pancreatitis with somatostatin. N Engl J Med 303:284, 1980.
170. Usadel K-H, Leuschner U, Uberla KK: Treatment of acute pancreatitis with somatostatin: A multicenter double-blind trial. N Engl J Med 303:999, 1980.
171. Rizza RA, Gerich JE: Somatostatin and diabetes. Med Clin North Am 62:735, 1978.
172. Fallucca F, Barbetti F, Maldonato A, et al: Effects of somatostatin on established induced ketosis. Horm Metab Res 14:512, 1982.
173. Greco AV, Ghirlanda G, Altomonte L, et al: Somatostatin and insulin infusion in the management of diabetic ketoacidosis. Horm Metab Res 13:310, 1981.
174. Bauer W, Briner U, Doepfner W, et al: SMS 201-995: A very potent and selective octapeptide analogue of somatostatin with prolonged action. Life Sci 31:1133, 1982.
175. Yalow RS, Berson SA: Immunoassay of endogenous plasma insulin in man. J Clin Invest 39:1157, 1960.

Section Ten

Appendix

1

Amino Acid Composition of Selected Substances

Felix Lluis, M.D.

The amino acid composition of gastrointestinal peptides is presented here in the usual three-letter code. However, a one-letter code for amino acids has evolved and is often used (Eur J Biochem 5:151, 1968) (Table A-1). Whenever possible, peptides are grouped in families according to their structural or biologic similarities.

Table A-1. One-letter code

One-Letter Symbol	*Three-Letter Symbol*	*Amino Acid*	*One-Letter Symbol*	*Three-Letter Symbol*	*Amino Acid*
A	Ala	Alanine	N	Asn	Asparagine
B	Asx	Aspartic acid or asparagine	P	Pro	Proline
			Q	Gln	Glutamine
C	Cys	Cysteine	R	Arg	Arginine
D	Asp	Aspartic acid	S	Ser	Serine
E	Glu	Glutamic acid	T	Thr	Threonine
pE	pGlu	Pyroglutamyl	V	Val	Valine
F	Phe	Phenylalanine	W	Trp	Tryptophan
G	Gly	Glycine	X	—	Unknown or "other"
H	His	Histidine			
I	Ile	Isoleucine	Y	Tyr	Tyrosine
K	Lys	Lysine	Z	Glx	Glutamic acid or glutamine
L	Leu	Leucine			
M	Met	Methionine			

GASTRIN-CHOLECYSTOKININ FAMILY

*Gastrin**

	Approx. M. W. *Gastrin:* I	II	
Little Gastrin (G-17)			
Man	2098	2178	pGlu-Gly-Pro-Trp-Leu-Glu-Glu-Glu-Glu-Glu-Ala-Tyr[a]-Gly-Trp-Met-Asp- Phe-NH_2
Hog	2116	2196	pGlu-Gly-Pro-Trp-Met-Glu-Glu-Glu-Glu-Glu-Ala-Tyr[a]-Gly-Trp-Met-Asp-Phe-NH_2
Dog	2058	2138	pGlu-Gly-Pro-Trp-Met-Glu-Glu-Glu-Ala-Glu-Ala-Tyr[a]-Gly-Trp-Met-Asp-Phe-NH_2
Cow and sheep	2026	2106	pGlu-Gly-Pro-Trp-Val-Glu-Glu-Glu-Glu-Ala-Ala-Tyr[a]-Gly-Trp-Met-Asp-Phe-NH_2
Cat	2040	2120	pGlu-Gly-Pro-Trp-Val-Glu-Glu-Glu-Ala-Glu-Ala-Tyr[a]-Gly-Trp-Met-Asp-Phe-NH_2

* Except where noted, the amino acid sequences for gastrins of different species are identical.
[a] Gastrin of each species exists in forms I and II; in form I, there is no SO_3H attached to Tyr in position 12.

Minigastrin (G-14-I, 5-17)		
Man	1833	Trp-Leu-Glu-Glu-Glu-Glu-Glu-Ala-Tyr-Gly-Trp-Met-Asp-Phe-NH_2
Big Gastrin (G-34-I)		
Man	3839	pGlu-Leu-Gly-Pro-Gln-Gly-Pro-Pro-His-Leu-Val-Ala-Asp-Pro-Ser-Lys-Lys-[b]Gln-Gly-Pro-Trp-Leu-Glu-Glu-Glu-Glu-Glu-Ala-Tyr-Gly-Trp-Met-Asp-Phe-NH_2
Hog	3883	pGlu-Leu-Gly-Leu-Gln-Gly-Pro-Pro-His-Leu-Val-Ala-Asp-Leu-Ala-Lys-Lys[b]-Gln-Gly-Pro-Trp-Met-Glu-Glu-Glu-Glu-Glu-Ala-Tyr-Gly-Trp-Met-Asp-Phe-NH_2
Pentagastrin		
	768	N-t-butyloxycarbonyl-β-Ala-Trp-Met-Asp-Phe-NH_2
Tetragastrin		
		-Trp-Met-Asp-Phe-NH_2
Trigastrin		
		-Met-Asp-Phe-NH_2

[b] Points of cleavage by trypsin.

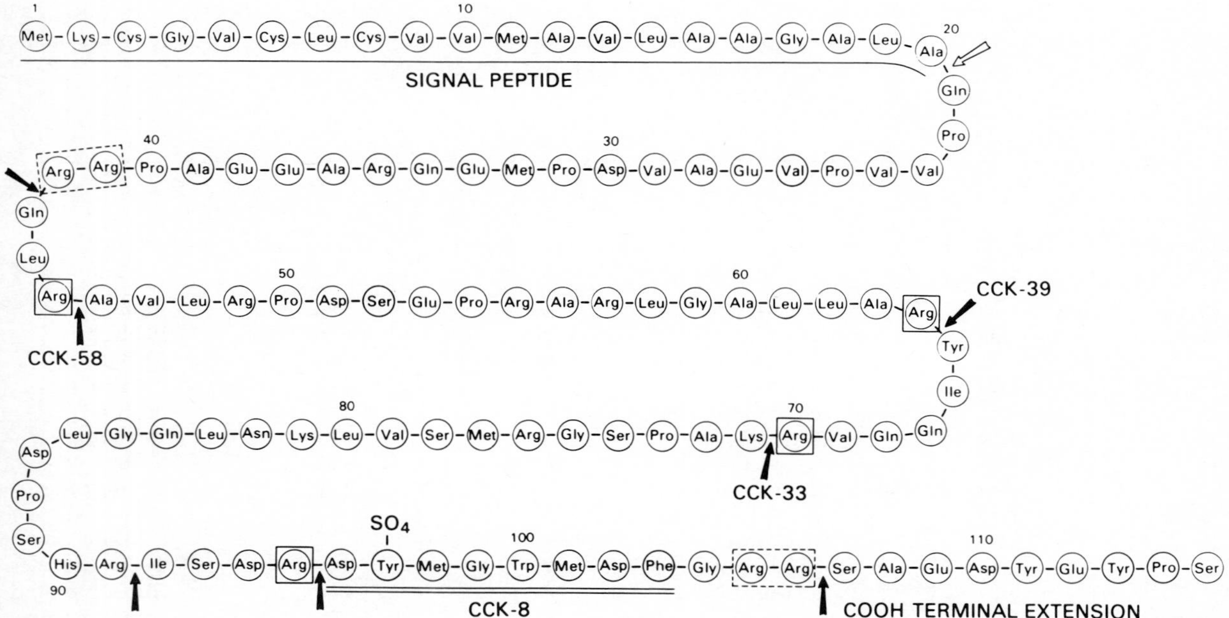

Figure A-1. The amino acid sequence of rat preprocholecystokinin has been deduced from the nucleotide sequence of cloned rat cDNA (Deschenes RJ et al: Ann NY Acad Sci 448:53, 1985). Arrows and boxes on the arginine indicate the predicted sites of proteolytic cleavage.

Cholecystokinin (CCK)

CCK-58 58 A.A. (Canine)

Ala-Val-Gln-Lys-Val-Asp-Gly-Glu-Pro-Arg-Ala-His-Leu-Gly-Ala-Leu-Leu-Ala-Arg-Tyr-Ile-Gln-Gln-Ala-Arg-Lys-Ala-Pro-Ser-Gly-Arg-Met-Ser-Val-Ile-Lys-Asn-Leu-Gln-Asn-Leu-Asp-Pro-Ser-His-Arg-Ile-Ser-Asp-Arg-Asp-Tyr-Met-Gly-Trp-Met-Asp-(Phe-NH_2)

CCK-39 M.W. = 4678, 39 A.A. (Porcine)

Tyr-Ile-Gln-Gln-Ala-Arg-Lys-Ala-Pro-Ser-Gly-Arg-Val-Ser-Met-Ile-Lys-Asn-Leu-Gln-Ser-Leu-Asp-Pro-Ser-His-Arg-Ile-Ser-Asp-Arg-Asp-Tyr-Met-Gly-Trp-Met-Asp-Phe-NH_2

CCK-33 M.W. = 3918, 33 A.A. (Porcine)

Lys-Ala-Pro-Ser-Gly-Arg-Val-Ser-Met-Ile-Lys-Asn-Leu-Gln-Ser-Leu-Asp-Pro-Ser-His-Arg-Ile-Ser-Asp-Arg-Asp-Tyr-Met-Gly-Trp-Met-Asp-Phe-NH_2

CCK-8 M.W. = 1143, 8 A.A.

-Asp-Tyr-Met-Gly-Trp-Met-Asp-Phe-NH_2

Caerulein M.W. = 1352, 10 A.A. (Frog)

pGlu-Glu-Asp-Tyr-Thr-Gly-Trp-Met-Asp-Phe-NH_2

SECRETIN-GLUCAGON FAMILY

Secretin M.W. = 3056, 27 A.A. (Porcine)

His-Ser-Asp-Gly-Thr-Phe-Thr-Ser-Glu-Leu-Ser-Arg-Leu-Arg-Asp-Ser-Ala-Arg-Leu-Gln-Arg-Leu-Leu-Gln-Gly-Leu-Val-NH_2

Glucagon M.W. = 3550, 29 A.A. (Human)

His-Ser-Gln-Gly-Thr-Phe-Thr-Ser-Asp-Tyr-Ser-Lys-Tyr-Leu-Asp-Ser-Arg-Arg-Ala-Gln-Asp-Phe-Val-Gln-Trp-Leu-Met-Asp-Thr

VIP (Vasoactive Intestinal Peptide) **M.W. = 3326, 28 A.A.** (Human, Porcine, Rat)

His-Ser-Asp-Ala-Val-Phe-Thr-Asp-Asn-Tyr-Thr-Arg-Leu-Arg-Lys-Gln-Met-Ala-Val-Lys-Lys-Tyr-Leu-Asn-Ser-Ile-Leu-Asn-NH_2

GIP (Gastric Inhibitory Peptide) **M.W. = 4976, 42 A.A.** (Porcine)

Tyr-Ala-Glu-Gly-Thr-Phe-Ile-Ser-Asp-Tyr-Ser-Ile-Ala-Met-Asp-Lys-Ile-Arg-Gln-Gln-Asp-Phe-Val-Asn-Trp-Leu-Leu-Ala-Gln-Lys-Gly-Lys-Lys-Ser-Asp-Trp-Lys-His-Asn-Ile-Thr-Gln

PHI (Peptide Histidine Isoleucine) **M.W. = 2996, 27 A.A.** (Porcine)

His-Ala-Asp-Gly-Val-Phe-Thr-Ser-Asp-Phe-Ser-Arg-Leu-Leu-Gly-Gln-Leu-Ser-Ala-Lys-Lys-Tyr-Leu-Glu-Ser-Leu-Ile-NH_2

GHRF (Growth Hormone-Releasing Factor) **M.W. = 5040, 44 A.A.** (Human)

Tyr-Ala-Asp-Ala-Ile-Phe-Thr-Asn-Ser-Tyr-Arg-Lys-Val-Leu-Gly-Gln-Leu-Ser-Ala-Arg-Lys-Leu-Leu-Gln-Asp-Ile-Met-Ser-Arg-Gln-Gln-Gly-Glu-Ser-Asn-Gln-Glu-Arg-Gly-Ala-Arg-Ala-Arg-Leu-NH_2

ENTERIC BOMBESIN-LIKE PEPTIDES

Bombesin M.W. = 1620, 14 A.A. (Frog)

pGlu-Gln-Arg-Leu-Gly-Asn-Gln-Trp-Ala-Val-Gly-His-Leu-Met-NH_2

GRP (Gastrin-Releasing Peptide) **M.W. = 2806, 27 A.A.** (Porcine)

Ala-Pro-Val-Ser-Val-Gly-Gly-Gly-Thr-Val-Leu-Ala-Lys-Met-Tyr-Pro-Arg-Gly-Asn-His-Trp-Ala-Val-Gly-His-Leu-Met-NH_2

GRP-10 (Neuromedin C) **M.W. = 1120, 10 A.A.** (Porcine)

Gly-Asn-His-Trp-Ala-Val-Gly-His-Leu-Met-NH_2

Neuromedin B M.W. = 1133, 10 A.A. (Porcine)

Gly-Asn-Leu-Trp-Ala-Thr-Gly-His-Phe-Met-NH_2

PANCREATIC POLYPEPTIDE FAMILY

PP M.W. = 4184, 36 A.A. (Human)

Ala-Pro-Leu-Glu-Pro-Val-Tyr-Pro-Gly-Asp-Asn-Ala-Thr-Pro-Glu-Gln-Met-Ala-Gln-Tyr-Ala-Ala-Asp-Leu-Arg-Arg-Tyr-Ile-Asn-Met-Leu-Thr-Arg-Pro-Arg-Tyr-NH_2

PP M.W. = 4226, 36 A.A. (Bovine)

Ala-Pro-Leu-Glu-Pro-Glu-Tyr-Pro-Gly-Asp-Asn-Ala-Thr-Pro-Glu-Gln-Met-Ala-Gln-Tyr-Ala-Ala-Glu-Leu-Arg-Arg-Tyr-Ile-Asn-Met-Leu-Thr-Arg-Pro-Arg-Tyr-NH_2

PP M.W. = 4238, 36 A.A. (Chicken, Avian)

Gly-Pro-Ser-Gln-Pro-Thr-Tyr-Pro-Gly-Asp-Asp-Ala-Pro-Val-Glu-Asp-Leu-Ile-Arg-Phe-Tyr-Asp-Asn-Leu-Gln-Gln-Tyr-Leu-Asn-Val-Val-Thr-Arg-His-Arg-Tyr-NH_2

PP M.W. = 36 A.A. (Ovine)

Ala-Ser-Leu-Glu-Pro-Gln-Tyr-Pro-Gly-Asp-Asp-Ala-Thr-Pro-Glu-Gln-Met-Ala-Gln-Tyr-Ala-Ala-Glu-Leu-Arg-Arg-Tyr-Ile-Asn-Met-Leu-Thr-Arg-Pro-Arg-Tyr-NH_2

PP M.W. = 36 A.A. (Porcine)

Ala-Pro-Leu-Glu-Pro-Val-Tyr-Pro-Gly-Asp-Asp-Ala-Thr-Pro-Glu-Gln-Met-Ala-Gln-Tyr-Ala-Ala-Glu-

Leu-Arg-Arg-Tyr-Ile-Asn-Met-Leu-Thr-Arg-Pro-Arg-Tyr-NH_2

PP M.W. = 4399, 36 A.A. (Rat)

Ala-Pro-Leu-Glu-Pro-Met-Tyr-Pro-Gly-Asp-Tyr-Ala-Thr-His-Glu-Gln-Arg-Ala-Gln-Tyr-Glu-Thr-Gln-Leu-Arg-Arg-Tyr-Ile-Asn-Thr-Leu-Thr-Arg-Pro-Arg-Tyr-NH_2

Peptide YY M.W. = 4241, 36 A.A. (Porcine)

Tyr-Pro-Ala-Lys-Pro-Glu-Ala-Pro-Gly-Glu-Asp-Ala-Ser-Pro-Glu-Glu-Leu-Ser-Arg-Tyr-Tyr-Ala-Ser-Leu-Arg-His-Tyr-Leu-Asn-Leu-Val-Thr-Arg-Gln-Arg-Tyr-NH_2

Neuropeptide Y M.W. = 4254, 36 A.A. (Porcine)

Tyr-Pro-Ser-Lys-Pro-Asp-Asn-Pro-Gly-Gly-Asp-Ala-Pro-Ala-Glu-Asp-Leu-Ala-Arg-Tyr-Tyr-Ser-Ala-Leu-Arg-His-Tyr-Ile-Asn-Leu-Ile-Thr-Arg-Gln-Arg-Tyr-NH_2

CALCIUM-RELATED REGULATORY PEPTIDES

Calcitonin M.W. = 3418, 32 A.A. (Human)

Cys-Gly-Asn-Leu-Ser-Thr-Cys-Met-Leu-Gly-Thr-Tyr-Thr-Gln-Asp-Phe-Asn-Lys-Phe-His-Thr-Phe-Pro-Gln-Thr-Ala-Ile-Gly-Val-Gly-Ala-Pro-NH_2

CGRP (Calcitonin Gene-Related Peptide)
M.W. = 3790, 37 A.A. (Human)

Ala-Cys-Asp-Thr-Ala-Thr-Cys-Val-Thr-His-Arg-Leu-Ala-Gly-Leu-Leu-Ser-Arg-Ser-Gly-Gly-Val-Val-Lys-Asn-Asn-Phe-Val-Pro-Thr-Asn-Val-Gly-Ser-Lys-Ala-Phe-NH_2

CGRP M.W. = 3807, 37 A.A. (Rat)

Ser-Cys-Asn-Thr-Ala-Thr-Cys-Val-Thr-His-Arg-Leu-Ala-Gly-Leu-Leu-Ser-Arg-Ser-Gly-Gly-Val-Val-Lys-Asp-Asn-Phe-Val-Pro-Thr-Asn-Val-Gly-Ser-Glu-Ala-Phe-NH_2

NON-PEPTIDE AGENTS

Histamine M.W. = 111

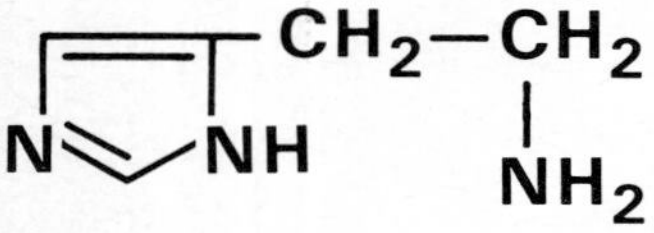

$CH_2—CH_2$, NH, N, NH_2

Serotonin M.W. = 176

HO, $CH_2—CH_2$, N, H, NH_2

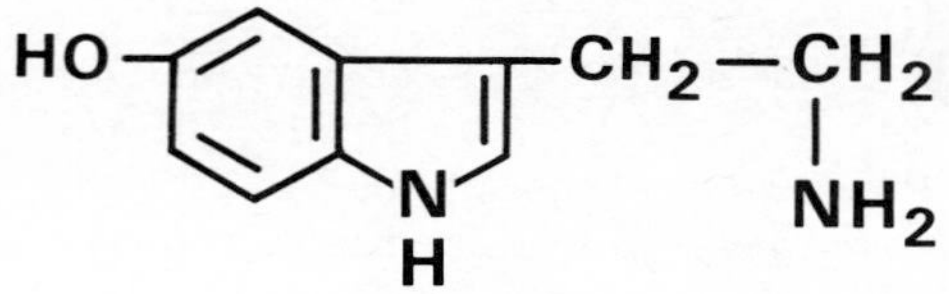

Prostaglandins (Prostanoic Acid) M.W. = 310

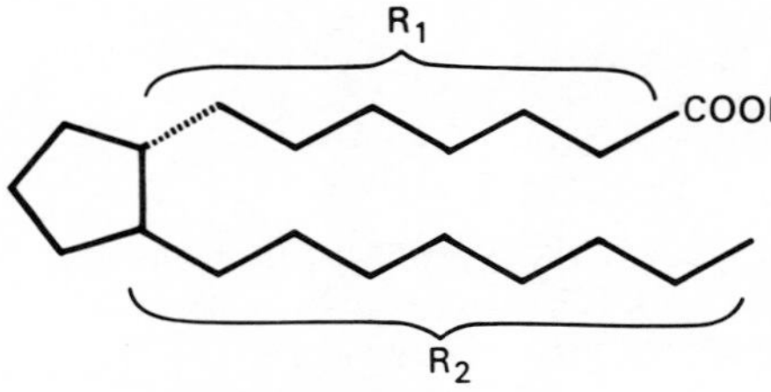

R_1, COOH, R_2

Prostanoic acid

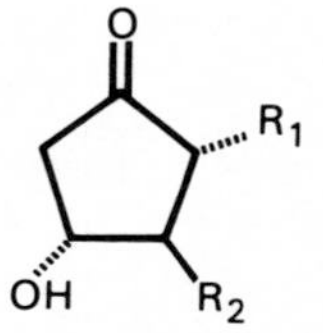

O, R_1, OH, R_2 — PGE

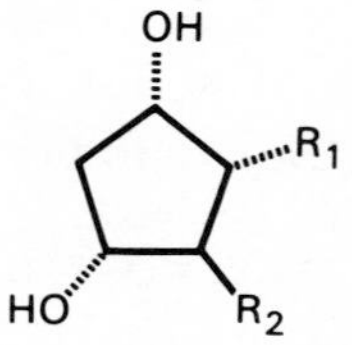

OH, R_1, HO, R_2 — PGF

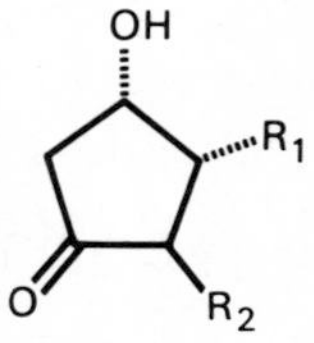

OH, R_1, O, R_2 — PGD_2

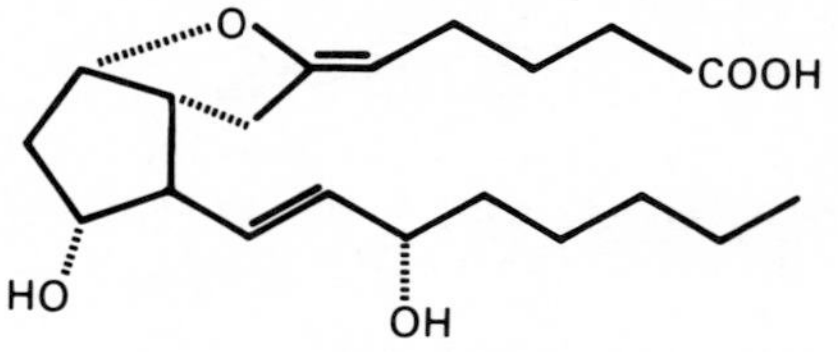

O, COOH, HO, OH

PGI_2
(prostacyclin)

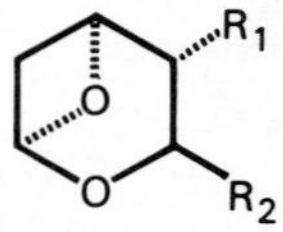

R_1, O, O, R_2

Thromboxane A_2

OTHER PEPTIDES

CRF (Corticotropin-Releasing Factor)
M.W. 4758, 41 A.A. (Human)

Ser-Glu-Glu-Pro-Pro-Ile-Ser-Leu-Asp-Leu-Thr-Phe-His-Leu-Leu-Arg-Glu-Val-Leu-Glu-Met-Ala-Arg-Ala-Glu-Gln-Leu-Ala-Gln-Gln-Ala-His-Ser-Asn-Arg-Lys-Leu-Met-Glu-Ile-Ile-NH_2

CRF M.W. 4671, 41 A.A. (Ovine)

Ser-Gln-Glu-Pro-Pro-Ile-Ser-Leu-Asp-Leu-Thr-Phe-His-Leu-Leu-Arg-Glu-Val-Leu-Glu-Met-Thr-Lys-

Ala-Asp-Gln-Leu-Ala-Gln-Gln-Ala-His-Ser-Asn-Arg-Lys-Leu-Leu-Asp-Ile-Ala-NH_2

Motilin M.W. = 2700, 22 A.A.

Phe-Val-Pro-Ile-Phe-Thr-Tyr-Gly-Glu-Leu-Gln-Arg-Met-Gln-Glu-Lys-Glu-Arg-Asn-Lys-Gly-Gln

Neurotensin M.W. = 1673, 13 A.A.

pGlu-Leu-Tyr-Glu-Asn-Lys-Pro-Arg-Arg-Pro-Tyr-Ile-Leu

Sauvagine M.W. = 4600, 39 A.A. (Frog)

pGlu-Gly-Pro-Pro-Ile-Ser-Ile-Asp-Leu-Ser-Leu-Glu-Leu-Leu-Arg-Lys-Met-Ile-Glu-Ile-Glu-Lys-Gln-Glu-Lys-Glu-Lys-Gln-Gln-Ala-Ala-Asn-Asn-Arg-Leu-Leu-Asp-Thr-Ile-NH_2

Somatostatin M.W. = 1638, 14 A.A.

Ala-Gly-Cys-Lys-Asn-Phe-Phe-Trp-Lys-Thr-Phe-Thr-Ser-Cys

Somatostatin M.W. = 2877, 28 A.A.

Ser-Ala-Asn-Ser-Asn-Pro-Ala-Met-Ala-Pro-Arg-Glu-Arg-Lys-Ala-Gly-Cys-Lys-Asn-Phe-Phe-Trp-Lys-Thr-Phe-Thr-Ser-Cys

Substance P M.W. = 1348, 11 A.A.

Arg-Pro-Lys-Pro-Gln-Gln-Phe-Phe-Gly-Leu-Met-NH_2

TRH (Thyrotropin-Releasing Hormone) M.W. = 362, 3 A.A.

pGlu-His-Pro-NH_2

CANDIDATE AGENTS

EGF (Epidermal Growth Factor) M.W. = 6045, 53 A.A.

Asn-Ser-Tyr-Pro-Gly-Cys-Pro-Ser-Ser-Tyr-Asp-Gly-Tyr-Cys-Leu-Asn-Gly-Gly-Val-Cys-Met-His-Ile-Glu-Ser-Leu-Asp-Ser-Tyr-Thr-Cys-Asn-Cys-Val-Ile-Gly-Tyr-Ser-Gly-Asp-Arg-Cys-Gln-Thr-Arg-Asp-Leu-Arg-Trp-Trp-Glu-Leu-Arg

Urogastrone M.W. = 6222, 53 A.A.

Asn-Ser-Asp-Ser-Glu-Cys-Pro-Leu-Ser-His-Asp-Gly-Tyr-Cys-Leu-His-Asp-Gly-Val-Cys-Met-Tyr-Ile-Glu-Ala-Leu-Asp-Lys-Tyr-Ala-Cys-Asn-Cys-Val-Val-Gly-Tyr-Ile-Gly-Glu-Arg-Cys-Gln-Tyr-Arg-Asp-Leu-Lys-Trp-Trp-Glu-Leu-Arg

OPIATE PEPTIDES

β-Endorphin (Human) M.W. = 3466, 31 A.A.

Tyr-Gly-Gly-Phe-Met-Thr-Ser-Glu-Lys-Ser-Gln-Thr-Pro-Leu-Val-Thr-Leu-Phe-Lys-Asn-Ala-Ile-Ile-Lys-Asn-Ala-Tyr-Lys-Lys-Gly-Glu-OH

β-Endorphin (1-27) (Human) M.W. = 3023, 27 A.A.

Tyr-Gly-Gly-Phe-Met-Thr-Ser-Glu-Lys-Ser-Gln-Thr-Pro-Leu-Val-Thr-Leu-Phe-Lys-Asn-Ala-Ile-Ile-Lys-Asn-Ala-Tyr-OH

β-Lipotropin 61-77 M.W. 1859, 17 A.A.

Tyr-Gly-Gly-Phe-Met-Thr-Ser-Glu-Lys-Ser-Gln-Thr-Pro-Leu-Val-Thr-Leu-OH

α-Endorphin (β-lipotropin 61-76) M.W. 1746, 16 A.A.

Tyr-Gly-Gly-Phe-Met-Thr-Ser-Glu-Lys-Ser-Gln-Thr-Pro-Leu-Val-Thr-OH

Methionine-enkephalin M.W. = 574, 5 A.A.

Tyr-Gly-Gly-Phe-Met

Leucine-enkephalin M.W. = 556, 5 A.A.

Tyr-Gly-Gly-Phe-Leu

Met-enkephalin-Arg-Phe M.W. = 877, 7 A.A.

Tyr-Gly-Gly-Phe-Met-Arg-Phe

Met-enkephalin-Arg-Gly-Leu M.W. = 900, 8 A.A.

Tyr-Gly-Gly-Phe-Met-Arg-Gly-Leu

α-Neo-endorphin M.W. = 1229, 10 A.A.

Tyr-Gly-Gly-Phe-Leu-Arg-Lys-Tyr-Pro-Lys

β-Neo-endorphin M.W. = 1100, 9 A.A.

Tyr-Gly-Gly-Phe-Leu-Arg-Lys-Tyr-Pro

Dynorphin 1-17 M.W. = 2148, 17 A.A.

Tyr-Gly-Gly-Phe-Leu-Arg-Arg-Ile-Arg-Pro-Lys-Leu-Lys-Trp-Asp-Asn-Gln

Leumorphin M.W. = 3528, 29 A.A.

Tyr-Gly-Gly-Phe-Leu-Arg-Arg-Gln-Phe-Lys-Val-Val-Thr-Arg-Ser-Gln-Glu-Asp-Pro-Asn-Ala-Tyr-Tyr-Glu-Glu-Leu-Phe-Asp-Val

Rimorphin M.W. = 1571, 13 A.A.

Tyr-Gly-Gly-Phe-Leu-Arg-Arg-Gln-Phe-Lys-Val-Val-Thr

2

Abbreviations Used in This Book

ABC, avidin-biotin-complex method
ACTH, adrenocorticotropin hormone
AP, aminopyrine
APP, avian PP
ATP, adenosine triphosphate
BBB, blood-brain barrier
BBS, bombesin
BLI, bombesin-like immunoreactivity
BOC, butyloxycarbonyl
BPP, bovine PP
BUI, brain uptake index
CCK, cholecystokinin
CCK-8, cholecystokinin-8
CCK-PZ, cholecystokinin-pancreozymin (now known as CCK alone)
CGRP, calcitonin gene-related peptide
CNS, central nervous system
CPP, canine PP
CRF, corticotropin releasing factor
CSF, cerebral spinal fluid
DAB, diaminobenzidine
DES, diethylstilbestrol
DFMO, difluoromethylornithine
2-DG, 2-deoxyglucose
DHT, 5-α-dihydrotestosterone
DMH, 1,2-dimethylhydrazine
DRC, dose-response curve
E_1, estrone
E_2, estradiol
E_3, estriol
EEG, electroencephalogram
EGF, epidermal growth factor
ENS, enteric nervous system
FSH, follicle stimulating hormone
G-17, gastrin-17
GHRF, growth hormone-releasing factor
GIP, gastric inhibitory polypeptide
GLI, glucagon-like immunoreactivity
GR, gastrin receptor
GRP, gastrin-releasing peptide
GRPP, glicentin-related pancreatic polypeptide
H^+, hydrogen ion
HCl, hydrochloric acid
HCO_3^-, bicarbonate
HPLC, high-pressure liquid chromatography
HPP, human PP
5-HT, serotonin
ICV, intracerebroventricular
ID, intraduodenal
IDM, infants of diabetic mothers
IgG, immunoglobulin
IMC, interdigestive migrating complex
IR, immunoreactive
IRG, immunoreactive glucagon
IR-GIP, immunoreactive GIP
IV, intravenous
LES, lower esophageal sphincter
LG, 15-leucine human gastrin
LH, luteinizing hormone
LT, leukotrienes
MCR, metabolic clearance rate
MEN, multiple endocrine neoplasia type I
MG, synthetic human gastrin
MMC, migrating motor complex
MNNG, N-methyl-N-nitro-N nitrosoguanidine
M_r, 120,000 molecular weight
MSH, melanocyte-stimulating hormone
NGS, normal goat serum
NorLG, 11-norleucine synthetic human gastrin-17-I
NPY, neuropeptide Y
NT, neurotensin
OPP, ovine PP
PAP, peroxidase-antiperoxidase
PHI, peptide histidine isoleucine
PP, pancreatic polypeptide
PPP, porcine PP
PSP, pancreatic spasmolytic polypeptide
PTH, parathyroid hormone
PYY, peptide YY
REM, rapid eye movement
RIA, radioimmunoassay
SC, subcutaneous
SCN, suprachiasmatic nuclei
TRH, thyrotropin releasing hormone
TSH, thyroid stimulating hormone
VIP, vasoactive intestinal peptide
V_d, volume of distribution
WDHA, watery diarrhea, hypokalemia, achlorhydria

Index